Reference Guide

for

Essential Oils

Connie and Alan Higley

This book has been designed to provide information to help educate the reader in regard to the subject matter covered. It is sold with the understanding that the publisher and the authors are not liable for the misconception or misuse of the information provided. It is not provided in order to diagnose, prescribe, or treat any disease, illness, or injured condition of the body. The authors and publisher shall have neither liability nor responsibility to any person or entity with respect to any loss, damage, or injury caused or alleged to be caused directly or indirectly by the information contained in this book. The information presented herein is in no way intended as a substitute for medical counseling. Anyone suffering from any disease, illness, or injury should consult a qualified health care professional.

Library of Congress Cataloging-in-Publication Data.

Higley, Connie.
    Reference guide for essential oils / Connie and Alan Higley
        p. ill. cm.
    Includes bibliographical references.
    1. Essences and essential oils–Therapeutic use–Handbooks, manuals, etc.
    2. Aromatherapy–Handbooks, manuals, etc. 00-500404

Published and distributed by:

Abundant Health
1460 N. Main St., #9
Spanish Fork, UT 84660

Phone: 1-888-718-3068 (toll-free) / 801-798-0642 (local)
Fax: 1-877-568-1988 (toll-free) / 801-798-0644 (local)

Internet: www.AbundantHealth4u.com
E-Mail: orders@abundanthealth4u.com

Printed and bound in the United States of America.

International Standard Book Number: 0-9706583-4-6

Dedication

We, the authors (compilers) of this information, were introduced to Young Living Essential Oils in 1995. At that time, there was no compiled information on the use of these valuable oils, so together with Pat Leatham, we set out to find what we could. We gathered notes from lectures and seminars by D. Gary Young, N.D. and product information from Young Living Essential Oils. Extensive research into the works of other aromatherapy experts have shown us that Dr. Young, through his own research and clinical study, not only supports, but expands their solid foundation of knowledge and expertise. When this book was first made available in 1996, we made a conscious decision to keep the names of D. Gary Young and Young Living Essential Oils out of this book so as to remove all possibility of recrimination or harm to Dr. Young or his company. However, all past, present, and future readers of this work need to understand that all of us, author and reader alike, are deeply indebted to Dr. Young for his brilliant insight, extensive research, and incredible vision of the healing power of essential oils.

We, therefore, dedicate this book to D. Gary Young, N.D. as a tribute to his vision of health for all who will embrace the oils and use them to their fullest potential. Dr. Young is one of the foremost experts on the organic cultivation, distillation, and clinical use of essential oils in North America. His unwavering passion for maintaining the highest quality in his products have produced some astounding healing results. We applaud his heroic and often solitary effort to continue proving, by clinical study, the efficacy of essential oils as indispensable tools for combating disease.

Acknowledgments

To our 5 young children who demonstrate much patience and responsibility with the freedom
they are given during the on-going compilation and updating of this book.

To the late Pat Leatham who provided the initial impetus for its creation.
Her many hours of research and meticulous note-taking will forever be appreciated.

And to all of you who are discovering, or re-discovering, for yourselves
the healing powers of essential oils. May this book provide quick access
to the information you need to help yourself, and those you love,
progress on the road to better health.

A special thanks goes to our families and to all of our "Essential Oil" friends! Without your love,
friendship, suggestions, support, patience, and prodding, we would have crumbled under the strain
of compiling a book such as this while trying to raise a family and have a life.

Contents

The section tabs shown on the right, correspond to each individual section listed below. By holding the spine of the book in the left hand and bending the right side back with the right hand, section markings become visible along the right edge. This should allow you quick and easy reference to any applicable section.

The sections on Personal Care Products, Bath Gels and Bar Soaps, Tinctures, Massage Oils, and Supplements and Vitamins list commercially available products that include pure essential oils either for additional therapeutic benefits or to enhance the bio-availability of the other ingredients.

Basic Information

BASIC FACTS ABOUT ESSENTIAL OILS

How long have essential oils been around?

Essential oils were mankind's first medicine. From Egyptian hieroglyphics and Chinese manuscripts, we know that priests and physicians have been using essential oils for thousands of years. In Egypt, essential oils were used in the embalming process and well preserved oils were found in alabaster jars in King Tut's tomb. Egyptian temples were dedicated to the production and blending of the oils and recipes were recorded on the walls in hieroglyphics. There is even a sacred room in the temple of Isis on the island of Philae where a ritual called "Cleansing the Flesh and Blood of Evil Deities" was practiced. This form of emotional clearing required three days of cleansing using particular essential oils and oil baths.

There are 188 references to essential oils in the Bible. Oils such as frankincense, myrrh, rosemary, hyssop, and spikenard were used for anointing and healing the sick. In Exodus, the Lord gave the following recipe to Moses for "an holy anointing oil":

> Myrrh ("five hundred shekels"— approximately 1 gallon)
> Sweet Cinnamon ("two hundred and fifty shekels"— approximately ½ gallon)
> Sweet Calamus ("two hundred and fifty shekels")
> Cassia ("five hundred shekels")
> Olive Oil ("an hin"— approximately 1 ⅓ gallons)

The three wise men presented the Christ child with essential oils of frankincense and myrrh. There are also accounts in the New Testament of the Bible where Jesus was anointed with spikenard oil; "And being in Bethany in the house of Simon the leper, as he sat at meat, there came a woman having an alabaster box of ointment of spikenard very precious; and she brake the box, and poured [it] on his head" (Mark 14:3). "Then took Mary a pound of ointment of spikenard, very costly, and anointed the feet of Jesus, and wiped his feet with her hair: and the house was filled with the odour of the ointment" (John 12:3). Some have even said that essential oils carry the consciousness of Christ.

What are *Pure, Therapeutic-Grade* essential oils?

Essential oils are the volatile liquids that are distilled from plants (including their respective parts such as seeds, bark, leaves, stems, roots, flowers, fruit, etc.). One of the factors that determine the purity and therapeutic value of an oil is its chemical constituents. These constituents can be affected by a vast number of variables including: the part(s) of the plant from which the oil was produced, soil condition, fertilizer (organic or chemical), geographical region, climate, altitude, harvest season and methods, and distillation process. For example, common thyme, or thyme vulgaris, produces several different chemotypes (biochemical specifics or simple species) depending on the conditions of its growth, climate, and altitude. One will produce high levels of thymol depending on the time of year it is distilled. If distilled during mid-summer or late fall, there can be higher levels of carvacrol which can cause the oil to be more caustic or irritating to the skin. Low pressure and low temperature are also keys to maintaining the purity, the ultimate fragrance, and the therapeutic value of the oil.

As we begin to understand the power of essential oils in the realm of personal, holistic health care, we comprehend the absolute necessity for obtaining the purest therapeutic-grade essential oils possible. No matter how costly pure therapeutic-grade essential oils may be, there can be no substitutes. Chemists can replicate some of the known individual constituents, but they have yet to successfully recreate complete essential oils in the laboratory.

The information in this book is based upon the use of pure, therapeutic-grade essential oils. Those who are beginning their journey into the realm of aromatherapy and essential oils, must actively seek for the purest quality and highest therapeutic-grade oils available. Anything less than pure, therapeutic-grade essential oil may not produce the desired results and can, in some cases, be extremely toxic.

Why is it so difficult to find *Pure, Therapeutic-Grade* essential oils?

Producing the purest of oils can be very costly because it may require several hundred pounds, or even several thousand pounds of plant material to extract one pound of pure essential oil. For example, one pound of pure melissa oil sells for $9,000 - $15,000. Although this sounds quite expensive, one must realize that three tons of plant material are required to produce that single pound of oil. Because the vast majority of all the oils produced in the world today are used by the perfume industry, the oils are being purchased for their aromatic qualities only. High pressure, high temperatures, rapid processing and the use of chemical solvents are often employed during the distillation process so that a greater *quantity* of oil can be produced at a faster rate. These oils may smell just as good and cost much less, but will lack most, if not all, of the chemical constituents necessary to produce the expected therapeutic results.

What benefits do *PURE, THERAPEUTIC-GRADE* essential oils provide?

1. Essential oils are the regenerating, oxygenating, and immune defense properties of plants.
2. Essential oils are so small in molecular size that they can quickly penetrate the skin.
3. Essential oils are lipid soluble and are capable of penetrating cell walls, even if they have hardened because of an oxygen deficiency. In fact, essential oils can affect every cell of the body within 20 minutes and are then metabolized like other nutrients.
4. Essential oils contain oxygen molecules which help to transport nutrients to the starving human cells. Because a nutritional deficiency is an oxygen deficiency, disease begins when the cells lack the oxygen for proper nutrient assimilation. By providing the needed oxygen, essential oils also work to stimulate the immune system.
5. Essential oils are very powerful antioxidants. Antioxidants create an unfriendly environment for free radicals. They prevent all mutations, work as free radical scavengers, prevent fungus, and prevent oxidation in the cells.
6. Essential oils are anti-bacterial, anti-cancerous, anti-fungal, anti-infectious, anti-microbial, anti-tumoral, anti-parasitic, anti-viral, and antiseptic. Essential oils have been shown to destroy all tested bacteria and viruses while simultaneously restoring balance to the body.
7. Essential oils may detoxify the cells and blood in the body.
8. Essential oils containing sesquiterpenes have the ability to pass the blood brain barrier, enabling them to be effective in the treatment of Alzheimer's disease, Lou Gehrig's disease, Parkinson's disease, and multiple sclerosis.
9. Essential oils are aromatic. When diffused, they provide **air purification** by:
   A. Removing metallic particles and toxins from the air;
   B. Increasing atmospheric oxygen;
   C. Increasing ozone and negative ions in the area, which inhibits bacterial growth;
   D. Destroying odors from mold, cigarettes, and animals; and
   E. Filling the air with a fresh, aromatic scent.
10. Essential oils help promote emotional, physical, and spiritual healing.
11. Essential oils have a bio-electrical frequency that is several times greater than the frequency of herbs, food, and even the human body. Clinical research has shown that essential oils can quickly raise the frequency of the human body, restoring it to its normal, healthy level.

What is frequency and how does it pertain to essential oils?

Frequency is a measurable rate of electrical energy that is constant between any two points. Everything has an electrical frequency. Bruce Tainio of Tainio Technology in Cheny, Washington, developed new equipment to measure the bio-frequency of humans and foods. Bruce Tainio and D. Gary Young, a North American expert on essential oils, used this bio-frequency monitor to determine the relationship between frequency and disease. Some of the results of their studies are show in the following table.

Human Brain	72-90 MHz	Processed/canned food	0 MHz
Human Body (day)	62-68 MHz	Fresh Produce	up to 15 MHz
Cold Symptoms	58 MHz	Dry Herbs	12-22 MHz
Flu Symptoms	57 MHz	Fresh Herbs	20-27 MHz
Candida	55 MHz	Essential Oils	52-320 MHz
Epstein Barr	52 MHz		
Cancer	42 MHz		
Death Begins	25 MHz		

Note: Due to the sensitivity of the instruments, these results are not easily duplicatable. What is important is the relativity of the numbers and the fact that the higher frequency of the essential oils can help raise the frequency of the human body to a more normal level.

Another part of this same study measured the frequency fluctuations within the human body as different substances were introduced. The chart shown below illustrates the frequency reaction of the human body to the introduction of coffee. The subsequent time necessary for the frequency to return to its original measurement was shown to be substantially reduced with the use of essential oils.

Frequency Reaction to Substance

☐ Held Cup of Coffee then Smelled Oil
■ Sip of Coffee and No Oil Used (3 days to recover)

Initially, the frequency of each of two different individuals—the first a 26 yr. old male and the second a 24 yr. old male—was measured at 66 MHz for both. The first individual held a cup of coffee (without drinking any) and his frequency dropped to 58 MHz in 3 seconds. He then removed the coffee and inhaled an aroma of essential oils. Within 21 seconds, his frequency had returned to 66 MHz. The second individual took a sip of coffee and his frequency dropped to 52 MHz in the same 3 seconds. However, no essential oils were used during the recovery time and it took 3 days for his frequency to return to the initial 66 MHz.

Another very interesting result of this study was the influence that thoughts have on our frequency as well. Negative thoughts lowered the measured frequency by 12 MHz and positive thoughts raised the measured frequency by 10 MHz. It was also found that prayer and meditation increased the measured frequency levels by 15 MHz.

How do *PURE, THERAPEUTIC-GRADE* essential oils affect the brain?

The blood-brain barrier is the barrier membrane between the circulating blood and the brain that prevents certain damaging substances from reaching brain tissue and cerebrospinal fluid. The American Medical Association (AMA) determined that if they could find an agent that would pass the blood-brain barrier, they would be able to cure Alzheimer's disease, Lou Gehrig's disease, multiple sclerosis, and Parkinson's disease. In June of 1994, it was documented by the Medical University of Berlin, Germany and Vienna, Austria that sesquiterpenes have the ability to go beyond the blood-brain barrier.

High levels of sesquiterpenes, found in the essential oils of frankincense and sandalwood, help increase the amount oxygen in the limbic system of the brain, particularly around the pineal and pituitary glands. This leads to an increase in secretions of antibodies, endorphins, and neurotransmitters.

Also present in the limbic system of the brain, is a gland called the amygdala. In 1989, it was discovered that the amygdala plays a major role in the storing and releasing of emotional trauma. The only way to stimulate this gland is with fragrance or the sense of smell. Therefore, with Aromatherapy and essential oils, we are now able to release emotional trauma.

What enables *PURE, THERAPEUTIC-GRADE* essential oils to provide such incredible benefits?

Essential oils are chemically very heterogenetic; meaning they are very diverse in their effects and can perform several different functions. Synthetic chemicals are completely opposite in that they have basically one action. This gives essential oils a paradoxical nature which can be difficult to understand. However, they can be compared to another paradoxical group—human beings. For example, a man can play many roles: father, husband, friend, co-worker, accountant, school teacher, church volunteer, scout master, minister. etc. and so it is with essential oils. Lavender can be used for burns, insect bites, headaches, PMS, insomnia, stress and so forth.

The heterogenetic benefits of an oil depend greatly on its chemical constituents; and not only on the existence of specific constituents, but also their amounts in proportion to the other constituents that are present in the same oil. Some individual oils may have anywhere from 200 to 800 different chemical constituents. However, of the possible 800 different constituents, only about 200 of those have so far been identified. Although not everything is known about all the different constituents, most of them can be grouped into a few distinct families, each with some dominant characteristics. The following section provides greater insights into these constituent families.

ESSENTIAL OIL CONSTITUENTS

As was mentioned previously, the chemical constituents of an oil are affected by a vast number of variables. However, most of these variables are controlled by the oil producers. One thing that the student of aromatherapy can do, is to ask questions about the company from which they are purchasing the oils. Some of the most important questions should be, "Does the company utilize gas chromatography (GC) in their quality control process?" "Does their GC equipment utilize a column of at least 50 to 60 meters in length in order to properly identify the hundreds of natural constituents found in an essential oil?" A gas chromatogram shows a pattern of the separated constituents of an oil and helps a trained technician determine its purity and therapeutic quality. The following information can help us understand the functions of some of the main chemical constituents.

In general, *pure* essential oil constituents can be subdivided into two distinct groups; the **hydrocarbons** which are made up almost exclusively of *terpenes* (monoterpenes, sesquiterpenes, and diterpenes), and the **oxygenated compounds** which are mainly *esters, aldehydes, ketones, alcohols, phenols,* and *oxides.*

Monoterpenes—occur in practically all essential oils and have many different activities. Most tend to inhibit the accumulation of toxins and help discharge existing toxins from the liver and kidneys. Some are antiseptic, anti-bacterial, stimulating, analgesic (weak), and expectorant, while other specific terpenes have anti-fungal, anti-viral, antihistaminic, antirheumatic, anti-tumor (antiblastic, anti-carcinogenic), hypotensive, insecticidal, purgative, and pheromonal properties. Monoterpenes, in general, have a stimulating effect and can be very soothing to irritated tissues as well. Most citrus oils (not bergamot) and pine oils, as well as Black pepper, nutmeg, and angelica, contain a high proportion of terpenes. Some common monoterpenes include the following:
Pinenes (α- & β-) have strong antiseptic, anti-bacterial, anti-fungal, and expectorant properties.
Camphene is an insect repellent and according to the Phytochemical Dictionary, it is "used to reduce cholesterol saturation index in the treatment of gallstones".
β-Myrcene is a cancer-preventative.
d-limonene is anti-cancerous, anti-bacterial, anti-fungal, antiseptic (5x phenol), and highly anti-viral. It can be found in 90% of the citrus oils.
Found as a Significant Constituent in ALL Essential Oils *Except*: Anise, basil, birch, calamus, cassia, cedarwood, German chamomile, cinnamon bark, clary sage, clove, Blue cypress, davana, geranium, jasmine, melissa, Lemon myrtle, onycha, palmarosa, patchouli, rosewood, sandalwood, vetiver, Western Red cedar, wintergreen, ylang ylang.

Sesquiterpenes are found in great abundance in essential oils. They are anti-bacterial, strongly anti-inflammatory, slightly antiseptic and hypotensive, and sedative. Some have analgesic properties while others are highly anti-spasmodic. They are soothing to irritated skin and tissue and are calming. They also work as liver and gland stimulants. Research from the universities of Berlin and Vienna show increased oxygenation around the pineal and pituitary glands. Further research has shown that sesquiterpenes have the ability to surpass the blood-brain barrier and enter the brain tissue. They are larger molecules than monoterpenes and have a strong aroma.

β-Caryophyllene is anti-edemic, anti-inflammatory, anti-spasmodic, and an insect and
    termite repellent. Found in high proportions in plants from the Labiatae family.

Chamazulene is very high in anti-inflammatory and anti-bacterial activity.

Farnesene is anti-viral in action.

Found as a Major Constituent In: Cedarwood, German chamomile, ginger, goldenrod,
    melissa, myrrh, patchouli, pepper, sandalwood, spikenard, vetiver, yarrow, ylang ylang.

Found as a Minor (but significant) Constituent In: Bergamot, carrot, cedar leaf, celery
    seed, Roman chamomile, cinnamon bark, clary sage, clove, cumin, cypress, Blue
    cypress, elemi, *Eucalyptus citriadora* (lemon eucalyptus), *Eucalyptus globulus*, Silver fir,
    White fir, frankincense, galbanum, geranium, helichrysum, hyssop, lavandin, lavender,
    ledum, lemongrass, *Melaleuca alternifolia* (Tea Tree), *Melaleuca ericifolia* (Rosalina),
    Melaleuca leucadendron (Cajeput), *Melaleuca quinquenervia* (Niaouli), peppermint,
    pine, rosewood, sage, Blue tansy, tsuga, valerian.

Alcohols—are commonly recognized for their anti-bacterial, anti-infectious, and anti-viral activities.
They are somewhat stimulating and help to increase blood circulation. Because of their high resistance to oxidation and their low toxicity levels, they have been shown to revert cells to normal function and activity in animal studies.   They create an uplifting quality and are regarded as safe and effective for young and old alike.

Monoterpene Alcohols (or Monoterpenols) stimulate the immune system, work as a
    diuretic and a general tonic, and are anti-bacterial and mildly antiseptic as well.

    Linalol can help relieve discomfort. It is anti-bacterial, anti-fungal, antiseptic (5x
        phenol), anti-spasmodic, anti-viral, and sedative.

    Citronellol is anti-bacterial, anti-fungal, antiseptic (3.8x phenol), and sedative.

    Geraniol is anti-fungal, antiseptic (7x phenol), cancer-preventative, and sedative.

    Farnesol is good for the mucous membranes and prevents bacterial growth from
        perspiration.

    Other terpene alcohols include borneol, menthol, nerol, terpineol (which Dr. Gattefosse
        considered to be a decongestant), vetiverol, and cedrol.

Sesquiterpene Alcohols (Sesquiterpenols) are anti-allergic, anti-bacterial, antiinflammatory,
    ulcer-protective (preventative), and a liver and glandular stimulant.

    Bisabolol is one of the strongest sesquiterpene alcohols. Others include nerolidol and
        zingiberol.

Found as a Significant Constituent in ALL Essential Oils *Except*: Anise, birch, calamus,
    cassia, celery seed, clove, cumin, davana, dill, *Eucalyptus polybractea*, Balsam
    fir, Silver fir, White fir, galbanum, goldenrod, grapefruit, hyssop, juniper, melissa,
    mugwort, Lemon myrtle, myrrh, onycha, oregano, pepper, pine, rosemary (CT

verbenon), spruce, Blue tansy, Idaho tansy, tarragon, tsuga, Western Red cedar, wintergreen, yarrow.

Esters—are the compounds resulting from the reaction of an alcohol with an acid (known as esterification). Esters are very common and are found in the mildest essential oils. Mostly free of toxicity and irritants, they tend to be the most calming, relaxing, and balancing of all the essential oil constituents. They are also anti-fungal and anti-spasmodic. They also have a balancing or regulatory effect, especially on the nervous system. Some examples are **linalyl acetate**, **geranyl acetate** (with strong anti-fungal properties), and **bornyl acetate** (effective on bronchial candida). Other esters include eugenyl acetate, lavendulyl acetate, and methyl salicylate.

> **Found as a Major Constituent In:** Birch, bergamot, cardamom, Roman chamomile (85%), clary sage, geranium, helichrysum, jasmine, lavandin, lavender, onycha, petitgrain, spruce, tsuga, valerian, wintergreen, ylang ylang.

> **Found as a Minor (but significant) Constituent In:** Angelica, carrot, cassia, cedar leaf, celery seed, cistus, clove, coriander, cypress, dill, *Eucalyptus citriadora* (lemon eucalyptus), Balsam fir, Douglas fir, Silver fir, White fir, fleabane, juniper, *Laurus nobilis*, lemon, lemongrass, mandarin, marjoram, melissa, myrtle, neroli, orange, palmarosa, rosemary (CT verbenon), sage lavender.

Aldehydes—are usually responsible for the fragrance of an oil. They exert powerful aromas and are often calming to the emotions. They are highly reactive and characterized by the group C-H-O (Carbon, Hydrogen, Oxygen). In general, they are anti-infectious, antiinflammatory, calming to the central nervous system, fever-reducing, hypotensive, and tonic. Some are antiseptic, anti-microbial, and anti-fungal, while others act as vasodilators. They can be quite irritating when applied topically (citrals being an example). However, it has been shown that adding an essential oil with an equal amount of d-limonene can negate the irritant properties of a high citral oil.

> **Citrals** (like neral, geranial, and citronellal) are very common with a distinctive antiseptic action. They also have an anti-viral application as with melissa oil when applied topically on herpes simplex.

> Other aldehydes include benzaldehyde, cinnamic aldehyde, cuminic aldehyde, and perillaldehyde.

> **Found as a Major Constituent In:** Cassia, cinnamon bark, cumin, *Eucalyptus citriadora* (lemon eucalyptus), lemongrass, Lemon myrtle, lemon verbena.

> **Found as a Minor (but significant) Constituent In:** Calamus, cistus, citronella, *Eucalyptus radiata*, grapefruit, lemon, lime, mandarin, myrrh, orange, tangerine.

Ketones—are sometimes mucolytic and neuro-toxic when isolated from other constituents. However, all recorded toxic effects come from laboratory testing on guinea pigs and rats. No documented cases exist where oils with a high concentration of ketones (such as mugwort, tansy, sage, and wormwood) have ever caused a toxic effect on a human being. Also, large amounts of these oils would have to be consumed for them to result in a toxic neurological effect. Ketones stimulate cell regeneration, promote the formation of tissue, and liquefy mucous. They are helpful with such conditions as dry asthma, colds, flu, and dry cough and are largely found in oils used for the upper respiratory system, such as hyssop, rosemary, and sage.

Thujone is one of the most toxic members of the ketone family. It can be an irritant and upsetting to the central nervous system and may be neuro-toxic when taken internally as in the banned drink *Absinthe*. Although oils containing thujone may be inhaled to relieve respiratory distress and may stimulate the immune system, they should usually be used in dilution (1-2%) and/or for short periods of time.

Jasmone (found in jasmine) and **fenchone** (found in fennel) are both non-toxic.

Other ketones include camphor, carvone, menthone, methyl nonyl ketone, and pinocamphone.

Found as a Major Constituent In: Calamus, cedar leaf, davana, dill, *Eucalyptus dives*, hyssop, rosemary (CT cineol), rosemary (CT verbenon), sage, sage lavender, spearmint, Idaho tansy, Western Red cedar.

Found as a Minor (but significant) Constituent In: Cedarwood, Roman chamomile, cistus, coriander, *Eucalyptus polybractea*, fennel, geranium, helichrysum, juniper, lavandin, lemongrass, melissa, mugwort, myrrh, peppermint, spikenard, Blue tansy, vetiver, yarrow.

Phenols—are the most powerful anti-bacterial, anti-infectious, and antiseptic constituents in the plant world. They are also very stimulating to both the nervous and immune systems. They contain high levels of oxygenating molecules and have antioxidant properties. However, they can be quite caustic to the skin and they present some concerns regarding liver toxicity. Essential oils that contain a high proportion of phenols should be diluted and/or used for short periods of time.

Eugenol is analgesic, anesthetic (in dentistry), anticonvulsant, anti-fungal, antiinflammatory, antioxidant, antiseptic, cancer-preventative, and sedative.

Thymol may not be as caustic as other phenols. It is anti-bacterial, anti-fungal, anti-inflammatory, antioxidant, anti-plaque, anti-rheumatic, antiseptic (20x phenol), anti-spasmodic, deodorant, expectorant.

Carvacrol is a product of auto-oxidation of d-limonene. It is anti-bacterial, anti-fungal, anti-inflammatory, antiseptic (1.5x phenol), anti-spasmodic, and an expectorant. Researchers believe it may possibly contain some anti-cancerous properties.

Others in the phenol family include methyl eugenol, methyl chavicol, anethole, and safrole.

Found as a Major Constituent In: Anise, basil, birch, cinnamon bark, clove, fennel, *Melaleuca alternifolia* (Tea Tree), Mountain savory, oregano, peppermint, tarragon, thyme, wintergreen.

Found as a Minor (but significant) Constituent In: Cassia, citronella, cumin, *Eucalyptus citriadora* (lemon eucalyptus), *Laurus nobilis*, marjoram, nutmeg, ylang ylang.

Oxides—According to *The American Heritage® Dictionary of the English Language*, an oxide is "a binary compound of an element or a radical with oxygen." They act as expectorants and are mildly stimulating.

   1,8-Cineol (or eucalyptol) is, by far, the most prevalent member of this family and virtually exists in a class of its own. It is anesthetic, antiseptic, and works as a strong mucolytic as it thins mucus in respiratory tract infections. Other oxides include linalol oxide, ascaridol, bisabolol oxide, and bisabolone oxide.

   Found as a Major Constituent In: Cardamom, German chamomile, *Eucalyptus globulus*, *Eucalyptus polybractea*, *Eucalyptus radiata*, *Laurus nobilis*, *Melaleuca leucadendron* (Cajeput), *Melaleuca quinquenervia* (Niaouli), myrtle, ravensara, rosemary (CT cineol).

   Found as a Minor (but significant) Constituent In: Basil, carrot, *Eucalyptus citriadora* (lemon eucalyptus), lavandin, lemongrass, lime, *Melaleuca alternifolia* (Tea Tree), *Melaleuca ericifolia* (Rosalina), melissa, mugwort, pepper, rosemary (CT verbenon), rosewood, sage, sage lavender, thyme, ylang ylang.

All pure essential oils have some anti-bacterial properties. They increase the production of white blood cells, which help fight infectious illnesses. It is through these properties that aromatic herbs have been esteemed so highly throughout the ages and so widely used during the onsets of malaria, typhoid, and of course, the epidemic plagues during the 16th century. Research has found that people who consistently use pure essential oils have a higher level of **resistance to illnesses**, colds, flues, and diseases than the average person. Further indications show that such individuals, after contracting a cold, flu, or other illness, will **recover 60-75 percent faster** than those who do not use essential oils.

THE ART OF BLENDING

Blending essential oils is an art and usually requires a little bit of training and experimentation. If you choose to create your own blends, it is important to understand that the order in which the oils are blended is key to maintaining the desired therapeutic properties in a synergistic blend. An alteration in the sequence of adding selected oils to a blend may change the chemical properties, the fragrance, and thus the desired results. The "Blend Classification", and "Blends With" listings under each oil in the Single Oils section of this book should assist one in the blending process. In general, oils that are from the same botanical family, usually blend well together. In addition, oils with similar constituents also mix well.

Another method utilizes four blending classifications. The following information explains the characteristics of each classification, the order in which they should be added to the blend (i.e. Personifiers first, Enhancers second, Equalizers third, and Modifiers fourth), and the amount of each type of oil as a percentage of the blend.

1st—The **Personifier** (1-5% of blend) oils have very sharp, strong and long-lasting fragrances. They also have dominant properties with strong therapeutic action.
  Oils in this classification may include: Angelica, birch, cardamom, cinnamon bark, cistus, Clary sage, clove, coriander, German chamomile, ginger, helichrysum, mandarin, neroli, nutmeg, orange, patchouli, peppermint, petitgrain, rose, spearmint, tangerine, tarragon, wintergreen, ylang ylang.

2nd—The **Enhancer** (50-80% of blend) oil should be the predominant oil as it serves to enhance the properties of the other oils in the blend. Its fragrance is not as sharp as the personifiers and is usually of a shorter duration.
  Oils in this classification may include: Basil, bergamot, birch, cajeput, cedarwood, cumin, dill, eucalyptus, frankincense, galbanum, geranium, grapefruit, hyssop, jasmine, lavender, lemon, lemongrass, lime, marjoram, *Melaleuca alternifolia* (Tea Tree), melissa, myrtle, orange, oregano, palmarosa, patchouli, petitgrain, ravensara, Roman chamomile, rose, rosemary, sage, spruce, thyme, wintergreen.

3rd—The **Equalizer** (10-15% of blend) oils create balance and synergy among the oils contained in the blend. Their fragrance is also not as sharp as the personifier and is of a shorter duration.
  Oils in this classification may include: Basil, bergamot, cedarwood, cypress, fennel, fir, frankincense, geranium, ginger, hyssop, jasmine, juniper, lavender, lemongrass, lime, marjoram, *Melaleuca alternifolia* (Tea Tree), melissa, myrrh, myrtle, neroli, oregano, pine, roman chamomile, rose, rosewood, sandalwood, spruce, tarragon, thyme.

4th—The **Modifier** (5-8% of blend) oils have a mild and short fragrance. These oils add harmony to the blend.

> **Oils in this classification may include:** Angelica, bergamot, cardamom, coriander, eucalyptus, fennel, grapefruit, hyssop, jasmine, lavender, lemon, mandarin, melissa, myrrh, neroli, petitgrain, rose, rosewood, sandalwood, tangerine, ylang ylang.

Depending upon the topical application of your blend, you will want to add some carrier/base oil. When creating a **therapeutic essential oil blend**, you may want to use about **28 drops of essential oil to ½ oz. of V-6 Mixing Oil**. When creating a **body massage blend**, you will want to use a total of about **50 drops of essential oils to 4 oz. of V-6 Mixing Oil**. Remember to store your fragrant creation in dark-colored glass bottles.

As essential oils can vary in thickness, the following are approximate measurements:

25-30 drops	= 1/4 teaspoon	= 1-2 milliliters	= 5/8 dram
45-50 drops	= 1/2 teaspoon	= 2-3 milliliters	= 1 dram
75-80 drops	= 3/4 teaspoon	= 3-4 milliliters	= 1/8 oz.
100-120 drops	= 1 teaspoon	= 5 milliliters	= 1/6 oz.
160 drops	= 1½ teaspoons	= 6-8 milliliters	= 1/4 oz.
320-400 drops	= 3 teaspoons	= 13-15 milliliters	= 1/2 oz.
600-650 drops	= 6 teaspoons	= 25-30 milliliters	= 1 oz.

Learn to trust your nose as it can help you decide which classification an oil should be in. More detailed information about these methods of blending is beyond the scope of this revision of the book. For additional information on using these classifications in your blending, we highly recommend Marcel Lavabre's <u>Aromatherapy Workbook</u>. Another very simple book about blending, with recipes and easy-to-follow guidelines, is Mindy Green's <u>Natural Perfumes</u>, which uses perfume notes (top, middle, base), odor, and odor intensity to help guide you in making your own fragrant blend creations (refer to the chart on the following page).

ESSENTIAL OILS ODOR CHART

(The following chart was compiled from the book <u>Natural Perfumes</u>, by Mindy Green, and various other sources. It lists essential oils by note types in order of odor intensity, 1-lightest to 5-strongest)

Essential Oil	Scent	Intensity	Essential Oil	Scent	Intensity
Top Notes	(5-20% of the blend)		**Middle Notes (continued)**	(50-80% of the blend)	
Orange	Fresh, citrusy, fruity, sweet, light	1	Helichrysum	Rich, sweet, fruity, slightly honey-like	3
Bergamot	Sweet, lively, citrus, fruity	2	Hyssop	Fresh, earthy, woody, fruity	3
Grapefruit	Clean, fresh, bitter, citrusy	2	Hyssop	Fresh, earthy, woody, fruity	3
Citronella	Citrusy, slightly fruity, fresh, sweet	3	Juniper	Sweet, musky, tenacious	3
Lemon	Sweet, sharp, clear, citrusy	3	Marjoram	Herbaceous, green, spicy	3
Lime	Sweet, tart, intense, lively	3	Melaleuca	Medicinal, fresh, woody, earthy	3
Mandarin	Very sweet, citrusy, fruity	3	Neroli	Floral, citrusy, semi-sweet, delicate	3
Petitgrain	Fresh, floral, citrusy, slightly woody	3	Niaouli	Earthy, musty, harsh	3
Ravensara	Slightly medicinal, eucalyptus-like	3	Black Pepper	Spicy, peppery, musky, warm	3
Spearmint	Minty, slightly fruity	3	Rosemary Cin.	Strong, camphorous, slightly woody	3
Tangerine	Fresh, sweet, citrusy	3	Rosewood	Sweet, woody, fruity, floral	3
Euc. Polybrac.	Fresh, woody, earthy	4	Spruce	Fresh, woody, earthy, sweet	3
Lemongrass	Grassy, lemony, pungent, earthy	4	Cardamom	Sweet, spicy, balsamic, slightly floral	4
Euc. Globulus	Fresh, medicinal, woody, earthy	5	G. Chamomile	Deep, rich, tenacious, cocoa-like	4
Galbanum	Warm, earthy, green, woody, spicy	5	R. Chamomile	Fresh, sweet, fruity, apple-like	4
Lemon Myrtle	Extremely lemony and crisp	5	Ginger	Sweet, spicy-woody, warm, fresh, sharp	4
Top to Middle Notes	(20-80% of the blend)		Nutmeg	Sweet, musky, spicy	4
Anise	Licorice-like, rich, sweet	3	Pine, Scotch	Fresh, woody, earthy, balsamic	4
Laurel	Sweet, fresh, spicy, medicinal	3	Thyme	Fresh, medicinal, herbaceous	4
Lavandin	Fresh, sweet, floral, herbaceous	3	Yarrow	Sharp, woody, herbaceous, slight floral	4
Myrtle	Sweet, slightly camphorous, floral hint	3	Oregano	Herbaceous, sharp	5
Palmarosa	Lemony, fresh, green, hints of rose	3	Peppermint	Minty, sharp, intense	5
Angelica	Earthy, peppery, green, spicy	4	**Middle to Base Notes**	(20-80% of the blend)	
Basil	Spicy, anise-like, camphorous, lively	4	Clary Sage	Spicy, hay-like, sharp, fixative	3
Fennel	Sweet, somewhat spicy, licorice-like	4	Rose	Floral, spicy, rich, deep, sensual, green	3
Middle Notes	(50-80% of the blend)		Clove Bud	Spicy, warming, slightly bitter, woody	5
Carrot Seed	Sweet, fruity, warm, earthy	2	Ylang Ylang	Sweet, heavy, narcotic, tropical floral	5
Dill	Fresh, sweet, herbaceous, slight earthy	2	**Base Notes**	(5-20% of the blend)	
Fir, Balsam	Fresh, clean, green, balsamic, sweet	2	Onycha	Rich, warm, slightly woody, creamy	1
Lavender	Floral, sweet, balsamic, slightly woody	2	Cedarwood	Warm, soft, woody	3
Melissa	Delicate, lemony	2	Cypress, Blue	Long-lasting, warm, woody, earthy	3
Cajeput	Fresh, camphorous, with fruity note	3	Frankincense	Rich, deep, warm, balsamic, sweet	3
Coriander	Woody, spicy, sweet	3	Sandalwood	Soft, woody, sweet, earthy, balsamic	3
Cypress	Fresh, herbaceous, slightly woody	3	Jasmine	Powerful, sweet, tenacious, floral	4
Elemi	Balsamic, fresh, citrusy, peppery, spicy	3	Myrrh	Warm, earthy, woody, balsamic	4
Euc Citriodora	Sweet, lemony, fresh, slightly woody	3	Patchouli	Earthy, sweet-balsamic, rich, wood-like	4
Euc. Radiata	Slightly camphorous, sweet, fruity	3	Vanilla	Sweet, balsamic, heavy, warm	4
Fir	Fresh, woody, earthy, sweet	3	Spikenard	Heavy, earthy, animal-like	5
Geranium	Sweet, green, citrus-rosy, fresh	3	Vetiver	Heavy, earthy, balsamic, smoky	5

METHODS OF APPLICATION

Topical Application

1. **Direct Application.** Apply the oils directly on the area of concern using one to six drops of oil. More oil is not necessarily better since a large amount of oil can trigger a detoxification of the surrounding tissue and blood. Such a quick detoxification can be somewhat uncomfortable. To achieve the desired results, one to three drops of oil is usually adequate. A few guidelines for direct application of the oils are as follows:
   - ✓ The feet are the second fastest area of the body to absorb oils because of the large pores. Other quick absorbing areas include behind the ears and on the wrists.
   - ✓ To experience a feeling of peace, relaxation, or energy, three to six drops per foot are adequate.
   - ✓ When massaging a large area of the body, always dilute the oils by 15% to 30% with the V-6 Mixing Oil.
   - ✓ When applying oils to infants and small children, dilute with V-6 Mixing Oil. Use one to three drops of an essential oil to one tablespoon (Tbs.) of V-6 Mixing Oil for infants and one to three drops of an essential oil to one teaspoon (tsp.) V-6 Mixing Oil for children from two to five years old.
   - ✓ <u>Do not mix</u> oil blends. Commercially available blends have been specially formulated by someone who understands the chemical constituents of each oil and which oils blend well. The chemical properties of the oils can be altered when mixed improperly, resulting in some undesirable reactions.
   - ✓ Layering individual oils is preferred over mixing your own blends. Layering refers to the process of applying one oil, rubbing it in, and then applying another oil. There is no need to wait more than a couple of seconds between each oil as absorption occurs quite rapidly. If dilution is necessary, the V-6 Mixing Oil may be applied on top. The layering technique is not only useful in physical healing, but also when doing emotional clearing.
   - ✓ The FDA has approved some essential oils for internal use and given them the designation of GRAS (Generally Regarded As Safe for internal consumption). *This designation is listed in the Single Oil Summary Information chart in the Appendix of this book under Safety Data.* **Oils without this designation should never be used internally.**

2. **Vita Flex Therapy.** A simple method of applying oils to contact points (or nerve endings) in the feet or hands. Then a series of hand rotation movements at those control points create a vibrational healing energy that carries the oils along the neuroelectrical pathways. The oils help increase the frequency of this healing energy and serve to either help remove any blockage along the pathways or travel the length of the pathway to benefit the particular organ. Refer to the following pages on Vita Flex Therapy for more details.

3.   **Raindrop Technique.** A simple application of dropping certain oils like little drops of rain from about six inches above the body along the entire length of the spine. It is also a tremendous boost to the immune system as it releases toxins and kills viruses and bacteria that have accumulated along the spine. See the pages on Raindrop Technique in this section of the reference guide for more details.

4.   **Auricular Therapy.** A method of applying the oils to the rim of the ears. This technique works extremely well for emotional clearing. Some physical benefits can also be obtained from this technique. See the pages on Auricular Therapy in this section of the reference guide for more details.

5.   **Perfume or Cologne.** Wearing the oils as a perfume or cologne can provide some wonderful emotional support, and physical support as well; not just a beautiful fragrance. (For some simple, yet exquisite perfume/cologne blends, refer to the book Natural Perfumes, by Mindy Green)

Compresses

1.   **Basin.** Fill a wash basin with two quarts of hot or cold water and add the desired essential oils. Stir the water vigorously then lay a towel on top of the water. Since the oils will float to the top, the towel will absorb the oils with the water. After the towel is completely saturated, wring out the excess water (leaving much of the oils in the towel) and place over the area needing the compress. For a **hot** compress, cover with a dry towel and a hot water bottle. For a **cold** compress, cover with a piece of plastic or plastic wrap. Finally, put another towel on top and leave for as long as possible (one to two hours is best).

2.   **Massage.** Apply a hot wet towel and a dry towel on top of an already massaged area. The moist heat will force the oils deeper into the tissues of the body.

Inhalations

1.   **Diffuser.** The easiest and simplest way of putting the oils into the air for inhalation is to use an aromatic diffuser. Diffusers that use a heat source (such as a light bulb ring) will alter the chemical make-up of the oil and its therapeutic qualities. A cold air diffuser uses room-temperature air to blow the oil up against some kind of a nebulizer. This breaks the oils up into a micro-fine mist that is then dispersed into the air, covering hundreds of square feet in seconds. The oils, with their oxygenating molecules, will then remain suspended for several hours to freshen and improve the quality of the air. The anti-viral, anti-bacterial, and antiseptic properties of the oils, kill bacteria and help to reduce fungus and mold. Essential oils, when diffused, have been found to reduce the amount of airborne chemicals and metallics as well as help to create greater spiritual, physical, and emotional harmony. The

greatest therapeutic benefit is received by diffusing oils for only 15 minutes out of an hour so that the olfactory system has time to recover before receiving more oils. The easiest way to do this is by using a timer that can be set in 15 minute increments over a 24 hour period. Abundant Health offers a variety of cold-air diffusers and timers for your convenience.

2.   **Cloth or Tissue.** Put one to three drops of an essential oil on a paper towel, tissue, cotton ball, handkerchief, towel, or pillow case and hold it close to your face and inhale.

3.   **Hot Water.** Put one to three drops of an essential oil into hot water and inhale. Again, heat reduces some of the benefits.

4.   **Vaporizer or Humidifier.** Put oil in a vaporizer or a humidifier. The cold air types are best since heat reduces some of the benefits.

5.   **Fan or Vent.** Put oil on a cotton ball and attach to ceiling fans or air vents. This can also work well in a vehicle as the area is so small.

Baths

1.   **Bath Water.** Begin by adding three to six drops of oil to the bath water while the tub is filling. Because the individual oils will separate as the water calms down, the skin will quickly draw the oils from the top of the water. People have commented that they were unable to endure more than six drops of oil. Such individuals may benefit from adding the oils to a bath and shower gel base first. Soak for 15 minutes.

2.   **Bath and Shower Gel.** Begin by adding three to six drops of oil to ½ oz. of a bath and shower gel base and add to the water while the tub is filling. The number of drops can be increased as described above under *Bath Water*. Adding the oils to a bath and shower gel base first allows one to obtain the greatest benefit from the oils as they are more evenly dispersed throughout the water and not allowed to immediately separate.

3.   **Wash Cloth.** When showering, add three to six drops of oil to a bath and shower gel base first before applying to a face cloth to effectively cover the entire body.

4.   **Body Sprays.** Fill a small spray bottle with distilled water and add 10-15 drops of your favorite oil blend or single oils. Shake well and spray onto the entire body just after taking a bath or shower.

> *I love to add a drop or 2 of lemon oil to the Joy blend! It's a wonderful perfume. If you want the blend to last longer and cool you off for the summer, fill a small spray bottle with distilled water and 10 drops of Joy, 2 drops of Lemon. I like to spray it on after I shower.*
>
> **-Submitted by Nancy Dutton (July 2004)**

Dishwater, Clothes Washers, And Dryers

The anti-bacterial properties of essential oils can effectively promote greater hygiene. Add a couple drops of Melrose or lemon to dishwater for clean dishes and a great smelling kitchen. Use lemon or another citrus oil to take gum out of clothes. A few drops of Purification in the wash water will kill bacteria and germs in clothes. Put Purification, Joy, or other oil on a wet rag and place in dryer, or mist from a spray bottle directly into the dryer.

Cooking

Essential oils can easily be incorporated into your cooking, as long as you remember that they are very concentrated. Usually only 1 drop is necessary, and sometimes even less. Use a toothpick to help control the addition of smaller amounts of oil, by dipping the toothpick into the oil (more oil on the toothpick = stronger flavor, etc.) then stirring it into the food. Here are a couple examples of recipes where people have used the essential oils for flavoring.

Lemon Tarragon Dressing

1 tablespoon fresh tarragon diced, or 1 teaspoon dried tarragon
1 tablespoon fresh or 1 teaspoon dried basil leaves
1 cup organic extra virgin cold pressed olive oil
dash of pepper
dash of red pepper
6 drops lemon essential oil

Mix well and drizzle on salad or fish or anything! Keep unused portion in the fridge.
-**Submitted by Jill Burk, Saginaw, Michigan (July 2004)**

Cream Cheese Icing

8 oz. package of cream cheese
1½ cups of powdered sugar
1 stick of butter
3 drops of tangerine essential oil

Cream together thoroughly the cream cheese, powdered sugar and butter with electric beater. Stir in the tangerine oil. Enjoy!
-**Submitted by Ellie Ayers (July 2004)**

Cleaning And Disinfecting

Put a few drops of **lemon, spruce, or fir** oil on a dust cloth or ten drops in water in a spray bottle to polish furniture and to clean and disinfect bathrooms and kitchens.

Painting

To effectively remove paint fumes and after smell, add one 15 ml. bottle of oil to any five gallon bucket of paint. The Abundance blend and citrus oils have been favorites. Either a paint sprayer or brush and roller may be used to apply the paint after mixing the oils into the paint by stirring vigorously. Oils may eventually rise to the top if using a water-based paint. Occasional stirring may be necessary to keep the oils mixed.

VITA FLEX THERAPY

Vita Flex Therapy is based on a small part of a complete system which was developed by Stanley Burroughs during a period of more than fifty years of research and application. Vita Flex uses the reflex system of internal body controls to release tensions, congestions, and maladjustments. When properly applied through specific application of hand rotation movements and control points, a vibrational healing energy is released along the neuro-electrical pathways to an exact point. This healing energy is created by the contact between the fingertips and the reflex (contact) points. The resulting spark of energy follows the neuro pathways of the nervous system to where there is a break in the electrical circuit. Upon reaching the break, any necessary changes are made automatically. This technique is believed to have originated in Tibet many thousands of years ago, long before acupuncture was ever discovered.

The Vita Flex Technique is a superior form of reflexology. Reflexology, as used today, has a tendency to ground out the electrical charge from constant compression and rotation, which causes cell separation, loss of oxygen to subdermal tissues, and further injury. With the Vita Flex technique people experience less discomfort. Using the thumb and all four fingers, the application is much more efficient. There are more than 5,000 Vita Flex points throughout the body (in the complete system as developed by Stanley Burroughs) in comparison to the 365 acupuncture points used in reflexology. With Vita Flex, the weakened or injured areas are corrected on reflected points, thereby preventing further injury.

Combining the electrical frequency of the oils and that of the person receiving the application creates rapid and phenomenal results. "Vita Flex" is derived from the term "vitality through the reflexes" and is a complete, workable system which, when combined with the healing properties of essential oils, can release an unlimited healing power.

Stanley Burroughs' book, Healing for the Age of Enlightenment, explains in detail the system that he designed over many years. For step-by-step instruction of the full Vita Flex treatment, refer to the video, Vita Flex Instruction with Tom Woloshyn. This video teaches the proper Vita Flex technique as developed by Stanley Burroughs, including the Atlas Adjustment (a non-chiropractic technique used to quickly and efficiently re-align the spine or any other misalignment in the body). Stanley Burroughs also designed the **Vita Flex roller**, or "Relax-a-Roller" to assist one in doing Vita Flex on themselves. This device is a special type of roller with staggered, fine-pointed pegs, placed close enough together so as not to dig in too deeply with heavy pressure. Yet, they are far enough apart to reach all Vita Flex points as one rolls both feet back and forth. With just a few minutes of use, tensions, drowsiness, weariness, and discomfort disappear. Also, by adding the desired oils to the feet and rolling them back and forth on the roller, one can easily achieve the benefits of Vita Flex Therapy. These rollers are produced in Canada and are available from Abundant Health.

<u>Key Principles</u>

1.   **To reduce any discomfort, fingernails should be cut and filed short**.

2.   Remove all jewelry and watches to prevent an interference of energy.

3.   Always **DROP** the oils into the palm of your non-dominant hand and use the dominant hand to stir the oils clockwise three times before application. This method will increase the electrical frequency of the oils and significantly improve the results. **To prevent contamination of the oils, do not touch the top of the bottle with any part of your body.**

4.   Put a drop of <u>White Angelica</u> on each of your shoulders to protect yourself against any negative energies from the person you are working on.

5.   Always start on the bottom of the feet. Put three to six drops of <u>Valor</u> on the bottom of each foot. Some may be applied to the brain stem if desired. Hold the bottoms of the feet with your hands; right hand to right foot and left hand to left foot. Continue holding the feet until you feel the body's energy balance. This usually feels like an energy pulse beating in both feet. Another way to balance, which may be preferable to some, is to put one drop of <u>Valor</u> on the wrists and hold the wrists crossed together for a few minutes, until you feel a pulse in the tips of the thumb and index finger.

6.   Use the Vita Flex charts (*shown on the next couple of pages*) to determine where the oils should be placed during the therapy. One to three drops of oil may be applied to the specific Vita Flex points of the foot. Vita Flex points on the hand can be used as an alternative to extremely sensitive or sore feet. Apply the oil(s).

7.   Apply the Vita Flex technique as follows: Starting with the fingers on their pads, curl the fingers up and over onto the nails (see photo examples on the next page). Increasing pressure is applied until the fingers are curled almost completely over on the nails. Pressure is then immediately released to create the spark of energy and send it on its way. The curling should be one continuous motion, not jerky, with medium to heavy pressure being placed on the contact point. Never press and hold while performing this technique. This may be done several times on the same spot to obtain the desired results. Some leverage can be achieved by placing the thumb of the same hand around to the other side of the foot or hand on which the Vita Flex is being performed. This allows the hand to operate in a fashion similar to a pipe wrench, which increases pressure on the pipe as it is twisted.

Vita Flex Start Position   Vita Flex Middle Position   Vita Flex End Position

VITA FLEX HAND CHART

Vita Flex points in this hand chart correspond to those in the feet. Occasionally the feet can be too sensitive for typical Vita Flex Therapy. Working with the hands will not only affect the specific body points, but may also help to provide some pain relief to the corresponding points on the feet. (Refer to Stanley Burroughs' book, Healing for the Age of Enlightenment, pg. 78 for a more detailed explanation.)

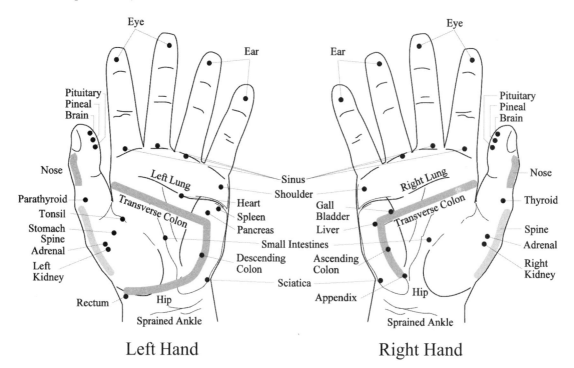

VITA FLEX FEET CHART

Right Foot   Left Foot

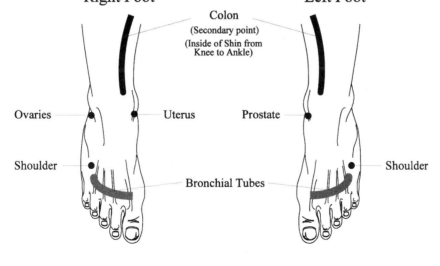

Note: This chart combines the work of Stanley Burroughs (Vita Flex Charting) and D. Gary Young (Electrical Frequency Tracing). Refer to their respective books, listed in the bibliography, for more detailed information.

AURICULAR INTERNAL BODY POINTS

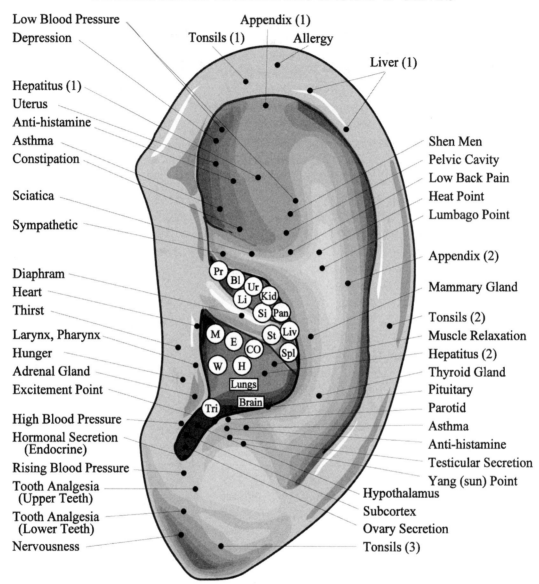

Low Blood Pressure
Depression
Appendix (1)
Tonsils (1)
Allergy
Liver (1)

Hepatitus (1)
Uterus
Anti-histamine
Asthma
Constipation

Sciatica

Sympathetic

Diaphram
Heart
Thirst

Larynx, Pharynx
Hunger
Adrenal Gland
Excitement Point

High Blood Pressure
Hormonal Secretion
(Endocrine)
Rising Blood Pressure
Tooth Analgesia
(Upper Teeth)
Tooth Analgesia
(Lower Teeth)
Nervousness

Shen Men
Pelvic Cavity
Low Back Pain
Heat Point
Lumbago Point

Appendix (2)

Mammary Gland

Tonsils (2)
Muscle Relaxation
Hepatitus (2)
Thyroid Gland
Pituitary
Parotid
Asthma
Anti-histamine
Testicular Secretion
Yang (sun) Point
Hypothalamus
Subcortex
Ovary Secretion
Tonsils (3)

M:	**Mouth**	**Pr:**	**Prostate**	**Liv:**	**Liver**
E:	**Esophagus**	**Bl:**	**Bladder**	**Spl:**	**Spleen**
CO:	**Cardiac Orifice**	**Ur:**	**Ureter**	**H:**	**Heart**
St:	**Stomach**	**Kid:**	**Kidney**	**W:**	**Windpipe,**
Si:	**Small Intestine**	**Pan:**	**Pancreas,**		**Trachea**
Li:	**Large Intestine**		**Gall Bladder**	**Tri:**	**Triple Warner**

RAINDROP TECHNIQUE

This application technique was developed by Dr. Don Gary Young, N.D. Aromatologist, and one of North America's leading experts on the art and science of aromatherapy. This technique involves dropping the oils directly onto the spine from about six inches above the body. The oils are then worked into the spine using light strokes with the fingers which stimulate energy impulses and disperse the oils along the nervous system throughout the entire body. In this way, the body can be brought into balance and the energy centers can be cleared and re-aligned. It will also help to reduce spinal inflammations and kill viruses that hibernate along the spinal column, as well as help to straighten any spinal curvatures. Although a session lasts for about 45 minutes to an hour, the oils will continue to work in the body for a week or more following the treatment. The Raindrop Technique that is explained below is an abbreviated form. The video entitled <u>Raindrop Technique</u> by D. Gary Young (*available from Abundant Health*) provides step-by-step instructions for this technique.

<u>Oils used in the Raindrop Technique</u>

VALOR—is the first and most important oil used in this technique because it helps balance the electrical energies within the body. It also helps create an environment where structural alignment can occur.

THYME—is used for its ability to support the immune system by attacking any bacteria, fungus, infection, or virus that may be present. It may also help one overcome fatigue and physical weakness after an illness.

OREGANO—works in conjunction with thyme to strengthen the immune system and to attack bacteria and viruses. It may also act as an antiseptic for the respiratory system, help balance metabolism, and strengthen the vital centers of the body.

CYPRESS—is used for its anti-bacterial, anti-infectious, antimicrobial, and diuretic properties. In addition, it may function as a decongestant for the circulatory and lymphatic systems.

BIRCH/WINTERGREEN—is great for removing discomfort associated with the inflammation of bones, muscles, and joints. It may also help cleanse the lymphatic system.

BASIL—is relaxing to spastic muscles and is stimulating to the nerves and the adrenal glands.

PEPPERMINT—is used to calm and strengthen the nerves, reduce inflammation, and is highly effective when dealing with conditions related to the respiratory system. It also has a synergistic and enhancing effect on all other oils.

MARJORAM—is used to relax spastic muscles, soothe the nerves, relieve cramps, aches, and pains, and to help calm the respiratory system.

AROMA SIEZ—may help to relax, calm, and relieve the tension of spastic muscles resulting from sports injury, fatigue, or stress.

ORTHO EASE—is the crowning oil to this application. It is used to help relax all the muscles of the back and legs and to help reduce any stress, arthritic pain, or tension that may exist.

V-6 MIXING OIL—is used to help dilute any of the oils that may be somewhat caustic to the skin. It should always be used with oregano and thyme and can be used with any of the other oils based upon the person's skin sensitivity.

Note: The oils used in this technique have many more benefits than those listed above. *For more specific information, please refer to the sections in this book on Singles and Blends.*

Raindrop Technique

1.   Remove all jewelry or metal to allow the energy to flow freely. Put a drop of **White Angelica** on each of your shoulders to protect you against any negative energies coming from the person receiving the treatment.

2.   Have the person lie face up on a table with their body as straight as possible on the table. The person receiving the treatment should be as comfortable as possible, so the arms can be resting along side the body or resting on the top of their hips, whichever they prefer (don't let their hands touch each other as this will tend to short circuit the flow of energy through their body). By covering the person with a sheet, their modesty can be protected as you roll them over and they can be kept warm as you alternate between working on the back and working on the legs and feet.

3.   Apply **three** drops of **Valor** on each shoulder as well as six drops on each foot. Hold right foot/shoulder with right hand and left foot/shoulder with left hand (crossing hands if necessary – see the photo illustration entitled, "Valor Balance on Feet") for five to ten minutes or until you can feel an energy pulse in the person's feet. For this part of the application, it works best if there is another person assisting in the treatment. If you are working by yourself, do the feet only. **Valor** is used to balance and it works well on the energy alignment of the body. **This is the most important oil that is used in this application.**

Valor Balance on Feet

4. First apply 2 drops of **thyme** to the Vita Flex spine points along the inside edge of each foot, working it in three times with the Vita Flex technique (*refer to Vita Flex Technique in this same section, Key Principle #7 and photo illustrations for an explanation of this technique*). Repeat this procedure with each of the following oils, one at a time: **Oregano**, **cypress**, **birch/wintergreen**, **basil**, and **peppermint**. Then, have the person roll over onto their stomach and perform steps 5 through 14 on their spine.

5. Hold the bottle of **thyme** about six inches from the spine and evenly space **four to five** drops from the sacrum (tailbone) to the neck. Work it in evenly along the curvature of the spine with gentle upward strokes. Apply **five** drops of **oregano** and work it in the same way. Then, apply **ten to fifteen** drops of **V-6 Mixing Oil** to prevent any discomfort since both these oils can be quite caustic.

6. Using the very tips of the fingers, alternate between left hand and right hand as you very lightly work up the spine from the sacrum to the base of the neck with short, brush-like strokes. Follow the curvature of the spine and repeat two more times.

7. Using your finger tips again, softly brush up a few inches from the sacrum then out to either side of the body; right hand to the right and left hand to the left.

    Repeat this step from the sacrum but go a few more inches up the spine then out to the sides. Then again from the sacrum, going up a few more inches then out. Then again, each time going further up the spine until you reach the base of the neck and flare out along the shoulders. This entire step should then be repeated two more times.

8. Using your finger tips again, start at the sacrum and in full-length strokes, lightly brush all the way up the spine to the base of the neck and then out over the shoulders. Repeat two more times.

9. Evenly space **four to five** drops of **cypress** from the sacrum to the neck. Work it in evenly along the curvature of the spine with gentle upward strokes. Then apply the oils of **birch/ wintergreen, basil, and peppermint** in the same manner.

10. Place both hands side by side (parallel to the spine) and using the tips of the fingers, massage in a circular, clock-wise motion, just off to one side of the spine, from the sacrum up to the neck. **Remember to never work directly on the spine**. Apply moderate pressure and move a finger's width at a time. This will help to loosen the muscles and allow the spine to straighten itself. After doing one side of the spine, move around the person and work the other side of the spine from the sacrum to the neck in the same manner. Repeat two more times on either side.

11. Using whichever hand is most comfortable to you, place the index and middle finger on either side of the spine at the sacrum. Place the other hand on top of the first, part way down the two fingers. Apply moderate pressure and with a quick, forward and back continued sawing motion of the hand on top, slide the fingers a little at a time up the spine to the skull. Move the fingers upward slowly during the sawing motion. Once the skull is reached, apply gentle but firm pressure to push the skull forward, stretching the spine. Return to the sacrum and repeat two more times.

12. Place the thumbs of each hand on either side of the spine at the sacrum and point them towards each other. Next, using the Vita Flex technique, roll the thumbs up and over onto the thumbnails, applying some pressure straight down during the roll. Then release and slide the thumbs up an inch or so and repeat the roll with pressure. Continue up to the base of the neck, then return to the sacrum and repeat two more times. This will become easier with practice.

13. Apply five to six drops of **marjoram** up the spine and work it in. Then apply five to six drops of <u>**Aroma Siez**</u> to each side and away from the spine. Gently massage these oils into the muscle tissue all over the back to soothe and relax the patient. After the oils have been massaged in well, you may cover the person with the sheet and rest for approximately five minutes. Apply **Ortho Ease** over the entire area of the back and gently massage it in. Then cover the person to keep them warm and massage **Ortho Ease** into the legs. This will help to relax the muscles that may be pulling on the spine.

14. Fold a hand towel, soak it in hot water, wring it out and lay it along the entire length of the spine. Take a dry bath towel and fold it in half lengthwise and place it over the hot wet towel. Be extremely sensitive to the feelings of the person as the heat may build along the spine. The heat will gradually build for five to eight minutes then cool right down to normal. If the heat becomes too uncomfortable, remove the towels and apply V-6 Mixing Oil. Then replace the towels and continue until the wet towel becomes cold. If the person's back is still hot, cover with a dry towel and allow the back to cool down slowly.

15. After the person's back begins to cool down, gently stretch the spine by crossing hands and straddle the spine with your hands, one pointing towards the top of the spine and the other towards the bottom as shown in the adjacent photo. Starting in the middle, gently press the hands downwards and apart towards opposite ends of the spine. Then move the hands apart more and repeat the stretch. Continue until the ends of the spine are reached.

16. Remove the wet towels and have the person roll over onto their back. Apply two to three drops of **birch/wintergreen** along the inside of each leg from the knee to the heel and up the inside of the foot to the big toe. Layer it in and apply the oils of **cypress, basil, and peppermint** in the same fashion. Then work the same area using the Vita Flex technique. The inside of the shin corresponds to the colon. By working this area, you are opening the colon and allowing it to expel any toxins released during the Raindrop Technique.

17. The final step is to perform another gentle stretching of the spine. If you are working alone, put your right hand behind the base of the head and your left hand under the chin. Very gently pull to create a slight tension and release. Do three times then move to the feet. Hold above the ankles and gently pull and release three times. If you have an assistant, one person can hold the head and the other hold the feet. Then together, apply a gentle tension and hold for a few minutes. This is then completed by the person at the head doing a very slight pull and release three times.

18.   If certain systems of the body need work, have the person roll back over onto their stomach and use the applicable blends and/or singles with the Vita Flex Technique on the spine. Refer to the chart of the autonomic nervous system to help with placement of the oils along the spine.

By stimulating the Central Nervous System, you have just given someone a total treatment, affecting every system in the body, including emotional release and support. Even though the oils continue to work in the body for a week or more, one application may last months or it may be necessary to repeat the application every week until the body begins to respond. The object is to develop a new memory in the tissues of the body and train it to hold itself in place. **(For a list of videos that effectively demonstrate this valuable application technique, refer to the** *Video Listing* **in the Bibliography section of this book.)**

Another aspect to the Raindrop Technique is the ability to **customize it** to the needs of the receiver. Each Raindrop Technique session should begin with the **Valor** essential oil blend, and the single oils of **oregano** (*Origanum compactum* CT carvacrol), and **thyme** (*Thymus vulgaris* CT thymol). However, after that, the remaining oils can be replace with others more specific to the condition or body system needing to be affected. To assist with this customization, the following chart is a partial list of single oils and oil blends under the particular body system which they affect. This chart is a condensed excerpt from the Body System Chart shown in the Appendix of this book

(Refer to the full chart in the Appendix for other products that can assist in strengthening a particular body system).

Cardiovascular System	Digestive System	Emotional Balance*	Hormonal System	Immune System	Nervous System	Respiratory System
anise	anise	angelica	anise	Abundance	angelica	anise
AromaLife	cardamon	Australian Blue	Clary sage	cistus	Brain Power	Aroma Siez
basil	celery seed	chamomile (both)	coriander	Citrus Fresh	carrot	cajeput
cajeput	clove	Chivalry	davana	clove	cedarwood	clove
carrot	coriander	fir, white	Dragon Time	cumin	celery seed	eucalyptus (all)
Christmas Spirit	cumin	frankincense	EndoFlex	cypress, Blue	chamomile (both)	fir (all)
clove	cypress, blue	Gathering	fennel	Exodus II	En-R-Gee	hyssop
cypress	Di-Gize	geranium	fleabane	frankincense	balsam fir	laurel
fleabane	fennel	jasmine	goldenrod	galbanum	frankincense	lavandin
goldenrod	ginger	juniper	jasmine	ImmuPower	hyssop	lemon
grapefruit	juniper	Lady Sclareol	Mister	laurel	juniper	melaleuca (all)
helichrysum	JuvaFlex	lavender	myrrh	ledum	lavender	Melrose
hyssop	Juva Cleanse	onycha	myrtle	lemon	myrrh	myrtle
lavandin	laurel	orange	nutmeg	lemongrass	nutmeg	peppermint
lavender	lemon	palmarosa	sage	lime	PanAway	pine
Longevity	mandarin	petitgrain	sage lavender	melaleuca	Peace & Calming	Raven
marjoram	myrtle	pine	SclarEssence	Mountain savory	pepper, black	ravensara
onycha	orange	sage lavender	Sensation	myrrh	peppermint	RC
palmarosa	peppermint	sandalwood	vetiver	nutmeg	sage lavender	rosemary ver-
rosemary	Purification	spikenard	yarrow	orange	sandalwood	banon
tsuga	rosemary	spruce	ylang ylang	ravensara	spruce	sage lavender
ylang ylang	SclarEssence	Valor		sage	tansy, blue	spruce
	spearmint	vetiver		Thieves	valerian	thyme linalol
	tarragon	ylang ylang		yarrow	vetiver	tsuga

The majority of the essential oil blends in this book deal with emotional balance and are therefore too numerous to list here. Refer to the Body Systems Chart in the Appendix for more possible blends.

The booklet, entitled <u>A Statistical Validation of Raindrop Technique</u>, by David Stewart, PhD, RA (available from Abundant Health), is the result of research conducted by the distribution of over 3,000 surveys to individuals that have either received a Raindrop Technique session, administered Raindrop Technique sessions to others, or both. The results of the survey were tabulated and the following are excerpts from these results, showing overwhelming evidence that "Raindrop is thought by the vast majority of its participants to benefit people in ways both objective and subjective, physical and emotional, social and spiritual."

	Perceived Results of Raindrop as Expressed by 416 clients receiving 3,584 Raindrops			Perceived Results of Raindrop as Expressed by Clients to the 265 Facilitators Responding to this Survey for 11,256 Raindrop Procedures Administered		
a.	Positive 97.0%	Neutral 2.5%	Negative 0.5%	Positive 96.3%	Neutral 3.5%	Negative 0.2%
b.	Pleasant 97.9%	Neutral 1.4%	Unpleasant 0.4%	Pleasant 96.4%	Neutral 3.0%	Unpleasant 0.6%
c.	Resulted in Healing 15.9%	No Perceptible Results 83.9%	Resulted in Harm or Injury 0.2%	Resulted in Healing 87.7%	No Perceptible Results 12.0%	Resulted in Harm or Injury 0.3%
d.	Felt Better Afterwards 97.7%	No Change in Feeling 1.4%	Felt Worse Afterwards 0.9%	Felt Better Afterwards 96.0%	No Change in Feeling 3.4%	Felt Worse Afterwards 0.6%
e.	Health Improved 89.1%	No Change in Health 10.9%	Health got Worse 0.0%	Health Improved 90.8%	No Change in Health 9.2%	Health got Worse 0.03%
f.	Emotional State Improved 86.2%	No Change in Emotions 13.4%	Emotional State Worsened 0.4%	Emotional State Improved 91.0%	No Change in Emotions 8.5%	Emotional State Worsened 0.5%
g.	Would Receive It Again 99.9%	Maybe So, Maybe Not 0.1%	Would Never Receive it Again 0.0%	Would Receive It Again 96.7%	Maybe So, Maybe Not 3.2%	Would Never Receive it Again 0.1%

–This information is included here with permission from the author, David Stewart

The following are some personal experiences with Raindrop Technique:

I was in a pitiful state. I had not been able to work for 5 years, lived on disability insurance, and then welfare. I depended on pharmaceuticals for pain management and depression. My social schedule consisted of doctor appointments and rest periods. I had been diagnosed with herniated disks and then fibromyalgia. I was a textbook case with all the symptoms and treatments which helped temporarily but didn't get rid of anything. Then a wonderful friend talked me into coming to see her to receive the Raindrop Technique. At first, I received the Raindrop Technique once a week for about 6 weeks, then once every other week, then once a month. After the first few sessions, I was feeling so very much better. Then I noticed that I would forget to take my medications and was doing just fine without them. After a while, I did not need to take anything anymore.

—Submitted by Pam Jones, Benton, Arkansas (July 2004)

Mom had worn a narcotic pain patch for the past two years for her "chronic back pain" due to osteoarthritis, spurring of the spine, and numerous back surgeries. By using PanAway, we were able to discontinue the pain patch. We continued to alternate PanAway with Wintergreen, Peppermint, Clove and V-6 oil to her back and feet with warm compresses once or twice a day as needed for complete relief. Six weeks after she started receiving weekly Raindrop massages, she no longer complained of back pain. She continues to receive weekly or bi-weekly Raindrop massages, and it's been 6 months since she has complained of back pain! Praise God!

—Submitted by E. Pinar (July 2004)

AUTONOMIC NERVOUS SYSTEM

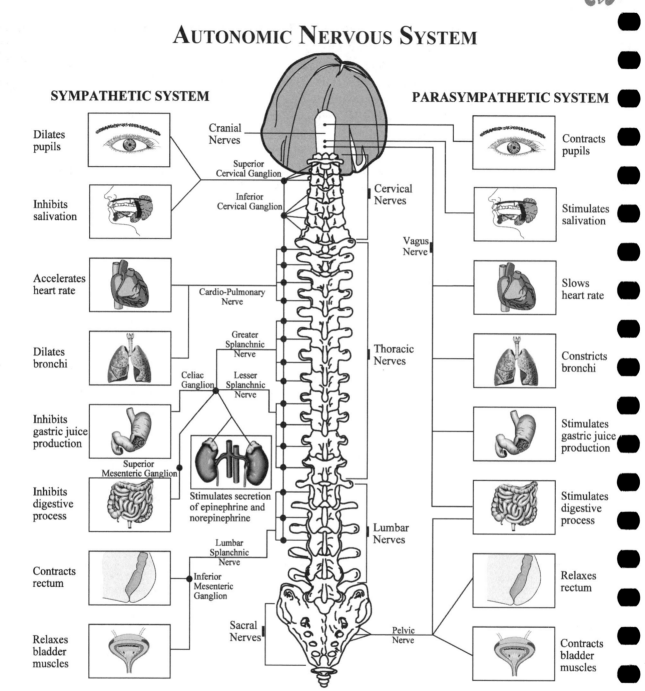

DIGESTIVE TRACT

"The gastrointestinal tract is a tube twenty-five to thirty-two feet long, that begins at the mouth and ends at the anus. It comprises the mouth, pharynx, esophagus, stomach, small intestine (duodenum, jejunum, and ileum), large intestine (cecum, ascending colon, transverse colon, and descending colon), rectum, and anus. Accessory organs—the liver, pancreas, and gallbladder—all play an important role in digestion.

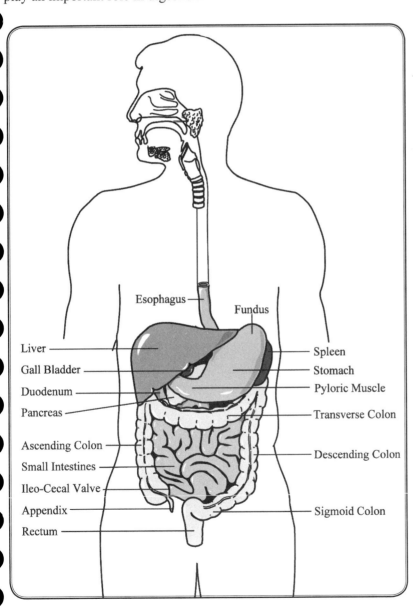

Esophagus
Fundus
Liver
Gall Bladder
Duodenum
Pancreas
Ascending Colon
Small Intestines
Ileo-Cecal Valve
Appendix
Rectum
Spleen
Stomach
Pyloric Muscle
Transverse Colon
Descending Colon
Sigmoid Colon

"Digestion begins when food mixes with enzymes in saliva. The process is then carried on in the stomach by hydrochloric acid (HCl) and pepsin. Food is liquefied in the stomach and passes into the small intestine, where it is further broken down by digestive enzymes from the pancreas (the enzyme protease digests proteins, the enzyme amylase digests carbohydrates, and the enzyme lipase digests fats). The gallbladder secretes bile, formed by the liver, to aid absorption of fats and fat-soluble vitamins.

"Most food absorption takes place in the small intestine, while water, electrolytes (essential body chemicals), and some of the final products of digestion are absorbed in the large intestine." (*Alternative Medicine—The Definitive Guide*, p. 680)

NOSE AND OLFACTORY SYSTEM

Cerebral Cortex

Hypothalamus

Pineal

Olfactory Bulb

Cilia (hairs) extending from Epithelium

Pituitary Gland

Amygdala

Caudate Nucleus

Thalamus

Cerebellum

Brain Stem

Odor molecules travel to the top of the nasal cavity and fit like little puzzle pieces into specific receptor cells on the cilia. The cilia are little bundles of six to eight tiny hairs which extend from each of about 10 million olfactory nerve cells. These millions of nerve cells (that are replaced every twenty eight days) make up a membrane which is known as the olfactory epithelium. The epithelium serves to transfer electric impulses from the cilia to the olfactory bulb, which it covers. The olfactory bulb, in turn, sends those impulses along to the amygdala (which is responsible for storing and releasing emotional trauma) and further on to the limbic system of the brain. Because the limbic system is directly connected to those parts of the brain that control heart rate, blood pressure, breathing, memory, stress levels, and hormone balance, essential oils can have some very profound physiological and psychological effects.

AURICULAR EMOTIONAL THERAPY

MOTHER: Geranium

Sexual Abuse: Geranium, Ylang Ylang
Abandonment: Geranium, Forgiveness, Acceptance

FATHER: Lavender

Sexual Abuse: Lavender, Ylang Ylang,
  Release
Male Abuse: Helichrysum, Lavender

DEPRESSION

Any of the following: Valor, Joy,
  Hope, White Angelica, Peace
  & Calming, Citrus Fresh,
  Christmas Spirit, Gentle Baby
Use whichever blend(s) work
  best for you.

OVERWHELMED

Use Hope and Acceptance

BEARING BURDENS OF THE WORLD

Use Release and Valor

ANGER & HATE

Use Joy to stimulate the pituitary.
Use Valor and Release to release the
  anger.

SELF EXPRESSION

Use Valor and Motivation. Take deep
  breaths to express oneself.

FEAR

Apply Valor, Release, Joy.

****If more than one oil/blend is
indicated, layer them one at a time. ****

**** When working on the ear, apply
Harmony and Forgiveness to the entire
ear and apply Valor on the feet. ****

SYMPATHY & GUILT

Use Joy and Inspiration.

SELF PITY

Use Acceptance.

REJECTION

Use Forgiveness and Acceptance.
  Work the rejection points on
  both ears. For rejection from
  Mother, use Geranium. For
  rejection from Father, use
  Lavender. While applying the
  oils, say "I choose to accept my
  Mother/Father for what they have
  done or not done. It is their life
  and not mine."

EYES and VISION

To improve eyesight, use 10
  Lemongrass, 5 Cypress, 3
  Eucalyptus, in ½ oz. of V-6
  Mixing Oil.
For Vision of goals, use Dream
  Catcher, Acceptance, and 3 Wise
  Men.

HEART

To strengthen the heart and lower
  blood pressure, use Aroma Life.
For self acceptance, apply Joy,
  Forgiveness, and Acceptance.

OPEN THE MIND

Apply 3 Wise Men.

EMOTIONAL RELEASE

Apply each of the following oils in the order suggested. Smell each oil before applying. If you find an oil repulsive, you may choose not to use it in this procedure.

1.   Apply three to six drops of <u>VALOR</u> to the bottom of the feet and balance by holding right foot in right hand and left foot in left hand. Continue to hold the feet until an energy pulse can be felt in both feet. <u>VALOR</u> helps balance electrical energies within the body, helps one overcome fear and opposition, and may give courage, confidence, and increase self esteem. Known as the "Chiropractor in a Bottle", it works best on the bottom of the feet, or on the spine (top and bottom, or entire length—raindrop style).

2.   Apply one drop of <u>HARMONY</u> either directly on the energy centers (chakras), or along the side of the body. <u>HARMONY</u> brings about a harmonic balance to the chakras (energy centers), allowing the energy to flow more efficiently through the body. It may reduce stress and create a general overall feeling of well being.

3.   Apply one drop of <u>3 WISE MEN</u> on the crown of the head in a clockwise motion. <u>3 WISE MEN</u> opens crown chakra and stimulates the pineal gland to release emotions and deep-seated trauma. It brings a sense of grounding and uplifting through memory recall. It also helps to keep negative energy and negative emotions from reattaching to the body.

4.   Apply one drop of <u>PRESENT TIME</u> on the thymus in a circular motion, close eyes and tap three times with energy fingers (pointer and middle). <u>PRESENT TIME</u> helps bring one into the moment. We must forget about the past and stop worrying about the future. We must live in the moment in order to heal.

5.   Apply one drop of <u>INNER CHILD</u> around the navel and nose. <u>INNER CHILD</u> may stimulate memory response and help one reconnect with their inner-self or their own identity. This is one of the first steps to achieving emotional balance.

6.   Apply one drop of <u>RELEASE</u> over the liver. <u>RELEASE</u> helps to enhance the release of memory trauma from the cells of the liver, where anger and hate emotions are stored. It may also help one let go of negative emotions so that progress is more effective and efficient.

7.   Apply one drop of <u>GROUNDING</u> to the brain stem, back of neck and sternum. <u>GROUNDING</u> may help one deal with the reality of their emotions in a peaceful way.

8.   Apply one drop of <u>FORGIVENESS</u> on the navel in a clockwise motion. <u>FORGIVENESS</u> may help one move past the barriers in life. It also helps to bring them into a higher spiritual

awareness of their needs and helps raise their frequency to the point where they feel almost compelled to FORGIVE, FORGET, LET GO, and go on with their lives.

9. Apply one drop of <u>HOPE</u> on the outer edge of the ears. <u>HOPE</u> helps support the body both physically and mentally. It may help one overcome suicidal depression and restore hope for tomorrow. By filling them with a feeling of strength and grounding, it empowers them to go forward with hope and achievement.

10. Apply one drop of <u>JOY</u> over the heart in a clockwise motion. <u>JOY</u> gives one a glorious feeling of self-love, confidence, and creates a frequency around oneself of the energy of love; the true source of all healing.

11. Apply one drop of <u>SARA</u> over the energy centers (chakras), navel, and chest. <u>SARA</u> may enable one to relax into a mental state and allow them to release the memories of traumatic experiences.

12. Apply one drop of <u>WHITE ANGELICA</u> Energy Centers on the crown and shoulders. <u>WHITE ANGELICA</u> strengthens and fortifies one's aura, generating a feeling of protection and an awareness of one's potential. As the final oil in this emotional clearing process, it supports all that has taken place and prepares one to search inward for the strength to proceed with life and to search upward for the true source of love and light.

13. Meditate for 20 minutes.

Comments: This procedure has been used successfully by many practitioners.

Note: Energy Centers are commonly known as Chakras. For a complete listing of the appropriate oils for each chakra, refer to the Personal Guide section of this book under Chakras.

Energy Centers

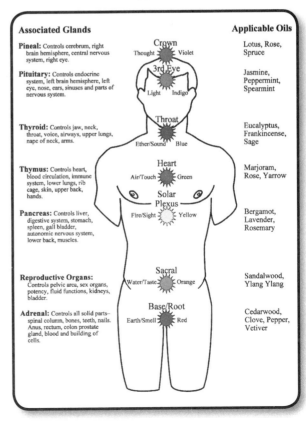

MUSIC AND AROMATHERAPY
Duets for Peaceful Emotional Healing
by Karyn Grant, Licensed Massage Therapist, Singer, Songwriter

Walking through life is like taking a journey. There are hidden treasures of knowledge along the path. There are precious traveling companions that enlighten our journey and make the way to healing more peaceful, more gentle, more beautiful. Music has become that traveling companion for me. It has never left my side.

I didn't realize it then, but I am aware now that it was as a youth that I learned that music was healing to the soul. I didn't know why I sang, I just sang. I found that through singing, my spirit was lifted and my mood was brightened. I began writing music by putting scriptures to simple guitar chords (I only knew three). Eventually, my own little handwritten verses became songs too. Just as the poetry of my heart turned to the lyrics of song, the simple everyday sorrows of a teenage girl turned into peaceful happy feelings. I was very happy as a youth. I took voice lessons, wrote songs, sang about everything from a stubbed toe to a broken heart. I didn't know exactly how it worked but I learned that when my heart was making music, I was the happiest. Music became for me, the peaceful way to handle any of life's problems.

I didn't understand then what was happening on a metaphysical level. I did not comprehend that music is a form of "light" and has healing vibrations of its own. I did not yet know what I now know; that music performs a massage on an atomic level in one's body and creates a way for less desirable energies to be transformed into more desirable ones. All I really knew was that when I sang, I got happy. When I wrote out my feelings and expressed them instead of holding them in, I got happy. And when I sang the heartfelt words I wrote, I got twice as happy. I had a quote on my wall at age sixteen that read, "I once wrote a poem that no one read, I once sang a song that no one heard, I once drew a picture that no one saw . . . and I was happy."

At nineteen, I was having my preschool class draw pictures as they listened to music blindfolded. I watched amused as they colored slower or scribbled faster to the tempos, rhythms and beats of the songs that I selected for them. I wondered how music could have such a powerful effect over someone so little? Their feelings and demeanors changed so quickly! Even then, I began learning, by exploring my own emotions and feelings, the mysterious power of music and the effect it had on myself and others.

As I reached my mid-twenties, the songs began coming again in the middle of the night. I learned that the combination of words and music could have a very softening effect on mind, heart, body and spirit. As my marriage grew more and more troubled, I realized that the gift of song was assuaging deep feelings of emotional isolation, spiritual bereavement and loneliness that I could not bear alone. I would arise at 3:00 a.m. every morning to nurse my baby girl back to sleep. Those became my own "feedings" too. That's when I began journeying with song again.

As the isolation grew in my marital relationship, so did the spiritual gift of singing. Singing the praises and sorrows of my heart literally took the ache from my heart and transformed grief into comfort, serenity and peace. I was able to focus on spiritual solutions for my less than desirable circumstance. The ability to express the innermost desires and feelings of my heart became easier. Not having developed the talent for writing the melodies, I sung them onto cassettes and hid them away in a drawer never imagining that these treasures would ever serve to bless other souls who were journeying through life carrying hidden wounds that could not be seen, diagnosed or solaced.

Not until years later, following my divorce, when I became a massage therapist, did I begin to understand the healing effect of music as therapy. I would work with clients during the day and would help them as best I could. Then, later in the night, I would be awakened with songs of comfort, courage and peace to sing to them at their next appointment. This I would do, and many wept tears of gratitude, saying that they never had anyone take the time to sing to them. N'Shama Sterling writes:

> When a woman in a certain African tribe knows she is pregnant, she goes out into the wilderness with a few friends and together they pray and meditate until they hear the song of the child. They recognize that every soul has its own vibration that expresses its unique flavor and purpose. When the women attune to the song, they sing it out loud. They then return to the tribe and teach the song of the child to the village.

> When the child is born, the community gathers and sings the child's song to him or her. Later, when the child enters education, the village gathers and chants the child's song. When the child passes through the initiation to adulthood, the people would again come together and sing. At the time of marriage, the person hears his or her song. Finally, when the soul is about to pass from this world, the family and friends gather at the person's bed, just as they did at their birth, and they sing the person to the next life.

> In this African tribe there is one other occasion upon which the villagers sing to the child. If at any time during his or her life, the person commits a crime or aberrant social act, the individual is called to the center of the village and the people in the community form a circle around them. They sing their song to them. The tribe recognized that the correction for antisocial behavior is not punishment; it is love and the remembrance of your true identity. When you recognize your own song, you have no desire or need to do anything that would hurt another.

A friend is someone who knows your song and sings it to you when you have forgotten it. Those who love you are not fooled by mistakes you have made or dark images you hold about yourself. They remember your beauty when you feel ugly; your wholeness when you are broken; your innocence when you feel guilty; and your purpose when you are confused. You may not have grown up in an African tribe that sings your song to you at crucial life transitions, but life is always reminding you when you are in tune with yourself and when you are not. When you feel good, what you are doing matches your song, and when you feel awful, it doesn't. In the end, we shall all recognize our song and sing it well. You may feel your voice is a bit "warbly" at the moment, but so have all the great singers at one time or another. Just keep singing.

I began learning that music was a vibrational soothing balm that could enter into places the physical ointment could not reach. Combining aromatherapy with the music began anchoring in the affirmations and imageries of the songs with scent. I instinctively knew that to reach those hidden wounds that are infected with the energies of loneliness, resentment, anger, despair, sadness, fear, doubt and other such emotions that are locked into the cellular memory of the glands, organs, tissues, and systems of the body, it would take the healing vibrations of touch, smell, visualization, and soothing sounds to transform those energies into positive and more joyful emotions.

From *The Book of Sound Therapy*, we read, "The human being is therefore likened to a very complex, unique, and finely-tuned musical instrument. Every atom, molecule, cell, tissue and organ of the body continually broadcasts the frequencies of physical, emotional, mental and spiritual life. The human voice is an indicator of its body's health on all these levels of existence. It establishes a relationship between the individual and the wondrous network of vibrations that is the cosmos."

In the ancient societies of Egypt, India, Greece, and China, to name a few, music played a vital role in just about everything, from health to architecture to politics. They believed that music was the bridge linking all things. Physical forms were considered manifestations of music, and it was held that life and health depended upon harmonic balance of rations and relationships. In ancient Greece, for instance, one could not become a physician until he had first become a musician, and prescriptions often included rhythmic singing and chanting from selected sacred melodic sequences.

If we could put a heart, broken and scarred, under a microscope and see the emotional aches manifesting themselves as rips and cuts and then pour the healing balm and vibrations of song and scent into those open and festering sores, I believe that we would watch in amazement as the rips began to mend and the cuts began to close in perfect alignment. For that is what I see in my mind's eye. I see song as living water. I see the vibrations of aromatherapy as more than just a scent, but as a healing balm for the soul. I see the wounds being cleansed and mending in perfect closure, having finally been acknowledged, addressed and administered to.

An anonymous quote reads, "Man of himself is an instrument of music; and when the chords of which he is composed are touched as sound salutes the ear, the sound appeals to his spirit and the sentiment to his understanding. If the strains are harmonious, he endorses and enjoys them with supreme delight. Whether the tones are from a human voice or from an instrument, they arrest his attention and absorb his whole being."

I have stood at the side of my massage table and beheld as countenances have changed from tearful torment into peaceful, blissful expressions of tranquil gratitude. For the hidden wounds of the heart and the spirit, there are no scalpels, no knives, no needles, no thread, no numbing medications. There is only beauty all around where there are flowers, where there are songs, where there are scents, where there is compassion, where there is pure touch, and where there is hope, but most of all where there is love. We only give the gifts which do the real healing.

Single Oils

This section provides concise information about many of the pure essential oils that are available for use by the general public. The listings of possible uses are meant for external application unless otherwise directed. The included safety data is also based on the external use of the oils and may differ from other published information that is based on oral application.

Other seeming discrepancies between sources of published safety data arise when one does not take into consideration the certain constituents of the oil being reviewed. One glaring example of this is thyme. A linalol type of oil does not have the same caustic/irritant effects that a thymol type would, but the particular application may require the added strength of the thymol type of oil. In this book, care has been taken to differentiate between the different types of essential oil for each application. Since pure essential oils are powerful healing agents, please remember to check the safety data before using an oil. Because there are several different oils that can help the same health condition, it should not be difficult to find one that will work for any particular situation. ***Also, for a listing of products that contain these individual oils, please refer to the Single Oil Summary section in the Appendix.***

ANGELICA
(Angelica archangelica)

Botanical Family: Apiaceae, Umbelliferae (parsley)

Extraction Method/Origin: Steam distillation of roots — France, Belgium

Chemical Constituents: Monoterpenes (up to 95%): d- and l-limonenes (up to 40%), α- and β-pinenes, α- and β-phellandrenes; Esters: bornyl acetate, verbenyl acetate; Terpene Alkaloids: bergaptene; Coumarins: umbelliferone.

Properties: Anti-coagulant, anti-inflammatory (intestinal wall), **calming, expectorant, sedative** (nervous system), **stomachic**, and **tonic**.

Folklore: One possible source for this oil's unique name comes from an old legend which states that during a terrible plague, an angel revealed this plant to a monk. History also records the use of the plant during the plague of 1660. The stems were chewed to prevent infection, and the seeds and roots were burned to help purify the air. The German people refer to the essence as the "oil of angels".

Esoteric Uses/Actions: Astrological: *Sun*; Body type: *Mesomorph*; Chakras: *links 7 to 8 and 7 to 1, also 8*; Character: *Yang*; Crystals: *Apophylite, green tourmaline (lifts 7^h to 8th chakra), moss*

agate, bloodstone (links crown to base chakra or 7ᵗʰ to 1ˢᵗ) ; Element: *Fire*; Oriental: *Cold & damp conditions*

Possible Uses: Angelica may help with **anorexia, appetite** (loss of), **bruises, colds, colic, coughs, flatulence, indigestion, menopause, pre-menstrual tension, respiratory infections**, and **rheumatic conditions**.

Body System(s) Affected: Emotional Balance, Nervous System.

Aromatic Influence: It may help one release and let go of negative feelings by bringing one's memory back to a point of origin before **trauma** or **anger** was experienced.

Application: Apply to **shoulders, vita flex points**, bottoms of **feet**, and/or directly on **area** of concern; Diffuse.

Oral Use As Dietary Supplement: Generally regarded as safe (GRAS) for internal consumption by the FDA. ***Dilute** one drop oil in 1 tsp. honey or 4 oz. of beverage (i.e. soy/rice milk). **Not for children under 6 years old; use with **caution** and in **greater dilution** for children 6 years old and over.***

Safety Data: *Avoid if **diabetic**. Use with caution during **pregnancy**. Avoid direct **sunlight** for up to 12 hours after use.*

Blend Classification: Personifier, Modifier.

Blends With: Clary sage, patchouli, vetiver, florals, woods, and most citrus oils.

Odor: Type: *Top to Middle Notes (20-80% of the blend)*; Scent: *Herbaceous, earthy, peppery, green, spicy*; Intensity: *4*

Frequency: Physical and Emotional; approximately 85 MHz.

ANISE
(Pimpinella anisum)

Botanical Family: Umbelliferae (dainty, white-flowered annual)

Extraction Method/Origin: Steam distillation from seeds (fruit) — Turkey

Chemical Constituents: Phenolic Ethers: anethol (up to 95%) and estragole (1-4%); Alcohols: anisol, linalol, α-terpineol; Phenols: p-anol; Aldehydes: anisicaldehyde.

Properties: Antiseptic, antispasmodic, estrogen-like, diuretic, stimulant (heart), and **tonic** (heart).

Esoteric Uses/Actions: Astrological: *Sun, Mercury, Pluto, and Jupiter*; Body type: *Mesomorph*; Character: *Yang*; Element: *Air*; Oriental: *Cold & damp conditions*

Historical Uses: This oil has been used for dry irritable **coughs, bronchitis**, and **whooping cough**.

Other Possible Uses: Alkalosis, blood oxygenation, bronchitis, colitis, constipation, digestion (accelerates), **diverticulitis, estrogen** (increases), **fertility, flatulence, hormonal imbalance, irritable bowel syndrome, menopause, parasites, pms, prostate cancer** (blend with frankincense), and **respiratory system** (strengthens).

Body System(s) Affected: Cardiovascular, Digestive, Hormonal, and **Respiratory Systems**.

Application: Apply to **Vita Flex Points** and directly on **area** of concern; Diffuse.

Oral Use As Dietary Supplement: Generally regarded as safe (GRAS) for internal consumption by the FDA. ***Dilute*** *one drop oil in 1 tsp. honey or 4 oz. of beverage (i.e. soy/rice milk).* ***Not for children under 6 years old; use with*** **caution** ***and in*** **greater dilution** *for children 6 years old and over.*

Safety Data: *Can irritate sensitive* **skin** *and has been known to cause* **dermatitis** *in some individuals. Best if used in moderation.*

Blend Classification: Difficult to use in blending. Use only in very small amounts.

Blends With: Bergamot, Blue tansy, fennel, ginger, juniper, lemongrass, patchouli, Black pepper, peppermint, tangerine, tarragon, and ylang ylang.

Odor: Type: *Top to Middle Notes (20-80% of the blend)*

BALSAM FIR
(See FIR, BALSAM)

BASIL
(Ocimum basilicum CT methyl chavicol)

Botanical Family: Lamiaceae or Labiatae (mint)

Extraction Method/Origin: Steam distillation of leaves, stems, and flowers — Egypt, India, Utah, France

Chemical Constituents: Phenolic Ethers: methyl chavicol (or estragole - up to 89%), methyl eugenol; Alcohols (up to 15%): linalol, citronellol, α-fenchol, α-terpineol; Oxides (up to 9%): 1,8 cineol, ocimene oxide; Esters (<5%); Monoterpenes (<4%); Ketones (<2%).

Properties: **Anti-bacterial, anti-infectious, anti-inflammatory, antiseptic** (stomach/intestinal), **antispasmodic** (powerful), **anti-viral, decongestant** (veins, arteries of the lungs, prostate), **stimulant** (nerves, adrenal cortex), and **uplifting**. Basil may also be anti-catarrhal, anti-depressant, energizing, and restorative.

Folklore: Considered by the ancient Greeks as the "king of plants", basil was used to anoint kings. Hindus placed sprigs of basil on the chests of deceased loved ones to protect them from evil and provide safe passage into the next life. Due to its supposed aphrodisiac qualities, Italian women displayed basil to alert possible suitors, and the men would present the women with basil sprigs.

Esoteric Uses/Actions: Astrological: *Mars*; Ayurvedic: *Vata*; Body type: *Endomorph*; Chakras: *2*; Character: *Yang*; Element: *Fire*; Number: *1*

Historical Uses: Basil was used anciently for respiratory problems, digestive and kidney ailments, epilepsy, poisonous insect or snake bites, fevers, epidemics, and malaria.

French Medicinal Uses: **Migraines** (especially from liver and gallbladder problems), **mental fatigue, menstrual periods** (scanty).

Other Possible Uses: This oil may be used for **aches/pains, anxiety, bronchitis, chronic colds, concentration**, nervous **depression, digestion, earache, fainting, fatigue**

(mental), **fever, gout, headaches, hemorrhoids, hiccoughs, insect bites** (soothing), **insect repellent, insomnia** (from nervous tension), **intestinal problems**, poor **memory**, chronic **mucus**, **muscle spasms**, **ovarian cysts**, **prostate problems**, **rhinitis** (inflammation of nasal mucus membranes), loss of **smell, snake bites, vomiting, wasp stings**, and **whooping cough**.

Body System(s) Affected: Cardiovascular System, Muscles and **Bones**.

Aromatic Influence: Helps one maintain an **open mind** and increases **clarity** of thought.

Application: Apply to **temples**, tip of **nose**, **Vita Flex Points**, and/or directly on **area** of concern; Diffuse. May also be added to food or water as a dietary supplement.

Oral Use As Dietary Supplement: Generally regarded as safe (GRAS) for internal consumption by the FDA. ***Dilute*** one drop oil in 1 tsp. honey or 4 oz. of beverage (i.e. soy/rice milk). ***Not for children under 6 years old; use with caution and in greater dilution for children 6 years old and over.***

Safety Data: *Avoid during* **pregnancy**. *Not for use by people with* **epilepsy**. *It may also irritate sensitive skin (test a small area first).*

Blend Classification: Enhancer and Equalizer

Blends With: Bergamot, birch, cypress, fir, geranium, helichrysum, lavender, lemongrass, marjoram, peppermint, spruce, wintergreen.

Odor: Type: *Top to Middle Notes (20-80% of the blend)*; Scent: *Herbaceous, spicy, anise-like, camphorous, lively*; Intensity: *4*

Frequency: Low (Physical); approximately 52 MHz.

BERGAMOT
(Citrus bergamia)

Botanical Family: Rutaceae (citrus)

Extraction Method/Origin: Solvent extraction or vacuum distilled; pressed from rind or peel; rectified and void of terpenes — Italy, Ivory Coast

Chemical Constituents: Monoterpenes: d-limonene (>30%), γ-terpinene, α & β-pinenes; Esters: linalyl acetate (usually around 20%); Alcohols: linalol, geraniol, nerol, α-terpineol; Sesquiterpenes: β-caryophyllene, β-bisabolene; Furanocoumarins; Aldehydes.

Properties: Analgesic, anti-bacterial (strep and staph infection), **anti-infectious, anti-inflammatory, anti-parasitic, antiseptic, antispasmodic, digestive, sedative**, and **uplifting**.

Folklore: Christopher Columbus is credited with bringing bergamot to Italy from the Canary Islands.

Esoteric Uses/Actions: Astrological: *Sun*; Body type: *Endomorph*; Chakras: *3, 4, & 5*; Character: *mildly Yang*; Crystals: *Watermelon tourmaline*; Element: *Fire*; Number: *2*; Oriental: *Qi stagnation (pts: Liv-3, GB-34)*

Historical Uses: Bergamot was used by the Italians to cool and relieve fevers, protect against malaria, and expel intestinal worms.

French Medicinal Uses: Agitation, appetite (loss of), **colic, depression, indigestion, infection, inflammation, insect repellent, insomnia, intestinal parasites, rheumatism, stress**, and **vaginal candida**.

Other Possible Uses: This oil may help **acne, anxiety,** regulate **appetite, boils, bronchitis, carbuncles, cold sores,** oily **complexion, coughs, cystitis, digestion, eczema, emotions, endocrine system, fever, gallstones, gonorrhea, infectious disease, insect bites,** soothe **lungs, psoriasis, respiratory infection, scabies, sore throat,** nervous **tension, thrush,** acute **tonsillitis, ulcers, urinary tract infection,** spot **varicose veins,** and **wounds**.

Body System(s) Affected: Digestive System, Emotional Balance, Skin.

Aromatic Influence: It may help to **relieve anxiety, depression, stress,** and **tension**. It is **uplifting** and **refreshing**. It helps to expand and open the **heart chakra**, and to radiate **love energy**.

Application: Apply to **forehead, temples, Vita Flex Points,** and/or directly on **area** of concern; Diffuse. May also be applied as a **deodorant** or added to food or water as a dietary supplement.

Oral Use As Dietary Supplement: Generally regarded as safe (GRAS) for internal consumption by the FDA. *Dilute one drop oil in 1 tsp. honey or 4 oz. of beverage (i.e. soy/rice milk).* **Not** *for children under 6 years old; use with **caution** and in **greater dilution** for children 6 years old and over.*

Safety Data: *Repeated use can result in extreme **contact sensitization**. Avoid direct **sunlight** or **ultraviolet light** for up to 72 hours after use.*

Blend Classification: Equalizer, Modifier, and Enhancer

Blends With: Chamomile, cypress, eucalyptus, geranium, jasmine, juniper, lavender, lemon, palmarosa, patchouli, and ylang ylang.

Odor: Type: *Top Note (5-20% of the blend)*; Scent: *Sweet, lively, citrusy, fruity*; Intensity: *2*

BIRCH (YELLOW BIRCH)
(Betula alleghaniensis)

Botanical Family: Betulaceae

Extraction Method/Origin: Steam distillation from wood — Canada, Scandinavia

Chemical Constituents: Phenolic Esters: methyl salicylate (89%); Carboxylic Acids; Oxides.

Properties: Analgesic, anti-inflammatory, anti-rheumatic, antiseptic, antispasmodic, disinfectant, diuretic, stimulant (bone, liver), and **warming**.

Historical Uses: Birch oil has a strong, penetrating aroma that most people recognize as wintergreen. Although birch (*Betula alleghaniensis* or *Betula lenta*) is completely unrelated to wintergreen (*Gaultheria procumbens*), they are almost identical in chemical constituents. The American Indians and early European settlers enjoyed a tea that was flavored with birch bark or wintergreen. According to Julia Lawless, "...this has been translated into a preference for 'root beer' flavourings [sic]." A synthetic methyl salicylate is now widely used as a flavoring agent, especially in 'root beer', chewing gum, toothpaste, etc.

French Medicinal Uses: **Rheumatism, muscular pain, cramps, arthritis, tendonitis, hypertension, inflammation**.

Other Possible Uses: This oil may be beneficial for **acne, bladder infection, cystitis, dropsy, eczema, edema**, reducing **fever, gallstones, gout, infection**, reducing discomfort in **joints, kidney stones**, draining and cleansing the **lymphatic system, obesity, osteoporosis, skin diseases, ulcers**, and **urinary tract disorders**. It is known for its ability to alleviate **bone pain**. It has a cortisone-like action due to the high content of methyl salicylate. For tissue pain, use Relieve It.

Body System(s) Affected: **Muscles** and **Bones**.

Aromatic Influence: It influences, elevates, opens, and increases **awareness** in **sensory system** (senses or sensations).

Application: Apply to **Vita Flex Points** and/or directly on **area** of concern; Diffuse. Apply topically on location and use only small amounts (dilute with V-6 Mixing Oil for application on larger areas).

Oral Use As Dietary Supplement: None.

Safety Data: *Avoid during* **pregnancy***. Not for use by people with* **epilepsy***. Some people are very allergic to methyl salicylate.* **Test a small area of skin first for allergies!**

Blend Classification: Personifier and Enhancer

Blends With: Basil, bergamot, chamomile, cypress, geranium, juniper, lavender, lemongrass, marjoram, peppermint, and rosewood.

BLACK PEPPER
(See PEPPER, BLACK)

BLUE CYPRESS
(See CYPRESS, BLUE)

CAJEPUT
(Melaleuca leucadendra)

Botanical Family: Myrtaceae (myrtle shrubs and trees)

Chemical Constituents: Oxides: 1,8 cineol (<50%); Alcohols: α-terpineol (>8%), viridiflorol, nerolidol; Monoterpenes: α- & β-pinenes, l-limonene; Sesquiterpenes: β-caryophyllene; Aldehydes: benzoicaldehyde; Esters: α-terpinyl acetate.

Properties: Analgesic (mild), **anti-catarrhal, anti-infectious, anti-inflammatory, antimicrobial, anti-neuralgic, antiseptic** (pulmonary, urinary, intestinal), **antispasmodic, expectorant, insecticidal**, and **tonic**.

Esoteric Uses/Actions: Chakra: *6*; Character: *Neutral*

Historical Uses: In Malaysia and other Indonesian islands, cajeput was considered valuable for cholera, colds, flu, headaches, rheumatism, throat infections, toothache, various skin conditions, and sore muscles.

Other Possible Uses: Cajeput may help with **acne, arthritis, asthma, bronchitis, bursitis, catarrh, colds, coughs, cystitis, dysentery, enteritis, flu, hay fever, headaches, infections** of the **urethra, insect bites, intestinal problems**, stiff **joints, laryngitis, pneumonia, psoriasis, respiratory infections, rheumatism, sinusitis, skin** (oily and spots), **sore throat, toothache, urinary complaints, viral infections**.

Body System(s) Affected: Cardiovascular and **Respiratory Systems**.

Application: Apply to **Vita Flex Points** and/or directly on **area** of concern. **Diffuse** for **respiratory infections**.

Oral Use As Dietary Supplement: Approved by the FDA for use as a Food Additive (FA) or Flavoring Agent (FL). ***Dilute*** *one drop oil in 1 tsp. honey or 4 oz. of beverage (i.e. soy/rice milk). Not for children under 6 years old; use with* **caution** *and in* **greater dilution** *for children 6 years old and over.*

Safety Data: *If not absolutely pure, cajeput could cause further blistering and skin eruptions! Even when pure, it can irritate sensitive* **skin**. *Use with* **caution.**

Blend Classification: Enhancer.

Blends With: Birch, eucalyptus, juniper, peppermint, and wintergreen.

Odor: Type: *Top Note (5-20% of the blend)*

CARAWAY
(Carum carvi)

Botanical Family: Umbelliferae (dainty, white-flowered annual)

Extraction Method/Origin: Steam distillation from seeds (fruit) — Netherlands

Chemical Constituents: Ketones: carvone (up to 60%); Monoterpenes: limonene (>45%), phellandrene, pinene, carvene; Monoterpene Alcohols (>6%): cis-carveol (<5%), furfurol, carvacrol, hydrocarveols; Coumarins: herniarine; Aldehydes: acetaldehyde, cuminic aldehyde.

Properties: Anti-parasitic, antihistamine, antimicrobial, antispasmodic, expectorant, diuretic, stimulant (circulatory, urinary), and **tonic** (digestive).

Esoteric Uses/Actions: Astrological: *Mercury*; Character: *Yang*; Element: *Air*

Historical Uses: Caraway is a very old, well known spice and has been used as far back as the Stone Age. Egyptians used it as food flavoring, the Romans used it in bread-making, and in the Middle Ages the Germans and Austrians used it in their cooking. Traditionally this herb is associated with sharp eyesight and sweet breath.

Other Possible Uses: Acne, appetite (aids poor), **asthma** (bronchial), **boils, bowels** (general complaints), **breath** (sweetens), **bronchitis** (acute catarrhal), **bruises, colic, colitis, cough, diarrhea, dizziness, dyspepsia, gas, indigestion, intestines** (calms muscle fibers), **laryngitis, liver** and **gallbladder** (promotes bile), **lymph** (stimulates flow), **menstrual period** (eases pains), **nursing** (increases milk), itchy **scalp, scabies, skin** (oily, stimulates pale skin), **toxins** (flushes), **urine** (increases), **vertigo, wounds**.

Body System(s) Affected: Digestive System.

Aromatic Influence: Caraway is **warming** to the **emotions**. It helps to ease **mental strain** and **fatigue** and helps one replenish lost **energy**.

Application: Apply to **Vita Flex Points** and directly on **area** of concern; **Diffuse**.

Oral Use As Dietary Supplement: Generally regarded as safe (GRAS) for internal consumption by the FDA. ***Dilute** one drop oil in 1 tsp. honey or 4 oz. of beverage (i.e. soy/rice milk). **Not for children under 6 years old; use with **caution** and in **greater dilution** for children 6 years old and over.***

Safety Data: *Avoid during* **pregnancy**. *Can irritate sensitive* **skin** *and has produced* **contact sensitivity**. *Best if used in moderation.*

Blend Classification: Difficult to use in blending. Use only in very small amounts.

Blends With: Basil, chamomile, coriander, frankincense, ginger, lavender, and orange.

Odor: Type: *Top Note (20-80% of the blend)*

CARDAMOM
(Elettaria cardamomum)

Botanical Family: Zingiberaceae (ginger)

Chemical Constituents: Esters (>40%): α-terpenyl acetate (30-45%), linalyl acetate (3%); Oxides: 1,8 cineol (up to 35%); Alcohols (7%): linalol, terpinen-4-ol, α-terpineol; Monoterpenes (6%): sabinene, myrcene, l-limonene; Aldehyde: geranial.

Properties: Anti-bacterial, anti-infectious, antiseptic, antispasmodic, aphrodisiac, digestive, diuretic, stomachic, and **tonic**.

Esoteric Uses/Actions: Astrological: *Venus & Mercury*; Body type: *Ectomorph*; Chakra: *1*; Character: *Yang*; Crystals: *Carnelian* ; Element: *Water & Air*; Number: *4*; Oriental: *Cold dampness (pts: Sp 9 & 6), Qi deficiency Spleen (pts: Sp-6)*

Historical Uses: Anciently, cardamom was used for epilepsy, spasms, paralysis, rheumatism, cardiac disorders, all intestinal illnesses, pulmonary disease, fever, and digestive and urinary complaints. It is said to be able to neutralize the lingering odor of garlic.

Other Possible Uses: Cardamom may help with **appetite** (loss of), **colic, coughs, debility, dyspepsia, flatulence, halitosis, headaches, mental fatigue, nausea, pyrosis** (or **heartburn**), **sciatica**, and **vomiting**. It may also help with **menstrual periods, menopause**, and nervous **indigestion**. *Note: Cardamom has the same properties as ginger but is less of an irritant.*

Body System(s) Affected: Digestive System.

Aromatic Influence: Cardamom is **uplifting, refreshing**, and **invigorating**. It may be beneficial for **clearing confusion**.

Application: Apply to **Vita Flex Points** and/or directly on **area** of concern. Dilute with base oil and **massage** over the stomach, solar plexus, and thighs. Excellent as a **bath** oil.

Oral Use As Dietary Supplement: Generally regarded as safe (GRAS) for internal consumption by the FDA. *Dilute one drop oil in 1 tsp. honey or 4 oz. of beverage (i.e. soy/rice milk).* **Not** *for children under 6 years old; use with* **caution** *and in* **greater dilution** *for children 6 years old and over.*

Blend Classification: Personifier and Modifier

Blends With: Bergamot, cedarwood, cinnamon bark, cistus, clove, neroli, orange, rose, and ylang ylang.

Odor: Type: *Middle Note (50-80% of the blend)*; Scent: *Sweet, spicy, balsamic, with floral undertones*; Intensity: *4*

CARROT
(Daucus carota)

Botanical Family: Umbelliferae (parsley)

Chemical Constituents: Alcohols: carotol (up to 50%), daucol (up to 5%), linalol; Monoterpenes: α- & β-pinenes, sabinene; Sesquiterpenes: β-bisabolene (10%), β-caryophyllene (4%), daucene; Oxides: epoxy β-caryophyllene; Esters: geranyl acetate; Phenols: β-asarone.

Properties: Carminative, hepatic (cleanses the liver), **stomachic**.

Historical Uses: Carrots have been used as a blood cleanser, for liver and skin problems, pulmonary conditions, allergies, inflammation of the intestines, as a tonic for the nervous system, and for eyesight. Carrots where used during the Second World War to help pilots with their night vision.

Other Possible Uses: Carrot oil may help with **anemia, colic** (with fennel), **constipation, diarrhea, eye problems, gallbladder problems, liver problems, rheumatism**, and **skin problems** (**aging skin, wrinkles, sunburn**, and **dryness**).

Body System(s) Affected: Cardiovascular and **Nervous Systems, Skin**.

Application: Apply to **Vita Flex Points** and/or directly on **area** of concern. To promote a healthy **suntan**, apply carrot oil (dilute with Hazelnut oil) for a few days before exposure to the sun.

Oral Use As Dietary Supplement: Generally regarded as safe (GRAS) for internal consumption by the FDA. *Dilute one drop oil in 1 tsp. honey or 4 oz. of beverage (i.e. soy/rice milk).* **Not** *for children under 6 years old; use with* **caution** *and in* **greater dilution** *for children 6 years old and over.*

Blend Classification: Considered as more of an active carrier oil (same as Vitamin E Oil and Wheatgerm Oil).

Blends With: Citrus oils, fennel, frankincense, geranium, spice oils.

Odor: Type: *Middle Note (50-80% of the blend)*; Scent: *Sweet, fruity, warm, earthy*; Intensity: *2*

CASSIA
(Cinnamomum cassia)

Botanical Family: Lauraceae (laurel)

Extraction Method/Origin: Steam distillation from bark — China

Chemical Constituents: Aldehydes: trans-cinnamaldehyde (up to 85%), benzaldehyde; Phenols (>7%): eugenol, chavicol, phenol, 2-vinyl-phenol; Esters: cinnamyl acetate, benzyl acetate.

Properties: Anti-bacterial, anti-fungal, anti-viral.

Esoteric Uses/Actions: Astrological: *Mercury & Sun*; Character: *Yang*

Historical Uses: Has been used extensively as a domestic spice. Medicinally, it has been used for colds, colic, flatulent dyspepsia, diarrhea, nausea, rheumatism, and kidney and reproductive complaints.

Other Possible Uses: This oil is best not used individually in aromatherapy as it can be extremely sensitizing to the dermal tissues. Can provide some powerful support to blends when used in very small quantities.

Application: None.

Oral Use As Dietary Supplement: Generally regarded as safe (GRAS) for internal consumption by the FDA. ***Dilute*** *one drop oil in 2 tsp. honey or 8 oz. of beverage (i.e. soy/rice milk). May need to increase dilution even more due to this oil's potential for irritating mucus membranes. Not for children under 6 years old; use with* **caution** *and in* **greater dilution** *for children 6 years old and over.*

Safety Data: *Repeated use can result in extreme* **contact sensitization.** *Avoid during* **pregnancy.** *Can cause extreme* **skin irritation.** *Diffuse with caution; it will irritate the nasal membranes if it is inhaled directly from the diffuser.*

Blend Classification: Personifier/Enhancer.

Odor: Type: *Middle Note (50-80% of the blend)*; Scent: *Spicy, warm, sweet*; Intensity: *5*

CEDAR, WESTERN RED
(Thuja plicata)

Botanical Family: Cupressaceae (conifer - cypress)

Extraction Method/Origin: Steam distillation from leaves and twigs — USA

Chemical Constituents: Ketones: α- & β-thujones (>60%), fenchone (<7%), camphor (<3%); Monoterpenes (<7%): sabinene, α- & β-pinenes; Esters: methyl thujate; Sesquiterpene Alcohols: muurolol.

Properties: Anti-bacterial and **antiseptic**.

Esoteric Uses/Actions: Astrological: *Mercury*; Chakra: *1 & 6*; Character: *Yin*; Element: *Earth & Ether*

Historical Uses: The Western Red cedar has been referred to as the "Tree of Life". It has been used by ancient civilizations to enhance their potential for spiritual communication during rituals and other ceremonies. It has also been used for coughs, fevers, intestinal parasites, cystitis, and venereal diseases.

Other Possible Uses: This oil may help with **hair loss, skin** (nourishing), **rheumatism, warts**, and **psoriasis**. It has powerful effects on the **subconscious** and **unconscious mind**.

Body System(s) Affected: Skin.

Aromatic Influence: It is **calming** and may help enhance **spiritual awareness** or **meditation**.

Application: Apply to **Vita Flex Points** and/or directly on **area** of concern. **Diffuse**.

Oral Use As Dietary Supplement: None.

Safety Data: *For Topical Use Only. Due to high Thujone content, use sparingly and dilute well with V-6 Mixing Oil.*

CEDAR LEAF (THUJA)
(Thuja occidentalis)

Botanical Family: Cupressaceae (conifer - cypress)

Extraction Method/Origin: Steam distillation from leaves, twigs, and bark — Canada, USA

Chemical Constituents: Ketones: α- & β-thujones (>60%), fenchone (up to 14%), camphor (<3%), piperitone; Monoterpenes: sabinene (<35%), l-limonene; Esters: bornyl acetate (up to 12%); Sesquiterpene Alcohols: occidentalol, occidol, α-, β-, & γ-eudesmols; Phenolic Alcohols: terpinen-4-ol (<6%).

Properties: Anti-rheumatic, astringent, expectorant, insect repellent, and stimulant (nerves, uterus and heart muscles).

Esoteric Uses/Actions: Astrological: *Mercury*; Chakra: *1 & 6*; Character: *Yin*; Element: *Earth & Ether*

Historical Uses: Has been used by ancient civilizations to enhance their potential for spiritual communication during rituals and other ceremonies. It has also been used for coughs, fevers, intestinal parasites, cystitis, and venereal diseases.

Other Possible Uses: May help with **rheumatism, warts**, and **psoriasis**.

Aromatic Influence: May help enhance **spiritual awareness** or **meditation**.

Application: Apply to **Vita Flex Points** and directly on **area** of concern. **Diffuse**.

Oral Use As Dietary Supplement: *Has been approved by the FDA for use as a Food Additive (FA) or Flavoring Agent (FL) as long as the finished food is thujone-free. (See 21CFR172.510) Best **not** to use this oil as a dietary supplement.*

Safety Data: *For Topical Use Only. Due to high Thujone content, use sparingly and dilute well with V-6 Mixing Oil.*

CEDARWOOD
(Cedrus atlantica)

Botanical Family: Pinaceae (conifer)

Extraction Method/Origin: Steam distillation from bark — Morocco, USA

Chemical Constituents: Sesquiterpenes (up to 90%): α-, β-, & γ-himachalenes (>55%), cadinene; Sesquiterpene Alcohols (up to 40%): alantol (<20%), α-caryophyllenol (<10%), β-cubenol (<10%), cedrol, cedrenol; Sesquiterpene Ketones (20%): α- & β-alantones.

Properties: Anti-fungal, anti-infectious, antiseptic (urinary and pulmonary), **astringent, diuretic, insect repellent**, and **sedative**.

Folklore: *Cedrus atlantica* is supposed to be the species most closely related to the biblical Cedars of Lebanon.

Esoteric Uses/Actions: Astrological: *Saturn, Sun, Jupiter, & Uranus*; Body type: *Mesomorph*; Chakra: *1 & 6*; Character: *Yang*; Crystals: *Lepidolite, amethyst, sapphire*; Element: *Fire, Light, & Air*; Number: *6*; Oriental: *Cold, dampness (pts: Sp-9 & 6), Qi deficiency (pts: Kid-3)*

Historical Uses: Cedarwood was used traditionally by the North American Indians to enhance their spiritual communication. It creates the symbolic effect of the umbrella protecting the earth and bringing energy in from the universe. At night the animals in the wild lie down under the tree for the protection, recharging, and rejuvenation the trees bring them.

French Medicinal Uses: Anger (calming effect), **arteriosclerosis, bronchitis, calming, cellulite, diuretic, hair loss, nervous tension, tuberculosis, urinary infections**.

Other Possible Uses: This oil is recognized for its **purifying** properties. It may also help **acne, anxiety, arthritis, congestion, coughs, cystitis, dandruff, psoriasis, purification, sinusitis, skin diseases**, and **water retention**. It may help **open** the **pineal gland**. It also helps to reduce **oily secretions**.

Body System(s) Affected: Nervous and **Respiratory Systems**.

Application: Apply to **Vita Flex Points** and/or directly on **area** of concern.

Oral Use As Dietary Supplement: None.

Safety Data: *Use with caution during **pregnancy.***

Blend Classification: Enhancer and Equalizer

Blends With: Bergamot, Clary sage, cypress, eucalyptus, floral oils, juniper, resinous oils, rosemary.

Odor: Type: *Base Note (5-20% of the blend)*; Scent: *Warm, soft, woody*; Intensity: *3*

Bible: Lev. 14:4, 6, 49, 51, 52

CELERY SEED
(Apium graveolens)

Botanical Family: Umbeliferae

Extraction Method/Origin: Steam distilled from seed — France

Chemical Constituents: Monoterpenes (up to 85%): d-limonene (>60%), ocimene (<11%), α & γ-terpinenes; Esters (<23%): carvyl acetate, geranyl acetate; Lactones (approx. 15%):

3-n-butylphthalide (up to 7%), sedanenolides (>1%), 4-dihydro-phthalide (1%), dihydro-ligustilide (3%); Sesquiterpenes (up to 12%): α- & β-selinenes; Ketones: d-carvone (<10%); Carboxylic Acids: sedanolic acid; Alcohols: α-terpineol.

Properties: Antioxidant, anti-rheumatic, antiseptic (urinary), **antispasmodic, hepatic** (stimulates drainage), **stimulant** (uterine), **tonic** (neuromuscular).

Esoteric Uses/Actions: Astrological: *Moon, Mercury, Sun*; Character: *Yin?*; Element: *Fire*; Color: *pale yellow*

Possible Uses: Celery seed may help with **arthritis, bloating, bronchitis, congestion** (respiratory), **cystitis, flatulence, glands** (swollen), **gout** (reduces uric acid), **hemorrhoids, indigestion, jaundice, kidney** detoxification (after illness), **lactation** (increases flow of breast milk), **liver** congestion (after infection), **lymphatic** drainage, **menstruation** (induces), **nervous** disorders, **neuralgia, rheumatism, sciatica, sexual** problems (minimizes), **skin** (puffiness, redness, spots, water-logged), **urine** flow (increases). It may help to balance the **endocrine system** to help with glandular problems. It is also a sedative and tonic for the **central nervous system** and may help provide a more **restful sleep**.

Body System(s) Affected: Digestive System, Muscle and **Bone, Nervous System**.

Aromatic Influence: Celery seed has a spicy, warm sweet, tenacious odor. It is fairly strong and long-lasting. The aroma is **calming** and **relaxing** to the mind and body.

Application: Apply to **Vita Flex Points** of the feet and directly on **area** of concern.

Oral Use As Dietary Supplement: Generally regarded as safe (GRAS) for internal consumption by the FDA. *Dilute one drop oil in 1 tsp. honey or 4 oz. of beverage (i.e. soy/rice milk). Not for children under 6 years old; use with caution and in greater dilution for children 6 years old and over.*

Safety Data: *Repeated use can possibly result in contact sensitization or skin irritation. Avoid during pregnancy.*

Blend Classification: Personifier. **Odor:** Type: *Middle Note (50-80% of the blend)*; Scent: *Spicy, warm, sweet, tenacious*; Intensity: *3*

CHAMOMILE, GERMAN (BLUE)
(Matricaria recutita)

Botanical Family: Compositae (daisy)

Extraction Method/Origin: Steam distillation from flowers — Egypt, Hungary, Utah

Chemical Constituents: Sesquiterpenes (up to 60%): α- & β-farnesenes (>20%), chamazulene (<20%), dihydrochamazulene I & II, cadinene, bisabolenes; Oxides: bisabolol oxide-A (>24%), bisabolone oxide (<20%), bisabolol oxide-B (<10%), 1,8 cineol (<5%); Sesquiterpene Alcohols: α-bisabolol (<8%), fanesol, spathulenol; Ethers; Monoterpenes.

Properties: Analgesic, anti-infectious, anti-inflammatory, antioxidant, antispasmodic, decongestant, digestive tonic, and is **hormone-like**.

Esoteric Uses/Actions: Astrological: *Venus, Moon, & Mercury*; Body type: *Ectomorph*; Chakra: *5*; Character: *Yin*; Crystals: *Blue tourmaline* ; Element: *Ether & Water*; Number: *7*; Oriental: *Excess heat (yang), rising heat, internal wind, (pts: Liv-2, He-3)*

Historical Uses: Native to Europe, it is no longer grown in Germany. It has a long history of use for all symptoms related to or resulting from tension.

French Medicinal Uses: Acne, cystitis, decongestant, digestive tonic, eczema, gallbladder, hormone-like, liver, ulcers.

Other Possible Uses: Chamomile neutralizes **allergies** and increases the ability of the **skin** to **regenerate**. It is a cleanser of the **blood** and also helps **open** the **liver, increase liver function** and **secretion**, and **support** the **pancreas**. This oil may be used for **abscesses, acne, boils, burns, cuts, cystitis, dermatitis, eczema, gallbladder,** chronic **gastritis, hair care, inflamed joints, ingrown nails** (infected), **insomnia, liver problems, menopausal problems, migraine headaches, open leg sores, rashes, skin disorders, stress related complaints, teething pains, toothaches, ulcers,** and **wounds**.

Body System(s) Affected: Emotional Balance, Nervous System, Skin.

Aromatic Influence: It can dispel **anger**, stabilize the **emotions**, and help to release emotions linked to the past. It may also be used to **soothe** and **clear** the **mind** creating an atmosphere of **peace** and **patience**.

Application: Apply to **Vita Flex Points** and directly on **area** of concern; Diffuse.

Oral Use As Dietary Supplement: Generally regarded as safe (GRAS) for internal consumption by the FDA. ***Dilute*** one drop oil in 1 tsp. honey or 4 oz. of beverage (i.e. soy/rice milk). ***Not for children under 6 years old; use with caution and in greater dilution for children 6 years old and over.***

Safety Data: *Use with caution during* **pregnancy**. *Can irritate sensitive* **skin**.

Blend Classification: Personifier

Blends With: Birch, fir, geranium, helichrysum, hyssop, lavender, lemongrass, marjoram, sandalwood, spearmint, spruce, melaleuca (Tea Tree), and wintergreen.

Odor: Type: *Middle Note (50-80% of the blend)*; Scent: *Deep, rich, tenacious, cocoa-like, herbaceous*; Intensity: *4*

Frequency: Emotional; approximately 105.

CHAMOMILE, ROMAN
(Chamaemelum nobile or Anthemis nobilis)

Botanical Family: Compositae (daisy)

Extraction Method/Origin: Steam distillation from flowers — Egypt, Utah

Chemical Constituents: Esters (up to 75%): isobutyl angelate (up to 25%), isoamyl methacylate (up to 25%), amyl butyrate (<15%), other angelate, butyrate, acetate, and tiglate esters; Monoterpenes (<35%): α- & β-pinenes (<20%), terpinenes, sabinene, camphene, d-limonene, p-cymene, myrcene; Ketones: pinocarvone (14%); Sesquiterpenes (up to 12%): β-caryophyllene, chamazulene; Alcohols (>7%): trans-pinocarveol, farnesol, nerolidol.

Properties: Anti-infectious, anti-inflammatory, anti-parasitic, antispasmodic, calming, and **relaxing**.

Esoteric Uses/Actions: Astrological: *Moon*; Body type: *Ectomorph*; Chakra: *5*; Character: *Yin/Yang*; Crystals: *Aquamarine, aqua aura, amazonite* ; Element: *Water*; Number: *5*; Oriental: *Excessive Yang (heat) (pts: Liv-2, He-3)*; Color: *Pale blue to clear*

Historical Uses: It was traditionally used by the ancient Romans to give them a **clear mind** and to empower them with **courage** for their battles. According to Roberta Wilson, "...chamomile was nicknamed the "plant's physician" because it supposedly cured any ailing plant placed near it."

French Medicinal Uses: Intestinal parasites, neuritis, neuralgia, shock (nervous).

Other Possible Uses: Chamomile neutralizes **allergies** and increases the ability of the **skin** to **regenerate**. It is a cleanser of the **blood** and also helps the **liver** to reject **poisons** and to discharge them. This oil may help with **allergies, bruises, cuts, depression, insomnia, muscle tension, nerves** (calming and promoting nerve health), **restless legs**, and **skin conditions** like, **acne, boils, dermatitis, eczema, rashes**, and **sensitive skin**. Chamomile is mild enough to use on **infants** and **children**. For centuries, mothers have used chamomile to **calm crying children**, ease **earaches**, fight **fevers**, soothe **stomachaches** and **colic**, and relieve **toothaches** and **teething pain**. It can safely and effectively reduce **irritability** and minimize **nervousness** in children, especially **hyperactive children**.

Body System(s) Affected: Emotional Balance, Nervous System, Skin.

Aromatic Influence: Because it is calming and relaxing it can combat **depression, insomnia**, and **stress**. It eliminates some of the emotional charge of **anxiety, irritability**, and **nervousness**. It can dispel **anger**, stabilize the **emotions**, and help to release emotions that are linked to the past. It may also be used to **soothe** and **clear** the **mind** creating an atmosphere of **peace** and **patience**.

Application: Apply to **Vita Flex Points** and/or directly on **area** of concern; Diffuse. Applied over the **throat**, it can help a person express his or her true feelings.

Oral Use As Dietary Supplement: Generally regarded as safe (GRAS) for internal consumption by the FDA. ***Dilute*** *one drop oil in 1 tsp. honey or 4 oz. of beverage (i.e. soy/rice milk).* ***Not for children under 6 years old; use with*** *caution and in* ***greater dilution*** *for children 6 years old and over.*

Safety Data: *Can irritate sensitive* ***skin***.

Blend Classification: Personifier.

Blends With: Lavender, rose, geranium, or Clary sage.

Odor: Type: *Middle Note (50-80% of the blend)*; Scent: *Fresh, sweet, fruity-herbaceous, apple-like, no tenacity*; Intensity: *4*

CINNAMON BARK
(Cinnamomum verum or C. zeylanicum)

Botanical Family: Lauraceae (laurel)

Extraction Method/Origin: Steam distillation from bark — India, Madagascar, Sri Lanka

Chemical Constituents: Aldehydes: trans-cinnamaldehyde (<50%), hydroxycinnamaldehyde, benzaldehyde, cuminal; Phenols (up to 30%): eugenol (<30%), phenol, 2-vinyl-phenol; Alcohols: linalol, cinnamic alcohol, benzyl alcohol, α-terpineol, borneol; Sesquiterpenes: β-caryophyllene; Carboxylic Acids: cinnamic acid.

Properties: Anti-bacterial (98% pathogenic bacteria, cocci gr +, bacillus gr -), **antidepressant, anti-fungal, anti-infectious** (intestinal, urinary), **anti-inflammatory, antimicrobial, antioxidant, anti-parasitic, antiseptic, antispasmodic** (light), **anti-viral, astringent, immune-stimulant, purifier, sexual stimulant**, and **warming**. It also **enhances** the action and activity of other oils.

Esoteric Uses/Actions: Astrological: *Sun & Mercury*; Ayurvedic: *Pitta*; Body type: *Endomorph*; Chakra: *1, 2, & 5*; Character: *Yang*; Crystals: *Tourmaline* ; Element: *Fire & Water*; Number: *2*; Oriental: *Yang deficiency (pts: St-36, Dir Ves-6)*

Historical Uses: This most ancient of spices was included in just about every prescription issued in ancient China. It was regarded as a tranquilizer, tonic, and stomachic and as being good for depression and a weak heart.

French Medicinal Uses: Sexual stimulant, tropical infection, typhoid, vaginitis.

Other Possible Uses: This oil may be beneficial for **circulation, colds, coughs, digestion, exhaustion, flu, infections, rheumatism**, and **warts**. This oil fights **viral** and **infectious diseases**, and testing has yet to find a **virus, bacteria**, or **fungus** that can survive in its presence.

Body System(s) Affected: Immune System.

Application: Apply to **Vita Flex Points** and directly on **area** of concern. Best diluted with V-6 Mixing Oil as the high amount of phenols can irritate the skin.

Oral Use As Dietary Supplement: Generally regarded as safe (GRAS) for internal consumption by the FDA. ***Dilute*** *one drop oil in 2 tsp. honey or 8 oz. of beverage (i.e. soy/rice milk). May need to increase dilution even more due to this oil's potential for irritating mucus membranes. Not for children under 6 years old; use with* **caution** *and in* **greater dilution** *for children 6 years old and over.*

Safety Data: *Repeated use can result in extreme* **contact sensitization.** *Avoid during* **pregnancy.** *Can cause extreme* **skin irritation.** *Diffuse with caution; it will irritate the nasal membranes if it is inhaled directly from the diffuser. Use* **extreme caution** *when* **diffusing** *cinnamon bark because it may burn the nostrils if you put your nose directly next to the nebulizer of the diffuser.*

Blend Classification: Personifier

Blends With: All citrus oils, cypress, frankincense, geranium, juniper, lavender, rosemary, and all spice oils.

Odor: Type: *Base Note (5-60% of the blend)*; Scent: *Spicy, warm, sweet*; Intensity: *5*
Frequency: Traditionally thought to have a frequency that attracted wealth.
Bible: Exod. 30:23, Prov. 7:17, Song. 4:14, Rev. 18:13

CISTUS (LABDANUM)
(Cistus ladanifer)

Botanical Family: Cistaceae
Extraction Method/Origin: Steam distillation from branches — France, Spain
Chemical Constituents: Monoterpenes (up to 65%): α-pinene (50%), camphene (4%), sabinene, myrcene, phellandrene, limonene, cymene; Alcohols: α-terpineol (>5%), pinocarveol, borneol; Esters: linalyle acetate, bornyl & geranyl acetates (3%), methyl benzoate, phenyl propanoate; Ketones: 2,2,6-trimethylcyclohexanone (2%), fenchone (1%); Aldehydes: benzaldehyde (>3%), neral; Carboxylic Acids.
Properties: **Antimicrobial, antiseptic, astringent, diuretic, expectorant**, and **tonic**.
Folklore: Anciently, cistus was among the first aromatic substances used.
Esoteric Uses/Actions: Astrological: *Pluto*; Chakra: *7*; Character: *Yang*; Element: *Earth*
Historical Uses: Used for catarrh, diarrhea, dysentery, and promoting menstruation.
Other Possible Uses: Cistus may help with **bleeding** (stop), **boils, bronchitis, colds, coughs, rhinitis, urinary infections, wounds**, and **wrinkles**.
Body System(s) Affected: Immune System. It may also assist the **auto-immune system**.
Aromatic Influence: Stimulating to the **senses** of touch, feeling, sight, and sound. It affects the upper part of the **brain**. It may also help quiet the **nerves**, calm the **insomniac**, and elevate the emotions in **meditation**.
Application: Apply to **Vita Flex Points** and/or directly on **area** of concern; Diffuse.
Oral Use As Dietary Supplement: Approved by the FDA for use as a Food Additive (FA) or Flavoring Agent (FL). **Dilute** *one drop oil in 1 tsp. honey or 4 oz. of beverage (i.e. soy/rice milk). Not for children under 6 years old; use with **caution** and in **greater dilution** for children 6 years old and over.*
Safety Data: *Use with caution during **pregnancy.***
Blend Classification: Personifier.
Blends With: Bergamot, calamus, chamomile, Clary sage, cypress, juniper, lavender, lavandin, patchouli, pine, sandalwood, and vetiver.

CITRONELLA
(Cymbopogon nardus)

Botanical Family: Gramineae (grasses)
Extraction Method/Origin: Steam distillation from grass — Egypt, Philippines, Sri lanka

Chemical Constituents: Alcohols (>35%): geraniol (>16%), citronnellol (8%), borneol (6%); Phenols: methyl ether (<10%), methyl isoeugenol (<10%), isoeugenol (7%); Monoterpenes: d-limonene (<10%); Aldehydes: citronnellal (<7%).

Properties: Anti-bacterial, anti-fungal, anti-inflammatory, antiseptic, antispasmodic, deodorant, and **insecticidal**.

Esoteric Uses/Actions: Astrological: *Venus*; Character: *Yang?*

Historical Uses: This oil belongs to the same family of aromatic, oil-rich tropical grasses as lemongrass and palmarosa. It has been used as an insecticide and for rheumatic problems or other aches and pains. The leaves of citronella have been utilized by many diverse cultures for fever, intestinal parasites, digestive and menstrual problems, and as a stimulant. This oil is hardly used alone in therapy, but because of its highly antiseptic and deodorizing properties, it is used a great deal in commercial preparations and some aromatherapy blends.

Other Possible Uses: Citronella may help with **colds, fatigue, flu, headaches**, minor **infections, migraine, neuralgia**, excessive **perspiration**, and **oily skin**. Can be used as an antiseptic to **sanitize** and **deodorize surfaces** where food has been prepared. Combined with cedarwood, it makes an excellent insect repellent.

Body System(s) Affected: Muscles and **Bones, Skin**.

Aromatic Influence: May increase the heart rate.

Application: Dilute and apply directly on **area** of concern.

Oral Use As Dietary Supplement: Generally regarded as safe (GRAS) for internal consumption by the FDA. ***Dilute*** *one drop oil in 1 tsp. honey or 4 oz. of beverage (i.e. soy/rice milk).* ***Not for children under 6 years old; use with*** *caution and in* ***greater dilution*** *for children 6 years old and over.*

Safety Data: *Repeated use can result in extreme* ***contact sensitization***. *Use with caution during* ***pregnancy***. *Can irritate sensitive* ***skin***. *Inhaling citronella can increase the heart rate.*

Blend Classification: Personifier.

Blends With: Bergamot, cedarwood, geranium, lemon, orange, and pine.

Odor: Type: *Top Note (5-20% of the blend)*; Scent: *Citrusy, slightly fruity, fresh, sweet*; Intensity: *3*

CLARY SAGE
(Salvia sclarea)

Botanical Family: Labiatae (mint)

Extraction Method/Origin: Steam distillation from flowing plant — France, Utah

Chemical Constituents: Esters (up to 75%): linalyl acetate (20-75%); Alcohols (20%): linalol (10-20%), geraniol, α-terpineol; Sesquiterpenes (<14%): germacrene-D (up to 12%), β-caryophyllene; Diterpene alcohols: sclareol (normally 0.5-2.5%, but 5-7% from double distillation in Utah); Monoterpenes: myrcene, α- and β-pinenes, l-limonene, ocimene, terpinolene; Oxides: 1,8 cineol, linalol oxide, sclareol oxide; Ketones: α- and β-thujone; Sesquiterpene alcohols; Aldehydes; Coumarins. *(More than 250 constituents)*

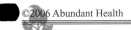
Properties: **Anti-convulsive, anti-fungal, antiseptic, antispasmodic, astringent, nerve tonic, sedative, soothing, tonic**, and **warming**.

Esoteric Uses/Actions: Astrological: *Mercury & Saturn*; Body type: *Ectomorph*; Chakras: *2 & 6*; Character: *Yang, with high Yin*; Crystals: *Malachite* ; Element: *Water, Light, & Earth*; Number: *7*

Historical Uses: Nicknamed "clear eyes", it was famous during the Middle Ages for its ability to clear eye problems. During that same time, it was widely used for female complaints, kidney/digestive/skin disorders, inflammation, sore throats, and wounds.

French Medicinal Uses: **Bronchitis, cholesterol, frigidity, genitalia, hemorrhoids, hormonal imbalance, impotence, infections, intestinal cramps, menstrual cramps, pms, pre-menopause, weak digestion**.

Other Possible Uses: This oil may be used for **amenorrhea, cell regulation, circulatory problems, depression, insect bites, insomnia, kidney disorders**, dry **skin, throat infection, ulcers**, and **whooping cough**.

Body System(s) Affected: **Hormonal System**.

Aromatic Influence: It may calm and enhance the **dream state**, helping to bring about a feeling of **euphoria**.

Application: Apply to **Vita Flex Points** and/or directly on **area** of concern; Diffuse.

Oral Use As Dietary Supplement: Generally regarded as safe (GRAS) for internal consumption by the FDA. **Dilute** *one drop oil in 1 tsp. honey or 4 oz. of beverage (i.e. soy/rice milk).* **Not** *for children under 6 years old; use with* **caution** *and in* **greater dilution** *for children 6 years old and over.*

Safety Data: *Use with caution during* **pregnancy**. *Not for babies. Avoid during and after consumption of* **alcohol.**

Blend Classification: Personifier

Blends With: Bergamot, cedarwood, citrus oils, cypress, geranium, juniper, and sandalwood.

Odor: Type: *Middle to Base Notes (5-60% of the blend)*; Scent: *Herbaceous, spicy, hay-like, sharp, fixative*; Intensity: *3*

CLOVE
(Syzygium aromaticum)

Botanical Family: Myrtaceae (shrubs and trees)

Extraction Method/Origin: Steam distillation from bud and stem — Madagascar, Spice Islands

Chemical Constituents: Phenols: eugenol (up to 85%), chavicol, 4-allylphenol; Esters: eugenyl acetate (up to 15%), styralyl, benzyl, terpenyl, ethyl phenyl acetates, methyl salicylate (tr.); Sesquiterpenes (up to 14%): β-caryophyllene (<12%), humulene, α-amorphene, α-muurolene, calamenene; Oxides (<3%): caryophyllene oxide, humulene oxide; Carboxylic Acids; Ketones.

Properties: Analgesic, anti-bacterial, anti-fungal, anti-infectious, anti-inflammatory, anti-parasitic, strong **antiseptic, anti-tumoral, anti-viral, disinfectant**, and **immune-stimulant**.

Folklore: Some old tales say that walking near clove trees while wearing a hat would frighten them into no longer bearing fruit. While the trees may have been afraid of hats, they were not afraid of viruses. History has it that the people of Penang (among the "Spice Islands") were free from epidemics until the sixteenth century, when Dutch conquerors destroyed the clove trees that flourished on those islands. Many of the islanders died from the epidemics that followed.

Esoteric Uses/Actions: Astrological: *Mars, Jupiter*; Ayurvedic: *Kapha*; Chakra: *1*; Character: *Yang*; Element: *Fire*

Historical Uses: Cloves were historically used for skin infections, digestive upsets, intestinal parasites, childbirth, and most notably for toothache. The Chinese also used cloves for diarrhea, hernia, bad breath and bronchitis.

French Medicinal Uses: Impotence, intestinal parasites, memory deficiency, pain, plague, toothache, wounds (infected).

Other Possible Uses: This oil may help **amebic dysentery, arthritis, bacterial colitis, bones, bronchitis, cholera, cystitis, dental infection, diarrhea, infectious acne, fatigue, flatulence** (gas), **flu, halitosis** (bad breath), tension **headaches, hypertension, infection** (wounds and more), **insect bites and stings, lupus, nausea, neuritis, nettles** and **poison oak** (takes out sting), **rheumatism, sinusitis, skin cancer**, chronic **skin disease, smoking** (removes desire), **sores** (speeds healing of mouth and skin sores), **tuberculosis, thyroid dysfunction**, leg **ulcers, viral hepatitis, vomiting**, and **warts**. (*See* **Warts** *in the Personal Guide section of this book.*)

Body System(s) Affected: Cardiovascular, Digestive, Immune, and **Respiratory Systems**.

Aromatic Influence: It may influence **healing**, improve **memory** (mental stimulant), and create a feeling of **protection** and **courage**. Septimas Piesse considered clove scent to **vibrate** in the **key** of **B** and in the color of **violet**. It can also cause a good sleep, generally culminating in stimulating dreams.

Application: Apply to **Vita Flex Points** and/or directly on **area** of concern. Rub directly on the **gums** surrounding an infected tooth. Place on **tongue** with finger to remove desire to smoke, or back of tongue for tickling cough. **Diffuse**.

Oral Use As Dietary Supplement: Generally regarded as safe (GRAS) for internal consumption by the FDA. ***Dilute*** *one drop oil in 1 tsp. honey or 4 oz. of beverage (i.e. soy/rice milk).* ***Not for children under 6 years old; use with* caution *and in* greater dilution *for children 6 years old and over.*

Safety Data: *Repeated use can result in extreme* **contact sensitization.** *Use with caution during* **pregnancy.** *Can irritate sensitive* **skin.**

Blend Classification: Personifier

Blends With: Basil, bergamot, cinnamon bark, Clary sage, grapefruit, lavender, lemon, nutmeg, orange, peppermint, rose, rosemary, and ylang ylang.

Odor: Type: *Middle to Base Notes (20-80% of the blend)*; Scent: *Spicy, warming, slightly bitter, woody, reminiscent of true clove buds, but richer*; Intensity: *5*

CORIANDER
(Coriandrum sativum L.)

Botanical Family: Umbelliferae (parsley)

Extraction Method/Origin: Steam distillation from seeds — India, Russia

Chemical Constituents: Alcohols (up to 80%): linalol (>30%), coriandrol (<30%), geraniol, terpinen-4-ol, borneol; Monoterpenes (up to 24%): α-pinene, γ-terpinene, l-limonene, p-cymene, myrcene, camphene; Esters: geranyl acetate, linalyl acetate; Ketones: camphor, carvone; Aldehydes: decanal.

Properties: **Analgesic, anti-bacterial, anti-fungal, antioxidant, anti-rheumatic, antispasmodic**, and **stimulant** (cardiac, circulatory, nervous systems). It also has **anti-inflammatory** and **sedative** properties.

Folklore: The seeds were found in the ancient Egyptian tomb of Rameses II.

Esoteric Uses/Actions: Astrological: *Mars*; Body type: *Endomorph*; Chakra: *2*; Character: *Yin?*; Element: *Fire & Water*; Number: *5*

Historical Uses: The Chinese have used coriander for dysentery, piles, measles, nausea, toothache, and painful hernias.

Other Possible Uses: Coriander may help with **anorexia, arthritis, colds, colic, diarrhea, digestive spasms, dyspepsia, flatulence, flu, gout, infections** (general), **measles, migraine, muscular aches and pains, nausea, nervous exhaustion, neuralgia, piles, poor circulation, rheumatism, skin** (oily skin, blackheads, and other impurities), and **stiffness**. Current research at Cairo University indicates that coriander lowers **glucose** levels by normalizing insulin levels and supporting the **pancreas function**. It may also help during **convalescence** and after a difficult childbirth. Because of its estrogen content, it may regulate and help control pain related to **menstruation**.

Body System(s) Affected: Digestive and **Hormonal Systems**.

Aromatic Influence: Coriander is a gentle stimulant for those with **low physical energy**. It also helps one relax during times of **stress, irritability, and nervousness**. It may also provide a **calming** influence to those suffering from **shock** or **fear**.

Application: Apply to **Vita Flex Points** and directly on **area** of concern; **Diffuse**.

Oral Use As Dietary Supplement: Generally regarded as safe (GRAS) for internal consumption by the FDA. ***Dilute*** *one drop oil in 1 tsp. honey or 4 oz. of beverage (i.e. soy/rice milk).* ***Not for children under 6 years old; use with*** *caution and in* ***greater dilution*** *for children 6 years old and over.*

Safety Data: *Use sparingly as coriander can be* ***stupifying*** *in large doses.*

Blend Classification: Personifier and Modifier

Blends With: Bergamot, cinnamon bark, citronella, Clary sage, cypress, ginger, jasmine, neroli, petitgrain, pine, sandalwood, and other spice oils.

Odor: Type: *Middle Note (50-80% of the blend)*; Scent: *Woody, spicy, sweet*; Intensity: *3*

CUMIN
(Cuminum cyminum)

Botanical Family: Umbelliferae (parsley)

Extraction Method/Origin: Steam distillation from seeds — Egypt

Chemical Constituents: Monoterpenes (up to 75%): α- and γ-terpinenes (<40%), β-pinene, p-cymene, camphene; Aldehydes (<60%): p-menthadienals (up to 35%), cuminal (up to 32%), dihydro-cuminal, p-mentha-3-en-7-ol; Phenols: p-cuminol; Sesquiterpenes: β-caryophyllene; Coumarins: scopoletin.

Properties: Anti-bacterial, antioxidant, anti-parasitic, antiseptic, antispasmodic, antitoxic, anti-viral, aphrodisiac, digestive, stimulant (heart, immune and nervous systems), and **tonic**.

Folklore: Cumin seeds were found in Egyptian tombs, and used by the Romans as a food preservative.

Esoteric Uses/Actions: Astrological: *Saturn & Mars*; Body type: *Endomorph*; Character: *Yin, with high Yang?*; Element: *Fire & Water*; Number: *3*; Perfume note: *Top*

Historical Uses: During biblical times it was used by the Hebrews as an antiseptic during their ceremony of circumcision. Traditionally one of the main ingredients in curry, it was also used to help with flatulence, the digestive system, for rheumatic conditions, the heart, and the nervous system.

Other Possible Uses: This oil may help with **cellulite**, poor **circulation, colic, deafness** following a bad viral **flu** infection, **digestive spasms, dyspepsia, flatulence, headaches, indigestion, lymphatic congestion, migraines**, and **nervous debility** and **exhaustion**.

Body System(s) Affected: Digestive and **Immune Systems**.

Aromatic Influence: Used by one source to encourage **bowel movements** in their child. It has also been used at dinner parties to **stimulate** the **appetite**.

Application: Apply to **Vita Flex Points** and directly on **area** of concern; **Diffuse**.

Oral Use As Dietary Supplement: Generally regarded as safe (GRAS) for internal consumption by the FDA. ***Dilute*** *one drop oil in 1 tsp. honey or 4 oz. of beverage (i.e. soy/rice milk).* ***Not for children under 6 years old; use with*** **caution** *and in* **greater dilution** *for children 6 years old and over.*

Safety Data: *Use with caution during* **pregnancy.** *Avoid direct* **sunlight** *for up to 12 hours after use.*

Blend Classification: Enhancer

Blends With: Cinnamon bark, jasmine, patchouli, rose, sandalwood, and ylang ylang.

CYPRESS
(Cupressus sempervirens)

Botanical Family: Cupressaceae (conifer - cypress)

Extraction Method/Origin: Steam distillation from branches — France, Spain

Chemical Constituents: Monoterpenes: α-pinene (>55%), δ-3-carene (<22%), l-limonene, terpinolene, sabinene, β-pinene; Sesquiterpene Alcohols: cedrol (up to 15%), cadinol; Alcohols: borneol (<9%), α-terpineol, terpinene-4-ol, linalol sabinol; Esters: α-terpinyl acetate (<5%), isovalerate, terpinen-4-yl acetate; Sesquiterpenes: δ-cadinene, α-cedrene; Diterpene Alcohols; labdanic alcohols, manool, sempervirol; Diterpene Acids; Oxides.

Properties: **Anti-bacterial, anti-infectious, antimicrobial, mucolytic, antiseptic, astringent, deodorant, diuretic, lymphatic** and **prostate decongestant, refreshing, relaxing**, and a **vasoconstrictor**.

Folklore: According to Roberta Wilson, "The evergreen branches of the cypress tree were considered symbolic of life after death. In fact, *sempervirens* means 'ever-living'."

Esoteric Uses/Actions: Astrological: *Saturn*; Body type: *Ectomorph*; Chakra: *5*; Character: *Yang*; Element: *Ether & Earth*; Number: *7*; Oriental: *Blood stagnation (pts: Sp-10 & 6)*

Historical Uses: It was used anciently for its benefits on the urinary system and other places where there is excessive loss of fluids, such as perspiration, diarrhea, and menstrual flow. The Chinese valued cypress for its benefits to the liver and respiratory system.

French Medicinal Uses: **Arthritis, bronchitis, circulation, cramps, hemorrhoids, insomnia, intestinal parasites, lymphatic decongestant, menopausal problems, menstrual pain, pancreas insufficiencies, pleurisy, prostate decongestant, pulmonary tuberculosis, rheumatism, spasms, throat problems, varicose veins, water retention**.

Other Possible Uses: This oil may be beneficial for **asthma**, strengthening **blood capillary walls**, reducing **cellulite, circulatory system, colds**, strengthening **connective tissue**, spasmodic **coughs, diarrhea, edema, energy, fever, gallbladder**, bleeding **gums, hemorrhaging, influenza, laryngitis, liver disorders, lung circulation, muscular cramps, nervous tension, nose bleeds, ovarian cysts**, increasing **perspiration, skin care, scar tissue, whooping cough**, and **wounds**.

Body System(s) Affected: **Cardiovascular System, Muscles** and **Bones**.

Aromatic Influence: It influences, strengthens, and helps ease the feeling of **loss**. It creates a feeling of **security, grounding**, and it helps to heal **emotions**.

Application: Apply to **Vita Flex Points** and directly on **area** of concern; **Diffuse**.

Oral Use As Dietary Supplement: None.

Safety Data: *Use with caution during* **pregnancy.**

Blend Classification: Equalizer

Blends With: Bergamot, Clary sage, juniper, lavender, lemon, orange, and sandalwood.

Odor: Type: *Middle Note (50-80% of the blend)*; Scent: *Fresh, herbaceous, slightly woody with evergreen undertones*; Intensity: *3*

CYPRESS, BLUE
(Callitris intratropica)

Botanical Family: Cupressaceae

Extraction Method/Origin: Steam distillation from the heartwood, which makes up 70% of the tree trunk — Australia

Chemical Constituents: Sesquiterpene Alcohols (up to 70%): guaiol (<26%), α- and β-eudesmols (<25%), bulnesol (<15%); Sesquiterpenes (<22%): β-elemene (<10%), β-selinene (<10%), δ-guaiazulene (<2%); Lactones.

Properties: Anti-inflammatory, anti-viral, insect repellent, and **stimulant** (to amygdalla, pineal gland, pituitary gland, and hypothalamus).

Historical Uses: Blue cypress has been used historically for incense, perfume and embalming. The resin was used for sores, cuts, and upset stomachs. The aboriginal Tiwi people of Australia would throw the wood onto the fire to drive away the mosquitoes and midges. The guaiazulene gives blue cypress oil its azure blue color.

Other Possible Uses: Blue cypress may help with **abdominal cramps, aches** and **pain** (minor), **brain** function (improves circulation and oxygenates), **cold sores, herpes simplex, herpes zoster,** and the **human papilloma virus (HPV).**

Body System(s) Affected: Digestive and **Immune Systems.**

Application: Apply to **Vita Flex Points** and directly on **area** of concern; Diffuse.

Oral Use As Dietary Supplement: None.

Safety Data: *None available.*

Blends With: Cedarwood, frankincense, helichrysum, lavender, melissa, and sandalwood.

Odor: Type: *Base Note (5-20% of the blend)*; Scent: *Long-lasting, warm, woody, earthy*; Intensity: *3*

Found In: Brain Power, Australian Blue, AromaGuard Mountain Mint Deodorant.

DAVANA
(Artemisia pallens)

Botanical Family: Compositae (daisy)

Extraction Method/Origin: Steam distillation of the stems and leaves — India

Chemical Constituents: Ketones: davanone (47-52%), nordavanone (<3%), artemone (<3%); Alcohols: nerol (10%), geraniol (5%), nerolidol (<3%), borneol, davanol, farnesol, linalol; Ethers: davana ether (<6%); Furanoids: davana furan (<4%); Terpenes: cadinene, para-cymene, camphene, sabinene; Carboxylic Acids: davanic acid (<3%); Esters: cinnamyl cinnamate (2%), ethyl davanate; Oxides: linalol oxide; Aldehydes: lilac aldehyde.

Properties: Anti-bacterial, anti-fungal, anti-infectious, nervine.

Historical Uses: Davana has been widely used in Iraqi and Indian folk medicine for the treatment of diabetes mellitus. According to one research study, "Oral administration of an aqueous/ methanolic extract from the aerial parts of the plants led to significant blood glucose lowering effect in glucose-fed hyperglycemic and alloxan-induced diabetic rabbits and rats" (Twaij HA and Al-Badr AA, 1988 and Subramoniam A et al 1996)

Possible Uses: This oil may help stimulate the **endocrine system**, improve **hormonal balance**, and soothe **rough, dry, and chapped skin**. It may also help with **coughing attacks** with **thick mucus** and **spasmodic coughs**, as well as help ease **anxious feelings** and **nervousness**.

Body System(s) Affected: Hormonal System.

Oral Use As Dietary Supplement: Approved by the FDA for use as a Food Additive (FA) or Flavoring Agent (FL). ***Dilute*** *one drop oil in 1 tsp. honey or 4 oz. of beverage (i.e. soy/rice milk).* ***Not for children under 6 years old; use with*** **caution** *and in* ***greater dilution*** *for children 6 years old and over.*

Safety Data: *Use with caution during* ***pregnancy.***

DILL
(Anethum graveolens)

Botanical Family: Umbelliferae (parsley)

Extraction Method/Origin: Steam distillation from whole plant — Austria, Hungary

Chemical Constituents: Monoterpenes (up to 65%): d-limonene (up to 25%), α- & β-pinenes (<30%), α- & β-phellandrenes, p-cymene; Ketones: d-carvone (<45%); Ethers (<11%).

Properties: Antispasmodic, anti-bacterial, expectorant, and **stimulant**.

Folklore: The dill plant is mentioned in the Papyrus of Ebers from Egypt (1550 B.C.). Roman Gladiators would rub it into their skin before a fight.

Possible Uses: This oil may help **bronchial catarrh, colic, constipation, dyspepsia, flatulence, headaches, indigestion, liver deficiencies, lower glucose levels, nervousness, normalize insulin levels, promote milk flow** in nursing mothers, and **support** the **pancreas function**.

Body System(s) Affected: Digestive System.

Aromatic Influence: It calms the autonomic nervous system and, when diffused with Roman chamomile, may help fidgety children

Application: Apply to **Vita Flex Points** and/or directly on **area** of concern; Diffuse. A drop or two on the **wrists** can help remove **addictions** to **sweets**.

Oral Use As Dietary Supplement: Generally regarded as safe (GRAS) for internal consumption by the FDA. ***Dilute*** *one drop oil in 1 tsp. honey or 4 oz. of beverage (i.e. soy/rice milk).* ***Not for children under 6 years old; use with*** **caution** *and in* ***greater dilution*** *for children 6 years old and over.*

Safety Data: *Use with caution if susceptible to* ***epilepsy***.

Blend Classification: Enhancer

Blends With: Nutmeg and citrus oils.

Odor: Type: *Middle Note (50-80% of the blend)*; Scent: *Fresh, sweet, herbaceous, slightly earthy*; Intensity: *2*

DOUGLAS FIR
(See FIR, DOUGLAS)

ELEMI
(Canarium luzonicum)

Botanical Family: Burseraceae

Extraction Method/Origin: Steam distillation from the gum of the tree — Philippines

Chemical Constituents: Monoterpenes (up to 90%): l-limonene (up to 70%), α- phellandrene (<24%), sabinene (<10%) β-phellandrene (5%), dipentene, terpinolene; Alcohols: elemol (up to 25%), α-terpineol; Ethers: elemicin; Sesquiterpenes: elemene; Ketones: d-carvone.

Properties: Anti-catarrhal, anti-depressant, anti-infectious, antiseptic, expectorant, and **sedative**.

Folklore: The name, elemi, comes from an Arabic phrase meaning "As above, so below". This helps us understand its action on both the emotional and spiritual planes. Because of the similar properties and uses, it has come to be known as the "poor man's frankincense".

Esoteric Uses/Actions: Astrological: *Sun*; Chakras: 7; Crystals: *Elestial, skeleton quartz* ; Color: *Yellow pale*

Historical Uses: Native to the Philippine Islands and the Moluccas, it is used locally for skin conditions and respiratory problems. Anciently, the Egyptians used the oil that was distilled from the resin in part of the embalming process.

Other Possible Uses: This oil may help with **bronchitis** (chronic), **chest infections, childbirth, coughs** (unproductive), **cuts** (infected), **gangrene, inflammation** (breast and uterus), **pregnancy, rashes** (allergic), **rejuvenation, skin** (chapped), **thymus gland, tissue** (builds), **ulcers, wounds** (infected), and **wrinkles**. *See frankincense and myrrh for other possible uses.*

Body System(s) Affected: Skin.

Aromatic Influence: When diffused, this oil may help with **nervous exhaustion, stress, sinusitis**, and other **bronchial infections**. During **meditation**, it may help to **calm** and Chakras (Energy Centers) **center** the individual. It may also help to bring the **mind, body**, and **spirit** into alignment with each other. It is psychologically **balancing** and **strengthening** as well as **fortifying** to the **psychic centers**.

Application: Apply to **Vita Flex Points** and/or directly on **area** of concern. May be used as a **compress** for infected **wounds** and **abscesses**. May also be diluted for use during a **massage**, or added to a **bath**.

Oral Use As Dietary Supplement: Approved by the FDA for use as a Food Additive (FA) or Flavoring Agent (FL). **Dilute** *one drop oil in 1 tsp. honey or 4 oz. of beverage (i.e. soy/rice milk).* **Not for children under 6 years old; use with** *caution* **and in** *greater dilution for children 6 years old and over.*

Blend Classification: Enhancer; the hint of lemon gives it more of a middle note.

Blends With: Cinnamon bark & other spices, frankincense, lavender, myrrh, rosemary, sage.
Odor: Type: *Middle Note (50-80% of the blend)*; Scent: *Balsamic, fresh, citrusy, peppery, spicy*; Intensity: *3*

EUCALYPTUS
(Eucalyptus globulus)

Botanical Family: Myrtaceae (Myrtle shrubs and trees)
Extraction Method/Origin: Steam distillation from leaves — Australia, Brazil
Chemical Constituents: Oxides: 1,8 cineol (up to 78%); Monoterpenes (>20%): α- & β-pinenes, l-limonene, ρ-cymene, α-phellandrene; Sesquiterpene Alcohols: globulol (>7%), trans-pinocarveol (<5%), ledol (>2%), linalol, terpinen-4-ol, eudesmol; Sesquiterpenes: aromadendrene (>7%), allo-aromadendrene (>2%), δ-guaiazulene, humulene; Ketones: pinocarvone, d-carvone, fenchone; Aldehydes: butyricaldehyde, caproicaldehyde, geranial, myrtenal, valericaldehyde; Phenols: myrtenol, p-cuminol; Alcohols: α-fenchol, α-terpineol; Esters: α-terpenyl acetate.
Properties: Analgesic, anti-bacterial, anti-catarrhal, anti-infectious, anti-inflammatory, antiseptic, anti-viral, diuretic, expectorant, insect repellent, and **stimulant**.
Esoteric Uses/Actions: Astrological: *Saturn & Mercury*; Ayurvedic: *Kapha*; Chakra: *4, 5, & 6*; Character: *Yang*; Crystals: *Aquamarine* ; Element: *Air & Earth*; Oriental: *Cold phlegm (pts: St-40, Sp-6)*
Historical Uses: Australian aborigines used the eucalyptus leaves to bind up serious wounds. This would not only prevent infection but also expedite healing.
French Medicinal Uses: Asthma, candida, coughs, diabetes, fever, hypoglycemia, lungs, measles, migraines, respiratory stimulant, sinusitis, tuberculosis, urinary stimulant.
Other Possible Uses: This oil may be used for **aches/pains, acne, allergies, bronchitis, burns, colds, cystitis, diarrhea, endometriosis**, increasing **energy, flu, gallstones, gonorrhea, hay fever, herpes, inflammation** of the **ear, inflammation** of the **iris, inflammation** of the **nasal mucous membrane, malaria, nasopharynx, rheumatism, skin infection/sores, sore throat, ulcers, vaginitis, viruses**, and **wounds**.
Body System(s) Affected: Muscles and **Bones, Respiratory System**.
Aromatic Influence: It promotes **health, well being, purification**, and **healing**.
Application: Apply to **Vita Flex Points** and/or directly on **area** of concern; *Diffuse. Apply under the nose and on each side of the nose for quick **sinus relief***.
Oral Use As Dietary Supplement: Approved by the FDA for use as a Food Additive (FA) or Flavoring Agent (FL). ***Dilute*** *one drop oil in 1 tsp. honey or 4 oz. of beverage (i.e. soy/rice milk).* ***Not for children under 6 years old; use with*** *caution **and in** greater dilution **for children 6 years old and over.***
Blend Classification: Enhancer

Blends With: Geranium, lavender, lemon, sandalwood, juniper, lemongrass, melissa, pine, thyme.
Odor: Type: *Top Note (5-20% of the blend)*; Scent: *Fresh, medicinal, woody, earthy*; Intensity: *5*

EUCALYPTUS CITRIODORA
(or LEMON EUCALYPTUS)
(Eucalyptus citriodora)

Botanical Family: Myrtaceae (Myrtle shrubs and trees)
Extraction Method/Origin: Steam distillation from leaves — China
Chemical Constituents: Aldehydes: citronellal (<80%); Alcohols: citronellol (<20%), geraniol, trans-pinocarveol, cis- & trans-p-menthane-3,8-diols; Phenols (<21%): isopulegol, eugenol, p-cuminol; Oxides (<18%): 1,8 cineol, linalol oxide, rose oxide; Esters (<12%): citronellyl acetate (<8%), citronellyl butyrate, citronellyl citronellate.
Properties: Anti-bacterial, anti-fungal, anti-infectious, anti-inflammatory, antirheumatic, antiseptic, anti-viral, deodorant, expectorant, and **insecticidal**.
Esoteric Uses/Actions: Astrological: *Mercury & Saturn*; Character: *Yin*; Element: *Air*; Oriental: *Hot wind, phlegm (pts: St-40, Sp-6)*
Historical Uses: *Eucalyptus citriodora* has been used to perfume the linen closet, and as an insect repellent, especially for cockroaches and silverfish.
Other Possible Uses: *Eucalyptus citriodora* may help with **asthma, athlete's foot** and other **fungal infections, colds, cuts, dandruff, fevers, herpes, infectious skin conditions** such as **chickenpox, infectious diseases, insect repellent, laryngitis, scabs, sore throat, sores, wounds**.
Body System(s) Affected: Respiratory System.
Application: Apply to **Vita Flex Points** and/or directly on **area** of concern.
Oral Use As Dietary Supplement: None.
Safety Data: *Repeated use can possibly result in* **contact sensitization**.
Odor: Type: *Middle Note (50-80% of the blend)*; Scent: *Sweet, lemony, fresh, with a woody hint;* Intensity: *3*

EUCALYPTUS DIVES
(Eucalyptus dives var. piperitone)

Botanical Family: Myrtaceae (Myrtle shrubs and trees)
Extraction Method/Origin: Steam distillation from leaves — Australia, Brazil
Chemical Constituents: Ketones: piperitone (up to 50%); Monoterpenes (<47%): α- & β-phellandrenes (<30%), p-cymene (<10%), α-thujene (<6%); Phenolic Alcohols: terpinen-4-ol (<6%); Sesquiterpenes (<4%): α-cubebene, β-caryophyllene, δ-cadinene, γ-elemene, longifolene; Alcohols (<3%): α-terpineol, linalol, piperitol; Oxides (<1%): α-pinene oxide, 1,8 cineol oxide.

Properties: Anti-bacterial (more specific than other varieties of eucalyptus oil)
Esoteric Uses/Actions: Astrological: *Mercury & Saturn*; Chakras: *4 & 6*; Character: *slightly Yang*; Element: *Air & Earth*
Possible Uses: See other varieties of eucalyptus for possible uses.
Body System(s) Affected: Respiratory System.
Application: Diffuse; Apply to **Vita Flex Points** and directly on **area** of concern.
Oral Use As Dietary Supplement: None.

EUCALYPTUS POLYBRACTEA
(Eucalyptus polybractea)

Botanical Family: Myrtaceae (Myrtle shrubs and trees)
Extraction Method/Origin: Steam distillation from leaves — Australia, Brazil
Chemical Constituents: Oxides: 1,8 cineol (up to 95%); Monoterpenes (<6%): l-limonene, α-pinene, p-cymene; Ketones: cryptone; Aldehydes: cuminal; Phenols: p-cuminol.
Properties: Anti-bacterial, anti-infectious, anti-inflammatory, anti-viral, expectorant, mucolytic, and **insecticidal**.
Esoteric Uses/Actions: Astrological: *Mercury & Saturn*; Character: *Neutral?*; Element: *Air & Earth*
Possible Uses: Acne, cystitis. See other varieties of eucalyptus for possible uses.
Body System(s) Affected: Respiratory System.
Application: Diffuse; Apply to **Vita Flex Points** and directly on **area** of concern.
Oral Use As Dietary Supplement: None.
Odor: Type: *Top Note (5-20% of the blend)*; Scent: *Fresh, woody, earthy*; Intensity: *4*

EUCALYPTUS RADIATA
(Eucalyptus radiata)

Botanical Family: Myrtaceae (Myrtle shrubs and trees)
Extraction Method/Origin: Steam distillation from leaves — Australia
Chemical Constituents: Oxides: 1,8 cineol (62-72%), caryophyllene oxide; Monoterpenes (up to 24%): α- & β-pinenes (<12%), l-limonene (<8%), myrcene, p-cymene; Alcohols (<19%): α-terpinol (14%), geraniol, borneol, linalol; Aldehydes (8%): myrtenal, citronellal, geranial, neral.
Properties: Anti-bacterial, anti-catarrhal, anti-infectious, anti-inflammatory, anti-viral, and **expectorant**.
Esoteric Uses/Actions: Astrological: *Saturn & Mercury*; Chakra: *6*; Character: *Yang*; Element: *Air & Earth*; Oriental: *Cools and quiets fire element of lungs - massage over chest, back, ribs, & over spleen/pancreas & lung meridians*
Other Possible Uses: This oil, when combined with bergamot, has been used effectively on **herpes simplex**. It may also help with **acne, bronchitis, ear** (inflammation), **endometriosis,**

flu, hay fever, iris (inflammation), **nasal mucous membrane** (inflammation), **sinusitis**, and **vaginitis**.

Body System(s) Affected: Respiratory System, Skin.

Application: Apply to **Vita Flex Points** and/or directly on **area** of concern; Diffuse.

Odor: Type: *Middle Note (50-80% of the blend)*; Scent: *Slightly camphorous, sweet, fruity*; Intensity: *3*

EUCALYPTUS STAIGERIANA
(Eucalyptus staigeriana)

Botanical Family: Myrtaceae (Myrtle shrubs and trees)

Extraction Method/Origin: Steam distillation from leaves — Brazil

Chemical Constituents: Aldehydes: citral (up to 40%), geranial (12%), neral; Monoterpenes: limonene (up to 25%), p-cymene (2%), many others; Alcohols: geraniol (6%), nerol; Oxides: 1,8 cineol (5%); Ester: geranyl acetate (4%), methyl geraniate.

Properties: Analgesic, anti-fungal, anti-infectious, anti-inflammatory, anti-viral, antiseptic (pulmonary, urinary), powerful **antispasmodic, purifying**, and **sedative** (CNS, heart).

Esoteric Uses/Actions: Character: *Yin*

Possible Uses: This oil may help with **bronchitis, colds, congestion, cystitis, dermatitis, fevers, infections, hypertension** (lowers blood pressure), **inflammation** (joint and muscle), **leucorrhea** (increases urine flow), **neck aches, solar plexus** (relaxes), **stress related disorders**, vaginitis, and it is very soothing and calming.

Body System(s) Affected: Muscles and **Bones, Respiratory System, Skin**.

Application: Apply to **Vita Flex Points** and/or directly on **area** of concern; Diffuse.

FENNEL
(Foeniculum vulgare)

Botanical Family: Umbelliferae (parsley)

Extraction Method/Origin: Steam distillation from the crushed seeds — Australia, Spain

Chemical Constituents: Phenolic Ethers (up to 80%): trans-anethole (70%), methyl chavicol (or estragole) (>3%); Monoterpenes (up to 50%): trans-ocimene (<12%), l-limonene (<12%), γ-terpinene (<11%), α- & β-pinenes (<10%), p-cymene, α- & β-phellandrenes, terpiolene, myrcene, sabinene; Alcohols (up to 16%): linalol (<12%), α-fenchol (<4%); Ketones (<15%): fenchone (12%), camphor; Oxides; Phenols.

Properties: Anti-parasitic, antiseptic, antispasmodic, anti-toxin, diuretic, and **expectorant**.

Folklore: During Medieval times, fennel was believed to ward off evil spirits and block spells cast by witches.

Esoteric Uses/Actions: Astrological: *Mercury*; Body type: *Lymphatic*; Chakra: *1*; Character: *Yang, Yin*; Element: *Air*; Oriental: *Cold damp (pts: Sp-9 & 6)*

Historical Uses: The ancient Egyptians and Romans awarded garlands of fennel as praise to victorious warriors because fennel was believed to bestow strength, courage, and longevity. It has been used for thousands of years for snakebite, to stave off hunger pains, to tone the female reproductive system, for earaches, eye problems, insect bites, kidney complaints, lung infections, and to expel worms.

French Medicinal Uses: Cystitis, sluggish **digestion, flatulence, gout, intestinal parasites, intestinal spasms**, increases **lactation, menopause problems, pre-menopause, urinary stones, vomiting**.

Other Possible Uses: Fennel oil may be used for **colic**, stimulating the **cardiovascular system, constipation, digestion** (supports the LIVER), balancing **hormones, kidney stones, nausea, obesity**, supporting **pancreatic function**, and PMS. It may break up **fluids** and **toxins**, and **cleanse** the **tissues**.

Body System(s) Affected: Digestive and **Hormonal Systems**.

Aromatic Influence: It influences and increases **longevity, courage** and **purification**.

Application: Apply to **Vita Flex Points** and directly on **area** of concern; Diffuse.

Oral Use As Dietary Supplement: Generally regarded as safe (GRAS) for internal consumption by the FDA. *Dilute* one drop oil in 1 tsp. honey or 4 oz. of beverage (i.e. soy/rice milk). *Not for children under 6 years old; use with **caution** and in **greater dilution** for children 6 years old and over.*

Safety Data: *Repeated use can possibly result in **contact sensitization**. Use with caution if susceptible to **epilepsy**. Use with caution during **pregnancy**.*

Blend Classification: Equalizer and Modifier

Blends With: Basil, geranium, lavender, lemon, rosemary, and sandalwood.

Odor: Type: *Top to Middle Notes (20-80% of the blend)*; Scent: *Sweet, somewhat spicy, licorice-like*; Intensity: *4*

FIR (SILVER FIR or FIR NEEDLE)
(Abies alba)

Botanical Family: Pinaceae (conifer)

Extraction Method/Origin: Steam distillation from needles — Balkans

Chemical Constituents: Monoterpenes (75-95%): l-limonene (34%), α-pinene (24%), camphene (21%), santene, δ-3-carene; Esters: bornyle acetate (up to 10%).

Properties: Analgesic, anti-arthritic, anti-catarrhal, antiseptic (pulmonary), **expectorant**, and **stimulant**.

Esoteric Uses/Actions: Astrological: *Jupiter*; Character: *Yang*

Historical Uses: The fir tree is the classic Christmas tree (short with the perfect pyramidal shape and silvery white bark). Though highly regarded for its fragrant scent, the fir tree has been prized through the ages for its medicinal virtues in regards to respiratory complaints, fever, muscular and rheumatic pain.

French Medicinal Uses: **Bronchitis, respiratory congestion, energy.**

Other Possible Uses: Fir creates the symbolic effect of the umbrella protecting the earth and bringing energy in from the universe. At night the animals in the wild lie down under the tree for the protection, recharging, and rejuvenation the trees bring them. It may be beneficial for reducing **aches/pains** from **colds** and the **flu**, fighting **airborne germs/bacteria, arthritis, asthma**, supporting the **blood, bronchial** obstructions, **coughs, fevers, oxygenating** the cells, **rheumatism, sinusitis**, and **urinary tract infections**.

Body System(s) Affected: **Respiratory System**.

Aromatic Influence: It creates a feeling of **grounding, anchoring**, and **empowerment**. It can **stimulate** the **mind** while allowing the body to relax.

Application: Apply to **Vita Flex Points** and/or directly on **area** of concern; Diffuse.

Oral Use As Dietary Supplement: Approved by the FDA for use as a Food Additive (FA) and Flavoring Agent (FL). *Dilute one drop oil in 1 tsp. honey or 4 oz. of beverage (i.e. soy/rice milk). Not for children under 6 years old; use with caution and in greater dilution for children 6 years old and over.*

Safety Data: *Can irritate sensitive skin.*

Blend Classification: Equalizer

Blends With: German chamomile, cedarwood, frankincense, lavender, myrtle, and rosewood.

Odor: Type: *Middle Notes (50-80% of the blend)*; Scent: *Fresh, woody, earthy, sweet*; Intensity: *3*

FIR, BALSAM (CANADIAN BALSAM)
(Abies balsamea)

Botanical Family: Pinaceae (conifer)

Extraction Method/Origin: Steam distillation from branches — Canada, USA

Chemical Constituents: Monoterpenes (up to 90%): α- & β-pinenes (<73%), δ-3-carene (<35%), camphene (<20%), l-limonene (<20%), β-phellandrene, bisabolene, dipentene; Esters (<23%): bornyl acetate (<23%), terpinyl acetate.

Properties: **Antiseptic** (genito-urinary, pulmonary), **astringent, diuretic, expectorant, sedative** (nerves), and **tonic**.

Esoteric Uses/Actions: Astrological: *Jupiter, Saturn*; Character: *Yang*; Element: *Air*

Historical Uses: This fir tree is tall and graceful with a perfect conical shape. Though highly regarded for its fragrant scent, the fir tree has been prized through the ages for its medicinal virtues in regards to respiratory complaints, fever, muscular and rheumatic pain. The oleoresin from the balsam fir tree has been used extensively for ritual purposes and for the external treatment of burns, sores, cuts, heart and chest pains, and for coughs.

Other Possible Uses: This oil may be beneficial for **asthma, bronchitis, burns, catarrh, chronic coughs, cuts, cystitis, depression, hemorrhoids, stress-related**

conditions, **sore throat, tension** (nervous), **urinary infections, wounds**. This oil may help with **anxiety, colds, flu, infections**, and **pain** (reduces). It may help enhance the production of hGH (human Growth Hormone) and reduce the levels of cortisol. It has been found to be very effective for soothing **overworked** or **tired muscles, ligaments, tendons,** and **joints**. It may also help with back pain.

Body System(s) Affected: Emotional Balance, Muscles and Bones, Nervous System, Respiratory System.

Aromatic Influence: It creates a feeling of **grounding, anchoring**, and **empowerment**. It can **stimulate** the **mind** while allowing the **body** to **relax**. It has been described as **appeasing, elevating**, and **opening**. It is also very **emotionally balancing**.

Application: Diffuse; Apply to **Vita Flex Points** and directly on **area** of concern.

Oral Use As Dietary Supplement: Approved by the FDA for use as a Food Additive (FA) and Flavoring Agent (FL). ***Dilute*** *one drop oil in 1 tsp. honey or 4 oz. of beverage (i.e. soy/rice milk). **Not for children under 6 years old; use with caution and in greater dilution for children 6 years old and over.***

Safety Data: *Can irritate sensitive **skin**. Avoid direct **sunlight** for 3 to 6 hours after use.*

Blend Classification: Equalizer

Blends With: German chamomile, cedarwood, cypress, frankincense, juniper, lavender, lemon, myrtle, pine, sandalwood, and rosewood.

Odor: Type: *Middle Note (50-80% of the blend)*; Scent: *Fresh, clean, green, balsamic, coniferous, sweet*; Intensity: *2*

FIR, DOUGLAS
(Pseudotsuga menziesii)

Botanical Family: Pinaceae (conifer)

Extraction Method/Origin: Steam distillation of leaves and twigs — Canada, USA

Chemical Constituents: Monoterpenes (up to 80%): α- & β-pinenes (<65%), l-limonene (<18%), δ-3-carene, camphene, terpinolene; Esters (up to 15%): bornyl acetate (<15%), geranyl acetate (<4%), bornyl & geranyl coproates; Alcohols (up to 10%): borneol (<6%), geraniol (<6%); Aldehydes: benzoicaldehyde, citrals; Ketones: camphor; Oxides: 1,8 cineol.

Properties: Antiseptic, astringent, diuretic, expectorant, sedative (joints, muscles, nerves), and **tonic**.

Historical Uses: Though highly regarded for its fragrant scent, the fir tree has been prized through the ages for its medicinal virtues in regards to respiratory complaints, fever, muscular and rheumatic pain.

Other Possible Uses: This oil may help with **anxiety, asthma, bronchitis, catarrh, colds, coughs, flu, infections, respiratory weakness, rheumatism, tension** (nervous), and **wounds**. It is very soothing for **sore muscles** and has been found to be very effective for calming **overworked** or **tired muscles** and **joints**.

Body System(s) Affected: Respiratory System, Muscles and Bones.

Aromatic Influence: It creates a feeling of **grounding, anchoring,** and **empowerment**. It can **stimulate** the **mind** while allowing the **body** to **relax**.

Application: Diffuse; Apply to **Vita Flex Points** and directly on **area** of concern.

Oral Use As Dietary Supplement: None.

Safety Data: *Can irritate sensitive skin.*

Blend Classification: Equalizer

Blends With: German chamomile, cedarwood, cypress, frankincense, juniper, lavender, lemon, myrtle, pine, sandalwood, and rosewood.

FIR, IDAHO BALSAM
(See FIR, BALSAM)

FIR, WHITE (or GIANT FIR)
(Abies grandis)

Botanical Family: Pinaceae (conifer)

Extraction Method/Origin: Steam distillation of leaves/twigs—Canada, France, USA

Chemical Constituents: Monoterpenes (up to 75%): α- & β-pinenes (<42%), β-phellandrene (<16%), camphene (<15%); Sesquiterpenes: δ-cadinene (<7%); Esters: bornyl acetate (<14%); Alcohols: borneol (<2%).

Properties: Analgesic, antiseptic, astringent, diuretic, expectorant, sedative (joints, muscles, nerves), and **tonic**.

Historical Uses: Though highly regarded for its fragrant scent, the fir tree has been prized through the ages for its medicinal virtues in regards to respiratory complaints, fever, muscular and rheumatic pain.

Other Possible Uses: This oil may help with **anxiety, asthma, bronchitis, catarrh, colds, coughs, flu, infections, respiratory weakness, rheumatism, tension** (nervous), and **wounds**. It has been found to be very effective for calming **overworked** or **tired muscles** and **joints** and for relieving **pain** resulting **from inflammation**.

Body System(s) Affected: Emotional Balance, Muscles and Bones, Respiratory System.

Aromatic Influence: It creates a feeling of **grounding, anchoring**, and **empowerment**. It can **stimulate** the **mind** while allowing the **body** to **relax**.

Application: Diffuse; Apply to **Vita Flex Points** and/or directly on **area** of concern.

Oral Use As Dietary Supplement: None.

Safety Data: *Can irritate sensitive skin.*

Blend Classification: Equalizer

Blends With: German chamomile, cedarwood, cypress, frankincense, juniper, lavender, lemon, myrtle, pine, sandalwood, and rosewood.

FLEABANE
(Conyza canadensis)

Botanical Family: Compositae (daisy)
Extraction Method/Origin: Steam distillation from stems, leaves, and flowers — Canada
Chemical Constituents: Monoterpenes (up to 83%): l-limonene (up to 75%), β-ocimene (<7%), β-pinene, myrcene; Furanocoumarins: α-bergamotene (<11%); Esters: methyl esters (<6%), methyl acetate; Alcohols: α-terpineol (<6%); Sesquiterpene Alcohols: nerolidol (<4%); Lactones; lachnophyllum lactone (<2%); Sesquiterpenes: β-farnesene.
Properties: Anti-rheumatic, antispasmodic, cardiovascular dilator, hormone-like.
French Medicinal Uses: Used by Daniel Pénoël, M.D. to treat children with **retarded puberty.**
Other Possible Uses: May help stimulate the **liver** and **pancreas**. It is a **mood enhancer** and promoter of hGH.
Body System(s) Affected: Cardiovascular and **Hormonal Systems**.
Application: Apply to **Vita Flex Points** and directly on **area** of concern; Diffuse.
Oral Use As Dietary Supplement: None.
Safety Data: *This oil is still under study. Best to dilute with V-6 Mixing Oil.*

FRANKINCENSE (OLIBANUM)
(Boswellia carterii or B. frereana)

Botanical Family: Burseraceae (resinous trees and shrubs)
Extraction Method/Origin: Steam distillation from gum/resin — Somalia
Chemical Constituents: Monoterpenes (up to 90%): α- & β-pinenes (43%), α-thujene (<22%), l-limonene (<16%), myrcene (<12%), sabinene (<7%), p-cymene (<5%), α-terpinene, camphene, α-phellandrene; Sesquiterpenes (<10%): β-caryophyllene (<8%), α-gurjunene, α-guaiene; Alcohols (<5%): incensol, borneol, olibanol, trans-pinocarveol, farnesol.
Properties: Anti-catarrhal, anti-depressant, anti-infectious, antiseptic, antitumoral, expectorant, immune-stimulant, and **sedative**.
Folklore: One of the gifts given to Christ at His birth. There are over 52 references to frankincense in the Bible (considering that "incense" is translated from the Hebrew/Greek "frankincense" and either refers to the same oil or to a mixture, of which frankincense was one of the ingredients).
Esoteric Uses/Actions: Astrological: *Sun & Saturn*; Body type: *Ectomorph*; Chakras: *Links 1 to 7, also 4, 5, & 6*; Character: *Yang-Hot 2nd degree*; Crystals: *Tiger's eye (links 1st to 7th chakra), Amber, Topaz*; Element: *Air, Ether, Light, & Fire*; Number: *3*
Historical Uses: Frankincense is a **holy oil** in the Middle East. As an ingredient in the holy incense, it was used anciently during sacrificial ceremonies to help improve communication with the **creator**.
French Medicinal Uses: Asthma, depression, ulcers.

Other Possible Uses: This oil may help with **aging, allergies, bites** (insect and snake), **bronchitis, cancer, carbuncles, catarrh, colds, coughs, diarrhea, diphtheria, gonorrhea, headaches, healing, hemorrhaging, herpes, high blood pressure, inflammation, jaundice, laryngitis, meningitis, nervous** conditions, **prostate** problems, **pneumonia, respiratory problems**, preventing **scarring, sciatic pain, sores, spiritual awareness, staph, strep, stress, syphilis, T.B., tension, tonsillitis, typhoid, wounds**, and **warts**. It contains sesquiterpenes, enabling it to go beyond the blood-brain barrier. It may also help **oxygenate** the **pineal** and **pituitary glands**. It increases the activity of **leukocytes** in defense of the body against infection. Frankincense may also help one have a better attitude, which may help to strengthen the **immune system**.

Body System(s) Affected: Emotional Balance, Immune and **Nervous Systems, Skin**.

Aromatic Influence: It increases **spiritual awareness** and **meditation**.

Application: Apply to **Vita Flex Points** and/or directly on **area** of concern; **Diffuse**.

Oral Use As Dietary Supplement: Approved by the FDA for use as a Food Additive (FA) and Flavoring Agent (FL). **Dilute** *one drop oil in 1 tsp. honey or 4 oz. of beverage (i.e. soy/rice milk).* ***Not for children under 6 years old; use with caution and in greater dilution for children 6 years old and over.***

Blend Classification: Enhancer and Equalizer

Blends With: All oils.

Odor: Type: *Base Note (5-20% of the blend)*; Scent: *Rich, deep, warm, balsamic, sweet, with incense-like overtones*; Intensity: *3*

Frequency: High (Spiritual)

Bible: Exod. 30:34, Lev. 2:1, 2, 15, 16; 5:11; 6:15; 24:7, Num. 5:15, Matt 2:11, Rev. 18:13

GALBANUM
(Ferula gummosa or F. galbaniflua)

Botanical Family: Umbelliferae (parsley)

Extraction Method/Origin: Steam distillation from resin derived from stems and branches — Iran, Turkey, Afghanistan, Lebanon

Chemical Constituents: Monoterpernes (up to 95%): α- & β-pinenes (<90%), δ-3-carene (<16%), myrcene, sabinene, camphene, tricyclene, limonene, terpinolene, β-phellandrene; Sesquiterpene Alcohols: α-, β-, & γ-eudesmols (=galbanol), guaiol, bulnesol, 10-γ-epijunenol, α-cadinol; Esters: fenchyl acetate, linalyl acetate, terpenyl acetate; Coumarins.

Properties: Analgesic, anti-infectious, anti-inflammatory, antimicrobial, antiseptic, antispasmodic, anti-viral, diuretic, expectorant, restorative, and **tonic**.

Esoteric Uses/Actions: Astrological: *Saturn & Venus*; Character: *Drying, preserving*; Color: *Green*; Odor: *Warm, earthy, green*

Historical Uses: Galbanum was used anciently as an incense and for embalming. It was also combined with frankincense as a holy incense (Exodus 30:34-38) and was only used in the tabernacle during sacrifices. It has also been used for treating wounds, inflammation, and skin disorders.

Other Possible Uses: Galbanum is similar to hyssop, oregano, and frankincense and is recognized for its **anti-viral**, body **strengthening** and **supporting** properties. It may also help with **abscesses, acne, asthma, boils, bronchitis, catarrh, chronic coughs, cramps, cuts, flatulence, indigestion, inflammation, muscular aches** and **pains, nervous tension**, the **pineal gland, poor circulation, rheumatism, scar tissue, skin** (tones), **stress related complaints, swollen glands, wrinkles**, and **wounds**. Some very interesting research is being done with galbanum. It has a low frequency, but when combined with other oils, such as frankincense or sandalwood, the frequency changes drastically. This oil is more than just a medicinal oil.

Body System(s) Affected: Immune System.

Aromatic Influence: It may help increase **spiritual awareness** and **meditation** and may have a **harmonizing** and **balancing** effect on the psyche.

Application: Apply to **Vita Flex Points** and directly on **area** of concern; **Diffuse**.

Oral Use As Dietary Supplement: Approved by the FDA for use as a Food Additive (FA) and Flavoring Agent (FL). ***Dilute*** *one drop oil in 1 tsp. honey or 4 oz. of beverage (i.e. soy/rice milk).* ***Not for children under 6 years old; use with*** **caution** ***and in*** **greater dilution** ***for children 6 years old and over.***

Blend Classification: Enhancer and Equalizer

Blends With: All oils.

Odor: Type: *Top Note (5-20% of the blend)*; Scent: *Warm, earthy, green, woody, spicy*; Intensity: *5*

Frequency: Low (Physical); approximately 56.

Bible: Exodus 30:34

GERANIUM
(Pelargonium graveolens)

Botanical Family: Geraniaceae

Extraction Method/Origin: Steam distillation from leaves — Egypt, India

Chemical Constituents: Alcohols (up to 70%): citronellol (>32%), geraniol (<23%), linalol (<14%), nerol, γ-eudesmol, α-terpineol, menthol; Esters (up to 30%): citronellyl formate (14%), geranyl formate & acetate (<12%), other propionates, butyrates, & tiglates; Ketones: isomenthone (<8%), menthone, piperitone; Sesquiterpenes: 4-guaiadiene-6,9, αcopaene, δ- & γ-cadinenes, δ-guaiazulene, β-farnesene; Aldehydes: geranial (<6%), neral, citronellal; Monoterpenes (<5%): α- & β-pinenes, l-limonene, myrcene, ocimene; Sesquiterpene Alcohols: farnesol (<3%).

Properties: Anti-depressant, antiseptic, astringent, diuretic, insect repellent, refreshing, relaxing, sedative, and **tonic**.

Folklore: During the 1600's, European gardeners would plant geraniums around their houses to keep the evil spirits out. However, this oil is not produced from the same geranium as the house plants.

Esoteric Uses/Actions: Astrological: *Venus*; Body type: *Endomorph*; Chakra: *2 & 5*; Character: *Yin*; Crystal: *Red Tourmaline*; Element: *Water & Ether*; Number: *4*; Oriental: *Yin deficiencies (pts: Kid-6, Sp-6)*

Historical Uses: Geranium oil has been used for dysentery, hemorrhoids, inflammations, heavy menstrual flow, and possibly even cancer (if the folk tale is correct). It has also been said to be a remedy for bone fractures, tumors, and wounds.

French Medicinal Uses: Diabetes, diarrhea, gallbladder, gastric ulcer, jaundice, liver, sterility, urinary stones.

Other Possible Uses: This oil may be used for **acne, bleeding** (increases to eliminate toxins, then stops), **burns, circulatory problems** (improves blood flow), **depression, digestion, eczema, hormonal imbalance, insomnia, kidney stones**, dilating biliary ducts for **liver detoxification, menstrual problems, neuralgia** (severe pain along the nerve), regenerating **tissue** and **nerves, pancreas** (balances), **ringworm, shingles, skin** (may balance the sebum which is the fatty secretion in the sebaceous glands of the skin that keep the skin supple. Good for expectant mothers, oily skin - as a cleanser, and may even liven up pale skin), **sores, sore throats**, and **wounds**. Geranium opens the **liver chakra** and discharges toxins from the liver that prevent us from having balance.

Body System(s) Affected: Emotional Balance, Skin.

Aromatic Influence: It may help to release **negative memories** and take us back to **peaceful, joyful moments**. It may also help **ease nervous tension** and **stress, balance** the **emotions, lift** the **spirit**, and foster **peace, well being**, and **hope**.

Application: Apply to **Vita Flex Points** and directly on **area** of concern; **Diffuse**.

Oral Use As Dietary Supplement: Generally regarded as safe (GRAS) for internal consumption by the FDA. **Dilute** *one drop oil in 1 tsp. honey or 4 oz. of beverage (i.e. soy/rice milk).* **Not** *for children under 6 years old; use with* **caution** *and in* **greater dilution** *for children 6 years old and over.*

Safety Data: *Repeated use can possibly result in some* **contact sensitization**.

Blend Classification: Enhancer and Equalizer

Blends With: All oils.

Odor: Type: *Middle Note (50-80% of the blend)*; Scent: *Sweet, green, citrus-rosy, fresh*; Intensity: *3*

GERMAN CHAMOMILE
(See CHAMOMILE, GERMAN)

GINGER
(Zingiber officinale)

Botanical Family: Zingiberaceae (ginger)

Extraction Method/Origin: Steam distillation from rhizomes — China, West Indies, and many others.

Chemical Constituents: Sesquiterpenes (up to 90%): zingiberene (up to 50%), α- & β-curcumene (<33%), β-farnesene (<20%), β-sesquiphellandrene (<9%), β- & γ-bisabolene (<7%), β-ylangene, β-elemene, α-selinene, germacrene-D; Monoterpenes: camphene (8%), β-phellandrene, l-limonene, p-cymene, α and β-pinenes, myrcene; Alcohols: nonanol (<8%), citronellol (<6%), linalol (<5%), borneol, butanol, heptanol; Sesquiterpene Alcohols: nerolidol (<9%), zingeberol, elemol; Ketones (<6%): heptanone, acetone, 2 hexanone; Aldehydes: butanal, citronellal, geranial; Sesquiterpene Ketones: gingerone.

Properties: **Antiseptic, laxative, stimulant, tonic**, and **warming**.

Esoteric Uses/Actions: Astrological: *Mars*; Body type: *Endomorph*; Chakra: *3 or 1, balances all*; Character: *Yang*; Crystal: *Rhodochrosite*; Element: *Fire*; Number: *8*; Oriental: *Yang deficiencies (pts: St-3, Dir Ves-6)*

Historical Uses: Anciently esteemed as a spice and recognized for its affinity for the digestive system, it has been used in gingerbread (up to 4,000 years ago in Greece), in Egyptian cuisine to ward off epidemics, in Roman wine (for its aphrodisiac powers), in Indian tea (to soothe upset stomachs), and in Chinese tonics (to strengthen the heart and relieve head congestion). It has also been used in Hawaii to scent the clothing, cook with and cure indigestion. They also added it to their shampoos and massage oils.

French Medicinal Uses: **Angina**, prevention of **contagious diseases, cooking, diarrhea, flatulence, impotence, rheumatic pain, scurvy**, and **tonsillitis**.

Other Possible Uses: Ginger may be used for **alcoholism**, loss of **appetite, arthritis, broken bones, catarrh** (mucus), **chills, colds, colic, congestion, coughs, cramps, digestive** disorders, **fevers, flu, impotence, indigestion, infectious diseases, memory, motion sickness, muscular aches/pains, nausea, rheumatism, sinusitis, sore throats**, and **sprains**. Also in **cooking**.

Body System(s) Affected: **Digestive** and **Nervous Systems**.

Aromatic Influence: The aroma may help influence physical energy, sex, love, money, and courage.

Application: Apply to **Vita Flex Points** and directly on **area** of concern; **Diffuse**.

Oral Use As Dietary Supplement: Generally regarded as safe (GRAS) for internal consumption by the FDA. **Dilute** *one drop oil in 1 tsp. honey or 4 oz. of beverage (i.e. soy/rice milk).* **Not** *for children under 6 years old; use with* **caution** *and in* **greater dilution** *for children 6 years old and over.*

Safety Data: *Repeated use can possibly result in* **contact sensitization.** *Avoid direct* **sunlight** *for 3 to 6 hours after use.*

Blend Classification: Personifier and Equalizer

Blends With: All spice oils, all citrus oils, eucalyptus, frankincense, geranium, myrtle, rosemary, and spearmint.

Odor: Type: *Middle Note (50-80% of the blend)*; Scent: *Sweet, spicy-woody, warm, tenacious, fresh, sharp*; Intensity: *4*

GOLDENROD
(Solidago canadensis)

Botanical Family: Asteraceae or Compositae (daisy)
Extraction Method/Origin: Steam distillation from stems, leaves, and flowers — Eastern Canada
Chemical Constituents: Monoterpenes (up to 55%): α-pinene (<18%), myrcene (<15%), l-limonene (<12%), sabinene (<11%), α-phellandrene (<2%); Sesquiterpenes (up to 35%): germacrene-D (<35%), isolongifolene; Alcohols: borneol; Esters: bornyl acetate, bornyl benzoate.
Properties: **Relaxing** and **calming**.
Esoteric Uses/Actions: Astrological: *Venus*; Element: *Air*
Traditional Uses: **Diphtheria, dyspepsia, hypertension, influenza, nervousness, respiratory mucus, tonsillitis** and **pharyngitis** (these uses have not been substantiated by modern clinical research).
Other Possible Uses: According to Franchomme (1990) and as mentioned in the Swiss Pharmacopia, *faltrank*, goldenrod supports the **circulatory system** including **cardiovascular problems** (like tachycardia and arrhythmia), **urinary tract**, and **liver function**. According to the University of Montreal in Canada, goldenrod shows great potential for help with **impotence**.
Body System(s) Affected: **Cardiovascular System, Hormonal System.**
Application: Apply to **Vita Flex Points** and/or directly on **area** of concern; **Diffuse**. According to literature from Young Living Essential Oils, may also be used as a dietary supplement by diluting one drop in 4 oz. of liquid (i.e. soy/rice milk or honey).
Oral Use As Dietary Supplement: None. *Although Young Living Essential Oils recommends the use of this oil as a dietary supplement, the FDA has **not yet** approved it for use as a food additive (FA) or flavoring agent (FL) (as of 07/01/2004 - see 21CFR172.510 and 21CFR182.20).*

GRAPEFRUIT
(Citrus x paradisi)

Botanical Family: Rutaceae (hybrid between *Citrus maxima* and *Citrus sinensis*)
Extraction Method/Origin: Cold pressed from rind — California
Chemical Constituents: Monoterpenes (up to 95%): d-limonene (<92%), myrcene, α-pinene, sabinene, β-phellandrene; Tetraterpenes: β-carotene, lycopene; Aldehydes (>2%): nonanal, decanal, citral, citronellal; Furanocoumarins: aesculetine, auraptene, bergaptole; Sesquiterpene Ketones (<2%): nootketone (used to determine harvest time); Alcohols: octanol.
Properties: **Anti-depressant, antiseptic, disinfectant, diuretic, stimulant,** and **tonic**.
Esoteric Uses/Actions: Astrological: *Sun*; Body type: *Ectomorph*; Chakra: *1*; Character: *Yang*; Number: *5*; Oriental: *Hot dampness (pts: Sp-9 & 6)*

French Medicinal Uses: Cellulite, digestion, dyspepsia, lymphatic decongestant, water retention.

Other Possible Uses: Grapefruit oil may help with **depression, drug withdrawal, eating** disorders, **fatigue, gallstones, jet lag, liver** disorders, **migraine headaches, obesity, pre-menstrual tension**, and **stress**. It may also have a cleansing effect on the **kidneys**, the **lymphatic system**, and the **vascular system**.

Body System(s) Affected: Cardiovascular System.

Aromatic Influence: It may help prevent one from drowning in their own negativity. It is **balancing** and **uplifting** to the mind, and may help to **relieve anxiety**.

Application: Apply to **Vita Flex Points** and/or directly on **area** of concern; **Diffuse**. Because grapefruit oil has many of the same uses as other citrus oils, it can be used in their place when immediate exposure to the sun is unavoidable. This is because grapefruit oil does not have the photosensitivity that the other citrus oils have.

Oral Use As Dietary Supplement: Generally regarded as safe (GRAS) for internal consumption by the FDA. ***Dilute*** one drop oil in 1 tsp. honey or 4 oz. of beverage (i.e. soy/rice milk). ***Not for children under 6 years old; use with caution and in greater dilution for children 6 years old and over.***

Blend Classification: Modifier and Enhancer.

Blends With: Basil, bergamot, cedarwood, chamomile, cypress, frankincense, geranium, juniper, lavender, peppermint, rosemary, rosewood, and ylang ylang.

Odor: Type: *Top Note (5-20% of the blend)*; Scent: *Clean, fresh, bitter, citrusy*; Intensity: *2*

HELICHRYSUM
(Helichrysum angustifolia var. italicum)

Botanical Family: Compositae

Extraction Method/Origin: Steam distilled from flowers — Yugoslavia, France, Italy *(Note: Since the supply of pure, therapeutic grade helichrysum can be somewhat erratic at times, similar therapeutic results have been achieved by using a blend of 3 oils as follows: 5 drops elemi, 5 drops Idaho tansy, 1 drop birch or wintergreen)*

Chemical Constituents: Esters (up to 60%): neryl acetate (up to 50%), neryl propionate & butyrate (<10%); Ketones: italidione (<20%), β-diketone; Sesquiterpenes: γ-curcumene (<15%), β-caryophyllene (<5%); Monoterpenes: l-limonene (<13%), α-pinene; Alcohols: nerol (<5%), linalol (<4%), geraniol; Oxides: 1,8 cineol; Phenols: eugenol.

Properties: Anti-catarrhal, anti-coagulant, antioxidant, antispasmodic, expectorant, and **mucolytic**.

Folklore: Helichrysum, as an ornamental dried flower, retains its fragrance, color, and shape almost forever. Hence the other names, "Everlasting" or "Immortelle", by which it is commonly known.

Esoteric Uses/Actions: Astrological: *Jupiter*; Chakra: *6*; Character: *Yin*

Historical Uses: Helichrysum has been used for asthma, bronchitis, whooping cough, headaches, liver ailments, and skin disorders.

French Medicinal Uses: Blood cleansing, chelating agent for **metallics, chemicals**, and **toxins**, viral **colitis, detoxification, gallbladder infection, hematoma, hypocholesterol, liver cell function stimulant, lymph drainage**, reduces **pain, pancreas stimulant, phlebitis, sciatica, sinus infection, skin conditions** (eczema, dermatitis, psoriasis), **stomach cramps, sun screen**.

Other Possible Uses: This oil may help **anger**, stop **bleeding, circulatory** functions, **gallbladder infection**, improve **hearing, hematoma** (swelling or tumor full of diffused blood), detoxify and stimulate the **liver** cell function, **lymph drainage, pain** (acute), relieve **respiratory** conditions, reduce **scarring, scar tissue**, reduce **tissue pain**, regenerate **tissue**, and **varicose veins**.

Body System(s) Affected: Cardiovascular System, Muscles and Bones.

Aromatic Influence: It is **uplifting** to the subconscious and may possess the ability to cut through **barriers** of anger, allowing one to forgive trespasses against them and move forward in life.

Application: Apply to **Vita Flex Points** and directly on **area** of concern; **Diffuse**.

Oral Use As Dietary Supplement: Generally regarded as safe (GRAS) for internal consumption by the FDA. *Dilute* one drop oil in 1 tsp. honey or 4 oz. of beverage (i.e. soy/rice milk). *Not for children under 6 years old; use with* **caution** *and in* **greater dilution** *for children 6 years old and over.*

Blend Classification: Personifier

Blends With: Geranium, Clary sage, rose, lavender, spice oils and citrus oils.

Odor: Type: *Middle Note (50-80% of the blend)*; Scent: *Rich, sweet, fruity, with tea and honey undertones*; Intensity: *3*

Frequency: High (Spiritual); approximately 181 MHz.

HYSSOP
(Hyssopus officinalis)

Botanical Family: Labiatae (mint)

Extraction Method/Origin: Steam distilled from stems/leaves — France, Hungary

Chemical Constituents: Ketones (>58%): isopinocamphone (>40%), pinocamphone (>12%), α and β-thujones, camphor; Monoterpenes (>25%); α- & β-pinenes (15-22%), l-limonene, ocimene, sabinene camphene, myrcene, p-cymene; Sesquiterpenes (<7%): germacrene-D, β-caryophyllene, aromadendrene, phellandrene; Phenols (4%): myrtenal methyl-ether, myrtenol, eugenol (methyl chavicol); Alcohols: borneol, linalol, nerolidol, geraniol; Esters: methyl myrtenate, bornyl acetate; Oxides: linalol oxide, 1,8 cineol.

Properties: Anti-asthmatic, anti-catarrhal, anti-infectious, anti-inflammatory, antioxidant, anti-parasitic, antiseptic, antispasmodic, anti-viral, astringent, decongestant, diuretic, mucolytic, and **sedative**.

Esoteric Uses/Actions: Astrological: *Jupiter*; Chakra: *4, 3*; Character: *Yang*; Crystals: *Lapis lazuli, Amethyst*; Element: *Fire*

Historical Uses: Hyssop is mentioned in Exodus Chapter 12 as the oil in lamb's blood. It was used to prevent the Plague, which may be similar to AIDS today.

Other Possible Uses: This oil may be beneficial for **anxiety**, restoring **appetite, arthritis, asthma, bruises, cleansing** and purifying, **colds, concentration** (alertness stimulating and clearing the mind), **coughs, cuts, dermatitis, digestion, fatigue** (strengthens and enlivens the body), **fever**, expelling **gas** from intestines, **gout, grief**, regulating **lipid metabolism**, raising **low blood pressure**, clearing **lungs**, promoting and regulating **menstrual flow**, discharging **mucus, nervous tension, parasites** (expelling worms), increasing **perspiration, rheumatism**, preventing **scarring, scar tissue, sore throats, stress** related conditions, **tonsillitis**, discharging **toxins, viral infections**, and **wounds**.

Body System(s) Affected: Cardiovascular, Nervous, and **Respiratory Systems**.

Aromatic Influence: It may help stimulate **creativity** and **meditation** and promote **centering**.

Application: Apply to **Vita Flex Points** and directly on **area** of concern; *Diffuse*.

Oral Use As Dietary Supplement: Generally regarded as safe (GRAS) for internal consumption by the FDA. *Dilute* one drop oil in 1 tsp. honey or 4 oz. of beverage (i.e. soy/rice milk). *However, due to high ketone content, extreme caution should be taken. Best avoided by children of any age.*

Safety Data: *According to some sources, the pinocamphone can cause toxic effects. Avoid during pregnancy. Avoid if dealing with high blood pressure. Not for use by people with epilepsy. Use extreme caution and dilute well when unsure!*

Blend Classification: Enhancer, Equalizer, and Modifier

Odor: Type: *Middle Note (50-80% of the blend)*; Scent: *Fresh, earthy, woody, fruity, slightly sweet*; Intensity: *3*

Bible: According to the Bible, hyssop *purges* and *cleanses*. See the following: Exodus 12:22; Lev. 14:4, 6, 49,51,52; Num. 19:6,18; 1 Kings 4:33; Psalms 51:7

IDAHO BALSAM FIR
(See FIR, BALSAM)

IDAHO TANSY
(See TANSY, IDAHO)

JASMINE
(Jasminum officinale)

Botanical Family: Oleaceae (olive)

Extraction Method/Origin: Absolute extraction from flowers (jasmine is actually an "essence" not an essential oil. The flowers must be picked at night to maximize the fragrance) — India

Chemical Constituents: Esters (up to 50%): benzyl acetate (<28%), benzyl benzoate (<21%), methyl anthranilate, methyl jasmonate; Diterpene Alcohols: phytol (<12%), isophytol (<7%); Alcohols: linalol (<8%), benzyl alcohol, farnesol; Triterpenes: squalene (<7%); Pyrroles: indole, scatole; Ketone: cis-jasmone.

Properties: Anti-catarrhal, anti-depressant, and **antispasmodic**.

Esoteric Uses/Actions: Astrological: *Moon & Jupiter*; Ayurvedic: *Pitta*; Body type: *Mesomorph*; Chakra: *2*; Character: *Yang (flowers-Yin, oil-Yang, Yin when diluted)*; Crystals: *Ruby, Red Jasper, Quartz, Moonstone, Sapphire*; Element: *Water & Fire*; Number: *9*; Oriental: *Cold & Dry*

Historical Uses: Known in India as the "queen of the night" and "moonlight of the grove", women have treasured it for centuries for its beautiful, aphrodisiac-like fragrance. According to Roberta Wilson, "In many religious traditions, the jasmine flower symbolizes hope, happiness, and love." Jasmine has been used for hepatitis, cirrhosis of the liver, dysentery, depression, nervousness, coughs, respiratory congestion, reproductive problems, and "to stimulate uterine contractions in pregnant women as childbirth approached." It was also used in teas, perfumes, and incense.

Other Possible Uses: This oil may help with **catarrh** (mucus), **conjunctivitis, coughs, dysentery, eczema** (when caused by emotions), **frigidity, hepatitis** (cirrhosis of the liver), **hoarseness, labor pains, laryngitis, lethargy** (abnormal drowsiness), **menstrual pain** and **problems, muscle spasms, nervous exhaustion** and **tension, pain relief, respiratory** conditions, **sex, skin care** (dry, greasy, irritated, and sensitive), **sprains**, and **uterine** disorders. Jasmine is an oil that affects the **emotions**; it penetrates the deepest layers of the soul, opening doors to our emotions. It produces a feeling of **confidence, energy, euphoria**, and **optimism**. It helps to reduce **anxiety, apathy, depression, dilemmas** that deal with **relationships, indifference**, and **listlessness**. As cologne, it increases feelings of **attractiveness**.

Body System(s) Affected: Emotional Balance, Hormonal System.

Aromatic Influence: It is very **uplifting** to the **emotions** and may help increase **intuitive** powers and **wisdom**. It may also help to promote powerful, inspirational **relationships**.

Application: Apply to **Vita Flex Points** and directly on **area** of concern; **Diffuse**.

Oral Use As Dietary Supplement: Generally regarded as safe (GRAS) for internal consumption by the FDA. **Dilute** *one drop oil in 1 tsp. honey or 4 oz. of beverage (i.e. soy/rice milk).* ***Not for children under 6 years old; use with caution and in greater dilution for children 6 years old and over.***

Blend Classification: Equalizer, Modifier, and Enhancer

Blends With: Bergamot, frankincense, geranium, helichrysum, lemongrass, mandarin, melissa, orange, palmarosa, rose, rosewood, sandalwood, spearmint.

Odor: Type: *Base Note (5-20% of the blend)*; Scent: *Powerful, sweet, tenacious, floral with fruity-herbaceous undertones*; Intensity: *4*

Note: *One pound of jasmine oil requires about 1,000 pounds of jasmine or 3.6 million fresh picked blossoms. The blossoms must be collected before sunrise, or much of the fragrance will have evaporated. The quality of the blossoms can also be compromised if they are squashed. A* *single 1 lb. can of pure jasmine oil can cost from $1,200 to $4,500. In contrast, synthetic jasmine oils can be obtained for $3.50 per pound, but they obviously do not possess the same therapeutic qualities as pure jasmine oil. The above mentioned properties and possible uses are based on pure jasmine oil, not synthetic oil.*

JUNIPER (or ROCKY MOUNTAIN JUNIPER)
(Juniperus osteosperma and/or J. scopulorum)

Botanical Family: Cupressaceae (conifer - cypress)

Extraction Method/Origin: Steam distilled from berries and twigs — Utah

Chemical Constituents: Monoterpenes (>50%): α-pinene (up to 40%), sabinene (<18%), myrcene (<8%), l-limonene (<6%); Esters: bornyl acetate (up to 20%); Ketones (up to 19%): camphor (<18%), junionone, pinocamphone; Sesquiterpenes: muurolene (<3%).

Properties: Antiseptic, antispasmodic, astringent, cleanser, detoxifier, diuretic, stimulant, and **tonic**.

Folklore: According to Roberta Wilson, "During biblical times, juniper was often used to banish evil spirits." Also, during Medieval times, "Bundles of juniper berries were hung over doors to ward off witches, and burning juniper wood supposedly deterred demons."

Esoteric Uses/Actions: Astrological: *Sun & Jupiter*; Ayurvedic: *Kapha*; Chakra: *3 & 6*; Character: *Yin*; Crystal: *Red Jasper*; Element: *Fire*

Historical Uses: Over the centuries, juniper has been used for embalming, for physical and spiritual purification, to cleanse infections and heal wounds, for liver complaints, to relieve arthritis and urinary tract infections, to ward off plagues, epidemics, and contagious diseases, for headaches, kidney and bladder problems, pulmonary infections, and fevers.

French Medicinal Uses: Acne, dermatitis, eczema.

Other Possible Uses: This oil may work as a **detoxifier** and a **cleanser** which may reduce **acne, dermatitis**, and **eczema**. It may also help **coughs, depression, energy, infection**, increase circulation through **kidneys, kidney stones, liver problems**, aching **muscles, nerve function** and **regeneration, obesity, rheumatism** (promotes excretion of uric acid and toxins), **ulcers, urinary infections, water retention**, and **wounds**.

Body System(s) Affected: Digestive System, Emotional Balance (aromatic), **Nervous System, Skin**.

Aromatic Influence: Juniper evokes feelings of **health, love**, and **peace** and may help to **elevate** one's **spiritual awareness**.

Application: Apply to **Vita Flex Points** and/or directly on **area** of concern; **Diffuse**. Juniper may also be applied to the **forehead** to enhance feelings of **optimism**, or on the **cheeks** for **confidence** and **euphoria**.

Oral Use As Dietary Supplement: *As of Oct. 30, 2006, the FDA has NOT given this variety of juniper the designation of GRAS (Generally Regarded As Safe for internal consumption) (see 21CFR182.20).* ***Not recommended for internal consumption.***

Blend Classification: Equalizer

Blends With: Bergamot, all citrus oils, cypress, geranium, lavender, melaleuca (tea-tree), <u>Melrose</u>, and rosemary.

Odor: Type: *Middle Note (50-80% of the blend)*; Scent: *Sweet, musky, tenacious*; Intensity: *3*

Frequency: Emotional; approximately 98 MHz.

Bible: Job 30:4

LAUREL (BAY or SWEET BAY)
(Laurus nobilis)

Botanical Family: Lauraceae

Extraction Method/Origin: Steam distilled from leaves — France

Chemical Constituents: Oxides: 1,8 cineol (up to 50%); Alcohols: linalol (>15%), α-terpineol (<10%), borneol, geraniol, cis-thujanol-4; Monoterpenes (up to 28%): α and β-pinenes (<18%), sabinene (>10%), limonene; Esters: α-terpinyl acetate (up to 10%), bornyl, geranyl & linalyl acetates (<10%); Phenols: eugenol (<9%), terpinen-4-ol (<3%); Lactones: costunolide (<2%), artemorine, laurensolide; Sesquiterpenes: β-caryophyllene, humulene, β-elemene, phellandrene.

Properties: Antiseptic, digestive, diuretic, anti-fungal.

Folklore: Ancient Greek and Roman generals would wear crowns of laurel leaves when victorious in battle. Both the Greeks and the Romans believed that the laurel tree had great powers of divination and prophecy, and that all one had to do to avoid thunder and lightning or evil spirits was to run under a laurel tree.

Esoteric Uses/Actions: Astrological: *Sun*; Body type: *Ectomorph*; Chakras: *2, 3, & 4*; Character: *Yin (medium)*; Element: *Fire*; Number: *1*

Historical Uses: Both the leaves and the black berries were also used to alleviate colic, indigestion, and loss of appetite. During the Middle Ages, it was used for angina pectoris, asthma, fever, gout, migraine, palpitations, and liver and spleen complaints. Laurel has also been used as a fragrance component in cosmetics and perfumes.

Other Possible Uses: Laurel oil is primarily produced in the country formerly known as Yugoslavia. Laurel may help with loss of **appetite, asthmatic conditions, chronic bronchitis, dyspepsia, flatulence, flu, hair loss** (after an infection), **pediculosis, scabies, viral infections**.

Body System(s) Affected: Digestive, Immune, and **Respiratory Systems**.

Application: Apply to **Vita Flex Points** and/or directly on **area** of concern.

Oral Use As Dietary Supplement: Generally regarded as safe (GRAS) for internal consumption by the FDA. ***Dilute*** *one drop oil in 1 tsp. honey or 4 oz. of beverage (i.e. soy/rice milk).* ***Not for children under 6 years old; use with*** *caution* ***and in*** *greater dilution for children 6 years old and over.*

Safety Data: *Repeated use can possibly result in* **contact sensitization**. *Moderate use is recommended. Avoid during* **pregnancy**.

Odor: Type: *Top to Middle Notes (20-80% of the blend)*; Scent: *Sweet, fresh, spicy, camphorous, medicinal*; Intensity: *3*

LAVANDIN
(Lavandula x hybrida)

Botanical Family: Labiatae

Chemical Constituents: Alcohols (up to 60%): linalol (> 40%), α-terpineol (<5%), borneol, geraniol, lavendulol, nerol; Esters (<55%): linalyl acetate (<50%), lavandulyl acetate, geranyl acetate, bornyl acetate, neryl acetate; Monoterpenes (up to 24%): β-ocimene (<16%), d-limonene (<7%), myrcene, camphene; Ketones: camphor (>5%); Oxides: 1,8 cineol (<10%), caryophyllene oxide, linalol oxide; Phenols: terpinen-4-ol (<6%); Coumarins.

Properties: **Anti-bacterial, anti-fungal**, and strong **antiseptic**. (See LAVENDER for additional properties.)

Esoteric Uses/Actions: Astrological: *Mercury*; Body type: *Endomorph*; Chakra: *4*; Character: *Almost neutral (leans Yang)*; Crystals: *Flourite, Amethyst*; Element: *Air*; Number: *7*

Historical Uses: Also known as *Lavandula x intermedia*, lavandin is a hybrid plant developed by crossing true lavender with spike lavender or aspic (*Lavandula Latifolia*). It has been used to sterilize the animal cages in veterinary clinics and hospitals throughout Europe. There is not a long history of the therapeutic use of lavandin as it was most often used to adulterate true lavender oils.

Other Possible Uses: Lavandin can be used in the same way as true lavender (see LAVENDER) *except NOT for burns*. It is more penetrating and has a much sharper scent than lavender. Some have even had success with using it to help reduce the itching and swelling associated with **insect bites** and **stings**.

Body System(s) Affected: Cardiovascular System, Muscles and Bones, Respiratory System.

Aromatic Influence: It has the same calming effects as lavender.

Application: Apply to **Vita Flex Points** and/or directly on **area** of concern; Diffuse.

Oral Use As Dietary Supplement: Generally regarded as safe (GRAS) for internal consumption by the FDA. *Dilute one drop oil in 1 tsp. honey or 4 oz. of beverage (i.e. soy/rice milk).* *Not for children under 6 years old; use with caution and in greater dilution for children 6 years old and over.*

Safety Data: *Use with caution if susceptible to* **epilepsy**. *Avoid during* **pregnancy**. *Do not use for burns!*

Blends With: Bergamot, cinnamon bark, citronella, clove, cypress, Clary sage, geranium, lime, patchouli, pine, rosemary, and thyme.

Odor: Type: *Top to Middle Notes (20-80% of the blend)*; Scent: *Fresh, sweet, floral, more herbaceous than Lavender*; Intensity: *3*

LAVENDER
(Lavandula angustifolia)

Botanical Family: Labiatae (mint)

Extraction Method/Origin: Steam distilled from flowering top — France, Idaho, Utah

Chemical Constituents: Alcohols (up to 58%): linalol (>41%), α-terpineol, borneol, lavendulol, geraniol, nerol; Esters (approx. 50%): linalyl acetate (up to 45%), lavendulyl & geranyl acetates, α-terpenyl acetate; Monoterpenes (up to 24%): β-ocimene (<16%), d-limonene (<5%), α- & β-pinenes, camphene, δ-3-carene; Sesquiterpenes: β-caryophyllene (<7%), χ-farnesene; Phenols: terpinen-4-ol (<6%); Aldehydes: benzaldehyde, cuminal, geranial, hexanal, myrtenal, neral; Oxides: 1,8 cineol, caryophyllene oxide, linalol oxide; Coumarins (<4%); Ketones: octanone (<3%), camphor; Lactones.

Properties: Analgesic, anti-coagulant, anti-convulsive, anti-depressant, anti-fungal, antihistamine, anti-infectious, anti-inflammatory, antiseptic, antispasmodic, antitoxic, cardiotonic, regenerative, and **sedative**.

Esoteric Uses/Actions: Astrological: *Mercury*; Body type: *Ectomorph*; Chakras: *4 & 7*; Character: *Neutral, Yin but leans Yang*; Crystals: *Flourite, Amethyst*; Element: *Air & Ether*; Number: *7*; Oriental: *Excess Yang (pts: Liv-2, He-3)*

Historical Uses: During Medieval times, people were obviously divided on the properties of lavender regarding love. Some would claim that it could keep the wearer chaste, while others claimed just the opposite–touting its aphrodisiac qualities. The list of uses is long.

French Medicinal Uses: Acne, allergies, burns (cell renewal), **cramps** (leg), **dandruff, diaper rash, flatulence, hair loss, herpes, indigestion, insomnia, lower blood pressure, lymphatic system drainage, menopausal conditions, mouth abscess, nausea, phlebitis, pre-menstrual conditions, scarring** (minimizes), **stretch marks, tachycardia, thrush, water retention**.

Other Possible Uses: Lavender is a universal oil that has traditionally been known to balance the body and to work wherever there is a need. If in doubt, use lavender. It may help **arthritis, asthma, balancing body systems, boils, bronchitis, bruises, carbuncles, cold sores, convulsions, depression, earaches, fainting, gallstones, hay fever**, relieve **headaches, heart** (irregularity), reduce **high blood pressure, hives** (urticaria), **hysteria, insect bites** and **bee stings, infection, influenza, injuries, laryngitis, migraine headaches, mouth abscess**, reduce **mucus, nervous tension, pineal gland** (activates), **respiratory function, rheumatism, skin conditions** (eczema, psoriasis, rashes), **sprains, stress, sunburns** (including lips), **sunstroke, tension, throat infections, tuberculosis, typhoid fever, whooping cough**, and **wounds**. One of our readers suggested putting a drop of lavender in the mascara bottle to thin it out and get more shine from eye lashes.

Body System(s) Affected: Cardiovascular System, Emotional Balance, Nervous System, Skin.

Aromatic Influence: It promotes **consciousness, health, love, peace** and a general sense of **well being**.

Application: Apply to **Vita Flex Points** and directly on **area** of concern; **Diffuse**.

Oral Use As Dietary Supplement: *As of Oct. 30, 2006, the FDA has NOT given this variety of lavender the designation of GRAS (Generally Regarded As Safe for internal consumption) (see 21CFR182.20).* ***Not recommended for internal consumption.***

Blend Classification: Enhancer and Modifier and Equalizer

Blends With: Most oils especially citrus oils, chamomile, Clary sage, and geranium.

Odor: Type: *Middle Note (50-80% of the blend)*; Scent: *Floral, sweet, herbaceous, balsamic, woody undertones*; Intensity: *2*

Frequency: Emotional and Spiritual; approximately 118.

LEDUM (or LABRADOR TEA)
(Ledum groenlandicum)

Botanical Family: Ericaceae (heather)

Extraction Method/Origin: Steam distilled from leaves — Canada

Chemical Constituents: Monoterpenes (up to 50%): l-limonene (up to 35%), p-menthatriene (<15%), α- and β-pinenes, sabinene, γ-terpinenes; Sesquiterpene Alcohols: p-menthadiene8-ol (<17%), ledol (<3%); Alcohols: α-terpineol; Aldehydes: myrtenal; Esters: bornyl acetate & butyrate; Sesquiterpene Ketones: germacrone; Sesquiterpenes: α-selinene, selinadiene; Phenols: terpinen-4-ol.

Properties: Anti-cancerous, anti-tumoral, anti-viral, nerve-stimulant, and **tonic**.

Historical Uses: Ledum tea has been used for all types of skin problems, kidney-related problems, coughs, and hoarseness. Some sources say it was used by the Eskimos of the arctic region to fight cancer. Other natives of North America have used ledum tea to fight scurvy for thousands of years. According to Laurie Lacey, "The Cree named this plant **muskeko-pukwan**, and used it to treat fevers, colds, and other conditions."

Other Possible Uses: This oil may be beneficial for **ADD, allergies, bronchitis, colds, edema, fever, hepatitis** (viral), **influenza, laryngitis, lymph nodes** (inflamed), **skin problems** (all kinds), and **thyroid regulation**. It may also be a wonderful support to the **urinary tract, respiratory system**, and **immune system**, as well as a powerful **liver** support and detoxifier (best when combined with JuvaTone). Research has indicated that this oil may contain more anti-cancerous and anti-tumoral properties than frankincense.

Body System(s) Affected: Digestive and **Immune Systems, Skin**.

Application: Diffuse or apply to **Vita Flex Points** and/or directly on **area** of concern. Best **diluted** in one teaspoon of V-6 Mixing Oil for topical application. According to literature from Young Living Essential Oils, may also be used as a dietary supplement by diluting one drop of oil in 4 oz. of liquid (i.e. soy/rice milk or honey).

Oral Use As Dietary Supplement: None. *Although Young Living Essential Oils recommends the use of this oil as a dietary supplement, the FDA has **not yet** approved it for use as a food additive (FA) or flavoring agent (FL) (as of 07/01/2004 - see 21CFR172.510 and 21CFR182.20).*

LEMON
(Citrus limon)

Botanical Family: Rutaceae (citrus)

Extraction Method/Origin: Cold pressed from rind (requires 3,000 lemons to produce a kilo of oil) — California, Italy

Chemical Constituents: Monoterpenes (up to 90%): d-limonene (up to 72%), α- & β-pinenes (<30%), α- & γ-terpinenes (7-14%), sabinene, p-cymene, terpinolene, α- & β-phellandrenes; Aldehydes (up to 12%): citral, citronellal, neral, geranial, heptanal, hexanal, nonanal, octanal, undecanal; Alcohols: hexanol, octanol, nonanol, decanol, linalol, αterpineol; Esters (<5%): geranyl acetate, neryl acetate, methyl anthranilate; Sesquiterpenes (<5%): β-bisabolene, β-caryophyllene; Tetraterpenes (<4%): β-carotene, lycopene; Phenols: terpinen-4-ol; Coumarins and Furocoumarins (<3%): umberlliferone, bergaptene, α-bergamotene, limettine, psoralen, bergamottin, bergaptole, citroptene scopoletin.

Properties: Antiseptic, anti-viral, astringent, invigorating, refreshing, and **tonic**.

Esoteric Uses/Actions: Astrological: *Saturn & Moon*; Body type: *Mesomorph*; Chakra: *3*; Character: *Yang*; Element: *Water & Fire*; Number: *7*; Oriental: *Blood stagnation (pts: Sp10 & 6), Hot phlegm (pts: St-40, S-6)*

Historical Uses: Lemon has been used to fight food poisoning, malaria and typhoid epidemics, and scurvy (in fact, sources say that Christopher Columbus carried lemon seeds to America– probably just the left overs from the fruit that was eaten during the trip). Lemon has also been used to lower blood pressure and to help with liver problems, arthritis, and muscular aches and pains.

French Medicinal Uses: Air disinfectant, anemia, asthma, cold, fever (reduces), **germicide, gout, heartburn, intestinal parasites, red blood cell formation, rheumatism, throat infection, ureter infections, varicose veins, water purification, white blood cell formation**.

Other Possible Uses: This oil may be beneficial for **anxiety, blood pressure**, soothing broken **capillaries**, dissolving **cellulite, clarity** of thought, **debility, digestive problems, energy, gallstones, hair** (cleansing), promoting **leukocyte formation, liver** deficiencies in children, **lymphatic system cleansing, memory improvement, nails** (strengthening and hardening), **nervous conditions, respiratory problems**, cleaning the **skin** of dirty kids, **sore throats**, and promoting a sense of **well being**. It works extremely well in **removing gum, wood stain, oil**, and **grease spots**. It may also brighten a pale, dull **complexion** by removing dead skin cells.

Body System(s) Affected: Digestive, Immune, and **Respiratory Systems**.

Aromatic Influence: It promotes **health, healing, physical energy**, and **purification**. Its fragrance is **invigorating, enhancing,** and **warming**.

Application: Apply to **Vita Flex Points** and directly on **area** of concern; **Diffuse**.

Oral Use As Dietary Supplement: Generally regarded as safe (GRAS) for internal consumption by the FDA. *Dilute* one drop oil in 1 tsp. honey or 4 oz. of beverage (i.e. soy/rice milk). *Not for children under 6 years old; use with* **caution** *and in* **greater dilution** *for children 6 years old and over.*

Safety Data: *Avoid direct* **sunlight** *for up to 12 hours after use. Can cause extreme* **skin irritation.**

Blend Classification: Modifier and Enhancer

Blends With: Chamomile, eucalyptus, fennel, frankincense, geranium, juniper, peppermint, sandalwood, and ylang ylang.

Odor: Type: *Top Note (5-20% of the blend)*; Scent: *Sweet, sharp, clear, citrusy*; Intensity: *3*

LEMONGRASS
(Cymbopogon flexuosus)

Botanical Family: Gramineae (grasses)

Extraction Method/Origin: Steam distilled from leaves — India, Guatemala

Chemical Constituents: Aldehydes (up to 80%): geranial (<42%), neral (<38%), farnesal (<3%), decanal; Alcohols (<15%): geraniol (<10%), α-terpineol (<3%), borneol (<2%), nerol, linalol, citronellol; Sesquiterpene Alcohols: farnesol (<13%); Esters (<11%): geranyl & linalyl acetates; Monoterpenes (<9%): myrcene (<5%), d-limonene (<3%), β-ocimene; Sesquiterpenes: β-caryophyllene (<6%); Oxides: caryophyllene oxide (<4%); Ketones: methyl heptanone (<3%).

Properties: **Analgesic, anti-inflammatory, antiseptic, insect repellent, revitalizer, sedative, tonic**, and **vasodilator**.

Historical Uses: Lemongrass has been used for infectious illnesses and fever, an insecticide, and as a sedative to the central nervous system.

French Medicinal Uses: Bladder infection (cystitis), **connective tissue** (regenerates), **digestive system, edema, fluid retention, kidney disorders, lymphatic drainage, parasympathetic nervous system** (regulates), **varicose veins, vascular walls** (strengthens).

Other Possible Uses: This oil may help improve **circulation**, improve **digestion**, improve **eyesight, fevers, flatulence, headaches**, clear **infections**, repair **ligaments**, wake up the **lymphatic system**, get the **oxygen** flowing, **purification, respiratory problems, sore throats, tissue regeneration**, and **water retention**.

Body System(s) Affected: Immune System, Muscles and Bones.

Aromatic Influence: It promotes **psychic awareness** and **purification**.

Application: Apply to **Vita Flex Points** or directly on **area** of concern; **Diffuse**.

Oral Use As Dietary Supplement: Generally regarded as safe (GRAS) for internal consumption by the FDA. ***Dilute*** *one drop oil in 1 tsp. honey or 4 oz. of beverage (i.e. soy/rice milk).* ***Not for children under 6 years old; use with*** **caution** *and in* **greater dilution** *for children 6 years old and over.*

Safety Data: *Can cause extreme* **skin irritation.**

Blend Classification: Enhancer and Equalizer

Blends With: Basil, cedarwood, Clary sage, eucalyptus, geranium, jasmine, lavender, melaleuca (Tea Tree), and rosemary.

Odor: Type: *Top Note (5-20% of the blend)*; Scent: *Grassy, lemony, pungent, earthy, slightly bitter*; Intensity: *4*

LIME
(Citrus aurantifolia)

Botanical Family: Rutaceae (citrus)

Extraction Method/Origin: Cold expressed from peel — India, Guatemala

Chemical Constituents: Monoterpenes (up to 80%): d-limonene (<65%), α- & β-pinenes (<17%), camphene, sabinene, p-cymene, myrcene, bisabolene, dipentene, phellandrene, cadinene; Oxides (<22%): 1,8 cineol (<20%), 1,4 cineol; Aldehydes (<20%): geranial (<8%), neral (<5%), citral, citronellal, octanal, nonanal, decanal, lauric aldehyde; Alcohols (4%): α-terpineol (<2%), borneol, α-fenchol, linalol; Coumarins: limettine; Furanoids: furfural, garanoxycoumarin.

Properties: Anti-bacterial, antiseptic, anti-viral, restorative, and **tonic**.

Esoteric Uses/Actions: Astrological: *Saturn, Mercury, & Sun*; Body type: *Endomorph*; Character: *Yang*; Element: *Fire*; Number: *1*

Historical Uses: For some time, lime was used as a remedy for dyspepsia with glycerin of pepsin. Was often used in place of lemon for fevers, infections, sore throats, colds, etc.

Other Possible Uses: This oil may be beneficial for **anxiety, blood pressure**, soothing broken **capillaries**, dissolving **cellulite, clarity** of thought, **debility, energy, fevers, gallstones, hair** (cleansing), promoting **leukocyte formation, liver** deficiencies in children, **lymphatic system cleansing, memory improvement, nails** (strengthening), **nervous conditions**, cleaning the **skin** of dirty kids, **sore throats, water** and **air purification**, and promoting a sense of **well being**. It works extremely well in **removing gum, wood stain, oil**, and **grease spots**. It may also help brighten a pale, dull **complexion** by removing the dead skin cells. Lime oil is capable of **tightening skin** and **connective tissue**.

Body System(s) Affected: Digestive, Immune, and **Respiratory Systems**.

Aromatic Influence: Lime oil has a fresh, lively fragrance that is **stimulating** and **refreshing**. It helps one overcome **exhaustion, depression**, and **listlessness**. Although unverifiable, some sources claim that inhaling the oil may stimulate the muscles around the eyes.

Application: Apply to **Vita Flex Points** and/or directly on **area** of concern; **Diffuse**. Excellent addition to **bath** and **shower gels, body lotions**, and **deodorants**.

Oral Use As Dietary Supplement: Generally regarded as safe (GRAS) for internal consumption by the FDA. ***Dilute*** *one drop oil in 1 tsp. honey or 4 oz. of beverage (i.e. soy/rice milk).* ***Not for children under 6 years old; use with* caution *and in* greater dilution** *for children 6 years old and over.*

Safety Data: *Avoid direct* **sunlight** *for up to 12 hours after use.*

Blend Classification: Enhancer and Equalizer

Blends With: Citronella, Clary sage, lavandin, lavender, neroli, rosemary, other citrus oils.

Odor: Type: *Top Note (5-20% of the blend)*; Scent: *Sweet, tart, intense, lively*; Intensity: 3

LIMETTE (or COMBAVA)
(Citrus hystrix)

Botanical Family: Rutaceae (citrus)

Extraction Method/Origin: Cold pressed from peel — Madagascar

Chemical Constituents: Aldehydes: citronellal (66%); Oxides: citronellol (up to 10%), nerol; Monoterpenes: limonene.

Properties: **Anti-infectious**, **antiseptic**, **decongestant** (liver), **stimulant** (gallbladder), **tonic** (nerves)

Historical Uses: Limette has been used to repel flies and other household pests.

Other Possible Uses: This oil may be beneficial for **anxiety, clarity** of thought, **debility, energy, memory improvement, nervous conditions**, **air purification, trauma**, and promoting a sense of **well being**.

Body System(s) Affected: **Nervous System**.

Aromatic Influence: Limette oil has a crisp, tart fragrance that is dominating and penetrating at first, but after a little getting used to, it becomes uniquely **refreshing** and **uplifting**. It helps one overcome **exhaustion, depression**, and **listlessness**.

Application: **Diffuse**.

Safety Data: *Avoid direct* **sunlight** *for up to 12 hours after use.*

Blends With: Orange, angelica, lemon, and jasmine.

MANDARIN
(Citrus reticulata)

Botanical Family: Rutaceae (citrus)

Extraction Method/Origin: Cold pressed from peel. — China, Italy, Madagascar

Chemical Constituents: Monoterpenes (up to 95%): d-limonene (up to 75%), γ-terpinene (<22%), α- & β-pinenes (<5%), p-cymene (<4%), myrcene, α-phellandrene, terpinolene; Alcohols (<10%): linalol (<6%), octanol, α-terpineol, citronellol, nonanol, geraniol; Tetraterpenes

(<8%): β-carotene (<6%), lycopene; Aldehydes (<4%): α-sinensal, decanal, perillaldehyde, octanal, citronellal; Esters: benzyl acetate, methyl anthranilate (>1%).

Properties: **Anti-fungal, antiseptic, antispasmodic, digestive, sedative** (nervous system), **stimulant** (digestive, lymphatic), **tonic**.

Folklore: The name of the fruit is said to have originated from a group of Imperial Chinese officials called the mandarins. The fruit was a traditional gift given to these officials.

Esoteric Uses/Actions: Astrological: *Saturn & Sun*; Body type: *Ectomorph*; Chakra: *2*; Character: *Yang/Yin?*; Crystals: *Pink and Gold Topaz*; Element: *Fire*; Number: *3*

Historical Uses: Mandarin has been used in children's remedies for indigestion, hiccoughs, etc. Also for the elderly to strengthen the digestive function and the liver.

Other Possible Uses: This oil may help with **acne, digestive problems, dyspepsia, fluid retention, hepatic duct function, hiccoughs, insomnia, intestinal problems, skin problems** (congested and oily skin, **scars, spots**, tones the skin), **stretch marks** (when combined with either jasmine, lavender, sandalwood, and/or frankincense), **nervous tension, obesity, restlessness**. Recommended for **children** and **pregnant women** because it is very gentle.

Body System(s) Affected: **Digestive System, Skin**.

Aromatic Influence: It is **appeasing, gentle**, and promotes **happiness**. It is also **refreshing, uplifting**, and **revitalizing**. Because of its sedative and slightly hypnotic properties, it is very good for **stress** and **irritability**.

Application: Apply to **Vita Flex Points** and/or directly on **area** of concern; **Diffuse**. During pregnancy, combine with Olive oil or Wheat Germ oil and **massage** on the **abdomen**.

Oral Use As Dietary Supplement: Generally regarded as safe (GRAS) for internal consumption by the FDA. ***Dilute*** *one drop oil in 1 tsp. honey or 4 oz. of beverage (i.e. soy/rice milk). **Not for children under 6 years old; use with caution and in greater dilution for children 6 years old and over.***

Safety Data: *Avoid direct **sunlight** for 3 to 6 hours after use.*

Blend Classification: Personifier and Modifier

Blends With: Lavender; neroli and other citrus oils; cinnamon bark, clove, nutmeg, and other spice oils.

Odor: Type: *Top Note (5-20% of the blend)*; Scent: *Very sweet, citrusy, fruity*; Intensity: *3*

MANUKA
(Leptospermum scoparium)

Botanical Family: Myrtaceae (Myrtle - shrubs and trees)

Extraction Method/Origin: Steam distilled from the leaves and branches — New Zealand

Chemical Constituents: Monoterpenes: pinenes; Sesquiterpenes: caryophyllene, humulene; Alcohols: linalol, geraniol; Cyclic Triketones (20-30%): leptospermone, iso-leptospermone, flavesone.

Properties: **Analgesic, anti-allergic, anti-fungal, anti-infectious, anti-viral, antihistamine, antiseptic, decongestant, insecticidal,** and highly **bactericidal (antimicrobial)** across a wide spectrum.

Historical Uses: This oil has a long history of use by the Maori people, for bronchitis, rheumatism and similar conditions. Also, Manuka oil has been used to treat a range of skin problems including chronic sores, ring worm, eczema, fungal infections (athlete foot and fungal nail infections), scalp itch and dandruff. A decoction of leaves was used for urinary complaints and to reduce fever. The leaves were boiled in water and inhaled for head colds, blocked sinuses, hay fever, even bronchitis and asthma. Leaves and bark were boiled together, and the warm liquid was rubbed on stiff backs and rheumatic joints. The leaves and young branches were put into vapor baths. The crushed leaves were applied as a poultice for many skin diseases and were directly applied to wounds and deep gashes to enhance healing and reduce the risk of infection. The young shoots were chewed and swallowed for dysentery. The bark, the sap, and the seed capsules of the Manuka were also used extensively for treating various ailments.

Other Possible Uses: This oil may help with **abrasions**, **acne**, **bronchitis**, **catarrh**, **chafing**, **colds**, **cuts**, **dandruff**, **fungal infections** (athletes foot, skin, and nails), **infections** (staph and strep), **insect bites** and **stings**, **muscle** and **joint pains**, **odor** (foot and body), **rashes**, **scratches**, oily **skin**, **skin irritation**, **sinusitis**, mild **sunburn**, **ulcers** (Active Manuka Honey, a unique honey produced from the blossoms of the Manuka tree, has been shown to naturally kill **Helicobacter pylori**).

Body System(s) Affected: **Muscles and Bones, Respiratory System, Skin.**

Aromatic Influence: Manuka helps to **calm oversensitive nerves** and **strengthen the psyche**, producing an almost sensual feeling of well-being. It's **stabilizing** and **calming** aroma makes it very good for combating **stress** and **irritability.**

Application: Apply to **Vita Flex Points** and/or directly on **area** of concern; **Diffuse**. Can also be used in the **bath** or as a **gargle.**

Blend Classification: Enhancer and Equalizer

Blends With: All citrus oils, cypress, eucalyptus, lavender, rosemary, and thyme.

MARJORAM
(Origanum majorana)

Botanical Family: Labiatae (mint)

Extraction Method/Origin: Steam distilled from leaves — France

Chemical Constituents: Monoterpenes (up to 60%): α- & γ-terpinenes (<30%), sabinene (<8%), myrcene (<7%), terpinolene, ocimene, δ-3-carene, p-cymene, α- and β-pinenes, δ-cadinene, α- & β-phellandrenes, l-limonene; Alcohols (<30%): α-terpineol (<15%), cis- & trans-thujanol-4 (<12%), linalol (<8%); Phenols: terpinen-4-ol (>21%), terpinen-1-ol-3; Esters: geranyl acetate (<7%), linalyl acetate, α-terpenyl acetate; Aldehydes: citral (<6%); Sesquiterpenes (<5%): β-caryophyllene, humulene; Phenolic Ethers: trans-anethole.

Properties: Anti-bacterial, anti-infectious, antiseptic, anti-sexual, antispasmodic, arterial vasodilator, digestive stimulant, diuretic, expectorant, sedative, and **tonic**.

Folklore: Known as the "herb of happiness" to the Romans and "joy of the mountains" to the Greeks, marjoram was used to decorate at both weddings and funerals. Not only would it warm both the body and the emotions, but many believed it would increase longevity. It was also grown on grave sites to comfort the departed soul.

Esoteric Uses/Actions: Astrological: *Mercury & Venus*; Ayurvedic: *Kapha*; Body type: *Mesomorph*; Chakra: *4*; Character: *Yang*; Element: *Air & Water*; Number: *9*

Historical Uses: Marjoram was used for poisoning, fluid retention, muscle spasms, rheumatism, sprains, stiff joints, bruises, obstructions of the liver and spleen, and respiratory congestions. According to Roberta Wilson, "Those curious about their futures anointed themselves with marjoram at bedtime so that they might dream of their future mates."

French Medicinal Uses: Aches, arthritis, asthma, bronchitis, colic, constipation, cramps, insomnia, intestinal peristalsis, migraine headache, muscles, neuralgia, pains, parasympathetic nervous system (tones), **blood pressure** (regulates), **rheumatism, sprains**.

Other Possible Uses: It may be **relaxing** and **calming** to the **muscles** that constrict and sometimes contribute to **headaches**. It may help **anxiety, boils, bruises, burns, carbuncles, celibacy** (vow not to marry), **colds, cold sores, cuts, fungus** and **viral infections, hysteria, menstrual problems**, calm **respiratory system, ringworm, shingles, shock, sores**, relieve **spasms, sunburns, tension**, and **water retention**.

Body System(s) Affected: Cardiovascular System, Muscles and Bones.

Aromatic Influence: It promotes **peace** and **sleep**.

Application: Apply to **Vita Flex Points** and directly on **area** of concern; **Diffuse**.

Oral Use As Dietary Supplement: Generally regarded as safe (GRAS) for internal consumption by the FDA. *Dilute* one drop oil in 1 tsp. honey or 4 oz. of beverage (i.e. soy/rice milk). *Not for children under 6 years old; use with* **caution** *and in* **greater dilution** *for children 6 years old and over.*

Safety Data: *Use with caution during* **pregnancy**.

Blend Classification: Enhancer and Equalizer

Blends With: Bergamot, cedarwood, chamomile, cypress, lavender, orange, nutmeg, rosemary, rosewood, ylang ylang.

Odor: Type: *Middle Note (50-80% of the blend)*; Scent: *Herbaceous, green, spicy*; Intensity: *3*

MELALEUCA (TEA TREE)
(Melaleuca alternifolia)

Botanical Family: Myrtaceae (Myrtle - shrubs and trees)

Extraction Method/Origin: Steam distilled from leaves — Australia

Chemical Constituents: Monoterpenes (up to 70%): α- & γ-terpinenes (<40%), p-cymene (<12%), α- and β-pinenes (<8%), terpinolene, l-limonene, sabinene, myrcene, α-thujene; Phenols: terpinen-4-ol (<40%); Sesquiterpenes (up to 20%): α- & δ-cadinenes (<8%), aromadendrene (<7%), viridiflorene (<5%), β-caryophyllene, α-phellandrene; Oxides: 1,8 cineol (<14%), 1,4 cineol (<3%), caryophyllene oxide; Alcohols: α- & β-terpineols (<8%); Sesquiterpene Alcohols (<5%): globulol, viridiflorol.

Properties: Analgesic, anti-bacterial, anti-fungal, anti-infectious, anti-inflammatory, antioxidant, anti-parasitic, a strong **antiseptic, anti-viral, decongestant, digestive, expectorant, immune-stimulant, insecticidal, neurotonic, stimulant**, and **tissue regenerator**.

Esoteric Uses/Actions: Character: *Yang*

Historical Uses: The leaves of the Melaleuca tree (or Tea Tree) have been used for centuries by the aborigines to heal cuts, wounds, and skin infections. With twelve times the antiseptic power of phenol, it has some strong immune building properties.

French Medicinal Uses: Athlete's foot, bronchitis, colds, coughs, diarrhea, flu, periodontal (gum) disease, rash, skin healing, sore throat, sunburn, tonsillitis, vaginal thrush.

Other Possible Uses: This oil may help **acne, burns, candida, cold sores, digestion, fungal infections, hysteria, infectious diseases, inflammation, shock, viral infections, warts**, and **wounds** (promotes healing).

Body System(s) Affected: Immune and **Respiratory Systems, Muscles and Bones, Skin**.

Aromatic Influence: It promotes **cleansing** and **purity**.

Application: Apply to **Vita Flex Points** and/or directly on **area** of concern; **Diffuse**.

Oral Use As Dietary Supplement: Approved by the FDA for use as a Food Additive (FA) or Flavoring Agent (FL). **Dilute** *one drop oil in 1 tsp. honey or 4 oz. of beverage (i.e. soy/rice milk). Not for children under 6 years old; use with **caution** and in **greater dilution** for children 6 years old and over.*

Safety Data: *Repeated use can possibly result in **contact sensitization**.*

Blend Classification: Enhancer and Equalizer

Blends With: All citrus oils, cypress, eucalyptus, lavender, rosemary, and thyme.

Odor: Type: *Middle Note (50-80% of the blend)*; Scent: *Medicinal, fresh, woody, earthy, herbaceous*; Intensity: *3*

MELALEUCA ERICIFOLIA (or ROSALINA)
(Melaleuca ericifolia)

Botanical Family: Myrtaceae (Myrtle - shrubs and trees)

Origin: Australia

Chemical Constituents: Alcohols (up to 52%): linalol (<45%), α-terpineol (<5%); Monoterpenes (up to 30%): β-phellandrene (up to 12%), α-pinene (<10%), p-cymene (<6%), l-limonene

(<2%), γ-terpinene (<2%); Oxides (up to 20%): 1,8 cineol (<19%), 1,4 cineol; Sesquiterpenes (up to 8%): aromandrene (<6%), viridiflorene (<2%); Phenols: terpinen-4-ol.

Properties: **Anti-bacterial, anti-fungal, anti-infectious**, powerful **antimicrobial, calming**, and **sedative**.

Other Possible Uses: Because this variety of melaleuca oil is **very gentle** and **nonirritating** to the skin, it is well suited for **youth** and others who may be more sensitive to the oils. Research by Dr. Daniel Pénoël, M.D. has shown this oil to help with **bronchitis, dermatitis, ear infections, eczema, influenza, insomnia, nervous tension, pneumonia**, and **sinusitis**.

Body System(s) Affected: Respiratory System, Skin.

Application: Apply to **Vita Flex Points** and/or directly on **area** of concern. May also be applied to the **chest, face, temples, throat**, or **wrists**. For a **full body massage**, dilute 4-8 drops of *Melaleuca ericifolia* oil in 30 ml. of a pure vegetable oil. May also be diffused or added to bath water. *Caution: Heating or burning this oil can cause it to lose all therapeutic value.*

Oral Use As Dietary Supplement: Approved by the FDA for use as a Food Additive (FA) or Flavoring Agent (FL). ***Dilute*** *one drop oil in 1 tsp. honey or 4 oz. of beverage (i.e. soy/rice milk).* ***Not for children under 6 years old; use with caution and in greater dilution for children 6 years old and over.***

Blend Classification: Personifier, Enhancer, Equalizer, and Modifier.

MELALEUCA LEUCADENDRON
(See CAJEPUT)

MELALEUCA QUINQUENERVIA (or NIAOULI)
(Melaleuca quinquenervia)

Botanical Family: Myrtaceae (Myrtle - shrubs and trees)

Extraction Method/Origin: Steam distilled from leaves and limbs — Australia

Chemical Constituents: Oxides: 1,8 cineol (>60%), 1,4 cineol; Monoterpenes (<29%): α- & β-pinenes (<21%), l-limonene (<8%), β-phellandrene, α- & γ-terpinenes; Sesquiterpene Alcohols (<22%): viridiflorol (>14%), nerolidol (<6%), globulol; Alcohols (<15%): α-terpineol (<12%), linalol; Sesquiterpenes (<4%): β- caryophyllene, aromadendrene, viridiflorene, δ-cadinene; Phenols: terpinen-4-ol (2%); Aldehydes: isovaleraldehyde, benzaldehyde.

Properties: Anti-bacterial, anti-fungal (very strong and powerful), **anti-inflammatory, antiseptic, anti-viral, digestive tonic, protector against radiation**, and a strong **tissue regenerator**.

Esoteric Uses/Actions: Astrological: *Mercury*; Character: *Neutral?*; Element: *Air*

Other Possible Uses: This oil may help with **respiratory allergies, infections, hemorrhoids**, and others as listed under MELALEUCA.

Body System(s) Affected: Muscles and Bones, Respiratory System.

Aromatic Influence: Some people may prefer this oil to melaleuca (*M. alternifolia*) because of its sweet, delicate scent. It aids in **concentration**, is **reviving**, and helps **clear** the **head**.

Application: Apply to **Vita Flex Points** and/or directly on **area** of concern; **Diffuse**. **Diffuse** for respiratory problems.

Oral Use As Dietary Supplement: Approved by the FDA for use as a Food Additive (FA) or Flavoring Agent (FL). ***Dilute** one drop oil in 1 tsp. honey or 4 oz. of beverage (i.e. soy/rice milk). **Not for children under 6 years old; use with **caution** and in **greater dilution** for children 6 years old and over.***

Safety Data: *Repeated use can possibly result in **contact sensitization**.* **Odor:** Type: *Middle Note (50-80% of the blend)*; Scent: *Earthy, musty, harsh*; Intensity: *3*

MELISSA (LEMON BALM)
(Melissa officinalis)

Botanical Family: Labiatae (mint)

Extraction Method/Origin: Steam distilled from leaves and flowers — France, Idaho, Utah

Chemical Constituents: Aldehydes (up to 65%): geranial (<35%), neral (<28%), citronellal (<3%), α-cyclocitral; Sesquiterpenes (<35%): β-caryophyllene (<19%), α-copaene (<5%), germacrene-D (<4%), β-bourbonene, δ- & γ-cadinenes, humulene, β-elemene; Oxides (<11%): caryophyllene oxide (<7%), 1,8 cineol (<4%); Alcohols (<7%): linalol, octen-3ol, nerol, geraniol, citronnellol, isopulegol, caryophyllenol, farnesol; Esters (<7%): methyl citronellate (<5%), citronellyl, geranyl, neryl, & linalyl acetates; Ketones (<7%): methyl heptanone (<5%), farnesylacetone, octanone; Monoterpenes (<3%): cis- & trans-ocimenes, l-limonene; Sesquiterpene Alcohols: elemol, α-cadinol; Furanocoumarins: aesculetine.

Properties: Anti-bacterial, anti-depressant, antihistamine, antimicrobial, antispasmodic, anti-viral, hypertensive, nervine, sedative, tonic, and **uterine**.

Folklore: Melissa, the "Elixir of Life", is one of the earliest known medicinal herbs.

Esoteric Uses/Actions: Astrological: *Jupiter*; Body type: *Endomorph*; Chakras: *4 & 3*; Character: *Yang with high Yin*; Element: *Fire*; Number: *1*

Historical Uses: Anciently, melissa was used for nervous disorders and many different ailments dealing with the heart or the emotions. It was also used to promote fertility. Melissa was the main ingredient in Carmelite water, distilled in France since 1611 by the Carmelite monks.

Other Possible Uses: Allergies, anxiety, asthma, bronchitis, chronic coughs, colds, cold-sore blisters (apply directly three times per day), **colic, depression, dysentery, eczema, erysipelas, fevers, heart conditions** (where there is overstimulation or heat), **hypertension, indigestion, insect bites, insomnia, menstrual problems, migraine, nausea, nervous tension, palpitations, shock, sterility** (in women), **throat infections, vertigo**, and **vomiting**. Dr. Dietrich Wabner, a professor at the Technical University of Munich, reported that a onetime application of true melissa oil led to complete remission of **herpes simplex lesions**. According to Robert Tisserand, "...Melissa is the nearest one can find to a rejuvenator—not something which will make us young again, but which helps to cushion, the effect of our mind and the world outside, on our body."

Body System(s) Affected: Emotional Balance, Skin.

Aromatic Influence: Melissa has a delicate, delightful, lemony scent that is unique among essential oils, providing a wonderful support to both body and mind. It has been known to bring out **gentle** characteristics within people. It is **calming** and **uplifting** and may help to **balance** the **emotions**. It may also help to remove **emotional blocks** and **instill** a **positive outlook** on **life**.

Application: Apply to **Vita Flex Points** and/or directly on **area** of concern.

Oral Use As Dietary Supplement: Generally regarded as safe (GRAS) for internal consumption by the FDA. ***Dilute*** one drop oil in 1 tsp. honey or 4 oz. of beverage (i.e. soy/rice milk). ***Not for children under 6 years old; use with caution and in greater dilution for children 6 years old and over.***

Blend Classification: Enhancer, Equalizer, and Modifier

Blends With: Geranium, lavender, and other floral and citrus oils.

Odor: Type: *Middle Note (50-80% of the blend)*; Scent: *Delicate, lemony*; Intensity: 2

Frequency: Emotional and Spiritual; approximately 102 MHz.

MOUNTAIN SAVORY (or WINTER SAVORY)
(*Satureja montana*)

Botanical Family: Labiatae (mint)

Extraction Method/Origin: Steam distilled from flowering plant — France

Chemical Constituents: Phenols (up to 58%): carvacrol (<35%), thymol (<24%), carvacrol methyl-ether (<9%), eugenol; Monoterpenes (<32%): p-cymene (<20%), α- & γ-terpinenes (20%); Alcohols (<25%): linalol (<11%), α-terpineol (<9%), cis- & trans-thujanol-4 (<4%), geraniol, borneol, myrtenol; Sesquiterpenes (<7%): β-caryophyllene (<7%); Oxides: 1,8 cineol (<1%), caryophyllene oxide; Ketones: camphor, damasceneone.

Properties: Anti-bacterial, anti-fungal, strong **anti-infectious** (genito-urinary & gastro-intestinal - superior to thyme, rosemary, and lavender), **anti-parasitic, anti-viral, immune-stimulant**, and a general **tonic** for the body.

Historical Uses: This oil has been used as a digestive remedy for colic and diarrhea.

Other Possible Uses: Due to its high phenol content, Mountain savory is a very strong antiseptic and has been used to hasten the **formation** of **scar tissue**, and to help with **abscesses, burns,** and **cuts**. It is also known to stimulate the **adrenal gland**.

Body System(s) Affected: Immune System.

Aromatic Influence: It may produce **strong psychological effects** and can help revitalize and stimulate the nervous system. It is a powerful **energizer** and **motivator**.

Application: Apply diluted to **Vita Flex Points** and on **area** of concern; **Diffuse**.

Oral Use As Dietary Supplement: Generally regarded as safe (GRAS) for internal consumption by the FDA. ***Dilute*** *one drop oil in 2 tsp. honey or 8 oz. of beverage (i.e. soy/rice milk). May need to increase dilution even more due to this oil's potential for irritating mucus membranes. Not for children under 6 years old; use with **caution** and in **greater dilution** for children 6 years old and over.*

Safety Data: *Robert Tisserand has classified Mountain savory as a dermal toxin, dermal irritant, and mucous membrane irritant. He recommends it never be used on the skin. However, other sources recommend its use but emphasize that it must always be used in dilution. Can cause extreme **skin irritation**. Avoid during **pregnancy** and use with **extreme caution**. Also, best if used for short duration, may be toxic to the liver during long term use.*

MUGWORT
(Artemisia vulgaris)

Botanical Family: Asteraceae or Compositae (daisy)

Extraction Method/Origin: Steam distillation from the leaves and root — Europe

Chemical Constituents: Monoterpenes (up to 45%): myrcene (up to 25%), sabinene (<14%), l-limonene (<3%), β-phellandrene (<3%), α- & β-pinenes, camphene, p-cymene, γ-cadinene; Ketones (<18%): α- & β-thujones (up to 12%), camphor (<2%); Oxide: 1,8 cineol; Lactones: vulgarin, pilostachyn.

Properties: Antiseptic, antispasmodic, calming, diuretic, expectorant.

Historical Uses: Having been associated with superstition and witchcraft, mugwort was seen as a protective charm against danger and evil. It has been used for painful or delayed menstruation, amenorrhea and dysmenorrhea, for hysteria and epilepsy, to expel worms, and control fever. According to some sources, mugwort was used by the Jews as one of the bitter herbs eaten during Passover.

Other Possible Uses: Mucus (expels), **nerves** (calms), **parasites** (blend with thyme)

Body System(s) Affected: Hormonal and **Nervous Systems.**

Aromatic Influence: This strongly aromatic oil was anciently believed to increase psychic powers.

Application: Apply to **Vita Flex Points** and/or directly on **area** of concern.

Oral Use As Dietary Supplement: *Has been approved by the FDA for use as a Food Additive (FA) or Flavoring Agent (FL) as long as the finished food is thujone-free. (See 21CFR172.510) Best **not** to use this oil as a dietary supplement.*

Safety Data: *For topical use only. Due to high Thujone content, use **sparingly** and **dilute well** with V-6 Mixing Oil. Avoid during **pregnancy** as it may contribute to a miscarriage.*

Blends With: Anise, German chamomile, ginger, peppermint, rosemary, tangerine, and tarragon.

Found In: ComforTone

MYRRH
(Commiphora myrrha)

Botanical Family: Burseraceae (resinous trees and shrubs)

Extraction Method/Origin: Steam distilled from gum/resin — Somalia

Chemical Constituents: Sesquiterpenes (up to 75%): lindestrene (up to 30%), β-, γ-, & δ-elemenes (<40%), α-copaene (<12%), β-bourbonene (<5%), muurolene, δ-cadinene, humulene, curzerene; Furanoids (<27%): methoxyfurogermacrene (<9%), furoendesmadiene (<8%), α-bergamotene (<5%), methylisopropenylfurone (<5%), furfural (<3%), furanodione (<2%), rosefuran; Ketones: (<20%): curzenone (<11%), methylisobutyl ketone (<6%), germacrone (<4%); Triterpenes (<7%): α-amyrin (<4%), α-amyrenone (<3%); Monoterpenes (<6%): ocimene, p-cymene, α-thujene, l-limonene, myrcene; Aldehydes: methylbutynal (<3%), cinnamaldehyde, cuminal; Arenes: xylene; Carboxylic Acids: acetic acid, formic acid, palmitic acid; Phenols: eugenol, cresol.

Properties: Anti-infectious, anti-inflammatory, antiseptic, astringent, and **tonic**.

Folklore: Well over 2,000 years before the baby Jesus received myrrh as a gift, it was one of the most desired and most expensive items in the world. According to Roberta Wilson, "In Greek mythology, Aphrodite forced the goddess Myrrha into an incestuous relationship with her father, Cinyras. Cinyras avenged the act by turning his daughter into a myrrh tree. When the tree sprouted its blooms, their child Adonis was born. The resinous drops that exude from cuts in the tree's bark were said to be Myrrha's tears."

Esoteric Uses/Actions: Astrological: *Saturn, Jupiter, & Sun*; Body type: *Ectomorph*; Chakras: *1 & 2*; Character: *Yang - Hot and Drying*; Crystals: *Hematite, Red Garnet, Pearl*; Element: *Water*; Number: *5*

Historical Uses: Myrrh was used as incense in religious rituals, in embalming, as a cure for cancer, leprosy, and syphilis. Myrrh, mixed with coriander and honey, was used to treat herpes.

French Medicinal Uses: Bronchitis, diarrhea, dysentery, hyperthyroidism, stretch marks, thrush, ulcers, vaginal thrush, viral hepatitis.

Other Possible Uses: This oil may help increase **appetite, asthma, athlete's foot, candida, catarrh** (mucus), **coughs, eczema, digestion, dyspepsia** (impaired digestion), **flatulence** (gas), **fungal infection, gingivitis, gum infection, hemorrhoids, mouth ulcers**, decongest **prostate gland, ringworm, sore throats, skin conditions** (chapped, cracked, and inflammation), **wounds**, and **wrinkles**.

Body System(s) Affected: Hormonal, Immune, and **Nervous Systems, Skin**.

Aromatic Influence: It promotes **spiritual awareness** and is **uplifting**.

Application: Apply to **Vita Flex Points** and/or directly on **area** of concern.

Oral Use As Dietary Supplement: Approved by the FDA for use as a Food Additive (FA) and Flavoring Agent (FL). ***Dilute*** *one drop oil in 1 tsp. honey or 4 oz. of beverage (i.e. soy/rice milk). **Not** for children under 6 years old; use with **caution** and in **greater dilution** for children 6 years old and over.*

Safety Data: *Use with caution during **pregnancy**.*

Blend Classification: Modifier and Equalizer
Blends With: Frankincense, lavender, patchouli, sandalwood, and all spice oils.
Odor: Type: *Base Note (5-20% of the blend)*; Scent: *Warm, earthy, woody, balsamic*; Intensity: *4*
Frequency: Emotional and Spiritual; approximately 105 MHz.
Comments: Myrrh is a true gift. When we open our **hearts** and **minds** to receive the gifts, they will be given.

MYRTLE
(Myrtus communis ssp. red)

Botanical Family: Myrtaceae (Myrtle - shrubs and trees)
Extraction Method/Origin: Steam distilled from leaves — Morocco, Tunisia
Chemical Constituents: Oxides (up to 48%): 1,8 cineol (<45%), caryophyllene oxide; Monoterpenes (up to 45%): α-pinene (>24%), l-limonene (<11%), β-pinene (<5%), camphene; Esters (<22%): myrtenyl acetate (<10%), geranyl acetate (<5%), terpenyl acetate (<3%), methyl myrtenate (<3%), also linalyl, neryl, bornyl, & trans-carvyl acetates; Alcohols (<18%): α-terpineol (<8%), linalol (<5%), myrtenol (<4%), nerol, geraniol; Aldehydes: myrtenal, decanal, hexanal, methylbutynal; Phenols: myrtenol, terpinen-4-ol; Furanoids: methylfuran, furfural; Lactones: myrtecommulone.
Properties: Anti-bacterial, anti-inflammatory, anti-parasitic, antiseptic, astringent, expectorant, decongestant, and **deodorizer**.
Folklore: According to Susanne Fischer-Rizzi, "...myrtle, considered the sacred plant of the goddess Aphrodite, was worshiped as a plant of mystery. Aphrodite, goddess of beauty and love, and born as a beautiful adult woman from sea foam, sought refuge in her newborn nakedness in a myrtle bush. That's why myrtle also stands for chaste beauty. Many brides today still wear myrtle as a symbol for innocence."
Esoteric Uses/Actions: Astrological: *Venus & Mercury*; Character: *Yang (with strong Yin)*; Element: *Water*
Historical Uses: Myrtle was used for diarrhea, dysentery, catarrhal conditions (asthma, bronchitis, chronic coughs, tuberculosis), lung and bladder infections, sinus infections, and skin care.
French Medicinal Uses: Bronchitis, coughs, flu, hypothyroidism, insomnia, ovaries (hormone-like effects), **prostate decongestant, sinus infection, tuberculosis, ureter infections**.
Other Possible Uses: This oil may help **anger, asthma, catarrh, children** (see comment), **colds, cystitis, diarrhea, dysentery, dyspepsia** (impaired digestion), **flatulence** (gas), **hemorrhoids**, support **immune system, infections, infectious diseases, pulmonary disorders, skin conditions** (acne, blemishes, bruises, oily skin, psoriasis, etc.), and **sinusitis**. Useful on **children** for **chest** complaints and **coughs**.
Body System(s) Affected: Digestive, Hormonal, and **Respiratory Systems, Muscles and Bones**.
Aromatic Influence: It is **elevating** and **euphoric**. It also soothes **anger**.

Application: Apply to **Vita Flex Points** or directly on **area** of concern; **Diffuse**.

Oral Use As Dietary Supplement: Approved by the FDA for use as a Food Additive (FA) and Flavoring Agent (FL). *Dilute one drop oil in 1 tsp. honey or 4 oz. of beverage (i.e. soy/rice milk). Not for children under 6 years old; use with **caution** and in **greater dilution** for children 6 years old and over.*

Blend Classification: Equalizer and Enhancer

Blends With: Bergamot, lavender, lemon, lemongrass, rosewood, rosemary, spearmint, thyme, and melaleuca (Tea Tree).

Odor: Type: *Top to Middle Notes (20-80% of the blend)*; Scent: *Sweet, slightly camphorous, with a floral hint*; Intensity: *3*

MYRTLE, LEMON
(Backhousia citriodora)

Botanical Family: Myrtaceae (Myrtle - shrubs and trees)

Extraction Method/Origin: Steam distilled from leaves — Australia

Chemical Constituents: Aldehydes (>90%): geranial (57%), neral (37%), citronellal; Alcohols (<4%): cis- & trans-verbenol (<3%), linalol, nerol. Other trace elements include linalyl acetate, myrcene, methylheptenone, and geranic acid.

Properties: Anti-bacterial, anti-fungal, antimicrobial, antiseptic, anti-viral, calming, corrective, and **sedative**.

Historical Uses: The leaves from the Lemon Myrtle trees have been dried and used as food flavoring for poultry and seafood as well as for air fresheners in wardrobes, shoe cabinets, and vehicles. Lemon myrtle is said to smell more "lemony than lemon". Research is showing that lemon myrtle oil has very good antibacterial activity and excellent anti-fungal activity, maybe even more so than *Melaleuca alternifolia*. Other tests have shown lemon myrtle to possess strong germicidal powers, twice that of *Eucalyptus citriodora* and even 19.5 times that of citral alone.

Other Possible Uses: This oil may help with **viral, bacterial**, and **fungal infections**. It has also been reported to help with sprained or torn **ligaments** and **tendons**. Due to its anti-bacterial, anti-fungal, and antimicrobial actions, it would work well as an additive to any natural cleaning product. And what a better way to clean than with the strong lemon scent from the oil.

Body System(s) Affected: Immune and Respiratory Systems, Muscles and Bones.

Aromatic Influence: It is **elevating** and **refreshing**.

Application: Apply to **Vita Flex Points** or directly on **area** of concern; **Diffuse**.

Odor: Type: *Top Note (5-20% of the blend)*; Scent: *Extremely lemony and crisp, more "lemony" than true lemon oil*; Intensity: *5*

NEROLI (or ORANGE BLOSSOM)
(Citrus aurantium bigaradia)

Botanical Family: Rutaceae (citrus)

Extraction Method/Origin: Absolute extraction from flowers of the orange tree — Morocco, Tunisia

Chemical Constituents: Alcohols (up to 53%): linalol (<44%), α-terpineol (<6%), geraniol (<3%), nerol; Sesquiterpene Alcohols (<7%): trans-nerolidol (<5%), farnesol (<2%); Monoterpenes (up to 40%); d-limonene (<18%), β-pinene (<17%), ocimene (<8%), myrcene (<4%) α-pinene, neptadecene, sabinene, camphene; Esters (>25%): linalyl acetate (<15%), methyl anthranilate (<10%), neryl & geranyl acetates; Aldehydes: decanal, benzaldehyde, vinylhexanal; Phenols: phenylethanol, benzyl alcohol; Pyrroles: indole, scatole.

Properties: **Anti-bacterial, anti-depressant, anti-infectious, anti-parasitic, antiseptic, antispasmodic, anti-viral, aphrodisiac, deodorant, sedative**, and **tonic**.

Folklore: The name of this oil is said to originate from a beloved princess of Nerola, Italy, who lavished it on everything. Brides adorned themselves and their bouquets with the orange blossoms, to signify their purity and beauty.

Esoteric Uses/Actions: Astrological: *Sun*; Body type: *Ectomorph*; Chakras: *4, 8 & Higher*; Character: *Yin with high Yang*; Crystals: *Selenite (best), Herkemer Diamond, Fluorite, Rutilated quartz, Diamond, &Chrysoprase, Chalcedony*; Element: *Air & Ether*; Number: *1*

Historical Uses: Neroli has been regarded traditionally by the Egyptian people for its great attributes for healing the **mind, body**, and **spirit**. It brings everything into the focus of one and at the moment.

Other Possible Uses: It may support the **digestive system** and fight **bacteria, infections, parasites**, and **viruses**. It may also help with **anxiety, chronic diarrhea, colic, depression, digestive spasms, fear, flatulence, headaches, heart** (regulates rhythm), **hysteria, insomnia, mature** and **sensitive skin, nervous dyspepsia, nervous tension, palpitations, pms, poor circulation, scars, shock, stress related conditions, stretch marks, tachycardia, thread veins**, and **wrinkles**. In support of the skin, it works at the cell level to help shed the old skin cells and **stimulate new cell growth**.

Body System(s) Affected: Digestive System, Skin.

Aromatic Influence: As a **natural tranquilizer**, neroli has some **powerful psychological effects**. It has been used successfully to treat **depression, anxiety**, and **shock**. It is **calming** and **relaxing** to body and spirit. It may also help to **strengthen** and **stabilize** the emotions, and **bring relief** to seemingly hopeless situations. It encourages **confidence, courage, joy, peace**, and **sensuality**. Neroli is said to vibrate in the 2nd and 4th chakra. In the words of one author, "Neroli offers the gift of strength and courage that helps us see life's beauty."

Application: Apply to **Vita Flex Points** and directly on **area** of concern; **Diffuse**.

Oral Use As Dietary Supplement: Generally regarded as safe (GRAS) for internal consumption by the FDA. ***Dilute** one drop oil in 1 tsp. honey or 4 oz. of beverage (i.e. soy/rice milk).* ***Not***

*for children under 6 years old; use with **caution** and in **greater dilution** for children 6 years old and over.*

Blend Classification: Equalizer, Modifier, and Personifier

Blends With: Rose, lavender, sandalwood, jasmine, cedarwood, geranium, lemon.

Odor: Type: *Middle Note (50-80% of the blend)*; Scent: *Floral, citrusy, sweet, delicate, slightly bitter*; Intensity: *3*

NIAOULI
(See MELALEUCA QUINQUENERVIA)

NUTMEG
(Myristica fragrans)

Botanical Family: Myristicaceae

Extraction Method/Origin: Steam distilled from fruits and seeds — Indonesia, Tunisia

Chemical Constituents: Monoterpenes (up to 80%): α- & β-pinenes (<46%), sabinene (25%), myrcene (<12%), d-limonene (<7%), α- & γ-terpinenes (<11%), p-cymene, δ-3-carene, terpinolene, camphene, α- & β-phellandrenes; Phenolic Ethers (<16%): myristicin (<12%), elemicin (<3%), safrole (<2%), eugenol; Phenols: terpinen-4-ol (<8%); Oxides: 1,8-cineol (<4%); Alcohols: α-terpineol (<2%); Sesquiterpenes: β-caryophyllene.

Properties: Anti-inflammatory, anti-parasitic, antiseptic, stimulant (cerebral, circulatory), **laxative**, and **tonic**.

Esoteric Uses/Actions: Astrological: *Jupiter*; Body type: *Ectomorph*; Chakra: *1*; Element: *Fire*; Number: *4*

Historical Uses: Nutmeg has been used for centuries for digestive and kidney problems.

French Medicinal Uses: Appetite (loss of), **chronic diarrhea, debility, digestion** (helps with starchy foods and fats), **gallstones, halitosis** (bad breath), **rheumatism**.

Other Possible Uses: This oil has adrenal cortex-like activity, which helps support the **adrenal glands** for **increased energy**. It may also help with **arthritis, bacterial infection, circulation**, revive **fainting, flatulence** (gas), **frigidity, gout, impotence, immune function** (support), **joints, menstruation** (regulates scanty periods and soothes pains), **muscles** (also muscle aches and pains), **nausea, nervous fatigue, neuralgia** (severe pain along nerve), support **nervous system**, and **vomiting**.

Body System(s) Affected: Hormonal, Immune, and **Nervous Systems**.

Application: Apply to **Vita Flex Points** and/or directly on **area** of Concern.

Oral Use As Dietary Supplement: Generally regarded as safe (GRAS) for internal consumption by the FDA. ***Dilute*** one drop oil in 1 tsp. honey or 4 oz. of beverage (i.e. soy/rice milk). *Not for children under 6 years old; use with **caution** and in **greater dilution** for children 6 years old and over.*

Safety Data: *Not for use by people with **epilepsy**. Use with caution during **pregnancy**. If over used (several undiluted drops at once), it may cause mental discomfort or delirium, and convulsions and could overstimulate the heart. Dilute well or use a single undiluted drop then wait for a period of time.*

Blend Classification: Personifier

Blends With: Cinnamon bark, clove, cypress, frankincense, lemon, orange, patchouli, rosemary, melaleuca, melissa.

Odor: Type: *Middle Note (50-80% of the blend)*; Scent: *Sweet, musky, spicy*; Intensity: *4*

ONYCHA (BENZOIN)
(Styrax benzoin)

Botanical Family: Styracaceae

Extraction Method/Origin: Absolute extraction from the resin (Onycha is actually an "essence" not an essential oil) — India, China, Laos, Thailand, or Vietnam.

Chemical Constituents: Non Volatile Fraction: Esters (<70%): coniferyl benzoate; **Volatile Fraction:** Carboxylic Acids: benzoic acid (up to 20%), cinnamic acid (<10%), hydroxyoleanic acid; Esters (<9%): cinnamyl benzoate & cinnamoate (<7%), propyl cinnamoate, benzyl cinnamate (tr.); Aldehydes: vanillin aldehyde; Alcohols: benzoresinol, siaresinotannol.

Properties: Anti-inflammatory, antiseptic, antioxidant, astringent, deodorant, diuretic, expectorant, and **sedative**.

Esoteric Uses/Actions: Astrological: *Mercury & Sun*; Chakra: *1*; Character: *Yang*; Element: *Air*; Oriental: *Cold dampness (pts. Sp-9 & 6)*

Historical Uses: Onycha (or benzoin), as either a resin or an absolute, has been used for thousands of years in the east for rituals and ceremonies as either incense or for anointings. It is mentioned in the Bible as one of the ingredients for an "Holy Anointing Oil" (Exodus 30:34). The Chinese used it for its heating and drying qualities and in the west it was used for respiratory complaints.

Other Possible Uses: This oil may help **arthritis, asthma, bleeding** (slow or stop), **bronchitis, chills, circulation** (poor), **colic, cuts, flatulence** (gas), **flu, gout, laryngitis, mucus** (helps remove), **nervous tension, rheumatism, skin** (lesions; chapped, inflamed, and irritated conditions), **stomach** (gripping pains), **stress** related conditions, **urinary tract infection**, and **wounds**. It is very **warming** which makes it good for **colds, coughs**, and **sore throats**.

Body System(s) Affected: Cardiovascular System, Emotional Balance, Skin.

Aromatic Influence: Onycha is **warming** and **soothing** to the **heart**. According to Marguerite Maury, "This essence creates a kind of euphoria; it interposes a padded zone between us and events." It may also help overcome **sadness, loneliness, depression**, and **anxiety**. When combined with rose, it can be very **comforting** and **uplifting**.

Application: Apply to **Vita Flex Points** and/or directly on **area** of concern; **Massage** (combine with rose and add to V-6 Mixing Oil). Because of its thick, resinous nature, thin heavily with lavender or peppermint oils for diffusion.

Oral Use As Dietary Supplement: Approved by the FDA for use as a Food Additive (FA) and Flavoring Agent (FL). *Dilute one drop oil in 1 tsp. honey or 4 oz. of beverage (i.e. soy/rice milk). Not for children under 6 years old; use with caution and in greater dilution for children 6 years old and over.*

Blend Classification: Enhancer and Equalizer

Blends With: Coriander, cypress, frankincense, jasmine, juniper, lemon, myrrh, rose, sandalwood, and other spice oils.

Odor: Type: *Base Note (5-20% of the blend)*; Scent: *Rich, warm, slightly woody, creamy, vanilla-like*; Intensity: *1*

ORANGE
(Citrus sinensis)

Botanical Family: Rutaceae (citrus)

Extraction Method/Origin: Cold pressed from rind. — USA, South Africa, Italy, China

Chemical Constituents: Monoterpenes (up to 95%): d-limonene (<90%), terpinolene, myrcene, α-pinene; Tetraterpenes (<8%): β-carotene (<6%), lycopene; Aldehydes (<8%): citral, decanal, citronellal, dodecanal, nonanal, octanal, α-sinensal; Alcohols (<6%): linalol, cis& trans-carveol, α-terpineol, geraniol; Ketones (<4%): l- & d-carvone (<3%), α-ionone; Esters (<3%): citronellyl acetate, geranyl acetate, linalyl acetate, methyl anthranilate; Furanoids: auraptene, bergaptole, imperatarine; Sesquiterpene Ketones: nootkatone.

Properties: **Anti-depressant, antiseptic, antispasmodic, digestive, sedative**, and **tonic**.

Folklore: According to Roberta Wilson, "From early times, oranges have been associated with generosity and gratitude. Once called 'golden apples', oranges symbolized innocence and fertility."

Esoteric Uses/Actions: Astrological: *Sun*; Ayurvedic: *Vata*; Body type: *Endomorph*; Chakra: *2*; Character: *Yin*; Element: *Fire*; Number: *1*

Historical Uses: Oranges, particularly the bitter orange, has been used for palpitation, scurvy, jaundice, bleeding, heartburn, relaxed throat, prolapse of the uterus and the anus, diarrhea, and blood in the feces.

French Medicinal Uses: **Angina** (false), **cardiac spasm, constipation, diarrhea** (chronic), **dyspepsia** (nervous), **insomnia, menopause, palpitation**.

Other Possible Uses: This oil may help **appetite, bones** (rickety), **bronchitis, colds, colic** (dilute for infants; helps them sleep), **complexion** (dull and oily), **dermatitis, digestive system, fever, flu**, lowers **high cholesterol, mouth ulcers, muscle soreness, obesity, sedation, tissue repair, water retention**, and **wrinkles**.

Body System(s) Affected: **Digestive** and **Immune Systems, Emotional Balance, Skin**.

Aromatic Influence: Orange brings **peace** and **happiness** to the **mind** and **body** and **joy** to the **heart**, which provide **emotional** support to help one overcome depression.

Application: Apply to **Vita Flex Points** and directly on **area** of concern; **Diffuse**.

Oral Use As Dietary Supplement: Generally regarded as safe (GRAS) for internal consumption by the FDA. ***Dilute** one drop oil in 1 tsp. honey or 4 oz. of beverage (i.e. soy/rice milk). **Not** for children under 6 years old; use with **caution** and in **greater dilution** for children 6 years old and over.*

Safety Data: *Avoid direct **sunlight** for up to 12 hours after use.*

Blend Classification: Enhancer and Personifier

Blends With: Cinnamon bark, frankincense, geranium, juniper, lavender, nutmeg, rosewood.

Odor: Type: *Top Note (5-20% of the blend)*; Scent: *Fresh, citrusy, fruity, sweet*; Intensity: 1

OREGANO

(Origanum compactum, CT Carvacrol)

Botanical Family: Labiatae

Extraction Method/Origin: Steam distilled from leaves — Morocco, France

Chemical Constituents: Phenols (up to 80%): carvacrol (<75%), thymol (<5%), terpinen-4-ol; Monoterpenes (<25%): p-cymene (<10%), γ-terpinene (<9%), myrcene (<3%), α and β-pinenes, camphene, l-limonene, α-terpinene; Sesquiterpenes (<6%): β-caryophyllene (<5%), β-bisabolene; Carboxylic Acids: rosmaric acid (<5%); Esters: linalyl acetate (<4%); Ketones: camphor, d-carvone; Alcohols: borneol, linalol, α-terpineol.

Properties: **Anti-bacterial, anti-fungal, anti-parasitic, antiseptic** to the respiratory system, **anti-viral**, and **immune-stimulant**.

Esoteric Uses/Actions: Astrological: *Mercury*; Chakra: *4*; Character: *Yang*; Element: *Air*; Number: *9*

French Medicinal Uses: **Asthma, bronchitis** (chronic), **mental disease, pulmonary tuberculosis, rheumatism** (chronic), **whooping cough**.

Other Possible Uses: This oil may help **colds, digestion problems**, balance **metabolism**, viral and bacterial **pneumonia**, and strengthen **vital centers**.

Body System(s) Affected: **Immune** and **Respiratory Systems, Muscles and Bones**.

Aromatic Influence: Strengthens one's feeling of **security**.

Application: Apply to **Vita Flex Points** and directly on **area** of concern; **Diffuse**.

Oral Use As Dietary Supplement: Generally regarded as safe (GRAS) for internal consumption by the FDA. ***Dilute** one drop oil in 1 tsp. honey or 4 oz. of beverage (i.e. soy/rice milk). **Not** for children under 6 years old; use with **caution** and in **greater dilution** for children 6 years old and over.*

Safety Data: *Can cause extreme **skin irritation**.*

Blend Classification: Enhancer and Equalizer

Blends With: Basil, fennel, geranium, lemongrass, myrtle, pine, thyme, rosemary.

Odor: Type: *Middle Note (50-80% of the blend)*; Scent: *Herbaceous, sharp*; Intensity: 5

PALMAROSA
(Cymbopogon martinii)

Botanical Family: Graminaceae

Extraction Method/Origin: Steam distilled from leaves — India, Conoros

Chemical Constituents: Alcohols (up to 90%): geraniol (<85%), linalol, nerol, citronellol (tr.), farnesol (tr.); Esters (<30%): geranyl formate, acetate, & isovalerate (<27%); Monoterpenes: d-limonene; Oxides: geranyl epoxide; Sesquiterpene Alcohols: elemol.

Properties: Anti-bacterial, anti-fungal, antimicrobial, antiseptic, anti-viral, hydrating, stimulant (digestive and circulatory), and **tonic**.

Folklore: Once known as Turkish Geranium oil or Indian Geranium oil, palmarosa was used for centuries by the Turks to adulterate the more costly Turkish Rose oil.

Esoteric Uses/Actions: Astrological: *Venus*; Body type: *Mesomorph*; Character: *Yang with high Yin*; Crystals: *Lapis Lazuli*; Element: *Water & Air*; Number: *2*

Historical Uses: Used to prevent infections and fight fever, palmarosa was also added to many culinary dishes to kill bacteria and aid digestion.

Other Possible Uses: This oil may be beneficial for **candida, circulation, digestion, fever, infection, nervous system**, and **rashes**. It is valuable for all types of **skin** problems because it stimulates new cell growth, regulates oil production, moisturizes and speeds healing.

Body System(s) Affected: Cardiovascular System, Emotional Balance, Skin.

Aromatic Influence: Strengthens one's feeling of **security**. It also helps to reduce **stress** and **tension**, and promotes recovery from **nervous exhaustion**. If uplifts the **emotions**, refreshes the **mind**, and clarifies **thoughts**. Inhaling palmarosa may also have a normalizing effect on the **thyroid gland**.

Application: Apply to **Vita Flex Points** and directly on **area** of concern; **Diffuse**.

Oral Use As Dietary Supplement: Generally regarded as safe (GRAS) for internal consumption by the FDA. ***Dilute*** *one drop oil in 1 tsp. honey or 4 oz. of beverage (i.e. soy/rice milk).* ***Not for children under 6 years old; use with*** *caution and in* ***greater dilution*** *for children 6 years old and over.*

Blend Classification: Enhancer and Equalizer.

Blends With: Basil, fennel, geranium, lemongrass, myrtle, pine, thyme, rosemary.

Odor: Type: *Top to Middle Notes (20-80% of the blend)*; Scent: *Lemony, fresh, green, with hints of rose and geranium*; Intensity: *3*

PALO SANTO ("HOLY WOOD")
(Bursera graveolens)

Botanical Family: Burseraceae (resinous trees and shrubs)

Extraction Method/Origin: Steam distilled from wood chips of dead heartwood — Ecuador.
Note: The wood must be dead for at least 2 years before the oil is pulled into the heartwood.

The wood must be cut into sawdust to get at the oil (9 kg of sawdust to produce 500 ml of oil). Also, this oil is distilled from the red wood that produced a much better quality oil.

Chemical Constituents: Monoterpenes: d-limonene (75-76%), α-pinene; Alcohols: α-terpineol; Sesquiterpenes: eudesmene; Ketones: carvone (<4%); Furanoids: menthofuran, agarofuran; Phenols: carvacrol, terpinen-4-ol; Sesquiterpene Alcohols: eudesmol.

Properties: Anti-infectious, antiseptic, antitumoral, immune-stimulant, and **sedative**.

Historical Uses: Palo Santo (also known as Holy Wood) is a natural wood aromatic incense. It has been used for centuries by the indigenous peoples of the Amazon in rituals and ceremonies for the purifying and cleansing of evil spirits, misfortune and calamity.

Other Possible Uses: This oil may help with **cancer, healing, muscle pain, nervous** conditions, acute **rheumatism**, and **spiritual awareness**.

Body System(s) Affected: Emotional Balance, Immune and **Nervous Systems**.

Aromatic Influence: It has a wonderfully **calming**, **soothing** aroma with a **powerful energy**. It may help to increase **spiritual awareness** and focus **meditation** while **clearing** the space of **negative energy**.

Application: Apply to **Vita Flex Points** and/or directly on **area** of concern; **Diffuse**. Some say that because it is a shamanic oil, the user must have a firm intention in mind before applying this oil to the **forehead** (3rd eye chakra) so that the oil can change the energy both inside and outside the person to assist in the fulfillment of that intention.

Blend Classification: Enhancer and Equalizer

Blends With: Benzoin, frankincense, myrrh, and sandalwood.

Odor: Type: *Base Note (5-20% of the blend)*; Scent: *Rich, citrusy, balsamic, sweet, with incense-like overtones*; Intensity: *4*

Frequency: High (Spiritual)

PATCHOULI (or PATCHOULY)
(Pogostemon cablin)

Botanical Family: Labiatae (mint)

Extraction Method/Origin: Steam distilled from leaves and flowers — Sumatra, Java, Malaysia, China, Brazil, Indonesia

Chemical Constituents: Sesquiterpenes (up to 63%): α-bulnesene (<20%), β-bulnesene (<16%), aromadendrene (<15%), α-gaiene (>12%), seychellene (6%), α-, β- & γ-patchoulenes (<12%), β-caryophyllene (<4%), δ-cadinene (<3%), β-gaiene, β-elemene, humulene; Sesquiterpene Alcohols (<38%): patchoulol (up to 35%), pogostol, bulnesol, guaiol, patchoulenol; Oxides (<5%): bulnesene oxide, caryophyllene oxide, guaiene oxide; Ketones: patchoulenone (<3%); Monoterpenes: α- & β-pinenes, l-limonene.

Properties: Anti-infectious, anti-inflammatory, anti-fungal, antiseptic, antitoxic, astringent, decongestant, deodorant, diuretic, insecticidal, stimulant (digestive), and **tonic**.

Esoteric Uses/Actions: Astrological: *Sun*; Body type: *Endomorph*; Chakras: *1 & 2*; Character: *Yang*; Crystals: *Green tourmaline, Black obsidian*; Element: *Fire & Earth*; Number: *1*

Historical Uses: For centuries, the Asian people used patchouli to fight infection, cool fevers, tone the skin (and entire body), and as an antidote for insect and snake bites. It was also used to treat colds, headaches, nausea, vomiting, diarrhea, abdominal pain, and halitosis (bad breath).

French Medicinal Uses: Allergies, dermatitis, eczema, hemorrhoids, tissue regeneration.

Other Possible Uses: This oil is a **digester** of **toxic material** in the body. It may also help **acne, appetite** (curbs), **bites** (**insect** and **snake**), **cellulite, congestion, dandruff, depression, digestive system**, relieve itching from **hives, skin conditions** (chapped and tightens loose skin), **UV radiation** (protects against), **water retention, weeping wounds, weight reduction**, and prevent **wrinkles**.

Body System(s) Affected: Skin.

Aromatic Influence: It is **sedating, calming**, and **relaxing** allowing it to reduce **anxiety**. It may have some particular influence on **sex, physical energy**, and **money**.

Application: Apply to **Vita Flex Points** and directly on **area** of concern; **Diffuse**.

Oral Use As Dietary Supplement: Approved by the FDA for use as a Food Additive (FA) and Flavoring Agent (FL). ***Dilute*** one drop oil in 1 tsp. honey or 4 oz. of beverage (i.e. soy/rice milk). *Not for children under 6 years old; use with **caution** and in **greater dilution** for children 6 years old and over.*

Blend Classification: Enhancer

Blends With: Bergamot, Clary sage, frankincense, geranium, ginger, lavender, lemongrass, myrrh, pine, rosewood, sandalwood.

Odor: Type: *Base Note (5-20% of the blend)*; Scent: *Earthy, herbaceous, sweet-balsamic, rich, with woody undertones*; Intensity: *4*

PEPPER, BLACK
(Piper nigrum)

Botanical Family: Piperaceae

Extraction Method/Origin: Steam distilled from berries — Egypt, India, Madagascar

Chemical Constituents: Monoterpenes (up to 70%): l-limonene (<15%), δ-3-carene (<15%), β-pinene (<14%), sabinene (<10%), α-phellandrene (<9%), α-pinene (<9%), α-thujene (<4%), γ- & α-terpinene (<7%), p-cymene (<3%), myrcene (<3%), terpinolene (<2%); Sesquiterpenes (up to 60%): β-caryophyllene (up to 35%), β-selinene (<8%), β-bisabolene (<5%), α-, β-, & δ-elemenes, β-farnesene, humulene, α-copaene, α-guaiene, α- & β-cubebenes; Oxides: caryophyllene oxide (<8%); Ketones (<2%): acetophenone, hydrocarvone, piperitone; Aldehydes: piperonal; Carboxylic Acids: piperonylic acid; Furanocoumarin: α-bergamotene.

Properties: Analgesic, anti-catarrhal, anti-inflammatory, antiseptic, antispasmodic, antitoxic, aphrodisiac, expectorant, laxative, rubefacient, and **stimulant** (nervous, circulatory, digestive),.

Folklore: Pepper was used by the Egyptians in mummification as evidenced by the discovery of Black pepper in the nostrils and abdomen of Ramses II. Indian monks ate several Black pepper corns a day to maintain their incredible stamina and energy.

Esoteric Uses/Actions: Astrological: *Mars*; Body type: *Mesomorph*; Chakras: *3, 4, & 1*; Character: *Yang*; Crystals: *Malachite, Bloodstone*; Element: *Fire*; Number: *2*

Historical Uses: Pepper has been used for thousands of years for malaria, cholera, and several digestive problems.

Other Possible Uses: This oil may increase **cellular oxygenation**, support **digestive glands**, stimulate **endocrine system**, increase **energy**, and help **rheumatoid arthritis**. It may also help with loss of **appetite, catarrh, chills, cholera, colds, colic, constipation, coughs, diarrhea, dysentery, dyspepsia, dysuria, flatulence** (combine with fennel), **flu, heartburn, influenza, nausea, neuralgia, poor circulation, poor muscle tone, quinsy, sprains, toothache, vertigo, viruses**, and **vomiting**.

Body System(s) Affected: **Digestive** and **Nervous Systems**.

Aromatic Influence: Pepper is considered to be good for the **1st chakra**. It is **comforting** and **stimulating**.

Application: Apply to **Vita Flex Points** and/or directly on **area** of concern; **Diffuse**. Mix very sparingly with juniper and lavender in a **bath** to help with **chills** or warm one up in the winter.

Oral Use As Dietary Supplement: Generally regarded as safe (GRAS) for internal consumption by the FDA. **Dilute** one drop oil in 1 tsp. honey or 4 oz. of beverage (i.e. soy/rice milk). **Not for children under 6 years old; use with caution and in greater dilution for children 6 years old and over.**

Safety Data: *Can cause extreme skin irritation.*

Blends With: Cumin, fennel, frankincense, lavender, marjoram, rosemary, sandalwood, and other spice oils.

Odor: Type: *Middle Note (50-80% of the blend)*; Scent: *Spicy, peppery, musky, warm, with herbaceous undertones*; Intensity: *3*

PEPPER, PINK (or BRAZILIAN PEPPERTREE)
(Schinus molle)

Botanical Family: Anacardiaceae

Extraction Method/Origin: Steam distilled from leaves — South America

Chemical Constituents: Monoterpenes: α- & β-pinenes, camphene, phellandrene; Sesquiterpenes: caryophyllene, and others; Phenols: carvacrol.

Properties: **Anti-bacterial, anti-fungal** (especially candida)**, anti-inflammatory, anti-tumoral, anti-viral, antimicrobial, antispasmodic, astringent, diuretic, stimulant** (digestive), **tonic,** and **wound healer**.

Historical Uses: According to Leslie Taylor, ND, "Virtually all parts of this tropical tree, including its leaves, bark, fruit, seeds, resin, and oleoresin (or balsam) have been used medicinally by indigenous peoples throughout the tropics."

Other Possible Uses: This oil may help with **bronchitis, gingivitis, gonorrhea, gout, heart problems** (hypertension and irregular heart beat), **inflammation** (general), **menstrual disorders** (excessive bleeding), **pain relief, rheumatism, sores, swellings, tuberculosis, tumors, ulcers, urethritis, urogenital disorders, venereal diseases, warts,** and **wounds**. According to Leslie Taylor, ND, "More recently, in 2002, researchers in Argentina documented that it was toxic in vitro against a human liver cancer cell line."

Body System(s) Affected: Immune and **Respiratory Systems, Skin**.

Application: Apply to **Vita Flex Points** and/or directly on **area** of concern.

Oral Use As Dietary Supplement: Generally regarded as safe (GRAS) for internal consumption by the FDA. **Dilute** *one drop oil in 1 tsp. honey or 4 oz. of beverage (i.e. soy/rice milk). Not for children under 6 years old; use with **caution** and in **greater dilution** for children 6 years old and over.*

Safety Data: *Avoid during* **pregnancy**.

PEPPERMINT
(Mentha piperita)

Botanical Family: Labiatae (mint)

Extraction Method/Origin: Steam distilled from leaves, stems, flower buds — North America

Chemical Constituents: Phenolic Alcohols (up to 44%): menthol (<44%), piperitols; Ketones (<25%): menthone (20-30% and up to 65% if distilled in September when flowering), pulegone (<5%), piperitone (<2%), carvone, jasmone; Monoterpenes (< 15%): α and β-pinenes (<6%), l-limonene (<6%), ocimene, myrcene, p-cymene, β-phellandrene, sabinene, α-terpinene, terpinolene, camphene; Sesquiterpenes (<10%): germacrene-D (<5%), β-bourbonene, ζ-bulgarene, γ-cadinene, β-caryophyllene, β-elemene, β-farnesene, muurolene; Esters (<9%): menthyl acetate (<9%), also menthyl butyrate & isovalerate; Oxides (<9%): 1,8 cineol (<5%), piperitone oxide, caryophyllene oxide; Furanoids: menthofuran (<8%); Phenols: terpinen-4-ol (<3%); Alcohols (<3%): α-terpineol, linalol; Sesquiterpene Alcohols: viridiflorol; Furanocoumarins: aesculetine; Sulphides: mint sulfide, di-menthyl sulfide.

Properties: Analgesic, anticarcinogenic, anti-inflammatory (prostate and nerves), **antiseptic, antispasmodic,** and **invigorating**.

Folklore: According to Roberta Wilson, "In Roman mythology, when Pluto professed his love for the nymph Mentha, his wife Persephone, afire with jealousy, crushed Mentha into dust on the ground. Pluto, unable to change her back, transformed her into a peppermint plant and gave her a fresh fragrance so she would smell sweet whenever stepped upon."

Esoteric Uses/Actions: Astrological: *Mercury & Venus*; Ayurvedic: *Pitta*; Chakras: *7, 2, & 6*; Character: *Yang*; Crystals: *Topaz, Chalcedony*; Element: *Air*

Historical Uses: For centuries, peppermint has been used to soothe digestive difficulties, freshen breath, and relieve colic, gas, headaches, heartburn, and indigestion.

French Medicinal Uses: Asthma, bronchitis, candida, diarrhea, digestive aid, fever (reduces), **flu, halitosis, heartburn, hemorrhoids, hot flashes, indigestion, menstrual irregularity, migraine headache, motion sickness, nausea, respiratory function** (aids), **shock, skin** (itchy), **throat infection, varicose veins, vomiting**.

Other Possible Uses: This oil may help **anger, arthritis, colic, depression, fatigue, food poisoning, headaches, hives, hysteria, inflammation, liver problems, morning sickness, nerves** (regenerate and support), **rheumatism**, elevate and open **sensory system**, soothe and cool **skin** (may help keep body cooler on hot days), **toothaches, tuberculosis**, and add flavor to **water**.

Body System(s) Affected: Digestive System, Muscles and Bones, Nervous and **Respiratory Systems, Skin**.

Aromatic Influence: It is **purifying** and **stimulating** to the **conscious mind**. Reduces **fevers**. Dr. Dembar of the University of Cincinnati discovered in a research study that inhaling peppermint oil **increased** the **mental accuracy** of the students by up to 28%.

Application: Apply to **Vita Flex Points** and/or directly on **area** of concern.

Oral Use As Dietary Supplement: Generally regarded as safe (GRAS) for internal consumption by the FDA. *Dilute one drop oil in 1 tsp. honey or 4 oz. of beverage (i.e. soy/rice milk). Not for children under 6 years old; use with **caution** and in **greater dilution** for children 6 years old and over.*

Safety Data: *Repeated use can possibly result in **contact sensitization**. Use with caution if dealing with **high blood pressure**. Use with caution during **pregnancy**.*

Blend Classification: Personifier

Odor: Type: *Middle Note (50-80% of the blend)*; Scent: *Minty, sharp, intense*; Intensity: *5*

Frequency: Physical; approximately 78.

PETITGRAIN
(Citrus aurantium)

Botanical Family: Rutaceae (citrus)

Extraction Method/Origin: Steam distilled from bitter orange tree leaves — Italy

Chemical Constituents: Esters (up to 65%): linalyl acetate (<55%), geranyl acetate (<5%), neryl & α-terpenyl acetates, methyl anthranilate; Alcohols (40%): linalol (<28%), α-terpineol (<8%), geraniol (<5%), nerol, citronellol; Monoterpenes (<28%): myrcene (<6%), β-cymene (<5%), cis- & trans-ocimenes (<5%), p-cymene (<3%), β-pinene, γ-terpinene, d-limonene, phellandrene, sabinene, terpinolene; Aldehydes: decanal, geranial, neral; Phenols: thymol, terpinen-4-ol; Furanocoumarins: bergaptene, citroptene.

Properties: Anti-bacterial, anti-infectious, anti-inflammatory, antiseptic, antispasmodic, deodorant, nervine, and **stimulant** (digestive, nervous).

Folklore: Petitgrain derives its name from the extraction of the oil, which at one time was from the green unripe oranges when they were still about the size of a cherry.

Esoteric Uses/Actions: Astrological: *Jupiter, Mars & Sun*; Body type: *Mesomorph*; Chakras: *2 & 4*; Character: *Yin?*; Element: *Fire*; Number: *1*

Historical Uses: Because of its very pleasing scent, petitgrain has been used extensively in high-quality perfumes and cosmetics.

Other Possible Uses: This oil may help re-establish **nerve equilibrium**. It may also help with **acne, dyspepsia, fatigue, flatulence, greasy hair, insomnia**, and excessive **perspiration**.

Body System(s) Affected: Emotional Balance.

Aromatic Influence: It is **uplifting** and **refreshing** and helps to refresh the **senses**, clear **confusion**, reduce **mental fatigue**, and reduce **depression**. It may also stimulate the **mind**, support **memory**, and gladden the **heart**.

Application: Apply to **Vita Flex Points** and directly on **area** of concern; **Diffuse**.

Oral Use As Dietary Supplement: Generally regarded as safe (GRAS) for internal consumption by the FDA. ***Dilute*** *one drop oil in 1 tsp. honey or 4 oz. of beverage (i.e. soy/rice milk).* ***Not for children under 6 years old; use with*** *caution* ***and in*** *greater dilution* ***for children 6 years old and over.***

Blend Classification: Enhancer, Modifier, and Personifier

Blends With: Bergamot, cistus, Clary sage, clove, geranium, jasmine, lavender, neroli, orange, palmarosa, and rosemary.

Odor: Type: *Top Note (5-20% of the blend)*; Scent: *Fresh, floral, citrusy, lighter in fragrance than neroli and slightly woody*; Intensity: *3*

PINE (or SCOTCH PINE)
(Pinus sylvestris)

Botanical Family: Pinaceae (conifer)

Extraction Method/Origin: Steam distilled from needles — Austria, Canada, Russia

Chemical Constituents: Monoterpenes (up to 80%): α-pinene (>41%), δ-3-carene (<17%), l-limonene (<16%), β-pinene (<15%), camphene, β-phellandrene, terpinolene, ocimene, p-cymene, γ-terpinene, sabinene; Sesquiterpenes (<12%): β-caryophyllene (<6%), γ-cadinene (<5%), α-copaene, β-guaiene, longifolene, muurolene; Alcohols: borneol (2%); Esters: bornyl acetate (<3%); Sesquiterpene Alcohols: α-cadinol, muurolol; Diterpenes: cembrene; Aldehydes: citronellal; Phenols: terpinen-4-ol.

Properties: Anti-bacterial, antimicrobial, anti-neuralgic, antiseptic (pulmonary, urinary, hepatic), **anti-viral, expectorant**, and **stimulant** (adrenal cortex, circulatory, nervous).

Folklore: In some cultures, pine branches were placed on coffins to signify immortality.

Esoteric Uses/Actions: Astrological: *Mars*; Body type: *Ectomorph*; Chakra: *6*; Character: *Yang*; Crystal: *Malachite*; Element: *Air & Light*; Number: *3*

Historical Uses: Pine was used by the American Indians to prevent scurvy. They also stuffed mattresses with pine to repel lice and fleas. It was used to treat pneumonia and lung infections and was even added to baths to revitalize people suffering from mental or emotional fatigue and nervous exhaustion.

French Medicinal Uses: Asthma, bronchitis, diabetes, infections (severe), **rheumatoid arthritis, sinusitis**.

Other Possible Uses: This oil may help dilate and open the **respiratory system**, particularly the **bronchial tract**. It may also help with **colds, coughs, cuts, cystitis, fatigue, feet** (excessive sweating), **flu, gout, lice, nervous exhaustion, scabies, skin parasites, sores, stress**, and **urinary infection**. Pine oil may also help increase **blood pressure** and **stimulate** the **adrenal glands** and the **circulatory system**. Pine is a good recommendation for any First Aid kit.

Body System(s) Affected: Emotional Balance, Respiratory System.

Aromatic Influence: It helps soothe **mental stress**, relieve **anxiety, freshen** and **deodorize** a room, and **revitalize** the entire body.

Application: Apply to **Vita Flex Points** and/or directly on **area** of concern; **Diffuse**. Pine is an excellent tonic when added to water and sprinkled on hot rocks in the **sauna**.

Oral Use As Dietary Supplement: Approved by the FDA for use as a Food Additive (FA) and Flavoring Agent (FL). **Dilute** one drop oil in 1 tsp. honey or 4 oz. of beverage (i.e. soy/rice milk). *Not for children under 6 years old; use with **caution** and in **greater dilution** for children 6 years old and over.*

Safety Data: *Repeated use can possibly result in **skin irritation**.*

Blends With: Cedarwood, eucalyptus, juniper, lemon, marjoram, melaleuca, and rosemary.

Odor: Type: *Middle Note (50-80% of the blend)*; Scent: *Fresh, woody, earthly, balsamic*; Intensity: *4*

RAVENSARA
(Ravensara aromatica)

Botanical Family: Lauraceae

Extraction Method/Origin: Steam distilled from leaves and branches — Madagascar

Chemical Constituents: Oxides: 1,8-cineol (up to 61%); Monoterpenes (<32%): sabinene (<15%), α and β-pinenes (<14%), l-limonene (<4%); Alcohols: α-terpineol (<7%); Phenols: terpinen-4-ol; Esters: α-terpenyl acetate; Sesquiterpenes: β-caryophyllene.

Properties: Anti-bacterial, anti-fungal, anti-infectious, antiseptic, powerful **antiviral**, and **expectorant**.

French Medicinal Uses: Bronchitis, cholera, herpes, infectious mononucleosis, insomnia, muscle fatigue, rhino pharyngitis, shingles, sinusitis, viral hepatitis.

Other Possible Uses: Ravensara is part of the Laurel family (akin to *Laurus nobilis*) and is another universal oil like lavender. It may help **asthma, bladder, bunions, burns** (healing), **cancer, colds, cuts, ears, flu, liver, lungs**, support the **nerves, pneumonia, scrapes,**

viral infections, and **wounds**. As a cross between clove and nutmeg, it may be very supportive to the **adrenal glands**.

Body System(s) Affected: Immune and **Respiratory Systems**.

Application: Apply to **Vita Flex Points** and/or directly on **area** of concern; **Diffuse**.

Blend Classification: Enhancer

Odor: Type: *Top Note (5-20% of the blend)*; Scent: *Slightly medicinal, eucalyptus-like, slightly sweet with a fruity hint*; Intensity: *3*

Frequency: High (Spiritual); approximately 134 MHz.

ROMAN CHAMOMILE
(See CHAMOMILE, ROMAN)

ROSALINA
(See MELALEUCA ERICIFOLIA)

ROSE (or BULGARIAN ROSE)
(Rosa damascena)

Botanical Family: Rosaceae

Extraction Method/Origin: Steam distilled from flowers (a two-part process) — Bulgaria, Turkey

Chemical Constituents: Alcohols (up to 70%): citronellol (up to 45%), geraniol (up to 28%), nerol (<9%), linalol, borneol, α-terpineol; Monoterpenes (<25%): stearoptene (<22%), α & β-pinenes, camphene, α-terpinene, l-limonene, myrcene, p-cymene, ocimene; Alkanes (<19%): nonadecane (<15%), octadecane, eicosane, and others; Esters (<5%): geranyl, neryl, & citronellyl acetates; Phenols (<4%): eugenol, phenylethanol; Sesquiterpene Alcohols: farnesol (<2%); Oxides: rose oxide; Ketones: α- & β-damascenone, β-ionone; Furanoids: rosefuran; Many other trace elements.

Properties: Anti-hemorrhaging, anti-infectious, and **aphrodisiac**.

Esoteric Uses/Actions: Astrological: *Venus*; Ayurvedic: *Pitta*; Body type: *Mesomorph*; Chakras: *2, 4, 6, & 7 (balances all)*; Character: *Yin; Cold and Dry in 2nd Degree*; Crystals: *Ruby (Chakra-2), Rose Quartz, Emerald (Chakra-4), Kunzite, Pink Calcite, Watermelon Tourmaline (Chakra-7)*; Element: *Water, Air, Light, & Ether*; Number: *6*; Oriental: *Yin deficiency (pts. Kid-6, Sp-6); Excess Yang (heat), (pts. Liv-2, He-3)*

Historical Uses: The healing properties of the rose have been utilized in medicine throughout the ages and still plays an important role in the East. It has been used for digestive and menstrual problems, headaches and nervous tension, liver congestion, poor circulation, fever (plague), eye infections, and skin complaints.

Other Possible Uses: This oil may help **asthma**, chronic **bronchitis, frigidity, gingivitis, hemorrhaging, herpes simplex, impotence, infections**, prevent **scarring, sexual**

debilities, **skin disease, sprains, thrush, tuberculosis, ulcers, wounds**, and **wrinkles**.

Body System(s) Affected: Emotional Balance, Skin.

Aromatic Influence: It is **stimulating** and **elevating** to the **mind**, creating a sense of **well being**. Its beautiful fragrance is almost intoxicating and **aphrodisiac-like**.

Application: Apply to **Vita Flex Points** and/or directly on **area** of concern; **Diffuse**.

Oral Use As Dietary Supplement: Generally regarded as safe (GRAS) for internal consumption by the FDA. **Dilute** *one drop oil in 1 tsp. honey or 4 oz. of beverage (i.e. soy/rice milk).* **Not** *for children under 6 years old; use with* **caution** *and in* **greater dilution** *for children 6 years old and over.*

Safety Data: *Use with caution during* **pregnancy.**

Blend Classification: Personifier, Enhancer, Equalizer, and Modifier.

Odor: Type: *Middle to Base Notes (20-80% of the blend)*; Scent: *Floral, spicy, rich, deep, sensual, green, honey-like*; Intensity: *3*

Frequency: Highest of all the oils (Spiritual); approximately 320 MHz. It enhances the frequency of every cell, bringing balance and harmony to the body.

ROSEHIP
(Rosa canina)

Botanical Family: Rosaceae

Properties: Regenerative

Possible Uses: Rosehip oil has been used effectively in the treatment of **skin conditions**. It promotes **tissue regeneration**, and may help heal **burns**, reduce **scarring**, retard **premature aging**, and soften **scar tissue**.

Application: Apply directly on **area** of concern.

Oral Use As Dietary Supplement: Generally regarded as safe (GRAS) for internal consumption by the FDA. **Dilute** *one drop oil in 1 tsp. honey or 4 oz. of beverage (i.e. soy/rice milk).* **Not** *for children under 6 years old; use with* **caution** *and in* **greater dilution** *for children 6 years old and over.*

ROSEMARY CINEOL
(Rosmarinus officinalis, CT 1,8 Cineol)

Botanical Family: Labiatae (mint)

Extraction Method/Origin: Steam distilled from flowering plant — France, Tunisia, USA

Chemical Constituents: Oxides: 1,8 cineol (up to 55%), caryophyllene oxide, humulene oxide; Monoterpenes: α-pinene (<14%), β-pinene (<9%), camphene (<8%), l-limonene, myrcene, p-cymene, α- & β-phellandrenes, α- & γ-terpinenes; Ketones (<32%): camphor (<30%), β-thujone, verbenone, d-carvone, hexanone, heptanone; Alcohols (<20%): borneol (<12%), α-terpineol (<5%), linalol, verbenol; Sesquiterpenes (<3%): β-caryophyllene, humulene; Phenols: terpinen-4-ol; Esters: bornyl & fenchyl acetates; Acids: rosemaric acid.

Properties: Anti-bacterial, anti-catarrhal, anti-infectious, and **expectorant**.

Esoteric Uses/Actions: Astrological: *Sun*; Body type: *Mesomorph*; Chakras: *3 & 6*; Character: *Yang*; Crystals: *Quartz Crystal, Sugalite*; Element: *Fire & Light*; Number: *6*

Historical Uses: The rosemary plant was regarded as sacred by many civilizations. It was used as a fumigant to help drive away evil spirits, and to protect against plague and infectious illness.

French Medicinal Uses: Arthritis, blood pressure (low), **bronchitis, cellulite, cholera, colds, dandruff, depression** (nervous), **diabetes, fatigue** (nervous/mental), **flu, fluid retention, hair loss, headache, hepatitis** (viral), **menstrual periods** (irregular), **sinusitis, tachycardia, vaginitis**.

Other Possible Uses: This oil may help **arteriosclerosis, bronchitis, chills, colds, colitis, cystitis, dyspepsia**, nervous **exhaustion, flu**, oily **hair, immune system** (stimulate), **otitis, palpitations**, prevent **respiratory infections, sinusitis**, sour **stomach, stress-related illness**. *Note: This chemotype is said to be best used for* **pulmonary congestion,** *slow* **elimination, candida,** *chronic* **fatigue,** *and* **infections** *(especially staph and strep).*

Body System(s) Affected: Immune, Respiratory, and **Nervous Systems**.

Aromatic Influence: Stimulates **memory** and opens the **conscious mind**.

Application: Apply to **Vita Flex Points** and/or directly on **area** of concern; **Diffuse**.

Oral Use As Dietary Supplement: Generally regarded as safe (GRAS) for internal consumption by the FDA. **Dilute** *one drop oil in 1 tsp. honey or 4 oz. of beverage (i.e. soy/rice milk).* **Not** *for children under 6 years old; use with* **caution** *and in* **greater dilution** *for children 6 years old and over.*

Safety Data: *Avoid during* **pregnancy**. *Not for use by people with* **epilepsy**. *Avoid if dealing with* **high blood pressure**.

Blend Classification: Enhancer.

Blends With: Basil, cedarwood, frankincense, lavender, peppermint, rosewood, eucalyptus, marjoram, pine.

Odor: Type: *Middle Note (50-80% of the blend)*; Scent: *Herbaceous, strong, camphorous, with woody-balsamic and evergreen undertones*; Intensity: *3*

ROSEMARY VERBENON
(Rosmarinus officinalis, CT Verbenon)

Botanical Family: Labiatae (mint)

Extraction Method/Origin: Steam distilled from flowering plant — Corsica

Chemical Constituents: Ketones (up to 50%): verbenon (<37%), camphor (<15%); Monoterpenes (<45%): α-pinene (<34%), camphene (<10%), l-limonene (<4%), β-pinene, myrcene, α-terpinene, terpinolene; Oxides: 1,8 cineol (<15%); Esters: bornyl acetate (<11%); Alcohols: borneol (<7%); Sesquiterpenes: β-caryophyllene, humulene.

Properties: Anti-bacterial, anti-catarrhal, anti-infectious, antispasmodic, cardiac regulator, **endocrine** regulator (pituitary - regulates ovaries and testicles), **expectorant, mucolytic**, and **nervous** regulator.

Esoteric Uses/Actions: (See Rosemary Cineol)

Historical Uses: (See Rosemary Cineol)

French Medicinal Uses: (See Rosemary Cineol)

Other Possible Uses: This oil may help **asthma, baldness, candida, cholesterol, circulation, gout**, balance **heart function**, support **immune system, injuries**, decongest the **liver, muscular aches/pains**, stimulate **nerves, obesity**, regulate **ovary** function, **respiratory functions, rheumatism, skin conditions**, energize **solar plexus, spinal, sprains**, regulate **testicular** function, **viruses**, and **wounds**. *Note: This chemotype is said to be best used for liver and gallbladder support, rejuvenation of skin (especially chronic dry skin), middle ear infections, and endocrine problems (regulates hypothalamic / pituitary / sexual glands).*

Body System(s) Affected: Digestive and **Hormonal Systems, Skin and Hair**.

Aromatic Influence: Stimulates **memory** and opens the **conscious mind**.

Application: Apply to **Vita Flex Points** and directly on **area** of concern; **Diffuse**.

Oral Use As Dietary Supplement: Generally regarded as safe (GRAS) for internal consumption by the FDA. *Dilute one drop oil in 1 tsp. honey or 4 oz. of beverage (i.e. soy/rice milk). Not for children under 6 years old; use with caution and in greater dilution for children 6 years old and over.*

Safety Data: *Avoid during* **pregnancy**. *Not for use by people with* **epilepsy**. *Avoid if dealing with* **high blood pressure.**

Blend Classification: Enhancer.

Blends With: Basil, eucalyptus, lavender, marjoram, peppermint, pine.

ROSEWOOD
(Aniba rosaeodora)

Botanical Family: Lauraceae

Extraction Method/Origin: Steam distilled from wood — Brazil

Chemical Constituents: Alcohols (up to 95%): linalol (<90%), α-terpineol (<7%), geraniol; Oxides (<6%): 1,8 cineol, linalol oxide; Sesquiterpenes: α-copaene; Ketones: heptanone.

Properties: Anti-bacterial, anti-fungal, anti-infectious, anti-parasitic, and **antiviral**.

Esoteric Uses/Actions: Astrological: *Sun, Venus*; Body type: *Mesomorph*; Chakras: *links 7 to 1; also 4*; Character: *Yang*; Crystals: *Rutilated smoky quartz, Apophylite (links 1st to 7th chakra)*; Element: *Earth*; Number: *3*

Historical Uses: According to Roberta Wilson, "The original site of production of *bois de rose*, as the French called rosewood, was French Guiana, on the northern coast of South America. So great was the demand among the French for rosewood oil, . . . that they depleted the colony's rosewood forests." Even now, this tropical, evergreen tree is one of the trees that is being extensively felled in the clearing of the South American rainforests.

French Medicinal Uses: Acne, candida, depression, eczema, oral infections, skin (dry), **vaginitis**.

Other Possible Uses: This oil may create **skin elasticity** and is **soothing** to the **skin**. It is recognized for its ability to get rid of **candida** of the **skin** and slow the **aging** process. It may also be beneficial for **cuts, nausea, tissue regeneration**, and **wounds**. It helps to create a synergism with all other oils.

Body System(s) Affected: Skin.

Aromatic Influence: It is **appeasing** to the **mind, relaxing** to the **body**, and creates a feeling of **peace** and **gentleness**.

Application: Apply to **Vita Flex Points** and/or directly on **area** of concern; **Diffuse**.

Oral Use As Dietary Supplement: Generally regarded as safe (GRAS) for internal consumption by the FDA. **Dilute** *one drop oil in 1 tsp. honey or 4 oz. of beverage (i.e. soy/rice milk)*. **Not** *for children under 6 years old; use with **caution** and in **greater dilution** for children 6 years old and over.*

Blend Classification: Modifier and Equalizer.

Odor: Type: *Middle Note (50-80% of the blend)*; Scent: *Sweet, woody, floral aroma*; Intensity: *3*

SAGE
(Salvia officinalis)

Botanical Family: Labiatae (mint)

Extraction Method/Origin: Steam distilled from leaves and flowers — Croatia, France, Spain

Chemical Constituents: Ketones (approx. 60%): α-thujone (<33%), camphor (<24%), β-thujone (<14%); Monoterpenes (<30%): camphene (<12%), α- & β-pinenes (<8%), l-limonene (<4%), p-cymene (<2%), myrcene, salvene, α- & β-phellandrene, sabinene, α- & γ-terpinenes, α-thujene; Alcohols (<28%): borneol (<14%), linalol (<11%), α-terpineol (<9%); Oxides: 1,8 cineol (<13%); Sesquiterpenes (<12%): β-caryophyllene (<7%), humulene (<5%), aromadendrene, α- & β-cadinenes, β-copaene, ledene, α-maalene; Sesquiterpene Alcohols: viridiflorol (<10%); Esters (<5%): bornyl, linalyl, & sabinyl acetates; Phenols: terpinen-4-ol (<4%), estragole, thymol; Diterpene Alcohols: sclareol.

Properties: Anti-bacterial, anti-cancerous, antiseptic, antispasmodic, decongestant, diuretic, and **disinfectant**. It contains estriol and has **estrogen-like properties**.

Folklore: Sage is recognized by the Lakota Indians as a purifier and as the master healer, and was called *herba sacra* or 'sacred herb' by the Romans.

Esoteric Uses/Actions: Astrological: *Jupiter*; Body type: *Ectomorph*; Chakras: *4, 2, & 3*; Character: *Yang*; Crystal: *Malachite*; Element: *Air*; Number: *7*; Perfume note: *Top*

Historical Uses: Sage has been used for respiratory infections, menstrual difficulties, digestive complaints, inflammations of the mouth, tongue, and throat, and to strengthen the senses.

French Medicinal Uses: Asthma, bronchitis (chronic), **digestion** (sluggish), **gingivitis, glandular disorders, lymphatic system, menopause, menstrual irregularity, night sweats**.

Other Possible Uses: This oil may help improve **estrogen** and **progesterone-testosterone balance**. It is believed to contain elements that contribute to the **secretion** of **progesterone-testosterone**. It activates the **nervous system** and **adrenal cortex** and may help with illness that is related to **digestion** and **liver problems**. It may also be beneficial for **acne, arthritis, bacterial infections, catarrh** (mucus), **dandruff, depression, eczema, fibrositis, hair loss, low blood pressure, mental fatigue, metabolism, respiratory problems, rheumatism, skin conditions, sores, sprains, tissue** (firms), and strengthening the **vital centers** of the body. It may also **balance** the **pelvic chakra** where negative emotions from denial and sexual abuse are stored.

Body System(s) Affected: Hormonal and **Immune Systems**.

Aromatic Influence: Helps to relieve **depression, mental fatigue**, and **strain**.

Application: Apply to **Vita Flex Points** and/or directly on **area** of concern; **Diffuse**.

Oral Use As Dietary Supplement: Generally regarded as safe (GRAS) for internal consumption by the FDA. ***Dilute*** *one drop oil in 2 tsp. honey or 8 oz. of beverage (i.e. soy/rice milk). However, due to thujone content, more dilution may be necessary.* ***Best avoided by children of all ages.***

Safety Data: *Classified by Robert Tisserand as an* **oral toxin** *due to thujone content. However, other sources indicate that for thujone to be toxic, undiluted oil in excess of 30 ml must be ingested in a short period of time. Therefore, use with caution. Best kept away from children. Avoid during* **pregnancy**. *Not for use by people with* **epilepsy**. *Avoid if dealing with* **high blood pressure.**

Blend Classification: Enhancer.

Blends With: Bergamot, lemon, lavender, peppermint, rosemary, lemongrass, pine.

SAGE LAVENDER (or SPANISH SAGE)
(Salvia lavandulafolia)

Botanical Family: Labiatae

Extraction Method/Origin: Steam distilled from flowering plant — Spain

Chemical Constituents: Monoterpenes (up to 43%): α- & β-pinenes (up to 34%), camphene (<10%), sabinene (<8%), limonene (<5%), myrcene (<5%), p-cymene (3%), α- & γ terpinenes (<3%), α-phellandrene, cis- & trans-ocimene, tricyclene, α-thujene; Ketones (<30%): camphor (<30%), α-thujone; Oxides (<26%): 1,8 cineol (<25%), caryophyllene oxide; Esters (<11%): α-terpenyl, linalyl, & bornyl acetates; Alcohols (<14%): α-terpineol (<6%), borneol (<5%), linalol (<3%), geraniol; Sesquiterpenes (<6%): β-caryophyllene, humulene, δ-cadinene, aromadendrene, bicyclogermacrene; Sesquiterpene Alcohols: viridiflorol, caryophyllenol; Phenols: terpinen-4-ol.

Properties: Anti-catarrhal, anti-depressant, anti-inflammatory, antimicrobial, antiseptic, anti-infectious, antispasmodic, astringent, analgesic, regulator (seborrhea), **stimulant** (liver, adrenal, and circulatory), **tonic**.

Esoteric Uses/Actions: Astrological: *Jupiter*; Body type: *Ectomorph*; Chakras: *4, 2, & 3*; Character: *Yang*; Crystal: *Malachite*; Element: *Air*; Number: *7*; Perfume note: *Top*

Possible Uses: Sage lavender may be beneficial for Alzheimer's Disease. It has been shown to inhibit cholinesterase activity and mimic **hormones** (increasing both estradiol and testosterone levels). It may also be beneficial for **aches/pains** (muscle), **acne, arthritis, asthenia, asthma, bronchitis, chills, circulation** (poor), **colds, coughs, cuts, dandruff, debility, dermatitis, eczema, exhaustion** (nervous), **fever, flu, gum** infections, **hair** loss, **headaches, jaundice, laryngitis, liver** congestion, **menstruation** (induces), **neuralgia, periods** (painful and difficult), **rheumatism, rhinitis, sinusitis, sterility, sweating** (excessive).

Body System(s) Affected: Emotional Balance, Hormonal System, Muscle and Bone, Nervous System, Respiratory System, Skin.

Aromatic Influence: Sage lavender helps improve **mood** and **memory**. It may also help **harmonize** and **balance** the **emotions** and reduce **stress-related** conditions.

Application: Apply to **Vita Flex Points** on feet and/or directly on **area** of concern; **Diffuse**.

Oral Use As Dietary Supplement: Generally regarded as safe (GRAS) for internal consumption by the FDA. **Dilute** *one drop oil in 1 tsp. honey or 4 oz. of beverage (i.e. soy/rice milk).* ***Not for children under 6 years old; use with*** *caution* ***and in*** *greater dilution* ***for children 6 years old and over.***

Blend Classification: Personifier and Equalizer.

Blends With: Clary sage, fennel, frankincense, geranium, sandalwood, ylang ylang.

SANDALWOOD
(Santalum album)

Botanical Family: Santalaceae (sandalwood)

Extraction Method/Origin: Steam distilled from wood — India, Indonesia

Chemical Constituents: Sesquiterpene Alcohols: α- & β-santalols (<80%); Sesquiterpenes : α & β-santalenes (<11%); Sesquiterpene Aldehydes: teresantalal (<3%); Carboxylic Acids : nor-tricyclo-eka-santalic acid (<2%).

Properties: Anti-depressant, antiseptic, aphrodisiac, astringent, calming, sedative, and **tonic**.

Folklore: Sandalwood purportedly awakens the latent life force energy during meditation, and frees the souls of the deceased at funerals. Many cultures still consider sandalwood to be sacred.

Esoteric Uses/Actions: Astrological: *Saturn, Moon, Jupiter & Uranus*; Ayurvedic: *Pitta*; Body type: *Mesomorph*; Chakras: *links 1 & 7, also 4, 5, & 1*; Character: *mildly Yang - Cold & Dry 2ⁿᵈ Degree*; Crystals: *Clear Calcite, Emerald, Turquoise, Citrine (links 2ⁿᵈ & 7ʰ chakras)*; Element: *Water, Fire, & Air*; Number: *6*; Oriental: *Hot dampness (pts: Sp-9 & 6)*

Historical Uses: Sandalwood was traditionally used as an incense during ritual work for enhancing meditation. The Egyptians also used sandalwood for embalming.

French Medicinal Uses: Bronchitis (chronic), **diarrhea** (obstinate), **hemorrhoids, impotence**.

Other Possible Uses: Sandalwood is very similar to frankincense in action. It may support the **cardiovascular system**, remove **negative programming** from **cells**, and relieve symptoms associated with **lumbago** and the **sciatic nerves**. It may also be beneficial for **acne**, regenerating **bone cartilage, catarrh, circulation** (similar in action to frankincense), **coughs, cystitis, depression, hiccoughs, lymphatic system, meditation, menstrual problems, nerves** (similar in action to frankincense), **nervous tension**, increasing **oxygen** around the **pineal** and **pituitary glands, skin infection** and **regeneration, tuberculosis**, and **yoga**.

Body System(s) Affected: Emotional Balance, Muscle and Bone, Nervous System, Skin.

Aromatic Influence: Slowly and powerfully **calms, harmonizes**, and **balances** the **emotions**. It helps one accept others with an open heart while diminishing one's own egocentricity. It may help **enhance meditation** by opening the third eye. It can also be stimulating as well as grounding as it is said to vibrate between the 7th and 1st chakra.

Application: Apply to **Vita Flex Points** of the feet and/or directly on **area** of concern; **Diffuse**.

Oral Use As Dietary Supplement: Approved by the FDA for use as a Food Additive (FA) and Flavoring Agent (FL). *Dilute one drop oil in 1 tsp. honey or 4 oz. of beverage (i.e. soy/rice milk). **Not for children under 6 years old; use with caution and in greater dilution for children 6 years old and over.***

Blend Classification: Modifier and Equalizer.

Blends With: Cypress, frankincense, lemon, myrrh, ylang ylang, patchouli, spruce.

Odor: Type: *Base Note (5-20% of the blend)*; Scent: *Soft, woody, sweet, earthy, balsamic, tenacious*; Intensity: *3*

Frequency: Physical and Emotional; approximately 96 MHz.

SPEARMINT
(Mentha spicata, CT Carvone)

Botanical Family: Labiatae (mint)

Extraction Method/Origin: Steam distilled from leaves — Utah, USA

Chemical Constituents: Ketones (up to 70%): l-carvone (<58%), dihydrocarvone (<10%), menthone (<2%), pulegone; Monoterpenes (<30%): l-limonene (<25%), myrcene (<3%), camphene, α- & β-pinenes, α-phellandrene; Alcohols (<10%): carveol (<3%), linalol, trans-thujanol-4, octanol, borneol; Sesquiterpenes (<5%): β-caryophyllene, β-bourbonene, α-elemene, β-farnesene; Esters: carvyl acetates (<4%); Oxides: 1,8 cineol (<3%); Sesquiterpene Alcohols: α-cadinol, farnesol, elemol; Phenolic Alcohols: menthol.

Properties: Anti-bacterial, anti-catarrhal, anti-fungal, anti-inflammatory, antiseptic, antispasmodic, hormone-like, insecticidal, and **stimulant**.

Esoteric Uses/Actions: Astrological: *Mercury & Venus*; Character: *Yang*; Element: *Air & Water*

Historical Uses: Spearmint has been used to relieve hiccough, colic, nausea, indigestion, flatulence, headaches, sores, and scabs.

French Medicinal Uses: Bronchitis, candida, cystitis, hypertension.

Other Possible Uses: This oil may balance and increase **metabolism**, which may help **burn up fats** and **toxins** in the body. It may aid the **glandular, nervous**, and **respiratory systems**. It may also help with **acne, appetite** (stimulates), **bad breath, balance, childbirth** (promotes easier labor), **constipation, depression, diarrhea, digestion, dry skin, eczema, fevers, headaches, intestines** (soothes), **kidney stones, menstruation** (slow, heavy periods), **migraines, nausea, sore gums, stomach** (relaxes muscles), s**urine retention, vaginitis, weight** (reduces), and bring about a feeling of **well being**.

Body System(s) Affected: Digestive System, Emotional Balance.

Aromatic Influence: Its **hormone-like** activity may help open and release emotional blocks to bring about a feeling of balance. It acts as an anti-depressant by relieving mental strain and fatigue, and by lifting one's spirits.

Application: Apply to **Vita Flex Points** and directly on **area** of concern; **Diffuse**.

Oral Use As Dietary Supplement: Generally regarded as safe (GRAS) for internal consumption by the FDA. ***Dilute*** *one drop oil in 1 tsp. honey or 4 oz. of beverage (i.e. soy/rice milk).* ***Not for children under 6 years old; use with*** *caution and in* ***greater dilution*** *for children 6 years old and over.*

Safety Data: *Use with caution during* **pregnancy**. *Not for use on babies.*

Blend Classification: Personifier.

Blends With: Basil, lavender, peppermint, rosemary.

Odor: Type: *Top Note (5-20% of the blend)*; Scent: *Minty, slightly fruity, less bright than peppermint*; Intensity: *3*

SPIKENARD
(Nardostachys jatamansi)

Botanical Family: Valerianaceae

Extraction Method/Origin: Steam distilled from roots — India

Chemical Constituents: Sesquiterpenes (up to 50%): β-gurjunene (<30%), β-maalene (<9%), aristoladiene (<7%), aristolene (5%), seychellene, dihydroazulene, β-patchoulene; Monoterpenes (up to 45%): calarene (<35%), β-ionene (<8%), α- & β-pinenes, limonene, aristolene; Sesquiterpene Alcohols (<11%): patchoulol (<7%), nardol, calarenol, maaliol, valerianol; Ketones (<10%): aristolenone (<7%), β-ionone, nardostachone, valerianone (=jatamansone); Phenolic Aldehydes: valerianal; Coumarins; Oxides: 1,8 cineol; Carboxylic Acids: jatamanshinic acid.

Properties: Anti-bacterial, anti-fungal, anti-inflammatory, deodorant, relaxing, and **skin tonic**.

Folklore: Spikenard has also been known as "nard" and "'false' Indian valerian root" oil. Prized in early Egypt, it was used in a preparation, called *kyphi*, with other oils like saffron, juniper, myrrh, cassia, and cinnamon. According to Roberta Wilson, "The Egyptians believed that in addition to appeasing the gods, Kyphi incense quelled fear and anxiety, improved meditation, and induced restful sleep with pleasant dreams."

Esoteric Uses/Actions: Astrological: *Saturn & Sun*; Chakras: *4 & 7*; Character: *Yin*; Element: *Fire & Ether*

Historical Uses: In India, spikenard was notably regarded as a perfume, medicinal herb, and as a skin tonic. Highly prized in the Middle East during the time of Christ, there are several passages in the Bible referring to spikenard. Spikenard was also used in the preparation of *nardinum*, a scented oil of great renown during ancient times.

Other Possible Uses: The oil is known for helping in the treatment of **allergic skin reactions**, and according to Victoria Edwards, "The oil redresses the skin's physiological balance and causes permanent regeneration." Spikenard may also help with **allergies, candida, flatulent indigestion, insomnia, menstrual difficulties, migraine, nausea, rashes, staph infections, stress, tachycardia, tension**, and **wounds** that will not heal.

Body System(s) Affected: Emotional Balance, Skin.

Aromatic Influence: Spikenard has a peaty, earthy, animal-like fragrance, reminiscent of goats. It is **balancing, soothing**, and **harmonizing**.

Application: Apply to **Vita Flex Points** and/or directly on **area** of concern.

Oral Use As Dietary Supplement: None.

Blends With: Cistus, lavender, patchouli, pine, and vetiver.

Odor: Type: *Base Note (5-20% of the blend)*; Scent: *Heavy, earthy, animal-like, similar to valerian*; Intensity: *5*

Bible: Song of Solomon 1:12, 4:13-14; Mark 14:3; John 12:3

SPRUCE (or BLACK SPRUCE)
(Picea mariana)

Botanical Family: Pinaceae (conifer) **Extraction Method/Origin:** Steam distilled from needles — Canada

Chemical Constituents: Monoterpenes (up to 55%): camphene (<25%), α-pinene (<19%), δ-3carene (<10%), β-pinene (<8%), l-limonene (<7%), santene, tricyclene; Esters: bornyl acetate (>35%); Alcohols: borneol, longiborneol; Sesquiterpenes: longifolene, longicyclene.

Properties: Anti-infectious, anti-inflammatory, antispasmodic, cortisone-like, disinfectant, and **tonic**.

Esoteric Uses/Actions: Chakras: *5, 6, & 3*; Character: *Yang*; Element: *Ether & Light*

Historical Uses: It was used by the Lakota Indians to enhance their communication with the Great Spirit.

French Medicinal Uses: Arthritis, candida, hyperthyroidism, immune-depression, prostatitis, rheumatism, solar plexus.

Other Possible Uses: Spruce oil creates the symbolic effect of the umbrella which protects the earth and brings energy in from the universe. At night the animals in the wild lie down under a tree for the protection, recharging, and rejuvenation the trees bring them. It may be beneficial for **bone pain, glandular system**, aching **joints**, opening the **pineal gland, sciatica pain**, and stimulating the **thymus** and **adrenal** glands.

Body System(s) Affected: Emotional Balance, Nervous and **Respiratory Systems**.

Aromatic Influence: Spruce oil **grounds** the body, creating the feeling of **balance** necessary to receive and to give. Helps release **emotional blocks**.

Application: Apply to **Vita Flex Points** and/or directly on **area** of concern.

Oral Use As Dietary Supplement: Approved by the FDA for use as a Food Additive (FA) and Flavoring Agent (FL). ***Dilute*** *one drop oil in 1 tsp. honey or 4 oz. of beverage (i.e. soy/rice milk). **Not for children under 6 years old; use with caution and in greater dilution for children 6 years old and over.***

Blend Classification: Equalizer and Enhancer

Blends With: Birch, eucalyptus, frankincense, helichrysum, ravensara, wintergreen.

Odor: Type: *Middle Note (50-80% of the blend)*; Scent: *Fresh, woody, earthy, sweet, with a hint of a fruity note*; Intensity: *3*

TAMANU
(Calophyllum inophyllum)

NOTE: This is a vegetal oil, not an essential oil. Listed here because of its value as a fixed oil in formulations. Only available through Creer Labs 801-418-8870.

Botanical Family: Gutiferae or Hypericaceae

Extraction Method/Origin: Cold pressed from the nut of the Polynesian Tamanu tree. — Tahiti

Chemical Constituents: Terpenic essences, benzoic & oxibenzoic acids, vitamin F, lipids, glycerides, saturated fatty acids, calophyllolide (3,4-dihydro-5-methoxyl-22-dimethyl-6), calophyllic acid, coumarin derivatives, and phospho-amino acids.

Properties: Antibacterial, anti-infectious, anti-inflammatory, anti-rheumatic.

Historical Uses: The natives of Tahiti believe that tamanu oil is a "sacred" gift of nature. The women use the oil as a natural moisturizing cosmetic on their faces and bodies. It was also used for protection against sunburns.

Other Possible Uses: Burns and **wounds** (when mixed with helichrysum), **hair** (creates healthy), and **natural sun screen**.

Body System(s) Affected: Skin

Aromatic Influence: Grounding and **soothing**. It has an earthly, musky smell, with a slight nutty odor.

Application: Apply directly on area of concern.

Oral Use As Dietary Supplement: None.

Safety Data: *Avoid if allergic to any kind of nuts.*
Blends With: Helichrysum (burns and wounds), rosemary camphor (hair growth)

TANGERINE
(Citrus nobilis or Citrus reticulata var. tangerine)

Botanical Family: Rutaceae (citrus)
Extraction Method/Origin: Cold pressed from rind — USA, Mexico, Brazil, South Africa
Chemical Constituents: Monoterpenes (up to 95%): d-limonene (<80%), γ-terpinene (<20%), myrcene (<4%), p-cymene, α- & β-phellandrenes, β-ocimene, α- & β-pinenes, terpinolene, cadinene; Tetraterpenes (<10%): β-carotene (<6%), lycopene (<4%); Alcohols: linalol, citronellol; Aldehydes: citral, neral.
Properties: **Anti-coagulant, anti-inflammatory, laxative**, and **sedative**.
Esoteric Uses/Actions: Astrological: *Sun*; Body type: *Nervous*; Chakra: *2*; Character: *Yang (some Yin)?*; Element: *Water*
Possible Uses: It may help dissolve **cellulite, circulation, constipation, diarrhea, digestive system disorders, fat digestion, dizziness, fear, flatulence, gallbladder, insomnia, intestinal spasms, irritability, limbs** (tired and aching), **liver problems**, decongest **lymphatic system** (helps to stimulate draining), **obesity, parasites, sadness, stomach** tonic, **stretch marks** (smooths when blended with lavender), **stress, swelling**, and alleviate **water retention (edema)**.
Body System(s) Affected: **Emotional Balance, Immune System, Skin**.
Aromatic Influence: Tangerine oil contains esters and aldehydes which are **sedating** and **calming** to the **nervous system**. When diffused together with marjoram, it can soothe emotions such as grief, anger, and shock.
Application: Apply to **Vita Flex Points** and directly on **area** of concern; **Diffuse**.
Oral Use As Dietary Supplement: Generally regarded as safe (GRAS) for internal consumption by the FDA. ***Dilute*** *one drop oil in 1 tsp. honey or 4 oz. of beverage (i.e. soy/rice milk).* ***Not for children under 6 years old; use with*** *caution and in* ***greater dilution*** *for children 6 years old and over.*
Blend Classification: Modifier and Personifier
Blends With: Basil, bergamot, chamomile, Clary sage, frankincense, geranium, grapefruit, lavender, lemon, orange.
Odor: Type: *Top Note (5-20% of the blend)*; Scent: *Fresh, sweet, citrusy*; Intensity: *3*

TANSY, BLUE
(Tanacetum annum)

Botanical Family: Compositae (daisy)
Extraction Method/Origin: Steam distilled from leaves and flowers — France, Morocco

Chemical Constituents: Monoterpenes (up to 65%): sabinene (<17%), myrcene (<13%), d-limonene (<11%), β-pinene (<10%), α-phellandrene (<10%), p-cymene (<8%); Ketones: camphor (<17%); Sesquiterpenes: chamazulene (<12%).

Properties: Analgesic, anti-bacterial, anti-inflammatory, antihistamine, hypotensive, hormone-like, and **nervine**.

Possible Uses: May help with **low blood pressure**, relieve **itching**, reduce **pain**, and sedate the **nerves**.

Body System(s) Affected: Nervous System.

Application: Apply to **Vita Flex Points** and/or directly on **area** of concern.

Safety Data: *This oil should only be used **externally and with caution.***

TANSY, IDAHO
(Tanacetum vulgare)

Botanical Family: Compositae (daisy)

Extraction Method/Origin: Steam distilled from leaves — Idaho, Washington

Chemical Constituents: Ketones: β-thujone (approx. 65%, can be as high as 81%), camphor (<8%), α-thujone (<5%), piperitone, artemisia ketone, davanone, isothujone, umbellulone, isopinocamphone; Monoterpenes (<10%): sabinene (<4%), α-pinene (<3%), camphene, α-terpinene; Sesquiterpenes: germacrene-D (<7%); Alcohols: borneol, α-terpineol, lyratol, chrysanthenol, vulgerol, thujyl alcohol; Sesquiterpene Lactones: artemarin, chrysanthemine, crispolid, parthenolide, santamarin, tatridin; Esters: bornyl, α-terpinyl, lyratyl, & chrysanthenyl acetates; Oxides: 1,8-cineol; Coumarins: scopoletin.

Properties: Anti-bacterial, anti-fungal, anti-infectious, anti-inflammatory, antispasmodic, anti-viral, nervine, and **stimulant**.

Carrier Oils: Some commercial companies will dilute this oil with almond oil.

Historical Uses: Wild tansy (similar in chemical make-up to Idaho tansy) was used historically among the gypsies as a sort of "cure all". It has been used for worms, colds, fever, miscarriage, dyspepsia, cramping pains, scabies, bruises, sprains, nervous disorders, and to keep flies and vermin away.

Other Possible Uses: Idaho tansy may be supportive to the **immune system** in helping to **fight colds, flu**, and **infections**. It may also be beneficial for **stomach** conditions, **arthritis** symptoms, and possibly **tumors**. It has been shown to soothe the **bowels** and tone the entire system,. The properties in this oil suggest that it may help with **aneurysms, bruises, diarrhea, dyspepsia, freckles, gout, heart disorders, inflamed eyes, irritable bowel syndrome, jaundice, kidneys, liver spots, menstruation** (promotes), **palpitations, respiratory infections, rheumatism, sciatica, sprains, sunburn, toothaches, tuberculosis**, and **vomiting**.

Body System(s) Affected: Immune System.

Aromatic Influence: It encourages an **uplifting feeling**, a **positive attitude** and a general feeling of **well being**.

Application: Apply to **Vita Flex Points** and/or directly on **area** of concern.

Oral Use As Dietary Supplement: None.

Safety Data: *Because Idaho tansy contains a high concentration of thujone, this oil has been classified (along with Wild tansy) as an **oral toxin** by Robert Tisserand. However, other sources indicate that for thujone to be toxic, undiluted oil in excess of 30 ml must be ingested in a short period of time. Best for this oil to only be used **externally** and with caution. Avoid during **pregnancy**. Not for use by people with **epilepsy**.*

Blends With: Most oils; perfumers in France have found that Wild tansy (similar in chemical make-up to Idaho tansy) has a greater fixative capability than any other oil.

Frequency: Emotional; approximately 105 MHz.

TARRAGON
(Artemisia dracunculus)

Botanical Family: Compositae

Extraction Method/Origin: Steam distilled from leaves — France, Slovenia

Chemical Constituents: Phenolic Ethers (up to 85%): methyl chavicol/estragole (<75%), anethole (<10%); Monoterpenes (<30%): cis- & trans-β-ocimenes (<24%), l-limonene (<6%), α- & β-pinenes, camphene; Coumarins: herniarin, scopoletin, scoparone, artemidin, esculetin; Also: nerol, thujone, cineol, and linalyl acetate in trace amounts.

Properties: Anti-bacterial, anti-cancerous, anti-infectious, anti-inflammatory, antiseptic, antispasmodic, anti-parasitic, anti-viral, diuretic, laxative, neuromuscular, and **stimulant**.

Folklore: The name is said to come from an ancient use as a remedy for bites from venomous creatures.

Esoteric Uses/Actions: Astrological: *Mars*; Character: *Yang, Yin*; Perfume note: *Top*

Historical Uses: Tarragon was used to induce appetite, for digestive and menstrual irregularities, and as a remedy for toothache.

French Medicinal Uses: Colitis, hiccoughs, intestinal spasms, parasites, rheumatic pain, sciatica.

Other Possible Uses: It may be beneficial for **abdominal discomfort** and **spasms, arthritis, dyspepsia** (impaired digestion), preventing **fermentation, genital urinary tract infection, kidneys, nausea, z** and **sluggish digestion, pre-menstrual** discomfort, and **weeping wounds**.

Body System(s) Affected: Digestive System. It may also help balance the **Autonomic Nervous System**.

Application: Apply to **Vita Flex Points** and/or directly on **area** of concern. Best to **dilute** with V-6 Mixing Oil.

Oral Use As Dietary Supplement: Generally regarded as safe (GRAS) for internal consumption by the FDA. ***Dilute** one drop oil in 1 tsp. honey or 4 oz. of beverage (i.e. soy/rice milk). **Not***

*for children under 6 years old; use with **caution** and in **greater dilution** for children 6 years old and over.*

Safety Data: *Avoid during **pregnancy**. Not for use by people with **epilepsy**.*

Blend Classification: Equalizer

Blends With: Chamomile, Clary sage, fir, juniper, lavender, pine, rosewood, orange, and tangerine.

THYME
(Thymus vulgaris, CT Thymol)

Botanical Family: Labiatae (mint)

Extraction Method/Origin: Steam distilled from leaves, stems, and flowers — Utah, Idaho, France

Chemical Constituents: Phenols (up to 60%): thymol (<55%), carvacrol (<10%); Monoterpenes (<54%): p-cymene (<28%), γ-terpinene (<11%), terpinolene (<6%), α-pinene (<6%), myrcene (<3%); Oxides: 1,8 cineol (<15%); Alcohols (<14%): linalol (<8%), borneol (<7%), thujanol, geraniol; Sesquiterpenes: β-caryophyllene (<8%); Carboxylic Acids: rosmaric acid (<2%), triterpenic acids (tr.); Ethers: methyl thymol (tr.), methyl carvacrol (tr.); Ketone: camphor (tr.); Also trace elements of menthone.

Properties: Highly **antimicrobial, anti-fungal, anti-viral, antiseptic**.

Esoteric Uses/Actions: Astrological: *Venus*; Chakras: *6 & 3*; Character: *Yang*; Crystals: *Pearl, Sodalite*; Element: *Fire & Water*; Oriental: *Cold phlegm (pts: St-40, Sp-6); Qi deficiencies (pts: Lu-9, St-36, Dir Ves-6); Hot phlegm (pts: St-40, Sp-6)*

Historical Uses: It was used by the Egyptians for embalming and by the ancient Greeks against infectious illnesses. It has also been used for respiratory problems, digestive complaints, the prevention and treatment of infection, dyspepsia, chronic gastritis, bronchitis, pertussis, asthma, laryngitis, tonsillitis, and enuresis in children.

French Medicinal Uses: Anthrax, asthma, bronchitis, colitis (infectious), **cystitis, dermatitis, dyspepsia, fatigue** (general), **pleurisy, psoriasis, sciatica, tuberculosis, vaginal candida**.

Other Possible Uses: This oil is a general **tonic** for the **nerves** and **stomach**. It may also help with **bacterial infections, colds, circulation, depression, digestion, physical weakness** after **illness, flu, headaches, immunological** functions, **insomnia, rheumatism, urinary infections, viruses** along the **spine**, and **wounds**.

Body System(s) Affected: Immune System, Muscles and Bones.

Aromatic Influence: It helps **supply energy** in times of **physical weakness** and **stress**. It has also been thought to increase **intelligence** and aid **concentration**. It is **uplifting** and helps to relieve **depression**.

Application: Apply to **Vita Flex Points** and/or directly on **area** of concern.

Oral Use As Dietary Supplement: Generally regarded as safe (GRAS) for internal consumption by the FDA. ***Dilute** one drop oil in 2 tsp. honey or 8 oz. of beverage (i.e. soy/rice milk). However, more dilution may be necessary due to this oil's potential for irritating mucus*

membranes. *Not for children under 6 years old; use with **caution** and in **greater dilution** for children 6 years old and over.*

Safety Data: *This type of thyme oil may be somewhat irritating to the mucous membranes and dermal tissues (skin). This type of thyme should be avoided during **pregnancy.** Use this type with caution when dealing with **high blood pressure.***

Blend Classification: Equalizer and Enhancer

Blends With: Bergamot, cedarwood, juniper, melaleuca, oregano, and rosemary.

Odor: Type: *Middle Note (50-80% of the blend)*; Scent: *Fresh, medicinal, herbaceous*; Intensity: *4*

THYME LINALOL
(Thymus vulgaris, CT Linalol)

Botanical Family: Labiatae (mint)

Extraction Method/Origin: Steam distilled from leaves, stems, and flowers — France

Chemical Constituents: Alcohols (up to 85%): linalol (<78%), thujanol (<4%), geraniol (<3%), α-terpineol; Monoterpenes (<21%): myrcene (<8%), p-cymene (<7%), γ-terpinene (<%); Phenols: terpinen-4-ol (<12%), thymol, carvacrol; Esters: linalyl acetate (<5%), geranyl acetate; Sesquiterpenes (tr.): β-caryophyllene, humulene; Also (tr.): 1,8 cineol, camphor.

Properties: Anti-bacterial, anti-fungal, anti-infectious, anti-inflammatory, antimicrobial, anti-parasitic, antiseptic, anti-viral, cardiotonic, neurotonic, and **uterotonic**.

Esoteric Uses/Actions: Astrological: *Venus*; Chakras: *3 & 6*; Character: *Yang*; Element: *Fire & Water*; Perfume note: *Top to Mid*

Historical Uses: It was used by the Egyptians for embalming and by the ancient Greeks against infectious illnesses. It has also been used for respiratory problems, digestive complaints, the prevention and treatment of infection, dyspepsia, chronic gastritis, bronchitis, pertussis, asthma, laryngitis, tonsillitis, and enuresis in children.

French Medicinal Uses: Anthrax, asthma, bronchitis, colitis (infectious), **cystitis, dermatitis, dyspepsia, fatigue** (general), **pleurisy, psoriasis, sciatica, tuberculosis, vaginal candida**.

Other Possible Uses: This oil is a general **tonic** for the **nerves** and **stomach**. It may also help with **bacterial infections, colds, circulation, depression, digestion, physical weakness** after **illness, flu, headaches, immunological** functions, **insomnia, rheumatism, urinary infections, viruses** along the **spine**, and **wounds**. *Note: This chemotype is said to be the best suited to kill **bacteria**, relieve discomfort in stomach or gut (**candida, parasites**), and nervous **fatigue.** It is nonirritating, especially for children, elderly, and the infirm.*

Body System(s) Affected: Respiratory System, Skin.

Aromatic Influence: It helps **supply energy** in times of **physical weakness** and **stress**. It has also been thought to increase **intelligence** and aid **concentration**. It is **uplifting** and helps to relieve **depression**.

Application: Apply to **Vita Flex Points** and/or directly on **area** of concern.

Oral Use As Dietary Supplement: Generally regarded as safe (GRAS) for internal consumption by the FDA. ***Dilute*** *one drop oil in 1 tsp. honey or 4 oz. of beverage (i.e. soy/rice milk).* ***Not for children under 6 years old; use with*** *caution and in* ***greater dilution*** *for children 6 years old and over.*

Safety Data: *Because this type of thyme oil is a 'linalol type', it is safe for use on the skin and with children. Other varieties of thyme oil can contain large amounts of thymol and carvacrol, making them somewhat toxic, irritating to the mucous membranes, and dermal (skin) irritants. While this type of thyme may be used during pregnancy, the other types should be avoided! Use this type with caution when dealing with* ***high blood pressure.***

Blend Classification: Equalizer and Enhancer

Blends With: Bergamot, citrus oil, cedarwood, juniper, melaleuca, oregano, and rosemary.

TSUGA (or HEMLOCK SPRUCE)
(Tsuga canadensis)

Botanical Family: Pinaceae (pine)

Extraction Method/Origin: Steam distilled from leaves and twigs — Idaho, Canada ***This oil is not to be confused with hemlock (Conium maculatum), which contains toxic alkaloids, and is not a source of essential oil.***

Chemical Constituents: Monoterpenes (up to 50%): α- & β-pinenes (<25%), camphene (<18%), l-limonene (<5%), tricyclene (<8%), α- & β-phellandrenes (<5%), myrcene (<3%); Esters: bornyl acetate (<38%); Sesquiterpenes (<14%): tricyclene (<8%), dipentene (<4%), δ-cadinene (<3%); Ketones: α-thujone (<3%).

Properties: Antimicrobial, antiseptic, astringent, diuretic, expectorant, nervine, tonic.

Esoteric Uses/Actions: Astrological: *Saturn*; Chakra: *6*; Element: *Light*; Perfume note: *Base*

Historical Uses: It has been used for diarrhea, cystitis, mucous colitis, leucorrhea, uterine prolapse, pharyngitis, stomatitis, gingivitis, wounds, sores, digestive disorders, diseases of the mouth and throat and scurvy.

Other Possible Uses: This oil may help with **anxiety, asthma, bronchitis**, poor **circulation, colds, coughs, flu, infections, muscular aches** and **pains, periodontal (gum) disease, respiratory weakness** (opens and dilates for better oxygen exchange), **rheumatism, stress-related conditions**, and **wounds**. It can also be used in **veterinary liniments**.

Body System(s) Affected: Cardiovascular and **Respiratory Systems**.

Aromatic Influence: It is **uplifting** to the **emotions** as it **opens** and **elevates** while **grounding** at the same time. Some have found it excellent for **yoga** and **meditation**.

Application: Diffuse. Apply to **Vita Flex Points** and/or directly on **area** of concern. For topical use, **dilute** in one teaspoon V-6 Mixing Oil.

Oral Use As Dietary Supplement: Approved by the FDA for use as a Food Additive (FA) or Flavoring Agent (FL) (see 21CFR172.510). ***Dilute*** *one drop oil in 1 tsp. honey or 4 oz. of* *beverage (i.e. soy/rice milk).* **Not for children under 6 years old; use with caution and in greater dilution for children 6 years old and over.**

Safety Data: *Repeated use can possibly result in skin irritation.*

Companion Products: Di-Gize, Essentialzyme, Fresh Essence Plus Mouthwash, K&B Tincture, Rose Ointment.

Blends With: Pine, cedarwood, galbanum, lavender, lavandin, and rosemary.

VALERIAN
(Valeriana officinalis)

Botanical Family: Valerianaceae

Extraction Method/Origin: Steam distilled from roots — Belgium, Croatia, France

Chemical Constituents: Esters (up to 50%): bornyl acetate (<44%), myrtenyl acetate (<5%), bornyl formate, butyrate, & isovalerate (responsible for odor & therapeutic effects), eugenyl isovalerate; Monoterpenes (<41%): camphene (<21%), α-fenchene (<13%), α-pinene (<8%), β-pinene (<6%); Alcohols (<6%): borneol, α-terpineol, geraniol, patchouli alcohol, valerianol; Sesquiterpenes (5%): vitivene, δ-cadinene, α-farnescene, valerazulene, β-caryophyllene; Sesquiterpene Aldehydes: valerianal; Sesquiterpene Ketones: valerianone, ionone; Carboxylic Acids: valerinic acid, isovaleric acid, chlorogenic acid, malic acid; Sesquiterpene Lactones: actinidine, valerianine.

Properties: Anti-bacterial, anti-dandruff, antispasmodic, depressant (central nervous system), **diuretic, hypnotic, regulator, sedative**.

Folklore: Once called "all heal", valerian has been treasured since medieval times.

Esoteric Uses/Actions: Astrological: *Venus*; Element: *Water*; Perfume note: *Base*

Historical Uses: Down through the centuries, valerian has been used for insomnia, migraine, dysmenorrhea, intestinal colic, rheumatism, cholera, epilepsy, skin complaints, backache, colds, menstrual problems, and sores. During that last few decades, it has been studied for its tranquilizing properties.

Other Possible Uses: Because of its effect on the nervous system, it may help with **insomnia, nervous indigestion, migraine, restlessness, sleep disturbances**, and **tension**. Valerian has also been shown to naturally inhibit the re-uptake of 5HT (serotonin). It also helps with the free-flow of blood platelets.

Body System(s) Affected: Nervous System.

Aromatic Influence: It may be useful in meditation as it helps cut through the tension and stress of our everyday lives to help us focus on our inner self, where true peace and calm can be found. It is profoundly **calming, relaxing, grounding**, and **balancing**.

Application: Apply to **Vita Flex Points** and/or directly on **area** of concern. May also be applied to the **wrists** or bottom of the **feet**. Is actually more effective when taken internally as a dietary supplement.

Oral Use As Dietary Supplement: Approved by the FDA for use as a Food Additive (FA) and Flavoring Agent (FL). **Dilute** *one drop oil in 1 tsp. honey or 4 oz. of beverage (i.e. soy/rice*

*milk). **Not for children under 6 years old; use with caution** and in **greater dilution for** children 6 years old and over.*

Safety Data: *Repeated use can possibly result in **contact sensitization**.*

Blends With: Cedarwood, lavender, mandarin, patchouli, petitgrain, pine, and rosemary.

VETIVER
(Vetiveria zizanoides)

Botanical Family: Gramineae (grasses)

Extraction Method/Origin: Steam distilled from roots — India, Haiti (best)

Chemical Constituents: Sesquiterpene Alcohols (up to 42%): isovalencenol (<15%), bicyclovetiverol (<13%), khusenol (<11%), tricyclovetiverol (<4%), vetiverol, zizanol, furfurol; Sesquiterpene Ketones (<22%): α- & β-vetivones (<12%), khusimone (<6%), nootkatone (<5%); Sesquiterpenes (<4%): vitivene, tricyclovetivene, vetivazulene, β- & δ-cadinenes; Sesquiterpene Esters: vetiveryl acetate; Carboxylic Acids: benzoic, palmitic, and vetivenic acids.

Properties: Antiseptic, antispasmodic, calming, grounding, immune-stimulant, rubefacient (locally warming), **sedative** (nervous system), **stimulant** (circulatory, production of red corpuscles).

Folklore: Known in India as "oil of tranquility", vetiver is distilled from the root of a scented grass native to India that is botanically related to citronella and lemongrass

Esoteric Uses/Actions: Astrological: *Venus & Saturn*; Body type: *Mesomorph*; Chakras: *1, 2, &* *3*; Character: *Intensely Yin (with rising Yang)*; Crystals: *Yellow Jasper, Black Tourmaline*; Element: *Earth & Water*; Number: *5*

Historical Uses: The distillation of vetiver is a painstaking, labor-intensive activity. The roots and rootlets of vetiver have been used in India as a perfume since antiquity.

Other Possible Uses: Vetiver may help **acne, anorexia, anxiety, arthritis, breasts** (enlarge), **cuts, depression** (including postpartum), **insomnia, muscular rheumatism, nervousness** (extreme), **skin care** (oily, aging, tired, irritated), **sprains**, and **stress**.

Body System(s) Affected: Emotional Balance, Hormonal and **Nervous Systems, Skin**.

Aromatic Influence: Vetiver has a heavy, smokey, earthy fragrance reminiscent of patchouli with lemon-like undertones. Because of its **psychologically grounding, calming**, and **stabilizing** properties, vetiver has also been valuable for relieving **stress** and helping people recover from **emotional traumas** and **shock**. As a natural tranquilizer, it may help induce a **restful sleep**. It is known to affect the **parathyroid gland**. According to Susanne Fischer-Rizzi, "Sexual energies become more peaceful and grounded."

Application: Apply to **Vita Flex Points** and/or directly on **area** of concern; **Diffuse**. Also excellent in **baths** or in **massage** blends. A very small amount of vetiver oil is all that is needed in most applications. Mix with geranium and ylang ylang to help with breast enlargement.

Oral Use As Dietary Supplement: Approved by the FDA for use as a Food Additive (FA) and Flavoring Agent (FL). **Dilute** *one drop oil in 1 tsp. honey or 4 oz. of beverage (i.e. soy/rice milk).* ***Not for children under 6 years old; use with*** **caution** ***and in*** **greater dilution** *for* ***children 6 years old and over.***

Safety Data: *Use with caution during* **pregnancy.**

Blends With: Clary sage, jasmine, lavender, patchouli, rose, sandalwood, ylang ylang.

Odor: Type: *Base Note (5-20% of the blend)*; Scent: *Heavy, earthy, balsamic, smoky, sweet undertones*; Intensity: *5*

VITEX
(Vitex negundo)

Botanical Family: Labiatae (mint)

Extraction Method/Origin: Steam distilled from the inner bark, small branches, and leaves of the Chaste tree (this essential oil is different from the extract of the chaste berry, which is used for PMS symptoms and hormone balance) — Turkey

Chemical Constituents: Sesquiterpenes (up to 65%): β-caryophyllene (<40%), germacrene-B (<10%), β-farnesene (<7%), logifolene (<6%), α-gurjunene (5%); Monoterpenes (<20%): sabinene (<15%), α-pinene (<6%), l-limonene (<3%); Oxides (<18%): caryophyllene oxide (<10%), 1,8 cineol (<8%); Esters: α-terpinyl acetate.

Historical Uses: Vitex has been historically used in Europe and Asia for its benefits relating to **rheumatism, hernias, deafness**, and **mental unrest**.

Other Possible Uses: Research is being conducted on the use of vitex oil for reversing the symptoms of Parkinson's Disease.

Oral Use As Dietary Supplement: None.

Safety Data: *Use with caution during* **pregnancy.**

WESTERN RED CEDAR
(See CEDAR, WESTERN RED)

WHITE FIR
(See FIR, WHITE)

WHITE LOTUS
(Nymphaea lotus)

Botanical Family: Nymphaeaceae **Extraction Method/Origin:** Steam distilled from flower — Egypt

(NOTE: This oil is only available periodically in very small amounts.)

Properties: Anti-cancerous.

Historical Uses: White lotus was traditionally used by the Egyptians for **spiritual, emotional**, and **physical** application; every recipe contained White lotus. Research in China found that White lotus contains **anti-cancerous** and strong **immune supporting** properties.

Other Possible Uses: Eyes (inflamed), **jaundice, kidneys, liver spots, menstruation** (promotes), **palpitations, rheumatism, sciatica, sprains, sunburn, toothaches, tuberculosis, vomiting**.

Body System(s) Affected: Immune System.

Aromatic Influence: White lotus has a euphoric fragrance that **lifts** and **stabilizes** the **emotions**, creating a powerful sense of **emotional, physical**, and **spiritual well being**.

Blends With: Most oils.

WINTERGREEN
(Gaultheria procumbens)

Botanical Family: Ericaceae (heather)

Extraction Method/Origin: Steam distillation from leaves — Canada

Chemical Constituents: Phenolic Esters: methyl salicylate (>90%); Carboxylic Acids: salicylic acid.

Properties: Analgesic, anti-inflammatory, anti-rheumatic, antiseptic, antispasmodic, disinfectant, diuretic, stimulant (bone), and **warming**.

Esoteric Uses/Actions: Astrological: *Mercury & Moon*; Character: *Yin?*; Element: *Earth*; Color: *Yellow, reddish, colorless*; Odor: *strong characteristics*

Historical Uses: Wintergreen oil has a strong, penetrating aroma. Wintergreen essential oil is almost identical in chemical constituents to birch essential oil (*Betula alleghaniensis*). The American Indians and early European settlers enjoyed a tea that was flavored with birch bark or wintergreen. According to Julia Lawless, "...this has been translated into a preference for 'root beer' flavourings [sic]." A synthetic methyl salicylate is now widely used as a flavoring agent, especially in 'root beer', chewing gum, toothpaste, etc. *In fact, the true essential oil is produced in such small quantities (compared to the very extensive uses of the synthetic methyl salicylate) that those desiring to use wintergreen essential oil for therapeutic uses should* **verify the source** *of their oil to make sure they have a true oil, not a synthetic one.*

French Medicinal Uses: Rheumatism, muscular pain, cramps, arthritis, tendonitis, hypertension, inflammation.

Other Possible Uses: This oil may be beneficial for **acne, bladder infection, cystitis, dropsy, eczema, edema**, reducing **fever, gallstones, gout, infection**, reducing discomfort in **joints, kidney stones**, draining and cleansing the **lymphatic system, obesity, osteoporosis, skin diseases, ulcers**, and **urinary tract disorders**. It is known for its ability to alleviate **bone pain**. It has a cortisone-like action due to the high content of methyl salicylate. For nerve or tissue pain, use <u>Relieve It</u>.

Body System(s) Affected: Muscles and Bones.

©2006 Abundant Health

Aromatic Influence: It influences, elevates, opens, and increases **awareness** in **sensory system** (senses or sensations).

Application: Apply to **Vita Flex Points** and/or directly on **area** of concern; **Diffuse**. Apply topically on location and use only small amounts (dilute with V-6 Mixing Oil for application on larger areas).

Safety Data: *Avoid during* **pregnancy**. *Not for use by people with* **epilepsy**. *Some people are very allergic to methyl salicylate.* **Test a small area of skin first for allergies!**

Blend Classification: Personifier and Enhancer

Blends With: Basil, bergamot, chamomile, cypress, geranium, juniper, lavender, lemongrass, marjoram, peppermint, and rosewood.

YARROW
(Achillea millefolium)

Botanical Family: Compositae (daisy)

Extraction Method/Origin: Steam distilled from flowering top — Utah

Chemical Constituents: Monoterpenes (up to 65%): sabinene (<40%), α- & β-pinenes (<16%), camphene (<6%), γ-terpinene; Sesquiterpenes (<55%): chamazulene (<30%), germacrene-D (<13%), trans-β-caryophyllene (<8%), humulene (<7%), dihydroazulenes; Ketones (<30%): camphor (<18%), isoartemisia ketone (<10%), thujone; Alcohols (<10%): borneol (<9%), terpineol; Oxides (<12%): 1,8 cineol (<10%), caryophyllene oxide; Phenols: terpinen-4-ol (<5%); Esters: bornyl acetate; Lactones: achillin; Sesquiterpene Alcohols: α-cadinol.

Properties: **Anti-inflammatory, antiseptic, astringent**, and **styptic**.

Folklore: The Greek Achilles, hero of the Trojan Wars, was said to have used yarrow to help cure the injury to his Achilles tendon. Yarrow was considered sacred by the Chinese, who recognized the harmony of the Yin and Yang energies within it. It has been said that the fragrance of yarrow makes possible the meeting of heaven and earth.

Esoteric Uses/Actions: Astrological: *Venus*; Character: *Yang (Yin when diluted), Hot to 2ⁿᵈ Degree*; Crystals: *Amethyst*; Element: *Water*; Oriental: *Rising heat, internal wind*

Historical Uses: Yarrow was used by Germanic tribes to treat battle wounds.

Other Possible Uses: It is a powerful decongestant of the **prostate** and helps to balance **hormones**. It may also help with **acne, amenorrhea, appetite** (lack of), **bladder** or **kidney weakness, cellulite, colds, catarrh, digestion** (poor), **dysmenorrhea, eczema, fevers, flatulence, gallbladder inflammation, gastritis, gout, hair** (promotes hair growth), **headaches, hemorrhoids, hypertension, injuries, kidney stones, liver, menopause problems, neuritis, neuralgia, open leg sores, pelvic infections, prostatitis, rheumatism, scarring** (reduces or prevents), **sprains, stomach flu, sunburn, thrombosis, ulcers, urinary infections, vaginitis, varicose veins**, and **wounds** (promotes healing).

Body System(s) Affected: **Hormonal** and **Immune Systems, Skin**.

Single Oils

Aromatic Influence: Balancing highs and lows, both external and internal, yarrow may allow us to have our heads in the clouds while our feet remain firm on the ground. Its **balancing** properties may also make it useful during **meditation**. It is **supportive** to **intuitive energies** and helps reduce **confusion** and **ambivalence**. One source suggests that it may help open our awareness to **cosmic energies**.

Application: Apply to **Vita Flex Points** and/or directly on **area** of concern; **Diffuse**. Also excellent for **baths** or **massage** blends.

Safety Data: *Repeated use can possibly result in* **contact sensitization.** *Use with caution during* **pregnancy.**

Blends With: Clary sage, hyssop, myrtle, pine, valerian, and vetiver.

Odor: Type: *Middle Note (50-80% of the blend)*; Scent: *Sharp, woody, herbaceous, with a slight floral undertone*; Intensity: *4*

YLANG YLANG
(Cananga odorata)

Botanical Family: Annonaceae (tropical trees and shrubs - custard-apple)

Extraction Method/Origin: Steam distilled from flowers — Commores, Madagascar, Indonesia, Philippines *(Flowers are picked early in the morning to maximize oil yield. The highest quality oil is drawn from the first hour of distillation.)*

Chemical Constituents: Sesquiterpenes (up to 55%): β-caryophyllene (<22%), germacrene-D (<20%), α-farnesene (<12%), humulene (<5%); Esters (<50%): benzyl acetate & benzoate (<25%), methyl salicylate & benzoate (<17%), farnesyl acetate (<7%), geranyl acetate (<4%), linalyl acetate; Alcohols (<45%): linalol (<40%), geraniol; Ethers: paracresyl methyl ether (<15%); Phenols (<10%): methyl p-cresol (<9%), methyl chavicol (estragole), eugenol, isoeugenol; Oxides: caryophyllene oxide (<7%); Sesquiterpene Alcohols: farnesol.

Properties: **Anti-depressant, antiseptic, antispasmodic, sedative**, and **tonic**.

Esoteric Uses/Actions: Astrological: *Venus*; Body type: *Ectomorph*; Chakras: *2 & 3*; Character: *Strongly Yin*; Crystals: *Kunzite*; Element: *Earth & Water*; Number: *7*

Historical Uses: Interestingly enough, the original wild flowers had no fragrance. Through selection and cloning, we have this unique fragrance today. Ylang ylang has been used to cover the beds of newlywed couples on their wedding night, for skin treatments, to soothe insect bites, and in hair preparations to promote thick, shiny, lustrous hair (it is also reported to help control split ends). It has also been used to treat colic, constipation, indigestion, stomachaches, and to regulate the heartbeat and respiration.

French Medicinal Uses: **Anxiety, arterial hypertension, depression, diabetes, fatigue** (mental), **frigidity, hair loss, hyperpnea** (reduces), **insomnia, palpitations, tachycardia.**

Other Possible Uses: Ylang ylang may help balance **male-female energies** so one can move closer towards being in spiritual attunement and allow them to focus their thoughts together, filtering out the ever-present garbage. It may help lower **blood pressure**, rapid **breathing**, balance **equilibrium, frustration**, balance **heart function, impotence, infection, intestinal problems, sex drive problems, shock**, and **skin problems**.

Body System(s) Affected: Emotional Balance, Cardiovascular and **Hormonal Systems**.

Aromatic Influence: It influences **sexual energy** and enhances **relationships**. It may help stimulate the adrenal glands. It is **calming** and **relaxing** and may also help with **anger** and possibly **rage** and **low self-esteem**. It brings back the feeling of **self-love, confidence, joy** and **peace**.

Application: Apply to **Vita Flex Points** and/or directly on **area** of concern; **Diffuse**. It may be beneficial when applied over the **thymus** (to help stimulate the immune system).

Oral Use As Dietary Supplement: Generally regarded as safe (GRAS) for internal consumption by the FDA. **Dilute** *one drop oil in 1 tsp. honey or 4 oz. of beverage (i.e. soy/rice milk).* ***Not for children under 6 years old; use with caution and in greater dilution for children 6 years old and over.***

Safety Data: *Repeated use can possibly result in* **contact sensitization.**

Blend Classification: Personifier and Modifier

Blends With: Anise, bergamot, cardamom, chamomile, cumin, geranium, grapefruit, lemon, marjoram, sandalwood, vetiver.

Odor: Type: *Middle to Base Notes (20-80% of the blend)*; Scent: *Sweet, heavy, narcotic, cloying, tropical floral, with spicy-balsamic undertones*; Intensity: *5*

I am so grateful to have these oils!

My daughter, Haley, at age 18 was ill one Sunday, and later in the evening was feeling quite worse. When we checked, she had a fever of 105 degrees. I filled a gel capsule with 10 drops of Clove oil and had her take it with some water. in 1/2 hour I checked her temperature and it was down to 102. I gave her 5 more drops in another capsule and in another 1/2 hour, her fever was totally gone!!

-Submitted by Sally Donahue, Wilsonville, Oregon

Goodbye to Fibroid Lumps

I had s uffered for 32 years with massive fibrocystic breast lumbs. They were so painful that I could not even hug my children when they were young. I took vitamin E during those years which seemed to help. Then I heard about the research done on therapeutic grade essential oils and breast cancer. I stopped using deodorants with aluminum. I also mixed 40 drops of frankincense essential oil with 4oz of pure apricot oil and applied t his mixture under my arms during the day as often as I would think about it. Every night before I went to bed, I applied 4-5 drops each of frankincense and lavender to both breasts. A little over 4 weeks later, all fibroid lumps, pain and tenderness were completely gone and have not returned.

-Submitted by Ann Gaither, Corpus Christi, Texas

Oil Blends

This section contains proprietary blends and detailed information about each. Other commercial blends exist on the market but the authors (and many others) find these blends to be superior in synergy and potency. An approximate frequency is indicated for many of the blends. However, please keep in mind that there are many variables involved in an oil's frequency. Consequently, these numbers may be difficult to duplicate. These product names are all trademarks of Young Living Essential Oils and although these product names appear throughout other sections of this book without the trademark symbol, they still refer to these same trademarked products.

ABUNDANCE™

This is a blend that was specifically designed to enhance **magnetic energy** and create the law of attraction through the magnetic field around us, to enhance one's thoughts through electrical stimulation of the somatides and the cells, and to put out a frequency charge of **prosperity** and **abundance**. It may **attract riches** to **oneself**. It also contains tremendous **anti-viral** and **anti-fungal** properties, which may make it a very powerful **support** to the **immune system**, possibly giving one an abundance of **health** as well.

Single Oils Contained In This Blend:
Myrrh—is part of the formula the Lord gave Moses (Exodus 30:22-27). It is a **true gift**. When we **open** our **hearts** and **minds** to receive the gifts, they will be given.

Frankincense—contains sesquiterpenes, which may help **oxygenate** the **pineal** and **pituitary glands**. It may help **promote** a **positive attitude**.

Patchouli—is **sedating, calming**, and **relaxing** allowing it to reduce **anxiety**. It may have some particular influence on **sex, physical energy**, and **money**.

Orange—brings **peace** and **happiness** to the **mind** and **body** and **joy** to the **heart**, which provide **emotional** support.

Clove—may influence **healing**, improve **memory**, and create a feeling of **protection** and **courage**.

Ginger—is **warming, uplifting**, and **empowering**. Emotionally, it may help influence **physical energy, love**, and **courage**. Because of its calming influence on the digestive system, it may help reduce feelings of **nausea**, and **motion sickness**.

Spruce—**grounds** the **body**, creating the **balance** and the **opening** necessary to **receive** and to **give**. It may help **dilate** the **bronchial tract** to **improve** the **oxygen exchange**. It also helps one release **emotional blocks**.

Body System(s) Affected: The oils in this blend may help it be effective for dealing with various problems related to the **Immune** and **Respiratory Systems**, and to **Emotional Balance**.

Aromatic Influence: When diffused, this oil creates harmonic energy around oneself.

Application: May be worn on the **wrists**, behind the **ears**, on the **neck** and **face**. Individuals with sensitive skin may want to blend with V-6 Mixing Oil, Genesis Hand and Body Lotion. May be worn as a **perfume** or **cologne** or placed on the **checkbook, car dash, computer, phone, wallet**, or in your **purse**. Try **cooking** with it. To create more business, one may want to add a ½ bottle of Abundance to 5 gallons of paint before painting the office.

Safety Data: *Repeated use can result in extreme* **contact sensitization.** *Can be irritating to sensitive* **skin.**

Companion Oils: Acceptance, Awaken, or Release may be used first to help release the emotions that stop us from receiving abundance. It may then be followed by Envision, Into the Future, Joy, Magnify Your Purpose, Motivation, or Live with Passion.

Frequency: Physical; approximately 78 MHz–same frequency as the brain.

Bible: "For as he thinketh in his heart, so [is] he . . ." (Proverbs 23:7). We can create the kind of abundance we want, even that of poverty by believing we can't receive.

ACCEPTANCE™

This blend was formulated to help stimulate the mind to open up and **accept new things** in **life**, enabling us to reach toward our higher potential. It may also be beneficial in helping one **overcome denial** or **procrastination** and to help create a feeling of **security**.

Single Oils Contained In This Blend:

Geranium—may help with **hormonal balance, liver** and **kidney functions** and the **discharge** of **toxins** from the **liver** that hold us back from having balance. Geranium **opens** the **liver chakra** (Solar Plexus). Note: The liver is the place where fear and anger are stored.

Blue Tansy—may help **cleanse** the **liver** and **calm** the **lymphatic system** to help rid one of **anger** and promote a feeling of **self-control**.

Frankincense—contains sesquiterpenes, which may help **oxygenate** the **pineal** and **pituitary glands**. As one of the ingredients for the holy incense, it was used anciently to help **enhance** one's **communication with the creator**. It may help **promote** a **positive attitude**.

Sandalwood—also, like frankincense, is high in sesquiterpenes, which were discovered to **increase** the amount of **oxygen** around the **pineal** and **pituitary glands**, thus helping to **improve** one's **attitude**. It **alleviates depression** and assists in the removal of **negative programming** from the cells of the body. It helps one **accept others** with an open heart while diminishing one's own egocentricity.

Neroli—has been regarded traditionally by the Egyptian people for its great attributes for **healing** the **mind, body** and **spirit**. It is **calming** and **relaxing** to body and spirit. It may also help to **strengthen** and **stabilize** the emotions, and **bring relief** to seemingly hopeless situations. It encourages **confidence, courage, joy, peace**, and **sensuality**.

Rosewood—is **soothing** to the **skin, appeasing** to the **mind, relaxing** to the **body**, and creates a feeling of **peace** and **gentleness**.

Carrier Oil Contained In This Blend: Almond Oil.

Body System(s) Affected: The oils in this blend may help it be effective for dealing with numerous problems related to the **Nervous System** and **Emotional Balance**. Even when dealing with a physical problem, emotional "acceptance" of the present situation, rather than denial, helps one move forward in the healing process.

Aromatic Influence: When inhaled or diffused, this blend may help **calm** a troubled mind and promote feelings of **confidence** and **courage**. By calming the raging storms of mental frustration, we are finally capable of viewing our true position in life. We can then accept where we are and move forward with confidence on our path to achieving loftier goals.

Application: Best when rubbed over the **liver** (when the liver is toxic, the mind and emotions are lethargic), behind the **ears**, on the **chest, face, heart, neck, thymus**, and **wrists**. It may also be applied over the **sacral chakra** (base) and worn as a **perfume** or **cologne**. It can be **diffused** for some great results.

Frequency: Physical and Emotional; approximately 102 MHz.

AROMA LIFE™

This is a blend of oils which, through some extensive research, were found to help **strengthen** and **improve** the **cardiovascular, lymphatic**, and **circulatory systems**. This blend may also help to lower **high blood pressure, reduce stress**, and **alleviate hemorrhoids**.

Single Oils Contained In This Blend:

Cypress—is **anti-infectious, mucolytic, antiseptic, lymphatic decongestant, refreshing**, and **relaxing**. It may help improve **lung circulation** and relieve other **respiratory problems**.

Marjoram—is **relaxing, calming**, and **appeasing** to the **muscles** that constrict and sometimes contribute to **headaches**.

Helichrysum—may help **cleanse** the **blood** and improve **circulatory functions**. It is **anti-catarrhal** in structure and nature. On a spiritual level, it may help one **let go of angry feelings** that prevent one from forgiving and moving forward in life.

Ylang Ylang—may help **balance** the **male-female energies** so one can move closer towards being in spiritual attunement and allow them to focus their thoughts together, filtering out the ever-present garbage.

Carrier Oil Contained In This Blend: Sesame Seed Oil.

Body System(s) Affected: The oils in this blend may help it be effective for dealing with various problems related to the **Cardiovascular System**.

Application: Best when massaged over the **heart** (left side of the chest). It can be diluted with V-6 Mixing Oil for a full body massage. It can also be applied to the **Vita Flex Heart Points**

including, under the **left ring finger** and the **left ring toe**, on the left arm just **above** the **elbow**, and on the **arteries** of the **neck**. It may also help to apply this blend along the spine from the 1st to the 4th thoracic vertebrae, which correspond to the cardiopulmonary nerves (*Refer to the Autonomic Nervous System chart in the Science and Application section of this book*).

Companion Oils: It may be beneficial to combine <u>Joy</u> with this blend when the heart is in stress or combine with <u>Valor</u> to give the heart courage. Adding some grapefruit oil to this blend may help improve circulation and dissolve fat more quickly. May also add helichrysum, rosemary, or ylang ylang.

Frequency: Physical; approximately 84 MHz.

Comments: This blend may work as a Natural Hemostat and Chelating agent. Red spots on the body may indicate a biotin deficiency. If so, using Super C may be beneficial.

AROMA SIEZ™

The oils in this blend were selected specifically for their ability to **relax, calm** and **relieve** the **tension** of **spastic muscles** resulting from **sports injury, fatigue** or **stress**. This blend may also help to relieve **headaches**.

Single Oils Contained In This Blend:

Basil—has **anti-inflammatory** and **antispasmodic** properties. It is relaxing to **spastic muscles**, including those that contribute to **headaches** and **migraines**.

Marjoram—is an **antispasmodic** and is **relaxing, calming**, and **appeasing** to the **muscles** that constrict and sometimes contribute to **headaches**. It has been useful for **muscle spasms, sprains, bruises, migraines**, and **sore muscles**.

Lavender—is an oil that has traditionally been known to **balance** the **body** and to work wherever there is a need. It has **antispasmodic** and **analgesic** properties. It may help with **sprains, sore muscles, headaches**, and general **healing**.

Peppermint—is an **anti-inflammatory** to the **nerves** and helps **reduce inflammation** in **damaged tissue**. It is **soothing, cooling**, and **dilating** to the **system**. It may help to **reduce fevers, candida, nausea, vomiting**, and strengthen the **respiratory system**.

Cypress—is **anti-infectious, mucolytic, antiseptic, lymphatic decongestant, refreshing**, and **relaxing**. It may help improve **lung circulation** as well as help relieve other **respiratory problems**. It may also help relieve **muscle cramps** and improve overall **circulation**.

Body System(s) Affected: The oils in this blend may help it be effective for dealing with various problems related to the **Respiratory System** and to **Muscles and Bones**.

Application: Best if applied on location for all **muscles** and on back of **neck** for **stress headaches**. It may also be applied over the **heart** or diluted with V-6 Mixing Oil for a full body **massage**. It is also beneficial when applied to the **Vita Flex points** on **feet** or placed in the **bath** water.

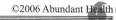

Companion Oils: Basil, birch, elemi, helichrysum, Idaho tansy, marjoram, spruce, wintergreen. Ortho Ease Massage Oil or Ortho Sport Massage Oil may also be used to enhance the effects of this blend.

Frequency: Low (Physical); approximately 64 MHz.

Australian Blue™

With a base of Blue cypress oil, this blend has an exotic, tropical scent that is **grounding** and **stabilizing**, yet **uplifting** and **inspiring**. Topically it may help relieve minor **aches** and **pains**. It may help calm **anger** and bring about **self-control** as it balances and stabilizes the **emotions**.

Single Oils Contained In This Blend:

Blue Cypress (*Callitris intratropica*)—is an abundant source of sesquiterpenes. It is the only oil obtained from wood that contains guaiol and guaiazulene, which gives it a deep blue color. It is grounding and stabilizing with a fragrance that uplifts and inspires.

Ylang Ylang—may help **balance** the **male-female energies** so one can move closer towards being in spiritual attunement and allow them to focus their thoughts together, filtering out the ever-present garbage.

Cedarwood—was used traditionally by the North American Indians to enhance their potential for **spiritual communication**. It may help **open** the **pineal gland**.

Blue Tansy—may help **cleanse** the **liver** and **calm** the **lymphatic system** to help rid one of **anger** and promote a feeling of **self-control**.

White Fir (*Abies grandis*)—creates a feeling of **grounding, anchoring**, and **empowerment**. It can **stimulate** the **mind** while allowing the **body** to **relax**. Topically it helps relieve **pain** from **inflammation**.

Body System(s) Affected: Emotional Balance.

Aromatic Influence: When diffused, this special blend of oils can be **calming** and **balancing** to the emotions. It may help **stress** and **anger**, relieve **anxiety** and **tension**, and help **relax** the entire body. Mentally it can be **stimulating** and **inspiring**.

Application: Diffuse, wear as **perfume** or **cologne**, or apply topically to areas of concern.

Safety Data: *Could possibly result in contact sensitization or skin irritation.*

Awaken™

This blend may help **awaken** one to the possibility of their **higher potential**, that they may make the necessary transitions in their lives to achieve greater things. This blend may also be beneficial for **spiritual** and/or **emotional enhancement**.

Oil Blends Contained In This Blend:

Joy—is a blend which may help to open the heart and promote feelings of **self-love** and **love for others** so one can experience ultimate joy.

Oil Blends

Forgiveness—is a blend which was formulated to help move people into a mental state which may help them to forgive and forget. Inhaling this blend may stimulate one to **forgive themselves** and **others** of **transgression**.

Dream Catcher—is an oil blend that was created to **open** the **mind**, to **enhance** ones **dreams**, to help one **visualize** their dreams and **hang onto** them until they become **reality**.

Present Time—is a blend of oils that was designed to bring one both mentally and emotionally into the **present time**. In order for us to **awaken** to **our higher potential**, we must be living in the moment **"now"**, not fretting about the past or daydreaming about the future.

Harmony—Without **harmony** none of the other states of mind would come to be. We must be in **harmony** with ourselves, with our creator, and with the world and all those around us. When we have harmony in our lives, then many other things will come to balance and fruition.

Carrier Oil Contained In This Blend: Almond Oil.

Body System(s) Affected: The oils in this blend may help it be effective for dealing with various problems related to **Emotional Balance**.

Aromatic Influence: We enjoy diffusing this blend while sleeping at night because it helps us wake up **invigorated** and **refreshed**.

Application: Best when applied on the **chest, heart, forehead, neck, sternum** (clearing allergies), **temples**, and **wrists**. It may be used as an **aftershave**, a **cologne**, or a **perfume**. It may also be diluted with V-6 Mixing Oil for a **full body massage** or added to the **bath** water. En-R-Gee may be put on the feet and Awaken on the temples or cheeks for one to feel like they have had eight hours of sleep.

Companion Oils: Dream Catcher, En-R-Gee, Envision, Harmony, Into the Future, Joy, Motivation, Live with Passion, Valor, White Angelica

Frequency: Physical; approximately 89 MHz.

BELIEVE™

This blend has been specifically formulated to calm the spirit while stimulating the mind, allowing us to believe in our own limitless potential to create and improve. It is **grounding** and **empowering**, helping to promote positive action toward the accomplishment of goals and fulfillment of dreams.

Single Oils Contained In This Blend:

Balsam Fir—creates a feeling of **grounding, anchoring**, and **empowerment**. It can **stimulate** the **mind** while allowing the **body** to **relax**. Topically it helps relieve **overworked** and **tired muscles** and **joints**.

Rosewood—may help improve **skin elasticity**. It is **soothing** to the **skin, appeasing** to the **mind, relaxing** to the **body**, and creates a feeling of **peace** and **gentleness**.

Frankincense—contains sesquiterpenes, which may help **oxygenate** the **pineal** and **pituitary glands**. As one of the ingredients for the holy incense, it was used anciently to help **enhance** one's **communication with the creator**. It may help **promote** a **positive attitude**.

Body System(s) Affected: The oils in this blend may help it be effective for dealing with various problems related to the **Nervous** and **Immune Systems, Muscles and Bones**, and to **Emotional Balance**.

Aromatic Influence: This blend of oils has a **calming, stabilizing** and **mentally energizing** aroma. Diffusing this blend may help to **release** the unlimited **potential** to **create** and **improve** our surroundings. The mentally uplifting and energizing aroma may help **promote belief** in ourselves and our capabilities.

Application: Diffuse or apply to the **forehead, temples**, and over the **heart**. May also be worn as a **perfume** or **cologne**.

Companion Oils: Humility, Gratitude, Grounding, Live with Passion, Motivation

BRAIN POWER™

This blend has been specifically formulated to include those oils that are high in sesquiterpene compounds. Research has shown that sesquiterpenes play a role in **dissolving petrochemicals** along the receptor sites near the **pituitary, pineal**, and **hypothalamus**. This helps to increase normal receptivity along those sites and increase the amount of oxygen in those areas. **Increased oxygen** around the pineal, pituitary, and hypothalamus can lead to **increased mental capacity, mental clarity**, and **reduced symptoms** of what has come to be known as **"brain fog"**.

Single Oils Contained In This Blend:

Cedarwood—was used traditionally by the North American Indians to enhance their potential for **spiritual communication**. It may help **open** the **pineal gland**.

Sandalwood—also, like frankincense, is high in sesquiterpenes, which were discovered to **increase** the amount of **oxygen** around the **pineal** and **pituitary glands**, thus helping to **improve** one's **attitude**. It **alleviates depression** and assists in the removal of **negative programming** from the cells of the body. It helps one **accept others** with an open heart while diminishing one's own egocentricity.

Frankincense—contains sesquiterpenes, which may help **oxygenate** the **pineal** and **pituitary glands**. As one of the ingredients for the holy incense, it was used anciently to help **enhance** one's **communication with the creator**. It may help **promote** a **positive attitude**.

Melissa—is an oil that is powerful as an **anti-viral** agent, yet it is very gentle and very delicate because of the nature of the plant. It has the ability to work with and enhance the gentle aspects of the human body. It is **calming** and **uplifting** and may also help to **balance** the **emotions**. It may also help to remove **emotional blocks** and **instill** a **positive outlook** on **life**.

Blue Cypress (*Callitris intratropica*)—comes from Australia and has been shown to improve circulation and increase the flow of oxygen to the brain.

Lavender—is an oil that has traditionally been known to **balance** the **body** and to work wherever there is a need. It has **antispasmodic** and **analgesic** properties. It may help with **sprains, sore muscles, headaches**, and general **healing**.

Helichrysum—may help **cleanse** the **blood** and improve **circulatory functions**. It is **anti-catarrhal** in structure and nature. On a spiritual level, it may help one **let go of angry feelings** that prevent one from forgiving and moving forward in life.

Body System(s) Affected: The oils in this blend may help it be effective for dealing with various problems related to the **Nervous System** and to **Emotional Balance**.

Aromatic Influence: This blend of oils has a **powerfully uplifting** and **mentally energizing** aroma. Diffusing this blend may help to provide **deep concentration** and **focus** during strenuous **mental activity**.

Application: May be applied to the **neck, throat**, under the **nose**, to the **roof** of the **mouth** using the thumb, or worn as a **perfume** or **cologne**. May also be applied **inside** the **mouth** with a finger, either **under** the **tongue** or on the **inside** of each **cheek** (*See SMELL in the Personal Guide section of this book*).

Companion Oils: Clarity, Envision, RC, Raven

Frequency: Physical; approximately 78 MHz–same frequency as the brain.

CHIVALRY™

This blend is a combination of four oil blends; Valor, Joy, Harmony, and Gratitude, each a value that is embodied in the word "chivalry". This blend was created to be **empowering** and **ennobling**. It helps to open the **energy centers** and promote feelings of **strength, peace, trustworthiness**, and **courage**.

Oil Blends Contained In This Blend:

Valor—is emotionally uplifting and helps to empower the physical and spiritual bodies. It helps to build **courage, confidence**, and **self-esteem** while promoting **calmness, peace**, and **relaxation**.

Joy—is a blend which may help to open the heart and promote feelings of **self-love** and **love for others** so one can experience ultimate joy.

Harmony—Without **harmony** none of the other states of mind would come to be. We must be in **harmony** with ourselves, with our creator, and with the world and all those around us. When we have harmony in our lives, then many other things will come to balance and fruition.

Gratitude—helps to **elevate, soothe**, and **appease** the **mind** while bringing **relief** and **relaxation** to the body.

Carrier Oil Contained In This Blend: Almond Oil.

Body System(s) Affected: Emotional Balance.

Aromatic Influence: When diffused or worn as perfume, this special blend of oils helps to **balance** the emotions. It may help **revitalize** and **empower** both body and mind promoting **courage, honor,** and **integrity**.

Application: Rub over the **heart**, and on **forehead**, and **temples**. **Diffuse** or wear as **perfume** or **cologne**.

Safety Data: *Use with caution during* **pregnancy***. Not for use by people with* **epilepsy***. Use with caution if dealing with* **high blood pressure***. Avoid exposure to* **direct sunlight** *for 3 to 6 hours after use.*

Companion Oils: Magnify Your Purpose, Live with Passion

CHRISTMAS SPIRIT™

This blend is effective for enhancing the **feeling** and **memory** of the beautiful times of **Christmas** and for enhancing the desire to be in that happy and joyful moment that Christmas brings. It may be very beneficial for **protecting** against **airborne viruses** and **bacteria** because it contains several very powerful **anti-viral** and **antiseptic** oils. It may also be quite **soothing** and **healing** to the **respiratory system**.

Single Oils Contained In This Blend:

Orange—spread a little sunshine on gloomy thoughts and depression. It may help encourage a positive outlook on life, bringing **peace** and **happiness** to the mind and body. Orange is **antiseptic** and **anti-depressant**.

Cinnamon Bark—is part of the formula the Lord gave Moses (Exodus 30:22-27). It has very specific purposes: (1) it is a **powerful purifier**, (2) it is a powerful **oxygenator**, and (3) it **enhances** the action and the activity of **other oils**. It may have a **stimulating** and **toning** effect on the whole body and particularly the circulatory system. It may also help bring about feelings of **joy**. It is **antiseptic, anti-bacterial**, and **anti-viral**.

Spruce—**grounds** the **body**, creating the balance and opening necessary to receive and to give. This oil is **warming, healing, uplifting**, and **soothing**. It may also help **relieve anxiety** and act as an **antiseptic**.

Body System(s) Affected: The oils in this blend may help it be effective for dealing with various problems related to the **Cardiovascular** and **Nervous Systems** and to **Emotional Balance**.

Aromatic Influence: This blend of oils has a delightful **fragrance** and is wonderful for creating the **feeling** of **security** that usually accompanies the **holiday season**. It is also nice for **air purification**.

Application: May be applied to the **crown** of the **head** or worn as a **perfume** or **cologne**. The beautiful fragrance of this blend can be further enhanced by placing it on pine boughs, pine cones, cedar chips, and on logs to burn in the fireplace. It makes an excellent addition to potpourri.

Safety Data: *Repeated use on the skin can result in extreme* **contact sensitivity.** *Can cause extreme* **skin irritation.**

Companion Oils: Mandarin, clove, and nutmeg.

Frequency: Emotional and Spiritual; approximately 104 MHz.

CITRUS FRESH™

Citrus Fresh is a blend which may help to enhance the **feeling** of **well being** in **children**. Because many of the oils contained in this blend are strong **antiseptics**, it may work well for **killing airborne bacteria**. It may be useful for **relaxing, calming**, and alleviating **insomnia**. It may also help to **balance** the **systems**. It is a fragrance that can be enjoyed by everyone. Flavoring ones water with this oil blend may help **open** the **lymphatic system** and **stimulate** the **immune system**.

Single Oils Contained In This Blend:

Orange—brings **peace** and **happiness** to the **mind** and **body** and **joy** to the **heart**, which provide **emotional** support to help one overcome depression.

Tangerine—contains esters and aldehydes which are **sedating** and **calming** to the **nervous system**. It is also a **diuretic** and a **decongestant** of the **lymphatic system**.

Mandarin—is **appeasing, gentle**, and promotes **happiness**. It is also **refreshing, uplifting**, and **revitalizing**. Because of its sedative and slightly hypnotic properties, it is very good for **stress** and **irritability**.

Grapefruit—is an **anti-depressant**, an **antiseptic**, and a **diuretic**. It is **balancing** and **uplifting** to the mind, and may help to **relieve anxiety**.

Lemon—promotes **health, healing, physical energy**, and **purification**. Its fragrance is **invigorating, enhancing**, and **warming**.

Spearmint—is **anti-fungal** and **antiseptic**. It also acts as an anti-depressant by relieving mental strain and fatigue, and by lifting one's spirits.

Body System(s) Affected: The oils in this blend may help it be effective for dealing with various problems related to the **Immune System** and to **Emotional Balance**.

Aromatic Influence: This blend of oils may create an enjoyable aromatic fragrance in the **home** or **work place**. Simple diffusion can be achieved by applying a few drops of this blend on a cotton ball and placing it on the desk at work or in an air vent.

Application: May be applied on the **ears, heart**, and **wrists** or worn as a **perfume** or **cologne**. It may be diluted with V-6 Mixing Oil for a **full body massage**. It may also be added to water for a **relaxing bath**. This blend can also help **purify drinking water**. Children may like to add this blend to water and freeze for **popsicles**. It is excellent for children, though dilution with V-6 Mixing Oil is highly recommended.

Safety Data: *Can cause extreme* **skin irritation.** *Avoid exposure to direct* **sunlight** *for up to 12 hours after use.*

Frequency: Physical and Emotional; approximately 90 MHz.

Comments: A university in Japan experimented with diffusing different oils in the office. When they diffused lemon there were 54% fewer errors, with jasmine there were 33% fewer errors, and with lavender there were 20% fewer errors. When oils are diffused while studying and smelled during a test via a hanky, cotton ball or plastic nasal inhaler, test scores may increase by as much as 50%. Different oils should be used for different tests, but the same oil should be used during the test as was used while studying for that particular test. The smell of the oil may help bring back the memory of what was studied.

CLARITY™

This blend may help with **memory retention** and **mental alertness**; it may even help **oxygenate** the **brain**. One may want to **study** with this blend, then smell it during a test to help recall what was studied earlier. It may also be a **stimulant** for **low energy** and may help keep one from going into **shock**.

Single Oils Contained In This Blend:

Basil—has been found beneficial for **alleviating mental fatigue**. It may help **sharpen** the **senses** and **encourage concentration**. It may also **stimulate** the **nerves** and the **adrenal cortex**.

Cardamom—is **uplifting, refreshing**, and **invigorating**. It may be beneficial for **clearing confusion**.

Rosemary verbenon—may help **balance heart function, energize** the **solar plexus**, and **reduce mental fatigue**. It also stimulates **memory** and opens the **conscious mind**.

Peppermint—is an **anti-inflammatory** to the **nerves** and helps **reduce inflammation** in **damaged tissue**. It is **soothing, cooling**, and **dilating** to the **system**. Dr. Dembar, of the University of Cincinnati, discovered in a research study that inhaling peppermint oil **increased** the **mental accuracy** of the students tested by up to 28%.

Rosewood—may help improve **skin elasticity**. It is **soothing** to the **skin, appeasing** to the **mind, relaxing** to the **body**, and creates a feeling of **peace** and **gentleness**.

Geranium—may help with **hormonal balance, liver** and **kidney functions** and the **discharge** of **toxins** from the **liver** that hold us back from having balance. Geranium **opens** the **liver chakra**.

Lemon—promotes **health, healing, physical energy**, and **purification**. Its fragrance is **invigorating, enhancing**, and **warming**.

Palmarosa—is valuable for all types of **skin** problems because it **stimulates** new **cell growth**, regulates oil production, **moisturizes** and **speeds healing**.

Ylang Ylang—may help **balance** the **male-female energies** so one can move closer towards being in spiritual attunement and allow them to focus their thoughts together, filtering out the ever-present garbage and establishing a sense of relaxation. It brings back the feeling of **self-love, confidence, joy** and **peace**.

Bergamot—is **soothing** to the **endocrine system** and the **hormones** of the body. It may **uplift** and **calm** the **emotions** to help relieve **anxiety, stress**, and **tension**.

Roman Chamomile—neutralizes **allergies** and helps to cleanse the **blood** and **expel toxins** from the **liver**.

Jasmine—is very **uplifting** to the **emotions**; it may produce a feeling of **confidence, energy, euphoria**, and **optimism**. As an **antispasmodic**, it has been used effectively for **menstrual** discomfort, **muscle spasms**, and **uterine** disorders.

Body System(s) Affected: The oils in this blend may help it be effective for dealing with various problems related to the **Nervous System** and to **Emotional Balance**.

Aromatic Influence: The oils in this blend are known for their ability to help increase **mental alertness**. Simple diffusion can be achieved by applying a few drops of this blend on a cotton ball and placing it on the desk at work or in an air vent. *Plastic nasal inhalers are also available from Abundant Health for more discreet, direct, long-lasting personal use.*

Application: Best when applied across the **brow**, on the back of the **neck**, on the **temples**, and on the **wrists**. This blend may be added to ones **bath** water or worn as a **perfume** or **cologne**.

Safety Data: *Can be irritating to sensitive **skin**. Use with caution during **pregnancy**. Avoid exposure to direct **sunlight** for up to 12 hours after use.*

Companion Oils: This blend and En-R-Gee together may help one stay awake while driving late at night. Others include Brain Power, lemon, and peppermint.

Frequency: Emotional; approximately 101 MHz.

Comments: Since this blend contains cardamom and high levels of transphenol, it may cause headaches when inhaled if there is petrochemical or heavy metal accumulation in the brain.

DI-GIZE™

This blend may be useful for **improving** the **digestive function**. The oils in this blend have been found to be beneficial in **digesting toxic material** and for **alleviating indigestion, stomach cramps, upset stomach, belching, bloating**, and **heartburn**. Placing a little of this blend behind the ears may help alleviate **morning sickness**. It has been found to rid animals and people of **parasites** by applying it to their feet. It has also been reported that this blend helps to alleviate discomfort from parasites by massage and compress application across the stomach.

Single Oils Contained In This Blend:

Tarragon—may help to reduce **anorexia, dyspepsia, flatulence, intestinal spasms, nervous** and **sluggish digestion**, and **genital urinary tract infection**.

Ginger—is **warming, uplifting**, and **empowering**. Emotionally, it may help influence **physical energy, love**, and **courage**. Because of its calming influence on the digestive system, it may help reduce feelings of **nausea**, and **motion sickness**.

Peppermint—is an **anti-inflammatory** to the **prostate** and **nerves**. It is **soothing, cooling** and **dilating** to the **system**. It may also be beneficial for **food poisoning,**

vomiting, diarrhea, constipation, flatulence, halitosis, colic, nausea, and **motion sickness**.

Juniper—has **antiseptic, cleansing**, and **detoxifying** properties. It may help to **improve circulation** through the **kidneys**.

Anise—may help **calm** and strengthen the **digestive system**.

Fennel—may help **support** the **digestive function** by **supporting** the **liver**. It may also help **balance** the **hormones**.

Lemongrass—is a **vasodilator, antiseptic, anti-bacterial, anti-inflammatory**, and **sedative**. It may help improve **circulation**, wake up the **lymphatic system**, and increase the flow of **oxygen**. It may also help to **lift** the **spirit**.

Patchouli—is **sedating, calming**, and **relaxing** allowing it to reduce **anxiety**. It is a digester of toxic material in the body.

Body System(s) Affected: The oils in this blend may help it be effective for dealing with various problems related to the **Digestive System**.

Application: May be applied to the **Vita Flex points** on the **feet** and **ankles**. It may also be applied topically over the **stomach**, as a **compress** on the **abdomen**, on other **Vita Flex points** on the **body**, and at the bottom of the **throat** (for gagging). As a **dietary supplement**, dilute one drop in 4 oz. of water or soy/rice milk and sip slowly. May also be used in a **retention enema** for ridding the **colon** of **parasites** and for combating **digestive candida**. Apply to **animal paws** for **parasites**.

Safety Data: *Use with caution during **pregnancy** (only a drop massaged on the outer ear for morning sickness). Not for use by people with **epilepsy**.*

Companion Oils: Peppermint and spearmint.

Companion Supplements: ComforTone, Essentialzyme, JuvaTone

Frequency: Emotional; approximately 102 MHz.

DRAGON TIME™

This is a blend of single oils that have historically been used to help **alleviate premenstrual** and **menstrual cramps** and discomfort. This blend may also help **men** with **prostate** problems.

Single Oils Contained In This Blend:

Clary Sage—is beneficial for **regulating cells** and **balancing** the **hormones**. It may help with **menstrual cramps, PMS**, and **pre-menopause** symptoms. It may also help with **circulatory problems**.

Fennel—may help **support** the **digestive function** by **supporting** the **liver**. It may also help **balance** the **hormones**.

Lavender—is an oil that has traditionally been known to **balance** the **body** and to work wherever there is a need. It may help with **PMS/menopausal problems, stress, stretch marks, tension**, and **water retention**.

Jasmine—is very **uplifting** to the **emotions**; it may produce a feeling of **confidence, energy, euphoria**, and **optimism**. As an **antispasmodic**, it has been used for **menstrual** discomfort, **muscle spasms**, and **uterine** disorders.

Yarrow—is a **powerful decongestant** of the **prostate** and a **hormone balancer**.

Body System(s) Affected: The oils in this blend may help it be effective for dealing with various problems related to the **Hormonal System** and to **Emotional Balance**.

Aromatic Influence: This blend of oils may be beneficial in times of **hormonal stress**. It may be diffused in the home or office, or put a few drops on a cotton ball and place in the car vent.

Application: May be applied to the **Vita Flex points** on the **feet** and around the **ankles**, both inside and out. It may be diluted with V-6 Mixing Oil for application on the other **Vita Flex points** on the **body**. It may also be applied as a hot **compress** or rubbed over the **abdomen**, across the **lower back**, or anywhere it **hurts**.

Safety Data: *Use with caution during* **pregnancy**.

Companion Oils: Combining this blend with <u>Mister</u> or <u>EndoFlex</u> may help **alleviate hot flashes (power surges)** in women.

Frequency: Physical; approximately 72 MHz.

Dream Catcher™

This blend may help to open the **mind**, to **enhance dreams**, and to help one **visualize** their **visions** and **hang onto** them until they become **reality**. It may also serve to **protect** one from the **negative dreams** that tend to steal our **vision**. Children love the smell of this blend and it may even help them to sleep more soundly. Our little girl asked for this blend every night for a while, until she felt comfortable with sleeping in her own bed. Later, if she was having a bad dream, she would come ask for some to be put on her forehead and would go right back to bed and sleep soundly for the rest of the night.

Single Oils Contained In This Blend:

Sandalwood—also, like frankincense, is high in sesquiterpenes, which were discovered to **increase** the amount of **oxygen** around the **pineal** and **pituitary glands**, thus helping to **improve** one's **attitude**. It **alleviates depression** and assists in the removal of **negative programming** from the cells of the body.

Bergamot—is **soothing** to the **endocrine system** and the **hormones** of the body. It may **uplift** and **calm** the **emotions** to help relieve **anxiety, stress**, and **tension**.

Ylang Ylang—may help **balance** the **male-female energies** so one can move closer towards being in spiritual attunement and allow them to focus their thoughts together, filtering out the ever-present garbage. It brings back the feeling of **self-love, confidence, joy** and **peace**.

Juniper—evokes feelings of **health, love**, and **peace** and may help to **elevate** one's **spiritual awareness**.

Blue Tansy—encourages an **uplifting feeling**, a **positive attitude**, and a general feeling of **well being**.

Tangerine—contains esters and aldehydes which are **sedating** and **calming** to the **nervous system**. It is also a **diuretic** and a **decongestant** of the **lymphatic system**.

Pepper, Black—may help **stimulate** the **endocrine system** and **increase energy**. May help **increase cellular oxygenation**.

Anise—may help **calm** and **strengthen** the **digestive system**.

Body System(s) Affected: The oils in this blend may help it be effective for dealing with various problems related to **Emotional Balance**.

Aromatic Influence: This blend may be diffused during the day, but seems to be most effective during sleep. This blend may also be useful during **meditation**.

Application: Best when applied to the **forehead** (**3rd eye** or **brow chakra**), **eye brows, temples,** behind the **ears**, and on the **throat chakra** (base of neck). It may be worn as a **perfume** or **cologne**. For a lasting aroma, place a drop under the **nose** or on the **pillow**. Add to **bath** water.

Safety Data: *Avoid exposure to direct* **sunlight** *for 3 to 6 hours after use.*

Companion Oils: To enhance **dream awareness**, put a couple drops of this blend on a **pillow**, Awaken on the **temples**, and Motivation on the **chest**. Other choices include Envision, Gathering, Into the Future, Live with Passion.

Frequency: Physical and Emotional; approximately 98 MHz.

Comments: Indian dream catchers have been used to help keep bad dreams away. This blend may accomplish the same purpose. However, if bad dreams do come, continued use of this oil may be necessary as something in the subconscious may need to be processed. Hold onto your dreams and visualize them into reality by bringing them from the mind to the heart to make them come true.

EGYPTIAN GOLD™

This special blend was formulated with oils that were used for various purposes in ancient Egypt, including mummification. Blended specifically to combat the "super bugs", the oils in this blend are highly anti-bacterial, anti-fungal, and antiviral. This blend may help stimulate the hypothalamus and pituitary glands. Its intoxicating fragrance is reminiscent of the grandeur of ancient Egypt. **Note**: The commercial availability of this blend may be somewhat erratic due to the occasional unavailability of some of the oils (i.e. hyssop).

Single Oils Contained In This Blend:

Frankincense—contains sesquiterpenes, which may help **oxygenate** the **pineal** and **pituitary glands**. As one of the ingredients for the holy incense, it was used anciently to help **enhance** one's **communication with the creator**. It was considered a prize possession and was given to Christ at his birth. It may help **promote** a **positive attitude**.

Lavender—is an oil that has traditionally been known to **balance** the **body** and to work wherever there is a need. It may help with **stress and tension**.

Balsam Fir—creates a feeling of **grounding, anchoring**, and **empowerment**. It can **stimulate** the **mind** while allowing the **body** to **relax**. Topically it helps relieve **overworked** and **tired muscles** and **joints**.

Myrrh—is part of the formula the Lord gave Moses (Exodus 30:22-27). It is a **true gift**. When we **open** our **hearts** and **minds** to receive the gifts, they will be given.

Spikenard—was highly prized in the Middle East during the time of Christ, and is referred to several times in the Bible. It is **anti-fungal, anti-inflammatory, relaxing, regenerative**, and helpful for allergic skin reactions.

Hyssop—was used by Moses during the Lord's Passover in Egypt (Exodus 12). It has **anti-inflammatory** and **anti-viral** properties. It may also have the ability to **open** up the **respiratory system** and **discharge toxins** and **mucus**.

Cedarwood—was used traditionally by the North American Indians to enhance their potential for **spiritual communication**. It may help **open** the **pineal gland**.

Rose—contains the highest frequency of the oils. It may help **enhance** the **frequency** of every cell, which could help bring **balance** and **harmony** to the body. It is thought by some to produce a magnetic energy that attracts **love** and enhances the frequency of **self-love**, bringing **joy** to the heart.

Cinnamon Bark—is part of the formula the Lord gave Moses (Exodus 30:22-27). It has very specific purposes: (1) it is a **powerful purifier**, (2) it is a powerful **oxygenator**, and (3) it **enhances** the action and the activity of **other oils**. It may have a **stimulating** and **toning** effect on the whole body and particularly the circulatory system. It is **antiseptic, anti-bacterial**, and **anti-viral**.

Body System(s) Affected: The oils in this blend may help it be effective for dealing with various problems related to the **Immune System** and to **Emotional Balance**.

Aromatic Influence: This blend of oils may help **lift** and **balance** one's **emotions**. It is also **stabilizing** and **empowering**. Simple diffusion can be achieved by applying a few drops of this blend on a cotton ball and placing it in the air vent of a car or on the heat registers of the home or hotel room.

Application: Best when applied on the **wrists** and behind and on the **ears**. It may also be massaged across the **base** of the **neck** and **temples**. Dilute with V-6 Mixing Oil to wear as a **perfume** or **cologne**.

Safety Data: *Could possibly result in **contact sensitization**. Use with caution if susceptible to epilepsy.*

Companion Oils: Sandalwood.

En-R-Gee™

En-R-Gee is a blend that may help **improve one's energy** in a natural way without overstimulating or creating problems that may be uncomfortable. It may also help with **mental alertness**.

Single Oils Contained In This Blend:

> **Rosemary cineol**—may help **balance heart function, energize** the **solar plexus**, and **reduce mental fatigue**.
>
> **Juniper**—has **antiseptic, cleansing**, and **detoxifying** properties. It may help to **improve circulation** through the **kidneys**.
>
> **Nutmeg**—has adrenal cortex-like activity, which helps support the **adrenal glands** for **increased energy**.
>
> **Fir**—may help create a feeling of **grounding, anchoring** and **empowerment**.
>
> **Pepper, Black**—may help **stimulate** the **endocrine system** and **increase energy**.
>
> **Lemongrass**—is a **vasodilator, antiseptic, anti-bacterial, anti-inflammatory**, and **sedative**. It may help improve **circulation**, wake up the **lymphatic system**, and increase the flow of **oxygen**. It may also help to **lift** the **spirit**.
>
> **Clove**—may influence **healing**, improve **memory**, and create a feeling of **protection** and **courage**. It may also help one overcome **fatigue**.

Body System(s) Affected: The oils in this blend may help it be effective for dealing with various problems related to the **Nervous System** and to **Emotional Balance**.

Aromatic Influence: This blend of oils may help boost one's **energy** when diffused. It is also **purifying**. Simple diffusion can be achieved by applying a few drops of this blend on a cotton ball and placing it in the air vent of a car or on the heat registers of the home or hotel room.

Application: Best when applied on the **wrists** and behind and on the **ears**. It may also be massaged across the **base** of the **neck, temples**, and rubbed on the **feet** in the morning. Dilute with V-6 Mixing Oil for **full body massage** or wear as a **perfume** or **cologne**.

Safety Data: *Can cause extreme **skin irritation**. Use with caution if susceptible to **epilepsy**.*

Companion Oils: One may feel like they have had eight hours of sleep by rubbing this blend on the feet and Awaken on **temples**. This blend and Clarity together may help one stay awake while driving late at night.

Frequency: Emotional; approximately 106 MHz.

ENDOFLEX™

This is a beautiful blend that may help provide overall **balance** and **support** to the **endocrine system** and may work to **improve** the **vitality** of the body. It may **support** the **pineal** and **pituitary** glands, **parathyroid, thymus**, and **adrenal** glands. It may also help to **alleviate hot flashes** and to **stimulate weight loss** by **improving** the **metabolic function**. It may support the **thyroid** for **metabolic** and **hormonal balance**.

Single Oils Contained In This Blend:

> **Spearmint**—is an oil that may balance and increase **metabolism**; helping to **burn up fats** and **toxins** in the body.

Sage—may help improve **estrogen** and **progesterone-testosterone balance**. It is believed to contain elements that contribute to the **secretion** of **progesterone-testosterone**.

Geranium—may help with **hormonal balance, liver** and **kidney functions** and the **discharge** of **toxins** from the **liver** that hold us back from having balance. Geranium **opens** the **liver chakra**.

Myrtle—may help **regulate thyroid function**. For **hypo-thyroid** it may **increase activity**, and **improve balance**.

Nutmeg—has adrenal cortex-like activity, which helps support the **adrenal glands** for **increased energy**.

German Chamomile—has been found to help **open** the **liver, increase liver function** and **secretion**, and **support** the **pancreas**.

Carrier Oil Contained In This Blend: Sesame Seed Oil.

Body System(s) Affected: The oils in this blend may help it be effective for dealing with various problems related to the **Hormonal (Endocrine) System.**

Application: May be applied over the **thyroid, kidneys, liver** (front right, 2" down from bra line), **pancreas** (front left), and all **glands**. It may also work well when applied to the **Vita Flex points** on the **feet** including under the **big toe** and on the **throat** or **endocrine gland locations**.

Safety Data: *Can be irritating to sensitive skin. Use with caution if susceptible to epilepsy.*

Frequency: Emotional and Spiritual; approximately 138 MHz.

ENVISION™

This blend is comprised of essential oils which provide powerful support and balance to the emotions. This type of emotional support is necessary for us to move forward with renewed faith in the future toward achieving our dreams and goals.

Single Oils Contained In This Blend:

Spruce—**grounds** the **body**, creating the **balance** and the **opening** necessary to **receive** and to **give**. It may help **dilate** the **bronchial tract** to **improve** the **oxygen exchange**. It also helps one release **emotional blocks**.

Sage—may help improve **estrogen** and **progesterone-testosterone balance**. It is believed to contain elements that contribute to the **secretion** of **progesterone-testosterone**.

Rose—contains the highest frequency of the oils. It may help **enhance** the **frequency** of every cell, which could help bring **balance** and **harmony** to the body. It is thought by some to produce a magnetic energy that attracts **love** and enhances the frequency of **self-love**, bringing **joy** to the heart.

Geranium—may help with **hormonal balance, liver** and **kidney functions** and the **discharge** of **toxins** from the **liver** that hold us back from having balance. Geranium **opens** the **liver chakra**.

Orange—brings **peace** and **happiness** to the **mind** and **body** and **joy** to the **heart**, which provide **emotional** support to help one overcome depression.

Lavender—is an oil that has traditionally been known to **balance** the **body** and to work wherever there is a need. It may help with **PMS/menopausal problems, stress, stretch marks, tension**, and **water retention**.

Body System(s) Affected: The oils in this blend may help it be effective for dealing with various problems related to **Emotional Balance**.

Aromatic Influence: This blend was structured specifically to **expel negative emotions, elevate** the **mind, balance, empower**, and **propel** one forward to achieve their desired goals.

Application: Apply to **Vita Flex points** on **feet** and/or directly on **area** of concern. This blend may also be **diffused**, applied to the **wrists** or **temples**, or added to warm **bath** water (best when first combined with a bath gel base). For an uplifting massage, dilute first with a pure carrier oil.

Safety Data: *Because this blend contains sage, it should be used with caution by those individuals who are susceptible to* **high blood pressure, epileptic seizures,** *or who are* **pregnant.**

Companion Oils: Acceptance, Clarity, Into the Future, Magnify Your Purpose, Motivation, Valor.

Frequency: Physical and Emotional; approximately 90 MHz.

EVERGREEN ESSENCE™

This blend is a combination of oils distilled from a variety of aromatic cedar, pine, and spruce trees. Now the **peace, serenity, grounding**, and even **sacred feelings** of the evergreen forests can be brought into the home or workplace. All of these oils are grounding to the body, creating the **balance** and **opening** necessary to receive and to give. This blend is **healing, uplifting**, and **soothing**. It may help **relieve anxiety** and facilitate the **release** of **emotional blocks**, as well as promote feelings of **protection, strength**, and **security**. *More detailed information for many of these oils is not readily available. In those cases, only the common names and the Latin names are listed.*

Single Oils Contained In This Blend:

Colorado Blue Spruce (*Picea pungens*)

Ponderosa Pine (*Pinus ponderosa*)

Pine—may help **dilate** and **open** the **respiratory system**, particularly the **bronchial tract**. It may also help **improve circulation throughout** the **lungs**. It helps soothe **mental stress**, relieve **anxiety**, and **revitalize** the entire body.

Red Fir (*Abies magnifica*)

Cedar (*Cedrus canadensis*)

White Fir (*Abies grandis*)—creates a feeling of **grounding, anchoring**, and **empowerment**. It can **stimulate** the **mind** while allowing the **body** to **relax**. Topically it helps relieve **pain** from **inflammation**.

Black Pine (*Pinus nigra*)

Piñon Pine (*Pinus edulis*)

Lodge Pole Pine (*Pinus contorta*)
May also contain Black spruce, fir, and cedarwood.
Body System(s) Affected: The oils in this blend may help it be effective for dealing with various problems related to **Emotional Balance**.
Aromatic Influence: When diffused, this blend of conifer oils, each with their own powerful antiseptic properties, helps to **freshen** and **deodorize** the air. It may help soothe **mental stress**, relieve **anxiety**, and **revitalize** the entire body. The individual oils in this blend have also been described as **appeasing, elevating**, and **opening**.
Application: Diffuse! Can also be sprinkled on logs in the fireplace or used to scent potpourri. Dilute well with V-6 Mixing Oil for any topical application.
Safety Data: *Could possibly result in **contact sensitization or skin irritation.***

Oil Blends

EXODUS II™

This blend is comprised of many powerful and precious essential oils that are mentioned many times in the Bible (see Exodus, chapter 30). The intent behind this particular blend of oils was to enhance the ability of the body to **expel disease** and **dead tissue**. It was also specifically designed to work with the **Exodus** food supplement to help build ones defenses.

Single Oils Contained In This Blend:

Cinnamon Bark—is part of the formula the Lord gave Moses (Exodus 30:22-27). It has very specific purposes: (1) it is a **powerful purifier**, (2) it is a powerful **oxygenator**, and (3) it **enhances** the action and the activity of **other oils**. It may have a **stimulating** and **toning** effect on the whole body and particularly the circulatory system. It is **antiseptic, anti-bacterial**, and **anti-viral**.

Cassia—is part of the formula the Lord gave Moses (Exodus 30:22-27). It is **antibacterial, anti-coagulant, anti-infectious** and **antimicrobial**.

Calamus—is part of the formula the Lord gave Moses (Exodus 30:22-27). It is **antibacterial, antiseptic**, and **antispasmodic**. It was once highly regarded as an aromatic stimulant and a tonic for the digestive system.

Myrrh—is part of the formula the Lord gave Moses (Exodus 30:22-27). It is a **true gift**. When we **open** our **hearts** and **minds** to receive the gifts, they will be given.

Hyssop—was used by Moses during the Lord's Passover in Egypt (Exodus 12). It has **anti-inflammatory** and **anti-viral** properties. It may also have the ability to **open** up the **respiratory system** and **discharge toxins** and **mucus**.

Frankincense—contains sesquiterpenes, which may help **oxygenate** the **pineal** and **pituitary glands**. As one of the ingredients for the holy incense, it was used anciently to help **enhance** one's **communication with the creator**. It was considered a prize possession and was given to Christ at his birth. It may help **promote** a **positive attitude**.

Spikenard—was highly prized in the Middle East during the time of Christ, and is referred to several times in the Bible. It is **anti-fungal, anti-inflammatory, relaxing, regenerative**, and helpful for allergic skin reactions.

Galbanum—combined with frankincense was used biblically to make a holy incense that would **enhance** ones **communication** with the **creator**. It is recognized for its **anti-viral** properties, its overall **strengthening** and **supporting** properties. It contains a low frequency in itself, but when combined with any other oils, such as frankincense or sandalwood, the frequency changes drastically.

Carrier Oil Contained In This Blend: Olive oil.

Body System(s) Affected: The oils in this blend may help it be effective for dealing with various problems related to the **Immune System**.

Application: Apply to **Vita Flex points** on **feet** and/or directly on **area** of concern. This blend may also be applied along the spine using the Raindrop Technique. **Dilution of this blend may be necessary due to the presence of cinnamon bark.**

Safety Data: *Repeated use on the skin can result in extreme **contact sensitization**. Can cause extreme **skin irritation**. Avoid during **pregnancy**.*

Companion Supplements: Exodus, ImmuneTune

Frequency: High (Spiritual); approximately 180 MHz.

Bible: "Purge me with Hyssop and I shall be clean" (Psalms 51:7). Several of the oils in this blend come from Chapter 30 in the book of Exodus.

FORGIVENESS™

The oils in this blend all have powerful emotional effects that may help people move past the barriers in life by bringing them into a **higher spiritual awareness** of their needs. This awareness leaves an angelic feeling in their soul that raises their frequency to the point where they are almost compelled to **forgive, forget, let go**, and go on with their lives.

Single Oils Contained In This Blend:

Frankincense—contains sesquiterpenes, which may help **oxygenate** the **pineal** and **pituitary glands**. As one of the ingredients for the holy incense, it was used anciently to help **enhance** one's **communication with the creator**. It may help **promote** a **positive attitude**.

Sandalwood—also, like frankincense, is high in sesquiterpenes, which were discovered to **increase** the amount of **oxygen** around the **pineal** and **pituitary glands**, thus helping to **improve** one's **attitude**. It **alleviates depression** and assists in the removal of **negative programming** from the cells of the body. It helps one **accept others** with an open heart while diminishing one's own egocentricity.

Lavender—is an oil that has traditionally been known to **balance** the **body** and to work wherever there is a need. It may help promote **consciousness, health, love, peace**, and a general sense of **well being**.

Melissa—is an oil that is powerful as an **anti-viral** agent, yet it is very gentle and very delicate because of the nature of the plant. It has the ability to work with and enhance the gentle aspects of the human body. It is **calming** and **uplifting** and may also help to **balance** the **emotions**. It may also help to remove **emotional blocks** and **instill** a **positive outlook** on **life**.

Angelica—may help one **release** and **let go** of **negative feelings**.

Helichrysum—may help **cleanse** the **blood** and improve **circulatory functions**. It is **anti-catarrhal** in structure and nature. On a spiritual level, it may help one **let go of angry feelings** that prevent one from forgiving and moving forward in life.

Rose—contains the highest frequency of the oils. It may help **enhance** the **frequency** of every cell, which could help bring **balance** and **harmony** to the body.

Rosewood—may help improve **skin elasticity**. It is **soothing** to the **skin, appeasing** to the **mind, relaxing** to the **body**, and creates a feeling of **peace** and **gentleness**.

Geranium—may help with **hormonal balance, liver** and **kidney functions** and the **discharge** of **toxins** from the **liver** that hold us back from having balance. Geranium **opens** the **liver chakra**.

Lemon—promotes **health, healing, physical energy**, and **purification**. Its fragrance is **invigorating, enhancing**, and **warming**.

Palmarosa—is valuable for all types of **skin** problems because it **stimulates** new **cell growth**, regulates oil production, **moisturizes** and **speeds healing**.

Ylang Ylang—may help **balance** the **male-female energies** so one can move closer towards being in spiritual attunement and allow them to focus their thoughts together, filtering out the ever-present garbage and establishing a sense of relaxation. It brings back feelings of **self-love, confidence, joy** and **peace**.

Bergamot—is **soothing** to the **endocrine system** and the **hormones** of the body. It may **uplift** and **calm** the **emotions** to help relieve **anxiety, stress**, and **tension**.

Roman Chamomile—neutralizes **allergies** and helps to cleanse the **blood** and **expel toxins** from the **liver**.

Jasmine—is very **uplifting** to the **emotions**; it may produce a feeling of **confidence, energy, euphoria**, and **optimism**. As an **antispasmodic**, it has been used effectively for **menstrual** discomfort, **muscle spasms**, and **uterine** disorders.

Carrier Oil Contained In This Blend: Sesame Seed Oil.

Body System(s) Affected: The oils in this blend may help it be effective for dealing with various problems related to **Emotional Balance**.

Aromatic Influence: When diffused, this blend of oils may stimulate one to feel the need to **forgive** themselves and others of transgression.

Application: Best when massaged clockwise over the **navel** (key area, lasts longer) and the **heart**, and also placed behind the **ears**, and on the **wrists**. It may also be worn as a **perfume** or **cologne**.

Companion Oils: <u>Valor</u> on the **feet, cheeks** and **face**; <u>Joy</u> on the **ears** and **chest**; <u>Gathering</u> on the **forehead**.

Frequency: High (Spiritual); approximately 192 MHz.
Bible: Matthew 6:14-15

GATHERING™

The oils in this blend may help **increase** the **oxygen** around the **pituitary** and **pineal glands**, bringing us more into a **harmonic frequency** to be a receptor of the communications that we desire to receive. As many of these single oils tend to move people in a profound way, this blend may help **bring people together** in **spiritual oneness** with **god**. This blend may also **help bring** not only the **physical** but also the **emotional** and **spiritual thoughts** and **feelings together** for **greater focus** and **clarity**. By helping to prevent the **fracturing** of **thought energy**, this blend may help one find a greater **peace** and **balance** in life. It may help to keep one **focused, grounded, connected**, and **clear**, and may even help **gather** ones **potential** for **self-improvement**. It may be a very powerful blend for **supporting** and **protecting** the **body** from **outside attacks**, especially when there has been a **lack** of **sleep**. Because it tends to act as an **amplifier**, refer to the comments below regarding its use.

Single Oils Contained In This Blend:

Galbanum—combined with frankincense was used biblically to make a holy incense that would **enhance** ones **communication** with the **creator**. It is recognized for its **anti-viral** properties, its overall **strengthening** and **supporting** properties. It contains a low frequency in itself, but when combined with any other oils, such as frankincense or sandalwood, the frequency changes drastically.

Frankincense—contains sesquiterpenes, which may help **oxygenate** the **pineal** and **pituitary glands**. As one of the ingredients for the holy incense, it was used anciently to help **enhance** one's **communication with the creator**. It was considered a prize possession and was given to Christ at his birth. It may help **promote** a **positive attitude**.

Sandalwood—also, like frankincense, is high in sesquiterpenes, which were discovered to **increase** the amount of **oxygen** around the **pineal** and **pituitary glands**, thus helping to **improve** one's **attitude**. It **alleviates depression** and assists in the removal of **negative programming** from the cells of the body. It helps one **accept others** with an open heart while diminishing one's own egocentricity.

Lavender—is an oil that has traditionally been known to **balance** the **body** and to work wherever there is a need. It may help promote **consciousness, health, love, peace**, and a general sense of **well being**.

Cinnamon Bark—is part of the formula the Lord gave Moses (Exodus 30:22-27). It has very specific purposes: (1) it is a **powerful purifier**, (2) it is a powerful **oxygenator**, and (3) it **enhances** the action and the activity of **other oils**. It may have a **stimulating** and **toning** effect on the whole body and particularly the circulatory system. It is **antiseptic, anti-bacterial**, and **anti-viral**.

Rose—contains the highest frequency of the oils. It may help **enhance** the **frequency** of every cell, which could help bring **balance** and **harmony** to the body.

Spruce—**grounds** the **body**, creating the **balance** and the **opening** necessary to **receive** and to **give**. It may help **dilate** the **bronchial tract** to **improve** the **oxygen exchange**. It also helps one release **emotional blocks**.

Geranium—may be **healing, calming** and **balancing** to the **skin**. It may help **balance** the **sebum** which is the fatty secretion in the sebaceous glands of the skin that **keep** the **skin supple**. It helps **open** and **elevate** the **mind**.

Ylang Ylang—may help **balance** the **male-female energies** so one can move closer towards being in spiritual attunement and allow them to focus their thoughts together, filtering out the ever-present garbage. It brings back the feeling of **self-love, confidence, joy** and **peace**.

Body System(s) Affected: The oils in this blend may help it be effective for dealing with various problems related to **Emotional Balance**.

Aromatic Influence: When diffused, this blend of oils may help one **gather** their **thoughts** so they can become focused. It may also help the **heart** and **mind** to work harmoniously, allowing **goals** and **dreams** to be **manifest** in **physical forms**.

Application: Best when applied to the **forehead, heart, right temple** across to the **left temple**, bottom front of the **neck, thymus, face, chest**, and on each side of the upper chest **near** the **shoulders**. It can be applied anywhere on the body or worn as a **perfume** or **cologne**.

Companion Oils: Forgiveness on the **navel**, Sacred Mountain on the **crown** (to bring a person with a negative attitude to a clear space). This blend also works well with Valor (on crown or feet), 3 Wise Men (crown), Clarity (temples), and Dream Catcher.

Frequency: Physical and Emotional; approximately 99 MHz.

Bible: Galbanum and frankincense are talked about in Exodus and were used by Moses as the holy incense. Cinnamon is part of the formula that the Lord gave Moses to help him "become single unto God".

Comments: Gathering has a specific purpose for each individual use. One must use this blend with the right intent as it may amplify negative as well as positive attitudes. Wear with caution when feeling negative because it may amplify the negative feelings. It may be necessary to use Sacred Mountain first in order to bring oneself to a clear space before using Gathering.

GENTLE BABY™

This is a wonderful blend, designed specifically for **expectant mothers** and **newborn babies**. It is **comforting, soothing**, and **relaxing**. It may help **relieve stress** during **pregnancy** and may even be **beneficial** during the **birthing process**. It helps to **enhance** the **youthful appearance** of the **skin** and may be beneficial for men to use on **chapped skin** and as an **aftershave**. It may also help with **skin elasticity** and **stretch marks**. Every oil in **Gentle Baby** is for **skin regeneration** and may help to **prevent** and **retard wrinkles**. This blend is so gentle and soothing to the skin that it could possibly be used for **diaper rashes** (dilute at least by ½).

Single Oils Contained In This Blend:

> **Rose Geranium** (*Pelargonium x asperum*)—may be **healing, calming** and **balancing** to the **skin**. It may help **balance** the **sebum** which is the fatty secretion in the sebaceous glands of the skin that **keep** the **skin supple**.

> **Rosewood**—may help improve **skin elasticity**. It is **soothing** to the **skin, appeasing** to the **mind, relaxing** to the **body**, and creates a feeling of **peace** and **gentleness**.

> **Palmarosa**—is valuable for all types of **skin** problems because it **stimulates** new **cell growth**, regulates oil production, **moisturizes** and **speeds healing**.

> **Lavender**—is an oil that has traditionally been known to **balance** the **body** and to work wherever there is a need. It may help prevent **scarring** and **stretch marks** and promote a general sense of **well being**.

> **Roman Chamomile**—neutralizes **allergies** and helps in **skin regeneration**. It may also help reduce **irritability** and minimize **nervousness** in children, especially **hyperactive children**.

> **Ylang Ylang**—may help **balance** the **male-female energies** so one can move closer towards being in spiritual attunement and allow them to focus their thoughts together, filtering out the ever-present garbage. It brings back the feeling of **self-love, confidence, joy** and **peace**.

> **Rose**—has a **beautiful fragrance** and contains the highest frequency of the oils. It may help **enhance** the **frequency** of every cell, which could help bring **balance** and **harmony** to the body.

> **Lemon**—promotes **health, healing, physical energy**, and **purification**. Its fragrance is **invigorating, enhancing**, and **warming**.

> **Bergamot**—is **soothing** to the **endocrine system** and the **hormones** of the body. It may **uplift** and **calm** the **emotions** to help relieve **anxiety, stress**, and **tension**.

> **Jasmine**—is very **uplifting** to the **emotions**; it may produce a feeling of **confidence, energy, euphoria**, and **optimism**.

Body System(s) Affected: The oils in this blend may help it be effective for dealing with various problems related to **Emotional Balance** and to the **Skin**.

Aromatic Influence: The aroma of this blend of oils is very **relaxing** and **calming**. It may also help one **create** a **space** for **being** in ones **childhood** again.

Application: Best when applied to the **Vita Flex points** on the **inner ankles**, across the **lower back** and **abdomen** (to reduce cramping and stretch marks), and on the **feet, face** and **neck** areas. Dilute with V-6 Mixing Oil for **full body massage** or wear as a **perfume** or **cologne**. It may also be added to **bath** water.

> BABY—When using on a baby dilute at least by ½. Dilute with V-6 Mixing Oil for **full body massage**. It may also be applied to the **feet, abdomen, lower back, face**, and **neck** areas.

> DELIVERY—Massage it on the **perineum** to help it **stretch** and possibly help **avoid** an **episiotomy**.

Frequency: High (Spiritual); approximately 152 MHz.

GLF™

This blend was formulated with specific oils to help encourage the proper functioning of the **gallbladder** and the **liver**. This blend makes a wonderful addition to other liver supporting supplements such as Juva Power and JuvaTone.

Single Oils Contained In This Blend:

Grapefruit—is an **anti-depressant**, an **antiseptic**, and a **diuretic**. It is **balancing** and **uplifting** to the mind, and may help to **relieve anxiety**.

Helichrysum—may help **cleanse** the **blood** and improve **circulatory functions**. It is **anti-catarrhal** in structure and nature. In the last few years, research has documented its **antioxidant** and **liver protective** properties.

Celery Seed—is **anti-oxidative** and **antiseptic** to the **urinary tract**. It helps **decongest** the **liver** by stimulating drainage. It has also been shown to aid **lymphatic drainage** and may help **balance** the **endocrine system**.

Ledum—has a long history of use as a tea by the natives of North America where it was used to fight **cancer, scurvy**, and **urinary problems**. It may be a wonderful support to the **urinary tract** and a powerful **liver** support and detoxifier.

Hyssop—was used by Moses during the Lord's Passover in Egypt (Exodus 12). It has **anti-inflammatory** and **anti-viral** properties. It may also have the ability to **open** up the **respiratory system** and **discharge toxins** and **mucus**.

Spearmint—is **anti-fungal** and **antiseptic**. It is an oil that may balance and increase **metabolism**; helping to **burn up fats** and **toxins** in the body.

Body System(s) Affected: The oils in this blend may help it be effective for dealing with various problems related to the **Digestive System** (especially the **gallbladder** and the **liver**).

Application: For topical use, dilute 1 part GLF with 1 part vegetable oil (e.g., olive oil, V-6 Enhanced Vegetable Oil Complex). Apply 4-6 drops **over liver** or on **Vita Flex points** on the **feet**. Avoid contact with eyes.

Safety Data: *Could possibly result in **skin irritation**. Use with caution during **pregnancy**. Avoid exposure to **direct sunlight** for 3 to 6 hours after use.*

Companion Products: JuvaFlex, Juva Cleanse, Juva Power, JuvaTone

GRATITUDE™

This blend was specifically formulated to **elevate, soothe**, and **appease** the **mind** while **bringing relief** and **relaxation** to the body. While the body is relaxing, the heart and mind can be opened to receive the gifts that are given each day.

Single Oils Contained In This Blend:

Balsam Fir—creates a feeling of **grounding, anchoring**, and **empowerment**. It can **stimulate** the **mind** while allowing the **body** to **relax**. Topically it helps relieve **overworked** and **tired muscles** and **joints**.

Frankincense—contains sesquiterpenes, which may help **oxygenate** the **pineal** and **pituitary glands**. As one of the ingredients for the holy incense, it was used anciently to help **enhance** one's **communication with the creator**. It was considered a prize possession and was given to Christ at his birth. It may help **promote** a **positive attitude**.

Rosewood—is **soothing** to the **skin, appeasing** to the **mind, relaxing** to the **body**, and creates a feeling of **peace** and **gentleness**.

Myrrh—is part of the formula the Lord gave Moses (Exodus 30:22-27). It promotes **spiritual awareness** and is a **true gift**. When we **open** our **hearts** and **minds** to receive the gifts, they will be given.

Galbanum—combined with frankincense was used biblically to make a holy incense that would **enhance** ones **communication** with the **creator**. It is recognized for its **anti-viral** properties, its overall **strengthening** and **supporting** properties. It contains a low frequency in itself, but when combined with any other oils, such as frankincense or sandalwood, the frequency changes drastically.

Ylang Ylang—may help **balance** the **male-female energies** so one can move closer towards being in spiritual attunement and allow them to focus their thoughts together, filtering out the ever-present garbage. It brings back the feeling of **self-love, confidence, joy** and **peace**.

Body System(s) Affected: The oils in this blend may help it be effective for dealing with various problems related to the **Nervous** and **Immune Systems, Muscles and Bones**, and to **Emotional Balance**.

Aromatic Influence: This blend of oils may help **soothe** and **appease** the **mind**. It is **relaxing** and **elevating**, promoting a sense of gratitude for blessings received.

Application: Rub over the **heart**, and on **forehead**, and **temples**. **Diffuse** or wear as **perfume** or **cologne**.

Companion Oils: Acceptance, Believe, Forgiveness, Inner Child, Inspiration, Peace & Calming

GROUNDING™

This blend may help to **stabilize** and **ground** us in order **to deal with reality** in a logical, peaceful manner. It can be easy for us to disconnect from reality. We are either excited about new ideas or want to escape into our own fantasy world. However, doing this allows us to make choices that can lead to some very unfortunate circumstances. This blend may **help us deal** with **reality**.

Single Oils Contained In This Blend:

Juniper—evokes feelings of **health, love**, and **peace** and may help to **elevate** one's **spiritual awareness**.

Angelica—may help one **release** and **let go** of **negative feelings**.

Ylang Ylang—may help **balance** the **male-female energies** so one can move closer towards being in spiritual attunement and allow them to focus their thoughts together, filtering out the ever-present garbage. It brings back the feeling of **self-love, confidence, joy** and **peace**.

Cedarwood—was used traditionally by the North American Indians to enhance their potential for **spiritual communication**. It may help **open** the **pineal gland**.

Pine—may help **dilate** and **open** the **respiratory system**, particularly the **bronchial tract**. It may also help **improve circulation throughout** the **lungs**. It helps soothe **mental stress**, relieve **anxiety**, and **revitalize** the entire body.

Spruce—**grounds** the **body**, creating the **balance** and the **opening** necessary to **receive** and to **give**. It may help **dilate** the **bronchial tract** to **improve** the **oxygen exchange**. It also helps one release **emotional blocks**.

Fir—may help create a feeling of **grounding, anchoring** and **empowerment**.

Body System(s) Affected: The oils in this blend may help it be effective for dealing with various problems related to **Emotional Balance**.

Aromatic Influence: The aroma of this blend may help **ground** and **balance** the **emotions**.

Application: Best when worn on the back of the **neck** and on the **temples**.

Safety Data: *Could possibly result in skin irritation.*

Frequency: Emotional and Spiritual; approximately 140 MHz.

HARMONY™

This blend may help to establish **spiritual** and **emotional harmony** within us. We must be in **harmony** with ourselves, our creator, others, and the world around us before we can truly feel and **overcome** our **negative emotions**. When we have **harmony** in our lives, many other things will come to balance and fruition. It may promote **physical** and **emotional healing** by bringing about a **harmonic balance** to the **chakras (energy centers)** of the **body**, allowing us to **relax** and feel **safe** and **secure**. Balancing and unblocking the **chakras** may allow the energy to flow more efficiently through the body, helping to **reduce stress** and create a general overall **feeling** of **well being**.

Single Oils Contained In This Blend:

Hyssop—was used by Moses during the Lord's Passover in Egypt (Exodus 12). It may help stimulate **meditation** and promote **centering**.

Spruce—**grounds** the **body**, creating the **balance** and the **opening** necessary to **receive** and to **give**. It also helps one release **emotional blocks**.

Lavender—is an oil that has traditionally been known to **balance** the **body** and to work wherever there is a need. It may help promote **consciousness, health, love, peace**, and a general sense of **well being**.

Frankincense—contains sesquiterpenes, which may help **oxygenate** the **pineal** and **pituitary glands**. As one of the ingredients for the holy incense, it was used anciently to help **enhance** one's **communication with the creator**. It was considered a prize possession and was given to Christ at his birth. It may help **promote** a **positive attitude**.

Geranium—may help with **hormonal balance, liver** and **kidney functions** and the **discharge** of **toxins** from the **liver** that hold us back from having balance. Geranium **opens** the **liver chakra** (Solar Plexus). Note: The liver is the place where fear and anger are stored.

Ylang Ylang—may help **balance** the **male-female energies** so one can move closer towards being in spiritual attunement and allow them to focus their thoughts together, filtering out the ever-present garbage. It brings back the feeling of **self-love, confidence, joy** and **peace**.

Orange—brings **peace** and **happiness** to the **mind** and **body** and **joy** to the **heart**, which provide **emotional** support to help one overcome depression.

Sandalwood—also, like frankincense, is high in sesquiterpenes, which were discovered to **increase** the amount of **oxygen** around the **pineal** and **pituitary glands**, thus helping to **improve** one's **attitude**. It **alleviates depression** and assists in the removal of **negative programming** from the cells of the body. It helps one **accept others** with an open heart while diminishing one's own egocentricity.

Angelica—may help one **release** and **let go** of **negative feelings**.

Sage Lavender—has been shown to increase both estradiol and testosterone levels. It may also help **harmonize** and **balance** the **emotions** and reduce **stress-related** conditions .

Rose—has a **beautiful fragrance** and contains the highest frequency of the oils. It may help **enhance** the **frequency** of every cell, which could help bring **balance** and **harmony** to the body.

Rosewood—may help improve **skin elasticity**. It is **soothing** to the **skin, appeasing** to the **mind, relaxing** to the **body**, and creates a feeling of **peace** and **gentleness**.

Lemon—promotes **health, healing, physical energy**, and **purification**. Its fragrance is **invigorating, enhancing**, and **warming**.

Palmarosa—is valuable for all types of **skin** problems because it **stimulates** new **cell growth**, regulates oil production, **moisturizes** and **speeds healing**.

Bergamot—is **soothing** to the **endocrine system** and the **hormones** of the body. It may **uplift** and **calm** the **emotions** to help relieve **anxiety, stress**, and **tension**.

Roman Chamomile—neutralizes **allergies** and helps in **skin regeneration**. It may also help reduce **irritability** and minimize **nervousness** in children, especially **hyperactive children**.

Jasmine—is very **uplifting** to the **emotions**; it may produce a feeling of **confidence, energy, euphoria**, and **optimism**.

Body System(s) Affected: The oils in this blend may help it be effective for dealing with various problems related to **Emotional Balance**.

Aromatic Influence: The fragrance of this blend of oils may help one establish and maintain a **positive attitude**, which is essential for **physical** and **emotional healing**.

Application: Best when applied on **each chakra** (or rub this blend between the hands in a circular, clockwise motion and place over the chakras), on the **ears, feet**, over the **heart**, and over areas of poor **circulation**. One may want to start at the **feet** and go up the **energy centers**

and then over the **crown**. Application of this blend to each chakra or "energy center" will help open them and balance the electrical fields surrounding the body. Wear it as **perfume** or **cologne**. If there is an **allergy** or irritation to the smell of an oil, do the following:

1. Rub this blend between both hands in a circular, clockwise motion.
2. Put one hand over the **navel** and the other hand over the **thymus** (above the heart). Hold for **20 seconds**. **Change hands** and **repeat**.

Safety Data: *Use with caution during **pregnancy**. Not for use by people with **epilepsy**. Use with caution if dealing with **high blood pressure**. Avoid exposure to **direct sunlight** for 3 to 6 hours after use.*

Frequency: Emotional; approximately 101 MHz.

HIGHEST POTENTIAL™

This blend contains the biblical oils of frankincense, galbanum, cedarwood, and sandalwood to help you tap into the divine power within yourself, **empowering** and **enabling** you to achieve your full potential. In addition, ylang ylang and lavender help to balance physical and emotional energies to help focus on the higher goal, while the emotionally uplifting scent of jasmine helps to promote confidence and energy to reach that goal. This unique blend of oils is **uplifting** and **inspiring** while promoting feelings of **stability** and **peace**.

Blends and Single Oils Contained In This Blend:

> **AUSTRALIAN BLUE**—is emotionally uplifting and helps to empower the physical and spiritual bodies. It helps to build **courage, confidence**, and **self-esteem** while promoting **calmness, peace**, and **relaxation**.
>
> **GATHERING**—helps to keep one **focused, grounded, connected**, and **clear**, and may even help **gather** ones **potential** for **self-improvement**.
>
> **Ylang Ylang**—may help **balance** the **male-female energies** so one can move closer towards being in spiritual attunement and allow them to focus their thoughts together, filtering out the ever-present garbage. It brings back the feeling of **self-love, confidence, joy** and **peace**.
>
> **Jasmine**—is very **uplifting** to the **emotions**; it penetrates the deepest layers of the soul, opening doors to our emotions. It produces feelings of **confidence, energy**, and **optimism**.

Body System(s) Affected: Emotional Balance.

Aromatic Influence: When diffused or worn as perfume, this special blend of oils helps to **balance** the emotions. It may help relieve **anxiety, revitalize** the entire body, and **empower** both mind and soul.

Application: Rub over the **heart**, and on **forehead**, and **temples**. **Diffuse** or wear as **perfume**.

Companion Oils: <u>Magnify Your Purpose</u>, <u>Live with Passion</u>, <u>Chivalry</u>

HOPE™

The single oils in this blend have the ability to help **support the body physically and mentally** to give us **hope**. These oils when inhaled together may give us the feeling of **going forward** with **hope** and **achievement**. It reconnects us with a feeling of **strength** and **grounding**. It may also help **relieve depression** and **suicidal thoughts**.

Single Oils Contained In This Blend:

Melissa—is an oil that is powerful as an **anti-viral** agent, yet it is very gentle and very delicate because of the nature of the plant. It has the ability to work with and enhance the gentle aspects of the human body. It is **calming** and **uplifting** and may help to **balance** the **emotions**. It may also help to remove **emotional blocks** and **instill** a **positive outlook** on **life**.

Myrrh—is part of the formula the Lord gave Moses (Exodus 30:22-27). It is a **true gift**. When we **open** our **hearts** and **minds** to receive, the gifts will be given.

Juniper—evokes feelings of **health, love**, and **peace** and may help to **elevate** one's **spiritual awareness**.

Spruce—**grounds** the **body**, creating the **balance** and the **opening** necessary to **receive** and to **give**. It may help **dilate** the **bronchial tract** to **improve** the **oxygen exchange**. It also helps one release **emotional blocks**.

Carrier Oil Contained In This Blend: Almond Oil.

Body System(s) Affected: The oils in this blend may help it be effective for dealing with various problems related to **Emotional Balance**.

Aromatic Influence: This blend of oils may be instrumental in giving one the feelings of **peace, security, hope** and **achievement**.

Application: Apply on **ears** (outer edge). It may also be placed on the **chest, heart, temples, solar plexus**, across the **nape** of the **neck** (in back), **feet, wrists**, or **any place** on the **body**. For **suicide thoughts**, use on **ears** and **wrists**. Wear as **perfume** or **cologne**.

Frequency: Physical and Emotional; approximately 98 MHz.

Comments: The first time this blend was used was for a lady in Arkansas for whom they could not find a diagnosis. She was dying from a mysterious disease. She was given Hope and her life was spared. At different times in our lives we may experience the feeling of hopelessness which can cause us to lose the vision of our goals and desires. Hope helps us reconnect with a feeling of strength and grounding, which may restore hope for tomorrow and help us go forward in life.

HUMILITY™

Having humility and forgiveness **helps us heal ourselves and our earth**. It is an integral ingredient in having forgiveness and seeking a closer relationship with God. Through its frequency and fragrance, you may find that special place where your own healing may begin.

Single Oils Contained In This Blend:

> **Geranium**—may help with **hormonal balance, liver** and **kidney functions** and the **discharge** of **toxins** from the **liver** that hold us back from having balance. Geranium **opens** the **liver chakra** (Solar Plexus). It may help **ease nervous tension** and **stress, balance** the **emotions, lift** the **spirit**, and foster **peace, well being**, and **hope**.
>
> **Ylang Ylang**—may help **balance** the **male-female energies** so one can move closer towards being in spiritual attunement and allow them to focus their thoughts together, filtering out the ever-present garbage. It brings back the feeling of **self-love, confidence, joy** and **peace**.
>
> **Frankincense**—contains sesquiterpenes, which may help **oxygenate** the **pineal** and **pituitary glands**. As one of the ingredients for the holy incense, it was used anciently to help **enhance** one's **communication with the creator**. It was considered a prize possession and was given to Christ at his birth. It may help **promote** a **positive attitude**.
>
> **Spikenard**—was highly prized in the Middle East during the time of Christ, and is referred to several times in the Bible. It is **anti-fungal, anti-inflammatory, relaxing, regenerative**, and helpful for allergic skin reactions.
>
> **Myrrh**—is part of the formula the Lord gave Moses (Exodus 30:22-27). It promotes **spiritual awareness** and is a **true gift**. When we **open** our **hearts** and **minds** to receive the gifts, they will be given.
>
> **Rose**—contains the highest frequency of the oils. It may help **enhance** the **frequency** of every cell, which could help bring **balance** and **harmony** to the body.
>
> **Rosewood**—is **soothing** to the **skin, appeasing** to the **mind, relaxing** to the **body**, and creates a feeling of **peace** and **gentleness**.
>
> **Melissa**—is an oil that is powerful as an **anti-viral** agent, yet it is very gentle and very delicate because of the nature of the plant. It has the ability to work with and enhance the gentle aspects of the human body. It is **calming** and **uplifting** and may help to **balance** the **emotions**. It may also help to remove **emotional blocks** and **instill** a **positive outlook** on **life**.
>
> **Neroli**—has been regarded traditionally by the Egyptian people for its great attributes for **healing** the **mind, body** and **spirit**. It is **calming** and **relaxing** to body and spirit. It may also help to **strengthen** and **stabilize** the emotions, and **bring relief** to seemingly hopeless situations. It encourages **confidence, courage, joy, peace**, and **sensuality**. It brings everything into the **focus** of one and at the moment.

Carrier Oil Contained In This Blend: Sesame Seed Oil.

Body System(s) Affected: The oils in this blend may help it be effective for dealing with various problems related to **Emotional Balance**.

Aromatic Influence: It may help one find that special, peaceful place where healing can begin.

Application: Rub over the **heart**, on **neck, temples**, etc.

Companion Oils: Acceptance, Envision, Forgiveness, Inner Child, Inspiration, Peace & Calming

Frequency: Physical and Emotional; approximately 88 MHz.

IMMUPOWER™

This is a powerful oil blend for **building, strengthening** and **protecting** the **body** and supporting its defense mechanism. This blend raises the frequency of the **immune system** which helps one overcome the **flu, colds, respiratory problems, infections**, etc. It should be worn and diffused in the home daily, especially during the seasons of cold and flu. It should be used to **protect** the **home environment**.

Single Oils Contained In This Blend:
> **Cistus**—has **anti-bacterial, anti-infectious**, and **anti-viral** properties. Because it is high in oxygenating molecules, it may assist the **auto-immune system**; it may help strengthen the **immune system**
>
> **Frankincense**—contains sesquiterpenes, which may help **oxygenate** the **pineal** and **pituitary glands**. As one of the ingredients for the holy incense, it was used anciently to help **enhance** one's **communication with the creator**. It may help **promote** a **positive attitude** and has **anti-infectious** and **antiseptic** properties.
>
> **Hyssop**—was used by Moses during the Lord's Passover in Egypt (Exodus 12). It has **anti-inflammatory** and **anti-viral** properties. It may also have the ability to **open** up the **respiratory system** and **discharge toxins** and **mucus**.
>
> **Ravensara**—is a powerful **anti-viral, anti-bacterial, anti-fungal**, and **anti-infectious** oil. It may help **dilate, open**, and **strengthen** the **respiratory system**. As a cross between clove and nutmeg, it may also help support the **adrenal glands**.
>
> **Mountain Savory**—has **immune-stimulant, anti-viral, anti-fungal, anti-infectious, antimicrobial**, and **anti-parasitic** properties.
>
> **Oregano**—has **anti-bacterial, anti-fungal, antiseptic, anti-viral**, and **immune-stimulant** properties. It strengthens one's feeling of **security**.
>
> **Clove**—is **anti-parasitic, anti-tumoral, anti-viral** and **immune-stimulant**.
>
> **Cumin**—is an **antiseptic** and an **immune-stimulant**.
>
> **Idaho Tansy**—is **anti-viral** and may help support the **immune system**.

Body System(s) Affected: The oils in this blend may help it be effective for dealing with various problems related to the **Immune System**.

Aromatic Influence: This blend of oils should be worn and diffused every other day (alternate with Thieves), especially during **cold** and **flu** season.

Application: To protect oneself from our chemical environment and during the cold and flu season, diffuse ImmuPower in the morning and again in the evening and apply Thieves to the feet. The next day, alternate with Thieves. Diffuse Thieves and apply ImmuPower to the **throat, chest, spine**, and **feet** (best to **dilute** for topical application - see Safety Data below). Apply two to three drops on **thymus** in a clockwise motion. Stimulate by tapping the Thymus with energy fingers (pointer and middle). Also apply oil on **jugular veins** in **neck** and on **arm pits**. Use ImmuPower by Raindrop Technique up the spine for a **fever, virus**, or to strengthen the **immune system**.

Safety Data: *Can be irritating to sensitive* **skin,** *best to* **dilute** *with V-6 Mixing Oil for topical application. Use with caution during* **pregnancy.** *Use with caution if susceptible to* **epilepsy.**

Companion Oils: Thieves or Exodus II (good to alternate with ImmuPower). Single oils that may be added for extra strength include the following: Cistus, clove, frankincense, melissa, Mountain savory, oregano, rosewood.

Companion Supplements: ComforTone, Essentialzyme, Exodus, ImmuneTune, Super C / Super C Chewable.

Frequency: Physical and Emotional; approximately 89 MHz.

INNER CHILD™

This blend has a fragrance that may **stimulate memory response** and help one **reconnect with** their inner-self or **own identity**, which is one of the first steps to finding **emotional balance**. When children have been abused and misused, they become disconnected from their inner child, or identity, which causes confusion. This can contribute to multiple personalties. These problems may not manifest themselves until early- to mid-adult years, often labeled as mid-life crisis.

Single Oils Contained In This Blend:

> **Orange**—is **uplifting** and **calming**. It brings **peace** and **happiness** to the **mind** and **body** and **joy** to the **heart**, which provide **emotional** support to help one overcome depression.

> **Tangerine**—contains esters and aldehydes which are **sedating** and **calming** to the **nervous system**. It is also a **diuretic** and a **decongestant** of the **lymphatic system**.

> **Jasmine**—is very **uplifting** to the **emotions**; it may produce a feeling of **confidence, energy, euphoria**, and **optimism**.

> **Ylang Ylang**—may help **balance** the **male-female energies** so one can move closer towards being in spiritual attunement and allow them to focus their thoughts together, filtering out the ever-present garbage. It brings back the feeling of **self-love, confidence, joy** and **peace**.

> **Spruce**—**grounds** the **body**, creating the **balance** and the **opening** necessary to **receive** and to **give**. It also helps one release **emotional blocks**.

> **Sandalwood**—also, like frankincense, is high in sesquiterpenes, which were discovered to **increase** the amount of **oxygen** around the **pineal** and **pituitary glands**, thus helping to **improve** one's **attitude**. It **alleviates depression** and assists in the removal of **negative programming** from the cells of the body. It helps one **accept others** with an open heart while diminishing one's own egocentricity.

> **Lemongrass**—is a **vasodilator, antiseptic, anti-bacterial, anti-inflammatory**, and **sedative**. It may help improve **circulation**, wake up the **lymphatic system**, and increase the flow of **oxygen**. It may also help to **lift** the **spirit**.

Neroli—has been regarded traditionally by the Egyptian people for its great attributes for **healing** the **mind, body** and **spirit**. It is **calming** and **relaxing** to body and spirit. It may also help to **strengthen** and **stabilize** the emotions, and **bring relief** to seemingly hopeless situations. It encourages **confidence, courage, joy, peace**, and **sensuality**. It brings everything into **focus** and into the moment.

Body System(s) Affected: The oils in this blend may help it be effective for dealing with various problems related to **Emotional Balance**.

Aromatic Influence: The oils in this blend are very **calming** to the **nerves** and **emotions** when diffused.

Application: Apply around **navel**, on **chest, temples**, and **nose**.

Safety Data: *Avoid exposure to direct **sunlight** for up to 12 hours after use. Could possibly result in **skin irritation.***

Companion Oils: <u>Acceptance</u>, <u>Awaken</u>, <u>Citrus Fresh</u>, <u>Envision</u>, <u>Forgiveness</u>, <u>Gentle Baby</u>, <u>Surrender</u>

Frequency: Physical and Emotional; approximately 98 MHz.

INSPIRATION™

This blend includes oils that have been combined to help **enhance** those desirous in **communicating with** and getting closer to the **creator** and enjoying the spiritual aspects of life. It **relieves negative thoughts** and **enhances spiritual awareness**. It creates a space for **prayer** and **inner awareness** during meditation and prayer.

Single Oils Contained In This Blend:

Cedarwood—was used traditionally by the North American Indians to enhance their potential for **spiritual communication**. It may help **open** the **pineal gland**.

Spruce—**grounds** the **body**, creating the **balance** and the **opening** necessary to **receive** and to **give**. It also helps one release **emotional blocks**. It was used by the Lakota Indians to enhance their communication with the Great Spirit. It may also **open** the **pineal gland**.

Rosewood—is **soothing** to the **skin, appeasing** to the **mind, relaxing** to the **body**, and creates a feeling of **peace** and **gentleness**.

Sandalwood—also, like frankincense, is high in sesquiterpenes, which were discovered to **increase** the amount of **oxygen** around the **pineal** and **pituitary glands**, thus helping to **improve** one's **attitude**. It **alleviates depression** and assists in the removal of **negative programming** from the cells of the body. It helps one **accept others** with an open heart while diminishing one's own egocentricity.

Frankincense—contains sesquiterpenes, which may help **oxygenate** the **pineal** and **pituitary glands**. As one of the ingredients for the holy incense, it was used anciently to help **enhance** one's **communication with the creator**.

Myrtle—is a **decongestant** of the **respiratory system**. It is **euphoric, elevating**, and may help to soother **anger**.

Mugwort (*Artemisia vulgaris*)—was seen as a protective charm against danger and evil and anciently believed to **increase psychic powers**.

Body System(s) Affected: The oils in this blend may help it be effective for dealing with various problems related to **Emotional Balance**.

Aromatic Influence: When diffused, this blend of oils is wonderful for creating a spiritual environment in the home during times of **prayer, meditation**, or when seeking **inspiration** and direction. Put on cotton ball near vent in the car.

Application: Apply to **horns** (right and left sides of **forehead**), **crown, shoulders**, along **spine**, and on back of **neck**.

Companion Oils: Acceptance, Forgiveness, Humility, Surrender, 3 Wise Men

Frequency: High (Spiritual); approximately 141 MHz.

INTO THE FUTURE™

This blend may help one leave the past behind in order to go forward with vision and excitement. The single oils contained in this blend are all invigorating and uplifting. So many times we find ourselves settling for mediocrity and sacrificing one's own potential and success because of the fear of the unknown and what the future may or may not hold. This blend was formulated to **support** the **emotions in** helping us create the feeling of **moving forward** and not being afraid to let determination and that pioneering spirit come through. Living on the edge with tenacity and integrity brings the excitement of the challenge and the joy of success.

Single Oils Contained In This Blend:

Frankincense—contains sesquiterpenes, which may help **oxygenate** the **pineal** and **pituitary glands**. As one of the ingredients for the holy incense, it was used anciently to **enhance communication** with the **creator**.

Jasmine—is very **uplifting** to the **emotions**; it may produce a feeling of **confidence, energy, euphoria**, and **optimism**.

Clary Sage—may be beneficial for **regulating cells** and **balancing** the **hormones**. It may calm and enhance the **dream state**, helping to bring about a feeling of **euphoria**.

Juniper—may help to **improve circulation** through the **kidneys**. It has **antiseptic, antispasmodic, astringent, cleansing, detoxifying, diuretic, stimulant**, and **tonic** properties.

Idaho Tansy—is **anti-viral** and may help support the **immune system.**

Fir—may help create a feeling of **grounding, anchoring** and **empowerment.**

Ylang Ylang—may help **balance** the **male-female energies** so one can move closer towards being in spiritual attunement and allow them to focus their thoughts together, filtering out the ever-present garbage. It brings back the feeling of **self-love, confidence, joy** and **peace**.

May also contain orange and cedarwood.

Carrier Oil Contained In This Blend: Almond Oil.

Body System(s) Affected: The oils in this blend may help it be effective for dealing with various problems related to **Emotional Balance**.

Aromatic Influence: Diffusing this blend of oils may helps **lift** the **spirit** and **stabilize** the **emotions** making it easier for one to recognize their own potential.

Application: Diffuse, put in **bath** water, over the **heart**, on **wrists, neck**, as a **compress**, and dilute with V-6 Mixing Oil for **full body massage**.

Companion Oils: Awaken, Clarity, Dream Catcher, Envision, Inspiration, Magnify Your Purpose, Live with Passion

Frequency: Physical and Emotional; approximately 88 MHz.

JOY™

This blend is a beautiful complimentary blend of oils. When inhaled, it brings back **memories** of **being loved, being held, sharing loving times**, feeling and opening those blocks in our lives where perhaps we have shut down to love or receiving love or love of self. When there is grief, the adenoids and the adrenal glands shut down; Joy opens these glands.

Single Oils Contained In This Blend:

Lemon—promotes **health, healing, physical energy**, and **purification**. Its fragrance is **invigorating, enhancing**, and **warming**.

Mandarin—is **appeasing, gentle**, and promotes **happiness**. It is also **refreshing, uplifting**, and **revitalizing**. Because of its sedative and slightly hypnotic properties, it is very good for **stress** and **irritability**.

Bergamot—is **soothing** to the **endocrine system** and the **hormones** of the body. It may **uplift** and **calm** the **emotions** to help relieve **anxiety, stress**, and **tension**.

Ylang Ylang—may help **balance** the **male-female energies** so one can move closer towards being in spiritual attunement and allow them to focus their thoughts together, filtering out the ever-present garbage. It brings back the feeling of **self-love, confidence, joy** and **peace**.

Rose—contains the highest frequency of the oils. It may help **enhance** the **frequency** of every cell, which could help bring **balance** and **harmony** to the body. It is thought by some to produce a magnetic energy that attracts **love** and enhances the frequency of **self-love**, bringing **joy** to the heart.

Rosewood—may help improve **skin elasticity**. It is **soothing** to the **skin, appeasing** to the **mind, relaxing** to the **body**, and creates a feeling of **peace** and **gentleness**.

Geranium—may help with **hormonal balance, liver** and **kidney functions** and the **discharge** of **toxins** from the **liver** that hold us back from having balance. Geranium **opens** the **liver chakra** (Solar Plexus). It may help **ease nervous tension** and **stress, balance** the **emotions, lift** the **spirit**, and foster **peace, well being**, and **hope**.

Palmarosa—is valuable for all types of **skin** problems because it **stimulates** new **cell growth**, regulates oil production, **moisturizes** and **speeds healing**.

Roman Chamomile—neutralizes **allergies** and helps in **skin regeneration**. It may also help reduce **irritability** and minimize **nervousness** in children, especially **hyperactive children**.

Jasmine—is very **uplifting** to the **emotions**; it may produce a feeling of **confidence, energy, euphoria**, and **optimism**.

Body System(s) Affected: The oils in this blend may help it be effective for dealing with various problems related to **Emotional Balance**.

Aromatic Influence: The fragrance of this blend of oils promotes the feelings of **love, self-love**, and **confidence**. Emotional blockages to love may produce a dislike to the fragrance of this blend (see *HARMONY; Application* for method of correcting fragrance dislikes). Remember, the **energy** of **love** is the true source of all healing!

Application: Rub over **heart, ears, neck, thymus, heart chakras, temples, across brow**, and **wrists**. Apply on **heart Vita Flex Point**. Put four drops in KidScents Lotion for an aftershave. Put in **bath** water. Use as **compress**; dilute with V-6 Mixing Oil for a full **body massage**. Place on **areas** of **poor circulation**. Wear as **perfume** or **cologne** especially over the heart. Put two drops on a wet cloth and put in the dryer for **great smelling clothes**.

Safety Data: *Avoid exposure to direct **sunlight** for up to 12 hours after use.*

Companion Oils: Hope, Magnify Your Purpose, Motivation, Live with Passion, Valor

Frequency: High (Spiritual); approximately 188 MHz.

JUVA CLEANSE™

In today's chemically polluted environment, there is a desperate need for natural, effective products that **cleanse** and **detoxify** the **liver**. This blend was created with three of the most powerful and effective liver cleansing oils.

Single Oils Contained In This Blend:

Helichrysum—may help **cleanse** the **blood** and improve **circulatory functions**. It is **anti-catarrhal** in structure and nature. In the last few years, research has documented its **antioxidant** and **liver protective** properties.

Celery Seed—is **anti-oxidative** and **antiseptic** to the **urinary tract**. It helps **decongest** the **liver** by stimulating drainage. It has also been shown to aid **lymphatic drainage** and may help **balance** the **endocrine system**.

Ledum—has a long history of use as a tea by the natives of North America where it was used to fight **cancer, scurvy**, and **urinary problems**. It may be a wonderful support to the **urinary tract** and a powerful **liver** support and detoxifier.

Body System(s) Affected: Digestive System.

Application: Apply to **Vita Flex points** on **feet** and especially over the **liver**.

Safety Data: *Can be irritating to sensitive **skin** (test first for sensitivity).*

Oil Blends

JUVAFLEX™

This blend contains oils that have been recognized medically and traditionally for aiding the body in **cleansing** the **liver** and **building** a **stronger system**. It may help **detoxify** the **lymphatic system** and provide **digestive support**. Anger and hate are stored in the liver, which creates extreme toxicity. Liver cancer is caused by solidified hate. JuvaFlex supports **getting off addictions**. The helichrysum contained in JuvaFlex is for chelating and may possess the ability to cut through **anger barriers**.

Single Oils Contained In This Blend:
> **Fennel**—may help **support** the **digestive function** by **supporting** the **liver**. It is an **antiseptic** and a **tonic** for the **liver**. It may break up **fluids** and **toxins** and help **cleanse** the **tissues** in the body. It may also help **balance** the **hormones**.
>
> **Geranium**—may help with **hormonal balance, liver** and **kidney functions** and the **discharge** of **toxins** from the **liver** that hold us back from having balance. Geranium **opens** the **liver chakra** (Solar Plexus). It may help **dilate** the **biliary ducts** for **liver detoxification**.
>
> **Rosemary cineol**—may help **balance heart function, energize** the **solar plexus**, and **reduce mental fatigue**. It is an **antiseptic** and may help decongest the **liver**.
>
> **Roman Chamomile**—**neutralizes allergies** and increases the ability of the **skin** to **regenerate**. It may help the **liver** to **reject** and **discharge poisons**. This oil is **soothing, relaxing, calming**, and may help **remove fears**.
>
> **Blue Tansy**—may help **cleanse** the **liver** and **calm** the **lymphatic system**.
>
> **Helichrysum**—may help **cleanse** the **blood** and improve **circulatory functions**. It is **anti-catarrhal** in structure and nature. On a spiritual level, it may help one **let go of angry feelings** that prevent one from forgiving and moving forward in life.

Carrier Oil Contained In This Blend: Sesame Seed Oil.

Body System(s) Affected: The oils in this blend may help it be effective for dealing with various problems related to the **Digestive System** and to **Emotional Balance**.

Application: Apply to **Vita Flex points** on **feet**, **spine** (using the Raindrop Technique), and especially over the **liver**. Also over the **entire body** (dilute with V-6 Mixing Oil).

Safety Data: *Can be irritating to sensitive skin.*

Companion Oils: Enhance results by using this blend with Di-Gize.

Companion Supplements: Use JuvaTone and ComforTone together with this blend for maximum results. Best taken an hour apart. Also Essentialzyme to help digest expelled toxins.

Frequency: Physical; approximately 82 MHz.

LADY FLASH

This blend was formulated by D. Gary Young to help with **hot flashes**. This blend is currently only available through Creer Labs at 801-418-8870.

Single Oils Contained In This Blend:

Geranium—may help with **hormonal balance, liver** and **kidney functions** and the **discharge** of **toxins** from the **liver**.

Fennel—may help **support** the **digestive function** by **supporting** the **liver**. It may also help **balance** the **hormones**.

Sage—may help improve **estrogen** and **progesterone-testosterone balance**. It is believed to contain elements that contribute to the **secretion** of **progesterone-testosterone**.

Clary Sage—is beneficial for **regulating cells** and **balancing** the **hormones**. It may help with **menstrual cramps, PMS**, and **pre-menopause** symptoms. It may also help with **circulatory problems**.

Ylang Ylang—may help **balance** the **male-female energies** so one can move closer towards being in spiritual attunement and allow them to focus their thoughts together, filtering out the ever-present garbage. It brings back the feeling of **self-love, confidence, joy** and **peace**.

Peppermint—is **antiseptic, antispasmodic**, and **anti-inflammatory**. It is **soothing, cooling**, and **dilating** to the **system**.

Cypress—is **anti-infectious, mucolytic, antiseptic, lymphatic decongestant, refreshing**, and **relaxing**. It may also help relieve **muscle cramps** and improve overall **circulation**.

Jasmine—is very **uplifting** to the **emotions**; it penetrates the deepest layers of the soul, opening doors to our emotions. It produces feelings of **confidence, energy**, and **optimism**.

Roman Chamomile—is **anti-inflammatory** and **antispasmodic**. It is **calming** and **relaxing** and helps to relieve **muscle tension** and **stress**. It may also help **neutralizes allergies**.

Bergamot—is **soothing** to the **endocrine system** and the **hormones** of the body. It may **uplift** and **calm** the **emotions** to help relieve **anxiety, stress**, and **tension**.

Rosewood—is **soothing** to the **skin, appeasing** to the **mind, relaxing** to the **body**, and creates a feeling of **peace** and **gentleness**.

Lemon—promotes **health, healing, physical energy**, and **purification**. Its fragrance is **invigorating, enhancing**, and **warming**. It is an **antiseptic** and is great for the **respiratory system**.

Palmarosa— helps to reduce **stress** and **tension**, and promotes recovery from **nervous exhaustion**. If uplifts the **emotions**, refreshes the **mind**, and clarifies **thoughts**. It may also have a normalizing effect on the **thyroid gland**.

Body System(s) Affected: Emotional Balance, and **Hormonal System**.

Application: Apply on **location** around ankles, use for **massage**, and add to your Bath and Shower Gel Base. May also be used with a **compress** over the abdomen. Wear as a **perfume**.

LADY LOVE

This blend was formulated by D. Gary Young to help create a feminine feeling and strengthen the female libido. This blend is currently only available through Creer Labs at 801-418-8870.

Single Oils Contained In This Blend:

Mandarin—is **appeasing, gentle**, and promotes **happiness**. It is also **refreshing, uplifting**, and **revitalizing**. Because of its sedative and slightly hypnotic properties, it is very good for **stress** and **irritability**.

Bergamot—is **soothing** to the **endocrine system** and the **hormones** of the body. It may **uplift** and **calm** the **emotions** to help relieve **anxiety, stress**, and **tension**.

Palmarosa— helps to reduce **stress** and **tension**, and promotes recovery from **nervous exhaustion**. If uplifts the **emotions**, refreshes the **mind**, and clarifies **thoughts**. It may also have a normalizing effect on the **thyroid gland**.

Geranium—may help with **hormonal balance, liver** and **kidney functions** and the **discharge** of **toxins** from the **liver**.

Sage—may help improve **estrogen** and **progesterone-testosterone balance**. It is believed to contain elements that contribute to the **secretion** of **progesterone-testosterone**.

Clary Sage—is beneficial for **regulating cells** and **balancing** the **hormones**. It may help with **menstrual cramps, PMS**, and **pre-menopause** symptoms. It may also help with **circulatory problems**.

Ylang Ylang—may help **balance** the **male-female energies** so one can move closer towards being in spiritual attunement and allow them to focus their thoughts together, filtering out the ever-present garbage. It brings back the feeling of **self-love, confidence, joy** and **peace**.

Jasmine—is very **uplifting** to the **emotions**; it penetrates the deepest layers of the soul, opening doors to our emotions. It produces feelings of **confidence, energy**, and **optimism**.

Roman Chamomile—is **anti-inflammatory** and **antispasmodic**. It is **calming** and **relaxing** and helps to relieve **muscle tension** and **stress**. It may also help **neutralizes allergies**.

Rosewood—is **soothing** to the **skin, appeasing** to the **mind, relaxing** to the **body**, and creates a feeling of **peace** and **gentleness**.

Lemon—promotes **health, healing, physical energy**, and **purification**. Its fragrance is **invigorating, enhancing**, and **warming**. It is an **antiseptic** and is great for the **respiratory system**.

Body System(s) Affected: Emotional Balance, and **Hormonal System**.

Application: Apply on over the **heart**, use for **massage**, and add to your Bath and Shower Gel Base. May also be used with a **compress** over the abdomen. Wear as a **perfume**.

LADY SCLAREOL™

This blend was formulated to have a **seductive** and **alluring** scent with oils that are beneficial for the **skin** as well.

Single Oils Contained In This Blend:

Rosewood—is **soothing** to the **skin, appeasing** to the **mind, relaxing** to the **body**, and creates a feeling of **peace** and **gentleness**.

Vetiver—is **antispasmodic** and locally **warming**. Vetiver has also been valuable for relieving **stress** and helping people recover from **emotional traumas** and **shock**. According to Susanne Fischer-Rizzi, "Sexual energies become more peaceful and grounded."

Geranium—may help with **hormonal balance, liver** and **kidney functions** and the **discharge** of **toxins** from the **liver**.

Orange—is rich in compounds noted for their **stress-reducing** effects. It brings **peace** and **happiness** to the **mind** and **body** and **joy** to the **heart**.

Clary Sage—is beneficial for **regulating cells** and **balancing** the **hormones**. It may help with **menstrual cramps, PMS**, and **pre-menopause** symptoms. It may also help with **circulatory problems**.

Ylang Ylang—may help **balance** the **male-female energies** so one can move closer towards being in spiritual attunement and allow them to focus their thoughts together, filtering out the ever-present garbage. It brings back the feeling of **self-love, confidence, joy** and **peace**.

Sandalwood—helps to **alleviate depression** and assists in the removal of **negative programming** from the cells of the body. It helps one **accept others** with an open heart while diminishing one's own egocentricity.

Sage Lavender—has been shown to increase both estradiol and testosterone levels. It may also help **harmonize** and **balance** the **emotions** and reduce **stress-related** conditions .

Jasmine—is very **uplifting** to the **emotions**; it penetrates the deepest layers of the soul, opening doors to our emotions. It produces feelings of **confidence, energy**, and **optimism**.

Idaho Tansy—is **anti-viral** and may help support the **immune system**. Its aroma is **uplifting** and promotes a general sense of **well-being**.

Body System(s) Affected: Emotional Balance, Skin.

Aromatic Influence: Because the aroma of this blend of oils is so **seductive** and **arousing**, it promotes feelings of **excitement** and **romance**.

Application: Apply on **location** (most effective when applied by the male partner), use for **massage**, and add to your Bath and Shower Gel Base. May also be used with a **compress** over the abdomen. **Diffuse** or wear as a **perfume**.

Oil Blends

LAZARUS

This blend was formulated by D. Gary Young to help relieve stress, boost energy, and revitalize body and mind. This blend is currently only available through Creer Labs at 801-418-8870.

Single Oils Contained In This Blend:

Peppermint—is **antiseptic, antispasmodic**, and **anti-inflammatory**. It is **soothing, cooling**, and **dilating** to the **system**.

Cardamom—is **uplifting, refreshing**, and **invigorating**. It may be beneficial for **clearing confusion**.

Basil—has **antidepressant, anti-inflammatory**, and **antispasmodic** properties. It is relaxing to **spastic muscles**, including those that contribute to **headaches** and **migraines**.

Ginger—is **warming, uplifting**, and **empowering**. Emotionally, it may help influence **physical energy, love**, and **courage**. Because of its calming influence on the digestive system, it may help reduce feelings of **nausea**, and **motion sickness**.

Juniper—evokes feelings of **health, love**, and **peace** and may help to **elevate** one's **spiritual awareness**.

Frankincense—contains sesquiterpenes, which may help **oxygenate** the **pineal** and **pituitary glands**. As one of the ingredients for the holy incense, it was used anciently to help **enhance** one's **communication with the creator**. It was considered a prize possession and was given to Christ at his birth by the three wise men. It may help **promote** a **positive attitude**.

Cinnamon Bark—is part of the formula the Lord gave Moses (Exodus 30:22-27). It has very specific purposes: (1) it is a **powerful purifier**, (2) it is a powerful **oxygenator**, and (3) it **enhances** the action and the activity of **other oils**. It may have a **stimulating** and **toning** effect on the whole body and particularly the circulatory system. It is **antiseptic, anti-bacterial**, and **anti-viral**.

Lemongrass—is a **vasodilator, antiseptic, anti-bacterial, anti-inflammatory**, and **sedative**. It may help improve **circulation**, wake up the **lymphatic system**, and increase the flow of **oxygen**. It may also help to **lift** the **spirit**.

Body System(s) Affected: Emotional Balance.

Application: Apply on over the **heart**, use for **massage**, and add to your Bath and Shower Gel Base. Wear as a **cologne or perfume**.

LEGACY™

(THE MASTER BLEND)

This is an incredible, comprehensive blend of 90 essential oils. Its exquisite aroma fine-tunes and energies the entire body.

Single Oils Contained In This Blend: (*Botanical names are found under each individual oil in the Single Oils section*)

Angelica	Fleabane	Oregano
Balsam Fir	Frankincense	Palmarosa
Basil	Galbanum	Patchouli
Bergamot	Geranium	Peppermint
Black Pepper	German Chamomile	Petitgrain
Blue Tansy	Ginger	Pine
Buplevere (*Bupleurum fruticosum)*	Goldenrod	Ravensara
	Grapefruit	Red Fir (*Abies magnifica)*
Cajeput	Helichrysum	Roman Chamomile
Cardamom	Hyssop	Rose
Carrot Seed	Idaho Balsam Fir	Rosehip (*Rosa canina)*
Cedar Leaf	Idaho Tansy	Rosemary cineol
Cedarwood	Jasmine	Rosewood
Cinnamon Bark	Juniper	Sage
Cistus	Laurel	Sandalwood
Citronella	Lavender	Spearmint
Clary Sage	Ledum	Spikenard
Clove	Lemon	Spruce
Coriander	Lemongrass	Tangerine
Cumin	Lime	Tarragon
Cypress	Mandarin	Thyme linalol
Dill	Marjoram	Tsuga
Douglas Fir	*Melaleuca alternifolia*	Valerian
Elemi	*Melaleuca ericifolia*	Vetiver
Eucalyptus citriodora	Melissa	White Fir
Eucalyptus dives	Mountain Savory	Wintergreen
Eucalyptus globulus	Myrrh	Yarrow
Eucalyptus polybractea	Myrtle	Yellow Pine (*Pinus ponderosa)*
Eucalyptus radiata	Neroli	
Fennel	Nutmeg	Ylang Ylang
	Orange	

Body System(s) Affected: The oils in this blend may help it be effective for dealing with various problems related to **Emotional Balance**.

Aromatic Influence: Because of all the oils contained in this blend, it is **empowering** and **energizing**, not just for the emotions, but for the entire body.

Application: Apply to **Vita Flex points** on **feet** and/or directly on **area** of concern. This blend may also be **diffused**.

Safety Data: *Because of the diversity of the oils that exist in this blend, it should be used with caution by those individuals who are susceptible to* **epileptic seizures** *or who are* **pregnant**. *Repeated use could possibly result in* **contact sensitization** *or* **skin irritation**. *For* **topical** *use only.*

Companion Oils: Every single oil.

LIVE WITH PASSION™

The oils in this blend are all **emotionally balancing** and **uplifting**, helping to enhance our **passion** for life. By **strengthening** and **stabilizing** the emotions, not only may this blend help **bring relief** to seemingly hopeless situations, but it may also help to instill a **positive attitude** that can bring back the passion in our lives to help **propel** us toward **accomplishing our goals**.

Single Oils Contained In This Blend:

Melissa—is an oil that is powerful as an **anti-viral** agent, yet it is very gentle and very delicate because of the nature of the plant. It has the ability to work with and enhance the gentle aspects of the human body. It is **calming** and **uplifting** and may help to **balance** the **emotions**. It may also help to remove **emotional blocks** and **instill** a **positive outlook** on **life**.

Helichrysum—may help **cleanse** the **blood** and improve **circulatory functions**. It is **anti-catarrhal** in structure and nature. As a powerful **anti-inflammatory**, it may even help reduce inflammation in the meninges of the brain. On a spiritual level, it may help one **let go of angry feelings** that prevent one from forgiving and moving forward.

Clary Sage—is beneficial for **regulating cells** and **balancing** the **hormones**. It may help with **menstrual cramps, PMS**, and **pre-menopause** symptoms. It may also help with **circulatory problems**.

Cedarwood—was used traditionally by the North American Indians to enhance their potential for **spiritual communication**. It may help **open** the **pineal gland**.

Angelica—is referred to by the German people as the "oil of angels". It may help one **release** and **let go** of **negative feelings**.

Ginger—is **warming, uplifting**, and **empowering**. Emotionally, it may help influence **physical energy, love**, and **courage**. Because of its calming influence on the digestive system, it may help reduce feelings of **nausea**, and **motion sickness**.

Neroli—has been regarded traditionally by the Egyptian people for its great attributes for **healing** the **mind, body** and **spirit**. It is **calming** and **relaxing** to body and spirit. It may also help to **strengthen** and **stabilize** the emotions, and **bring relief** to seemingly hopeless situations. It encourages **confidence, courage, joy, peace**, and **sensuality**. It brings everything into the **focus** of one and at the moment.

Sandalwood—also, like frankincense, is high in sesquiterpenes, which were discovered to **increase** the amount of **oxygen** around the **pineal** and **pituitary glands**, thus helping to **improve** one's **attitude**. It **alleviates depression** and assists in the removal of **negative programming** from the cells of the body.

Patchouli—is **sedating, calming**, and **relaxing** allowing it to reduce **anxiety**.

Jasmine—is very **uplifting** to the **emotions**; it may produce a feeling of **confidence, energy, euphoria**, and **optimism**.

Body System(s) Affected: The oils in this blend may help it be effective for dealing with various problems related to the **Nervous System** and to **Emotional Balance**.

Aromatic Influence: This blend is **uplifting, empowering**, and **stabilizing** to the emotions. It may help to improve one's **attitude** by encouraging **confidence** and **courage**.

Application: Apply on the **wrists, temples, chest area**, and **forehead**. Add two to four drops in **bath** water. May also be worn as **perfume** or **cologne**.

Companion Oils: Acceptance, Clarity, Gathering, Harmony, Inspiration, Magnify Your Purpose, Motivation, 3 Wise Men

Frequency: Physical and Emotional; approximately 89 MHz.

LONGEVITY™

This blend contains oils that have powerful antioxidant properties. As measured on the ORAC (oxygen radical absorbent capacity) scale, this blend has scored near 150,000! When taken as a dietary supplement, it may help to promote longevity and prevent premature aging. *For easier supplement use, refer to Longevity Capsules in the Supplements section of this book.*

Single Oils Contained In This Blend:

Thyme CT Thymol—has been shown in studies to **dramatically boost glutathione levels** in the heart, liver, and brain. Because it can also help to **prevent** the **oxidation** of **fats** in the body, it may help to slow the aging process. It is also **anti-fungal** and **anti-viral**.

Orange—is rich in compounds noted for their **stress-reducing** effects; lipid-soluble traits; **antioxidant** properties which **enhance vitamin absorption**.

Clove—has one of the highest ORAC (oxygen radical absorbent capacity) scores. It is **anti-bacterial, anti-fungal, anti-infectious, anti-parasitic**, a strong **antiseptic, anti-viral**, and an **immune stimulant**; helps preserve integrity of fatty acids. Clove may also influence **healing** and help improve **memory**.

Frankincense—has powerful **anti-tumoral** and **anti-inflammatory** properties. It has been used in several clinical applications for fighting cancer. Frankincense also contains sesquiterpenes, which may help **oxygenate** the **pineal** and **pituitary glands**.

Body System(s) Affected: The oils in this blend may help it be effective for dealing with various problems related to the **Cardiovascular System**.

Application: Can be taken as a dietary supplement by diluting one drop in 4 oz. of liquid (i.e. soy/rice milk); Diffuse. This blend of oils has been put into gel capsules for easier consumption as a dietary supplement (*refer to Longevity Capsules in the Supplements section of this book*).

Safety Data: *Repeated use can possibly result in contact sensitization. Can be irritating to sensitive skin. Avoid eye contact. Avoid exposure to direct sunlight for 3 to 6 hours after use.*

M-Grain™

This blend contains single oils that have traditionally been proven to help **relieve migraine** and **stress headaches**. This blend may also help with **nausea** and **depression**.

Single Oils Contained In This Blend:
Basil—has **antidepressant, anti-inflammatory**, and **antispasmodic** properties. It is relaxing to **spastic muscles**, including those that contribute to **headaches** and **migraines**.

Marjoram—is **relaxing, calming**, and **appeasing** to the **muscles** that constrict and sometimes contribute to **headaches**.

Lavender—is an oil that has traditionally been known to **balance** the **body** and to work wherever there is a need. It has **antispasmodic** and **analgesic** properties. It may help with **sprains, sore muscles, headaches**, and general **healing**.

Peppermint—is **anti-inflammatory** to the **nerves**. It has a **soothing** and **cooling effect** on **headaches**. It is **purifying** and **stimulating** to the **conscious mind**.

Roman Chamomile—is **anti-inflammatory** and **antispasmodic**. It is **calming** and **relaxing** and helps to relieve **muscle tension** and **stress** that can lead to migraine headaches.

Helichrysum—may help **cleanse** the **blood** and improve **circulatory functions**. It is **anti-catarrhal** in structure and nature. As a powerful **anti-inflammatory**, it may even help reduce inflammation in the meninges of the brain. On a spiritual level, it may help one **let go of angry feelings** that prevent one from forgiving and moving forward.

Body System(s) Affected: The oils in this blend may help it be effective for dealing with various problems related to the **Nervous System** and to **Muscles and Bones**.

Aromatic Influence: It is very effective for clearing **headaches** when inhaled.

Application: It is most effective when **inhaled**; for **migraines**, place two drops in **palms** of **hands** then cup over nose and **inhale**. **Massage** along the **brain stem** or through the **thumbs**. Have someone cross their hands and rub your thumbs using their middle finger to push toward your hand. Also put on **forehead, crown, shoulders, back** of **neck, temples**, and **Vita Flex points** on the **feet**.

Companion Oils: Aroma Siez, Clarity, PanAway.

Frequency: Physical; approximately 72 MHz.

Magnify Your Purpose™

The emotionally uplifting properties of the single oils in this blend make it excellent for helping us to **overcome negative emotions** and such self-defeating behaviors as procrastination and self-pity. By helping us to deal with belittling feelings like abandonment, rejection, and betrayal, we are able to more fully understand and **magnify** our life's purpose.

Single Oils Contained In This Blend:

Sandalwood—also, like frankincense, is high in sesquiterpenes, which were discovered to **increase** the amount of **oxygen** around the **pineal** and **pituitary glands**, thus helping to **improve** one's **attitude**. It **alleviates depression** and assists in the removal of **negative programming** from the cells of the body. It helps one **accept others** with an open heart while diminishing one's own egocentricity.

Nutmeg—has adrenal cortex-like activity, which helps support the **adrenal glands** for **increased energy**.

Rosewood—is **soothing** to the **skin, appeasing** to the **mind, relaxing** to the **body**, and creates a feeling of **peace** and **gentleness**.

Cinnamon Bark—is part of the formula the Lord gave Moses (Exodus 30:22-27). It has very specific purposes: (1) it is a **powerful purifier**, (2) it is a powerful **oxygenator**, and (3) it **enhances** the action and the activity of **other oils**. It may have a **stimulating** and **toning** effect on the whole body and particularly the circulatory system. It is **antiseptic, anti-bacterial**, and **anti-viral**.

Ginger—is **warming, uplifting**, and **empowering**. Emotionally, it may help influence **physical energy, love**, and **courage**. Because of its calming influence on the digestive system, it may help reduce feelings of **nausea**, and **motion sickness**.

Sage—may help improve **estrogen** and **progesterone-testosterone balance**. It is believed to contain elements that contribute to the **secretion** of **progesterone-testosterone**.

Body System(s) Affected: The oils in this blend may help it be effective for dealing with various problems related to the **Nervous System** and to **Emotional Balance**.

Aromatic Influence: Because of the oils contained in this blend, it is **empowering** and **uplifting**, helping us to rise above our negative emotions.

Application: Apply to **Vita Flex points** on **feet** and/or directly on **area** of concern. This blend may also be **diffused**, applied to the **wrists** or **temples**, or added to warm **bath** water (best when first combined with a bath gel base). For an uplifting massage, dilute first with a pure carrier oil.

Safety Data: *Because of the existing contra-indications for nutmeg, cinnamon bark, and sage, this blend should be used with caution by those individuals who are susceptible to epileptic seizures or who are pregnant. Repeated use could possibly result in contact sensitization or skin irritation.*

Companion Oils: Clarity, Harmony, Gathering, Into the Future, Live with Passion, Sensation

Frequency: Physical and Emotional; approximately 99 MHz.

MELROSE™

The strong antiseptic properties of the single oils in this blend make it excellent for cleansing and healing **cuts, bruises, scrapes, insect bites**; but primarily, for helping with **tissue regeneration** from damage or injury. It also helps with **skin abrasions, burns, rashes, earaches, gums, cold sores, canker sores**, and **candida**. It fights **infection** and kills

anaerobic bacteria and **fungus**. It has been used to help horses (and other animals) with skin cuts. *Avoid use on cats.*

Single Oils Contained In This Blend:
Melaleuca—has **anti-bacterial, anti-fungal, anti-infectious, anti-viral, strong antiseptic**, and **tissue regenerating** properties.

Melaleuca quinquenervia—is a very strong, very powerful **anti-fungal, anti-viral** and **anti-bacterial** oil. It may help **protect** against **radiation** and is a **strong tissue regenerator**.

Rosemary cineol—may help **balance heart function, energize** the **solar plexus**, and **reduce mental fatigue**. It has **analgesic, antiseptic**, and **anti-infectious** properties.

Clove—is **anti-bacterial, anti-infectious, anti-inflammatory**, a **strong antiseptic, disinfectant, immune-stimulant**, and **topical anesthetic**.

Body System(s) Affected: The oils in this blend may help it be effective for dealing with various problems related to the **Respiratory System** and to the **Skin**.

Aromatic Influence: Dispels **odors**.

Application: Rub across **brow, thumb Vita Flex points**, and **liver**. Apply topically on **cuts, scrapes, burns, rashes**, or **any infection**. Put one to two drops on a piece of cotton and place in the **ear** for earaches.

Safety Data: *Repeated use can possibly result in* **contact sensitization.** *Can be irritating to sensitive* **skin.**

Companion Oils: *Melaleuca ericifolia.*

Companion Products: Rose Ointment (delays evaporation of oil and promotes healing)

Frequency: Very Low (Physical); approximately 48 MHz.

MISTER™

This blend was initially formulated to help **balance male energy** and help **regulate prostate function**. However, it has also been used successfully in eliminating **hot flashes for women**. Generally, Mister is good for **women age 30-45**, while EndoFlex is for **women age 45+** and Dragon Time is for **women** up to **age 30**.

Single Oils Contained In This Blend:
Sage—may help improve **estrogen** and **progesterone-testosterone balance**. It is believed to contain elements that contribute to the **secretion** of **progesterone-testosterone**.

Fennel—may help **support** the **digestive function** by **supporting** the **liver**. It may also help **balance** the **hormones**.

Lavender—is an oil that has traditionally been known to **balance** the **body** and to work wherever there is a need. It is **anti-inflammatory** and may help reduce inflammation of the **prostate**.

Myrtle—is a **decongestant** of the **prostate** and **respiratory system.**
Yarrow—is a **powerful decongestant** of the **prostate** and a **hormone balancer.**
Peppermint—is **anti-inflammatory** to the **prostate.**
Carrier Oil Contained In This Blend: Sesame Seed Oil.
Body System(s) Affected: The oils in this blend may help it be effective for dealing with various problems related to the **Hormonal System.**
Application: Apply to **Vita Flex points** on **ankles, lower pelvis** as a **compress** and **Vita Flex points** on **body.** Use directly on area of concern. Use on **prostate** (may want to dilute).
Safety Data: *Avoid during pregnancy. Use with caution if susceptible to epilepsy.*
Companion Oils: Dragon Time is a good companion with Mister for ladies. Single oils may include sage and Clary sage.
Companion Supplements: FemiGen (capsules), Estro (tincture)
Frequency: High (Spiritual); approximately 147 MHz.

MOTIVATION™

The single oils in this blend were combined to help people overcome **fear** and **procrastination** and take action in their lives. The authors of this book have used this blend several times to help push us through the difficult tasks of reformatting and editing.

Single Oils Contained In This Blend:
Roman Chamomile—was used by the ancient Romans traditionally to **empower** them to go into battle. It was also to give them a **clear mind.** This oil is **soothing, relaxing, calming,** and may help **remove fears.**
Ylang Ylang—may help **balance** the **male-female energies** so one can move closer towards being in spiritual attunement and allow them to focus their thoughts together, filtering out the ever-present garbage. It brings back the feeling of **self-love, confidence, joy** and **peace.**
Spruce—**grounds** the **body,** creating the **balance** and the **opening** necessary to **receive** and to **give.** This is **empowering, anchoring** and **encouraging.**
Lavender—is an oil that has traditionally been known to **balance** the **body** and to work wherever there is a need. It may help promote **consciousness, health, love, peace,** and a general sense of **well being.**
Body System(s) Affected: The oils in this blend may help it be effective for dealing with various problems related to the **Nervous System** and to **Emotional Balance.**
Aromatic Influence: This blend of oils is wonderful for helping to **overcome** the **fear** of **achieving goals** and **dreams** and for **motivating** the **body** and **mind** into action.
Application: Wear on the **chest** or the **nape** of the **neck** to stimulate the mind to want to take action. Place on **solar plexus, sternum** (key area), **feet** (especially the **big toe**), **navel** area, **ears** (on and behind), **wrist, palms** of **hands,** and **under nose** (sniff). Wear as **perfume** or **cologne.**
Frequency: Emotional; approximately 103 MHz.

PANAWAY™

Due to the aspirin-like properties of wintergreen and the powerful anti-inflammatory properties of the other oils, this blend helps to **reduce pain**. It also **stimulates quicker healing** by the **induction** of **oxygen** into the **tissue site**. It has been used to **relieve pain during surgery** with no anesthetic (helichrysum and clove were also used). It alleviates the symptoms of **sciatica**, relieves **bone pain, arthritis, rheumatism**, and promotes **healthy circulation**. It also helps with **sports injuries, sprains, muscle spasms, bumps**, and **bruises**.

Single Oils Contained In This Blend:
Wintergreen—contains 99% methyl salicylate which gives it cortisone-like properties. It may be beneficial for **arthritis, rheumatism, tendinitis**, and any other discomfort that is related to the inflammation of **bones, muscles**, and **joints**.

Helichrysum—may help **cleanse** the **blood** and improve **circulatory functions**. It is **anti-catarrhal** in structure and nature. As a powerful **anti-inflammatory**, it may even help reduce inflammation in the meninges of the brain. On a spiritual level, it may help one **let go of angry feelings** that prevent one from forgiving and moving forward.

Clove—is **anti-infectious, anti-inflammatory**, a **strong antiseptic, disinfectant, immune-stimulant**, and **topical anesthetic**. It is also good for **arthritis, infection**, and **rheumatism**.

Peppermint—is **anti-inflammatory** to the **prostate** and to **damaged tissues**. It has a **soothing** and **cooling** effect which may help with **arthritis** and **rheumatism**.

Body System(s) Affected: The oils in this blend may help it be effective for dealing with various problems related to the **Nervous System** and to **Muscles and Bones**.

Application: Apply as a **compress** on **spine** and to **Vita Flex points** on **feet**. Apply on location for **muscles, cramps, bruises**, or any place that hurts.

Companion Oils: Add helichrysum (to enhance), birch/wintergreen (for bone pain), or use with Ortho Ease or Ortho Sport Massage Oil. For deep tissue pain use Relieve It.

Frequency: Emotional; approximately 112 MHz.

PEACE & CALMING™

The oils in this blend have historically been used to help reduce **depression, anxiety, stress** and **tension**. This blend may help **hyperactive children** get off **ritalin**. It may also help children with **hypertension**. It may be useful at the end of a stressful day to promote **relaxation** and **peace** or to relieve **insomnia**.

Single Oils Contained In This Blend:
Tangerine—contains esters and aldehydes which are **sedating** and **calming** to the **nervous system**. It is also a **diuretic** and a **decongestant** of the **lymphatic system**.

Orange—brings **peace** and **happiness** to the **mind** and **body** and **joy** to the **heart**, which provide **emotional** support to help overcome depression.

Ylang Ylang—may help **balance** the **male-female energies** so one can move closer towards being in spiritual attunement and allow them to focus their thoughts together, filtering out the ever-present garbage. It brings back the feeling of **self-love, confidence, joy** and **peace**.

Patchouli—is **sedating, calming**, and **relaxing** allowing it to reduce **anxiety**.

Blue Tansy—may help **cleanse** the **liver** and **calm** the **lymphatic system**.

Body System(s) Affected: The oils in this blend may help it be effective for dealing with various problems related to the **Nervous System** and to **Emotional Balance**.

Aromatic Influence: This blend of oils is perfect for **calming** the **nerves** or **emotions** at the end of a long day or in times of stress. It may help one **relax** before going to bed. By helping the body relax, more blood is able to circulate to the brain, allowing **goals** and **dreams** to be visualized more vividly and accurately.

Application: Apply **under nose**, back of **neck, back** (dilute with V-6 Mixing Oil), and **feet**. Put in **bath** water. Apply to **navel, feet**, or **back** of **neck** for **insomnia**. Wear as **perfume** or **cologne**.

Safety Data: *Avoid exposure to direct **sunlight** for 3 to 6 hours after use.*

Companion Oils: Lavender (add for INSOMNIA), chamomile (for calming)

Frequency: Emotional; approximately 105 MHz.

PRESENT TIME™

This blend was specifically created to helped **bring people** into the **moment**. We must live in the moment in order to heal. We cannot live yesterday; we cannot live tomorrow; we have to live **today**.

Single Oils Contained In This Blend:

Neroli—has been regarded traditionally by the Egyptian people for its great attributes for **healing** the **mind, body** and **spirit**. It is **calming** and **relaxing** to body and spirit. It may also help to **strengthen** and **stabilize** the emotions, and **bring relief** to seemingly hopeless situations. It encourages **confidence, courage, joy, peace**, and **sensuality**. It brings everything into the **focus** of one and at the moment.

Spruce—**grounds** the **body**, creating the **balance** and the **opening** necessary to **receive** and to **give**. It also helps one release **emotional blocks**. It was used by the Lakota Indians to enhance their communication with the Great Spirit.

Ylang Ylang—may help **balance** the **male-female energies** so one can move closer towards being in spiritual attunement and allow them to focus their thoughts together, filtering out the ever-present garbage. It brings back the feeling of **self-love, confidence, joy** and **peace**.

Carrier Oil Contained In This Blend: Almond Oil.

Body System(s) Affected: The oils in this blend may help it be effective for dealing with various problems related to **Emotional Balance**.

Application: It is most effective when rubbed clockwise over the **thymus** (down the sternum—middle front of ribs) in a circular motion, close eyes and tap three times with energy fingers (pointer and middle). Also apply to **neck** and **forehead**.

Companion Oils: Harmony, Hope.

Frequency: Physical and Emotional; approximately 98 MHz.

PURIFICATION™

The individual oils in this blend have some powerful antiseptic, anti-bacterial, anti-fungal, and sanitizing properties. This blend is therefore useful for **killing odors** and their **bacteria, molds** and **fungus**. It **kills anaerobic bacteria**. It **purifies** and **cleanses bacteria** in the **air**, neutralizes **mildew, cigarette smoke**, and other noxious **odors**. It **repels bugs, insects**, and **mice** that like to live in homes, offices, and other confined areas. It has also been beneficial in **neutralizing poison from insect bites**; such as **spiders, bees, hornets**, and **wasps**. It is good for first-aid in sterilizing **wounds** and **cuts**.

Single Oils Contained In This Blend:

Citronella—has **antiseptic, anti-bacterial, antispasmodic, anti-inflammatory, deodorizing, insecticidal, purifying**, and **sanitizing** properties.

Lemongrass—is a **vasodilator, antiseptic, anti-bacterial, anti-inflammatory**, and **sedative**. It may help improve **circulation**, wake up the **lymphatic system**, and increase the flow of **oxygen**. It may also help to **lift** the **spirit**.

Rosemary cineol—may help **balance heart function, energize** the **solar plexus**, and **reduce mental fatigue**. It may **improve circulation** and help **stimulate** the **nerves**. It is **antiseptic** and **anti-infectious**.

Melaleuca—may help **balance heart function** and act as a **cleanser** and **detoxifier** of the **blood**. It has **anti-bacterial, anti-fungal, anti-infectious, antiseptic, anti-viral**, and **immune-stimulant** properties.

Lavandin—is an **anti-fungal**, an **anti-bacterial**, a **strong antiseptic**, and a **tissue regenerator**.

Myrtle—is a **decongestant** of the **respiratory system**. It may help **improve oxygenation** and work as an **expectorant** in **discharging mucus**. It is **antiseptic** and **anti-bacterial**, and is **euphoric** and **elevating**.

Body System(s) Affected: The oils in this blend may help it be effective for dealing with various problems related to the **Digestive System**, to **Emotional Balance**, and to the **Skin**.

Aromatic Influence: This blend is great for **air purification** when diffused. When illness is in the **home**, diffuse for one hour then wait for two. Repeat this pattern as desired. **Diffuse** in the **office, barn, garbage areas**, or put on cotton ball and place in an air vent to freshen the **car**.

Application: Apply to **Vita Flex points** of the **body, ears, feet**, and **temples**. Apply topically for infections and cleansing. Put on cotton balls and place in air vents for an **insect repellent** at home or at work. Can also be added to **paint** to help **reduce fumes**.

Safety Data: *Repeated use can possibly result in **contact sensitization**. Can be irritating to sensitive **skin**.*

Companion Oils: Citrus Fresh, Melrose, Thieves

Frequency: Very Low (Physical); approximately 46 MHz.

RAVEN™

The properties of the individual oils in this blend make it well suited to help alleviate the symptoms of **tuberculosis** and **pneumonia**. It goes beyond RC for **upper respiratory problems** and is especially useful for **viral** infections. It has been very beneficial for alleviating the symptoms of **asthma**.

Single Oils Contained In This Blend:

> **Ravensara**—is a powerful **anti-viral, anti-bacterial, anti-fungal**, and **anti-infectious** oil. It may help **dilate, open**, and **strengthen** the **respiratory system**. As a cross between clove and nutmeg, it may also help support the **adrenal glands**.

> *Eucalyptus radiata*—may have a profound **anti-viral** effect upon the **respiratory system**. It may also help reduce **inflammation** of the **nasal mucous membrane**.

> **Peppermint**—is **antiseptic, antispasmodic**, and **anti-inflammatory**. It is **soothing, cooling**, and **dilating** to the **system**.

> **Wintergreen**—contains 99% methyl salicylate which gives it cortisone-like properties. It may be beneficial for **arthritis, rheumatism, tendinitis**, and any other discomfort that is related to the inflammation of **bones, muscles**, and **joints**. It is also a **lymphatic cleanser**.

> **Lemon**—promotes **health, healing, physical energy**, and **purification**. Its fragrance is **invigorating, enhancing**, and **warming**. It is an **antiseptic** and is great for the **respiratory system**.

Body System(s) Affected: The oils in this blend may help it be effective for dealing with various problems related to the **Respiratory System** and to the **Skin**.

Aromatic Influence: This blend of oils is excellent for opening the **respiratory system** when diffused or inhaled.

Application: Apply to **Vita Flex points** of the **body**. Apply topically to **lungs** and **throat**. Put on pillow at night. It was traditionally used in **suppository** or **enema** application with V-6 Mixing Oil and retained throughout the night. This method of application can directly benefit the **lungs** within seconds.

Safety Data: *Can be irritating to sensitive **skin**.*

Companion Oils: Melrose, RC, Thieves.

Frequency: Physical; approximately 70 MHz.

RC™

Although not as powerful against viral infections as <u>Raven</u>, the properties of the oils in this blend make it extremely effective against **allergies, colds, bronchitis, respiratory congestion, flu, cold sores, pneumonia, sinusitis, sore throat, mucus**, and **bone spurs**.

Single Oils Contained In This Blend:

Eucalyptus (four types including *E. globulus*, *E. radiata*, *E. australiana*, and *E. citriodora*)—may have a profound **anti-viral** effect upon the **respiratory system**. They also have **strong anti-bacterial, anti-catarrhal**, and **antiseptic** properties.

Myrtle—is a **decongestant** of the **respiratory system**. It may help **improve oxygenation** and work as an **expectorant** in **discharging mucus**. It is **antiseptic** and **anti-bacterial**, and is **euphoric** and **elevating**.

Marjoram—is **relaxing, calming**, and **appeasing** to the **muscles** that constrict and sometimes contribute to **headaches**. As an **antispasmodic**, it may help relieve spasms in the **respiratory system**.

Pine—may help **dilate** and **open** the **respiratory system**, particularly the **bronchial tract**. It may also help **improve circulation throughout** the **lungs**.

Cypress—is **anti-infectious, mucolytic, antiseptic, lymphatic decongestant, refreshing**, and **relaxing**. It may help improve **lung circulation** as well as help relieve other **respiratory problems**.

Lavender—is an oil that has traditionally been known to **balance** the **body** and to work wherever there is a need. It may help promote **consciousness, health, love, peace**, and a general sense of **well being**.

Spruce—**grounds** the **body**, creating the **balance** and the **opening** necessary to **receive** and to **give**. It may help **dilate** the **bronchial tract** to **improve** the **oxygen exchange**. It also helps one release **emotional blocks**.

Peppermint—is **antiseptic, antispasmodic**, and **anti-inflammatory**. It is **soothing, cooling**, and **dilating** to the **system**.

Body System(s) Affected: The oils in this blend may help it be effective for dealing with various problems related to the **Respiratory System**.

Aromatic Influence: <u>RC</u> is very beneficial in the diffuser to **decongest** and **relieve allergy-type** symptoms such as **coughs, sore throat**, and **lung congestion**.

Application: Diffuse. Dilute with V-6 Mixing Oil and **massage** on the **chest, back**, and **feet**. It can be used as a **compress** over the **chest** and **back**. Put on **sinuses** and **nasal passages** (put oil on a Q-tip and rub on inside of **nasal passages**). Rub around **ears, feet, neck**, and **throat**. Apply to **Vita Flex points** on **body**. It can be exchanged and alternated effectively with <u>Raven</u>.

Companion Oils: <u>Raven</u> on feet, <u>RC</u> on throat and chest, alternate morning and night. Run hot steaming water in sink, put <u>Raven</u>, <u>RC</u> and birch/wintergreen in water, put towel over head and **inhale** to open sinuses for **flu, colds** or **pneumonia**. Also <u>Thieves</u>.

Frequency: Physical; approximately 75 MHz.

RELEASE™

This is a powerful blend for enhancing the **release** of **memory trauma** from the cells of the liver, where anger and hate emotions are stored. The frequency of the oils in Release may aid in the **letting go** of **negative emotions** so one can progress in a more effective and efficient way. It helps to **release frustration**.

Single Oils Contained In This Blend:
> **Ylang Ylang**—may help **balance** the **male-female energies** so one can move closer towards being in spiritual attunement and allow them to focus their thoughts together, filtering out the ever-present garbage. It brings back the feeling of **self-love, confidence, joy** and **peace**.
> **Lavandin**—is an **anti-fungal**, an **anti-bacterial**, a **strong antiseptic**, and a **tissue regenerator**.
> **Geranium**—may help with **hormonal balance, liver** and **kidney functions** and the **discharge** of **toxins** from the **liver** that hold us back from having balance. Geranium **opens** the **liver chakra** (Solar Plexus). It may help **dilate** the **biliary ducts** for **liver detoxification**. It may also help foster **peace, well being**, and **hope**.
> **Sandalwood**—also, like frankincense, is high in sesquiterpenes, which were discovered to **increase** the amount of **oxygen** around the **pineal** and **pituitary glands**, thus helping to **improve** one's **attitude**. It **alleviates depression** and assists in the removal of **negative programming** from the cells of the body. It helps one **accept others** with an open heart while diminishing one's own egocentricity.
> **Blue Tansy**—may help **cleanse** the **liver** thereby helping to release **anger** and **negative emotions**.

Carrier Oil Contained In This Blend: Olive Oil.
Body System(s) Affected: The oils in this blend may help it be effective for dealing with various problems related to **Emotional Balance**.
Application: Apply over **liver** or as a **compress**. Put on **ears**, bottom of **feet**, especially **Vita Flex points** of **feet**. Wear as **perfume or cologne**.
Companion Oils: Put Valor on **feet** first, then put Harmony (for balance) on **feet**, JuvaFlex on **feet**, Release on **liver**, rotate the oil used each day.
Frequency: Emotional; approximately 102 MHz.

RELIEVE IT™

The pepper oil along with the other deep penetrating oils in this blend, make it effective for the relief of **deep tissue pain**. This extraordinary blend, with its high **anti-inflammatory** action, seems to go beyond **PanAway** in some pain applications, especially when alternated with **PanAway** and/or helichrysum. It may also help with **sciatica** and **arthritic pain** (Try birch or wintergreen too!) **PanAway** is more for **bone pain**.

Single Oils Contained In This Blend:

Spruce—**grounds** the **body**, creating the **balance** and the **opening** necessary to **receive** and to **give**. It may help **dilate** the **bronchial tract** to **improve** the **oxygen exchange**. It also helps one release **emotional blocks**.

Pepper, Black—may help **stimulate** the **endocrine system** and **increase energy**. It is an **anti-inflammatory** and was traditionally used for **rheumatoid arthritis**. It may also help **increase cellular oxygenation**.

Hyssop—was used by Moses during the Lord's Passover in Egypt (Exodus 12). It has **anti-inflammatory** and **antispasmodic** properties. It may also have the ability to **open** up the **respiratory system** and **discharge toxins** and **mucus**.

Peppermint—is **antiseptic**, **antispasmodic**, and **anti-inflammatory**. It is **soothing, cooling**, and **dilating** to the **system**.

Body System(s) Affected: The oils in this blend may help it be effective for dealing with various problems related to **Muscles and Bones**.

Application: Apply on location, anywhere there is **deep tissue pain.**

Safety Data: *Can be irritating to sensitive skin. Use with caution during* **pregnancy.** *Use with caution if susceptible to* **epilepsy** *or* **high blood pressure.**

Companion Oils: PanAway is a great companion to Relieve It, especially when there is **bone pain**. Other companion oils may include Aroma Siez, Melrose, cypress, and helichrysum.

Frequency: Very Low (Physical); approximately 56 MHz.

SACRED MOUNTAIN™

The predominance of conifer oils in this blend creates a feeling of **protection, empowerment**, and **grounding**. This blend may help one find **security** and **sacredness** within **oneself**. In addition, it is **anti-bacterial** and very **soothing** to the **respiratory system**.

Single Oils Contained In This Blend:

Spruce—**grounds** the **body**, creating the **balance** and the **opening** necessary to **receive** and to **give**. It also helps one release **emotional blocks**. It was used by the Lakota Indians to enhance their communication with the Great Spirit.

Ylang Ylang—may help **balance** the **male-female energies** so one can move closer towards being in spiritual attunement and allow them to focus their thoughts together, filtering out the ever-present garbage. It brings back the feeling of **self-love, confidence, joy** and **peace**.

Balsam Fir—may help create a feeling of **grounding, anchoring** and **empowerment**.

Cedarwood—was used traditionally by the North American Indians to enhance their potential for **spiritual communication**. It may help **open** the **pineal gland**.

Body System(s) Affected: The oils in this blend may help it be effective for dealing with various problems related to **Emotional Balance**.

Aromatic Influence: The aroma of this blend of oils creates a feeling of **strength, empowerment, grounding**, and **protection**.

Application: Diffuse. Apply to **solar plexus, brain stem, crown** of **head**, back of **neck**, behind **ears, thymus**, and **wrists**. Wear as **perfume** or **cologne**.

Safety Data: *Can be irritating to sensitive skin.*

Frequency: High (Spiritual); approximately 176 MHz.

Comments: The three conifer oils have been traditionally used by the North American Indians symbolically to represent the umbrella they create in protecting the earth and bringing energy in from the universe. At night the animals in the wild lie under a tree for the protection, recharging and rejuvenation the trees bring to them.

SARA™

The oils in this blend produce such a beautiful fragrance as may allow one to relax into a mental state whereby they may be able to **release** and let go of the **negative emotions** and **memory** of **traumatic experiences**. Although created specifically for relief from the **memory trauma** of **sexual** and/or **ritual abuse**, it may also work well for other traumatic experiences.

Single Oils Contained In This Blend:

Blue Tansy—may help **cleanse** the **liver** and **calm** the **lymphatic system**.

Rose—has a **beautiful fragrance** and contains the highest frequency of the oils. It may help **enhance** the **frequency** of every cell, which could help bring **balance** and **harmony** to the body. It is thought by some to produce a magnetic energy that attracts **love** and enhances the frequency of **self-love**, bringing **joy** to the heart.

Lavender—is an oil that has traditionally been known to **balance** the **body** and to work wherever there is a need. It may help promote **consciousness, health, love, peace**, and a general sense of **well being**.

Geranium—may help with **hormonal balance, liver** and **kidney functions** and the **discharge** of **toxins** from the **liver** that hold us back from having balance. Geranium **opens** the **liver chakra** (Solar Plexus). It may help **dilate** the **biliary ducts** for **liver detoxification**. It may also help foster **peace, well being**, and **hope** by promoting the release of **negative memories**.

Orange—brings **peace** and **happiness** to the **mind** and **body** and **joy** to the **heart**, which provide **emotional** support to help overcome depression.

Cedarwood—was used traditionally by the North American Indians to enhance their potential for **spiritual communication**. It may help **open** the **pineal gland**.

Ylang Ylang—may help **balance** the **male-female energies** so one can move closer towards being in spiritual attunement and allow them to focus their thoughts together, filtering out the ever-present garbage. It brings back the feeling of **self-love, confidence, joy** and **peace**.

White Lotus—was traditionally used by the Egyptians for spiritual, emotional, and physical applications. It has a euphoric fragrance that **lifts** and **stabilizes** the **emotions**, creating a powerful sense of **emotional, physical**, and **spiritual well being**.

Body System(s) Affected: The oils in this blend may help it be effective for dealing with various problems related to **Emotional Balance**.

Aromatic Influence: The aroma of this blend of oils creates a feeling of **peace** and **freedom** to move forward in life with **joy**.

Application: Apply over **energy centers**, on **Vita Flex points**, **temples, nose**, and **areas** of **abuse**.

Companion Oils: Forgiveness, Hope, Inner Child, Inspiration, Joy, Magnify Your Purpose, 3 Wise Men, Trauma Life, Valor, White Angelica

Frequency: Emotional; approximately 102 MHz.

Comments: One individual muscle tested positive for this oil for the purpose of overcoming the emotions related to having a twin brother die early in gestation, but remain in the womb until full-term delivery.

SclarEssence™

This blend was formulated to support the **hormones** and increase estradiol and testosterone levels. When taken as a dietary supplement, it may also help improve **digestion**, reduce **bloating**, and help balance the body's pH.

Single Oils Contained In This Blend:

Clary Sage—is beneficial for **regulating cells** and **balancing** the **hormones**. It may help with **menstrual cramps, PMS**, and **pre-menopause** symptoms. It may also help with **circulatory problems**.

Peppermint—is an **anti-inflammatory** to the **prostate** and **nerves**. It is **soothing** to the **stomach, cooling**, and **dilating** to the **system**.

Sage Lavender—has been shown to increase both estradiol and testosterone levels. It may help **harmonize** and **balance** the **emotions** and reduce **stress-related** conditions. It may also help decongest the **liver**.

Fennel—may help **support** the **digestive function** by **supporting** the **liver**. It may also help **balance** the **hormones**.

Body System(s) Affected: Hormonal and **Digestive Systems**.

Oral Use As Dietary Supplement: *Put 1-20 drops in a capsule. Ingest 1 capsule daily as needed. Not recommended for children.*

Sensation™

Because of the incredibly beautiful aromas of ylang ylang, rosewood, and jasmine, this blend is extremely **uplifting, refreshing**, and **arousing**. It is very beneficial for **skin problems** of any kind as it is very nourishing and hydrating for the skin.

Single Oils Contained In This Blend:

    Rosewood—is **soothing** to the **skin, appeasing** to the **mind, relaxing** to the **body**, and creates a feeling of **peace** and **gentleness**.

    Ylang Ylang—may help **balance** the **male-female energies** so one can move closer towards being in spiritual attunement and allow them to focus their thoughts together, filtering out the ever-present garbage. It brings back the feeling of **self-love, confidence, joy** and **peace**.

    Jasmine—is very **uplifting** to the **emotions**; it may produce a feeling of **confidence, energy, euphoria**, and **optimism**. Body System(s) Affected: The oils in this blend may help it be effective for dealing with various problems related to the **Hormonal System** and to **Emotional Balance**.

Aromatic Influence: Because the aroma of this blend of oils is so **uplifting** and **arousing**, it creates a feeling **excitement** and **romance** which may help move one to new heights of **self-expression** and **awareness**.

Application: Apply on **location**, use for **massage**, and add to your Sensation Bath and Shower Gel. May also be used with a **compress** over the abdomen, or just worn as a **cologne** or **perfume**.

Companion Oils: <u>Awaken</u>, <u>Dream Catcher</u>, <u>Into the Future</u>, <u>Joy</u>, <u>Live with Passion</u>

Frequency: Physical and Emotional; approximately 88 MHz.

SURRENDER™

    Most of the single oils in this blend are **calming, relaxing**, and **balancing** to the emotions, making it effective for those with **dominant personalities** who at times may become **unfocused** or **overbearing**. By **balancing** the **emotions, clearing** the **mind**, and reducing feelings of **anxiety** and **stress**, this blend may help such individuals recover **equilibrium**, and calm **inner strength**.

Single Oils Contained In This Blend:

    Lavender—is an oil that has traditionally been known to **balance** the **body** and to work wherever there is a need. It may help promote **consciousness, health, love, peace**, and a general sense of **well being**.

    Roman Chamomile—eliminates some of the emotional charge of **anxiety, irritability**, and **nervousness**. Because it is **calming** and **relaxing**, it can combat **stress**.

    German Chamomile—can dispel **anger**, stabilize the **emotions**, and help release emotions liked to the past. It may also help to **soothe** and **clear** the **mind** creating an atmosphere of **peace** and **patience**.

    Angelica—is referred to by the German people as the "oil of angels". It may help one **release** and **let go** of **negative feelings**.

    Mountain Savory—has **immune-stimulant, antimicrobial**, and **anti-parasitic** properties. It is also a powerful **energizer** and **motivator**.

Lemon—promotes **health, healing, physical energy**, and **purification**. Its fragrance is **invigorating, enhancing**, and **warming**.

Spruce—**grounds** the **body**, creating the **balance** and the **opening** necessary to **receive** and to **give**. It may help **dilate** the **bronchial tract** to **improve** the **oxygen exchange**. It also helps one release **emotional blocks**.

Body System(s) Affected: The oils in this blend may help it be effective for dealing with various problems related to the **Nervous System** and to **Emotional Balance**.

Aromatic Influence: May help to reduce **anxiety** and calm **nervousness** and **irritability**. It may also help to **balance** the **emotions** and **clear** the **mind**.

Application: Apply on the **forehead**, along the **rim** of the **ears**, at the **nape** of the **neck**, on the **chest**, and on the **solar plexus**. May also be added to **bath** water.

Safety Data: *Because of some of the oils contained within this blend, it should be used with caution by individuals who are* **pregnant***. Repeated use could possibly result in* **skin irritation.**

Companion Oils: Clarity, Forgiveness, Grounding, Peace & Calming, Sacred Mountain

Frequency: Physical and Emotional; approximately 98 MHz.

THIEVES®

The highly anti-viral, antiseptic properties of the single oils contained in this blend help protect the body from the onset of **flu, candida, colds**, etc. It may also help with **sinusitis, bronchitis, pneumonia, coughs, strep, sore throats, periodontal (gum) disease, teething, cold sores, canker sores, bruises, cuts, infection, slivers and splinters** (pulls to surface). It is considered **anti-plague** as it was used by thieves in England to protect them from the plague when stealing from the sick and dying.

Single Oils Contained In This Blend:

Clove—is **anti-bacterial, anti-fungal, anti-infectious, anti-parasitic**, a **strong antiseptic, anti-viral**, and an **immune stimulant**. It may influence **healing** and help create a feeling of **protection** and **courage**.

Lemon—promotes **health, healing, physical energy**, and **purification**. Its fragrance is **invigorating, enhancing**, and **warming**. It is an **antiseptic** and is great for the **respiratory system**.

Cinnamon Bark—is part of the formula the Lord gave Moses (Exodus 30:22-27). It has very specific purposes: (1) it is a **powerful purifier**, (2) it is a powerful **oxygenator**, and (3) it **enhances** the action and the activity of **other oils**. It may have a **stimulating** and **toning** effect on the whole body and particularly the circulatory system. It is **anti-bacterial, anti-fungal, anti-infectious, anti-inflammatory, antimicrobial, anti-parasitic, antiseptic, antispasmodic, anti-viral, astringent, immune-stimulant, sexual stimulant**, and **warming**.

Eucalyptus radiata—may have a profound **anti-viral** effect upon the **respiratory system**. It also has **strong anti-bacterial, anti-catarrhal**, and **antiseptic** properties.

Rosemary cineol—may help **balance heart function, energize** the **solar plexus**, and **reduce mental fatigue**. It may **improve circulation** and help **stimulate** the **nerves**. It is **antiseptic** and **anti-infectious**.

Body System(s) Affected: The oils in this blend may help it be effective for dealing with various problems related to the **immune system**.

Aromatic Influence: Diffuse this blend of oils periodically for 20-25 minutes at a time to help protect the body against the onset of **flu, colds**, and **viruses**.

Application: Massage bottom of **feet, throat, stomach**, and **intestines**. Dilute one drop of Thieves in 15 drops of V-6 Mixing Oil and massage the **thymus** to stimulate the **immune system** and massage **under** the **arms** to stimulate the **lymphatic system**. It is best applied to the bottom of the feet as it may be caustic to the skin. **Always dilute with V-6 Mixing Oil.**

Safety Data: *Repeated use can result in extreme **contact sensitization**. Can cause extreme **skin irritation**. Use with caution during **pregnancy**.*

Companion Oils: Put <u>ImmuPower</u> on the **throat** and <u>Thieves</u> on the **feet**, then alternate by putting <u>Thieves</u> on the **throat** and <u>ImmuPower</u> on the **feet**. Can also alternate <u>ImmuPower</u> with <u>Exodus II</u>.

Frequency: Emotional and Spiritual; approximately 150 MHz.

Comments: Studies conducted by Weber State University (Ogden, UT) during 1997 showed the antibacterial effectiveness of this blend (<u>Thieves</u>) against airborne microorganisms. One study showed a 90% reduction in the number of gram positive *Micrococcus luteus* organisms after diffusing <u>Thieves</u> for 12 minutes. After diffusing <u>Thieves</u> for a total of 20 minutes, there was a 99.3% reduction. Another study against the gram negative *Pseudomonas aeruginosa* showed a kill rate of 99.96% after just 12 minutes of diffusion.

3 WISE MEN™

The highly spiritual nature of the oils in this blend allow it to **open** the **crown chakra** and facilitate the release of negative emotions. This blend brings a sense of **grounding** and **uplifting** through **memory recall**. It also keeps negative energy and negative emotions from reattaching to the body.

Single Oils Contained In This Blend:

Sandalwood—also, like frankincense, is high in sesquiterpenes, which were discovered to **increase** the amount of **oxygen** around the **pineal** and **pituitary glands**, thus helping to **improve** one's **attitude**. It **alleviates depression** and assists in the removal of **negative programming** from the cells of the body. It helps one **accept others** with an open heart while diminishing one's own egocentricity.

Juniper—evokes feelings of **health, love**, and **peace** and may help to **elevate** one's **spiritual awareness**.

Frankincense—contains sesquiterpenes, which may help **oxygenate** the **pineal** and **pituitary glands**. As one of the ingredients for the holy incense, it was used anciently to help **enhance** one's **communication with the creator**. It was considered a prize possession and was given to Christ at his birth by the three wise men. It may help **promote** a **positive attitude**.

Spruce—**grounds** the **body**, creating the **balance** and the **opening** necessary to **receive** and to **give**. It also helps one release **emotional blocks**. It was used by the Lakota Indians to enhance their communication with the Great Spirit.

Myrrh—is part of the formula the Lord gave Moses (Exodus 30:22-27). It promotes **spiritual awareness** and is a **true gift** (one of the gifts that was brought for the Christ child). When we **open** our **hearts** and **minds** to receive the gifts, they will be given.

Carrier Oil Contained In This Blend: Almond Oil.

Body System(s) Affected: The oils in this blend may help it be effective for dealing with various problems related to **Emotional Balance**.

Aromatic Influence: Diffusing this blend of oils may help to create a feeling of **reverence** and heightened **spiritual consciousness**.

Application: Apply to the **crown** of the **head** in a clockwise motion to create an energy of opening and releasing, followed by receiving the energy of the oils to **fill** the **new void**. Put on **neck, eye brow, solar plexus**, and **thymus** (clockwise). Wear as **perfume** or **cologne**.

Companion Oils: Frankincense, myrrh, sandalwood, juniper, and spruce.

Frequency: Physical; approximately 72 MHz.

Comments: When all or any of the companion oils are combined with 3 Wise Men, a sense of **grounding** and **upliftment** come through the release of memory recall. In addition, when the oil is placed on the crown, it elevates ones spiritual consciousness.

TRANSFORMATION™

Many of the oils in this blend are powerfully **energizing** and **stimulating** to the **conscious mind** allowing for the **support** necessary when making changes, especially **mental** and **emotional changes**.

Single Oils Contained In This Blend:

Lemon—promotes **health, healing, physical energy**, and **purification**. Its fragrance is **invigorating, enhancing**, and **warming**.

Peppermint—is **anti-inflammatory** to the **nerves**. It has a **soothing** and **cooling effect** on **headaches**. It is **purifying** and **stimulating** to the **conscious mind**.

Sandalwood—also, like frankincense, is high in sesquiterpenes, which were discovered to **increase** the amount of **oxygen** around the **pineal** and **pituitary glands**, thus helping to **improve** one's **attitude**.

Frankincense—contains sesquiterpenes, which may help **oxygenate** the **pineal** and **pituitary glands**. As one of the ingredients for the holy incense, it was used anciently to help **enhance** one's **communication with the creator**. It may help **promote** a **positive attitude**.

Clary Sage—may calm and enhance the **dream state**, helping to bring about a feeling of **euphoria**.

Balsam Fir—creates a feeling of **grounding, anchoring**, and **empowerment**. It can **stimulate** the **mind** while allowing the **body** to **relax**.

Rosemary cineol—may help **balance heart function, energize** the **solar plexus**, and **reduce mental fatigue**. It may **improve circulation** and help **stimulate** the **nerves**.

Cardamom—is **uplifting, refreshing**, and **invigorating**. It may be beneficial for **clearing confusion**.

Body System(s) Affected: The oils in this blend may help it be effective for dealing with various problems related to **Emotional Balance**.

Aromatic Influence: When diffused or worn as perfume, this blend of oils may help **stimulate** one's mind and **strengthen** one's resolve when dealing with difficult decisions, especially when related to a change in **attitude** or a change in one's **belief system**.

Application: Diffuse or apply to the **forehead** ("third eye" chakra) and over the **heart**, helping to unite heart and mind.

Companion Oils: Hope, Humility, Into the Future.

Frequency: Physical and Emotional; approximately 92 MHz.

TRAUMA LIFE™

Many of the oils in this blend are powerfully **calming** and **grounding**, helping **purge** the **stress** and **uproot** the **traumas** that are often at the heart of our physical fatigue and overburdened immune system. Others are **spiritually uplifting**, bringing us closer to our **creator** and helping us to see our **trials** from the **proper perspective**. Sometimes, physical and mental difficulties are a result of unreleased trauma. For example, our one year old daughter would continuously babble until she fell down a flight of stairs. Although she was not physically hurt from the fall, we soon noticed that the babbling had stopped. One application of this blend brought back the constant babbling.

Single Oils Contained In This Blend:

Limette (*Citrus hystrix*)—is very high in aldehydes and esters, making it very **sedating** and **calming**.

Davana—is **anti-infectious** and may stimulate the **endocrine system** and improve **hormonal balance**.

Geranium—may help with **hormonal balance, liver** and **kidney functions** and the **discharge** of **toxins** from the **liver** that hold us back from having balance. Geranium **opens** the **liver chakra** (Solar Plexus). It may help **dilate** the **biliary ducts** for **liver detoxification**, which may help one let go of **anger** and **negative emotions**.

Spruce—**grounds** the **body**, creating the **balance** and the **opening** necessary to **receive** and to **give**. It may help **dilate** the **bronchial tract** to **improve** the **oxygen exchange**. It also helps one release **emotional blocks**.

Helichrysum—may help **cleanse** the **blood** and improve **circulatory functions**. It is **anti-catarrhal** in structure and nature. As a powerful **anti-inflammatory**, it may even help reduce inflammation in the meninges of the brain. On a spiritual level, it may help one **let go of angry feelings** that prevent one from forgiving and moving forward.

Rose—contains the highest frequency of the oils. It may help **enhance** the **frequency** of every cell, which could help bring **balance** and **harmony** to the body. It is thought by some to produce a magnetic energy that attracts **love** and enhances the frequency of **self-love**, bringing **joy** to the heart.

Sandalwood—also, like frankincense, is high in sesquiterpenes, which were discovered to **increase** the amount of **oxygen** around the **pineal** and **pituitary glands**, thus helping to **improve** one's **attitude**.

Frankincense—contains sesquiterpenes, which may help **oxygenate** the **pineal** and **pituitary glands**. As one of the ingredients for the holy incense, it was used anciently to help **enhance** one's **communication with the creator**. It may help **promote** a **positive attitude**.

Lavender—is an oil that has traditionally been known to **balance** the **body** and to work wherever there is a need. It may help promote **consciousness, health, love, peace**, and a general sense of **well being**.

Valerian—has a powerful sedative effect. It is also **antispasmodic, depressant** to the central nervous system, and somewhat **hypnotic**. It may help minimize the shock, the feeling of anxiety, and the stress that accompanies traumatic situations.

Body System(s) Affected: The oils in this blend may help it be effective for dealing with various problems related to **Emotional Balance**.

Aromatic Influence: When diffused, this blend of oils may help promote the **calming** and **balancing** effect that is necessary in overcoming **trauma**.

Application: Best when applied to the **spine** using the Raindrop Technique. It is also beneficial when placed on the bottom of the **feet**, on the **chest**, behind the **ears**, on the nap of the **neck**, or in the center of the **forehead** ("third eye" chakra).

Companion Oils: Peace & Calming, Joy, Hope, Into the Future.

Frequency: Physical and Emotional; approximately 92 MHz.

Valor™

This blend has been used to help **empower** the **physical** and **spiritual bodies**. It helps us **overcome fear** and **opposition** so we can stand tall during adversity. It may help build **courage, confidence**, and **self-esteem**. It brings a feeling of **calmness, peace** and **relaxation**. It may be used in place of Peace & Calming for **hyperactivity** and **attention deficit disorder** in **children**. It has been found beneficial in helping to **align** the **physical structure** of the **body, relieving pain** along **spine**. It also **balances** and **aligns electrical energies** within the **body**. It is best

applied with six drops on each foot or massaged in along the spine using the Raindrop Technique._
Valor has been touted as a **chiropractor** in a bottle. It has improved **scoliosis** in as little as 30
minutes, though this should not be considered normal. Some individuals require several months of
application before any improvement is seen. *Valor has also been shown to change anaerobic mutated
cells back to their aerobic natural state.*

Single Oils Contained In This Blend:
> Spruce—**grounds** the **body**, creating the **balance** and the **opening** necessary to
>> **receive** and to **give**. It may help **dilate** the **bronchial tract** to **improve** the **oxygen
>> exchange**. It also helps one release **emotional blocks**.
> Rosewood—is **soothing** to the **skin, appeasing** to the **mind, relaxing** to the **body**, and
>> creates a feeling of **peace** and **gentleness**.
> Blue Tansy—may help **cleanse** the **liver** and **calm** the **lymphatic system** to help rid one
>> of **anger** and promote a feeling of **self-control**.
> Frankincense—contains sesquiterpenes, which may help **oxygenate** the **pineal** and
>> **pituitary glands**. As one of the ingredients for the holy incense, it was used anciently
>> to help **enhance** one's **communication with the creator**. It may help **promote** a
>> **positive attitude**.

Carrier Oil Contained In This Blend: Almond Oil.

Body System(s) Affected: The oils in this blend may help it be effective for dealing with various
problems related to **Muscles and Bones, Skin**, the **Nervous System**, and **Emotional
Balance**.

Aromatic Influence: This blend of oils may help **balance** the **electrical energies** in the body.
Diffuse wherever and whenever possible.

Application: It **works best** on **bottom** of **feet**. Put six drops of Valor on **bottom** of **feet**. Put
Valor on **heart, throat chakra, wrists, solar plexus** from **neck** to **thymus**. To **balance
left** and **right brain**, put Valor on **left fingers** and rub on **right temple** or put Valor
on **right fingers** and rub on **left temple or cross arms** and rub **Vita Flex points** on
bottom of **feet**. To **relieve pain** along the **spine**, apply Valor to **Vita Flex points** on **feet**
and on **spine** using the **raindrop technique**. Wear as **perfume** or **cologne**.

Companion Oils: Balance with Valor and **protect** with White Angelica.

Frequency: Very low to balance and align the physical body; aligns the skeletal system;
approximately 47 MHz.

Comments: This blend is the most important oil in any application. It helps balance electrical
energies within the body, giving courage, confidence, and self-esteem. Most importantly, it
builds the bridge between the body and the oils allowing higher frequency oils to raise the
frequency of the body thus promoting physical, emotional, and spiritual well being. (*Refer
to the Vita Flex Therapy part of the Science and Application section of this book for the
importance of using this blend and how to use it to balance the body's energy*).

WHITE ANGELICA™

This unique blend of 10 different oils helps create a frequency field to **ward off** the **bombardment** of **negative energy**. It is important for use in **emotional cleansing**. It may help **increase** the **aura** around the body, bringing a delicate sense of **strength** and **protection** and a greater **awareness** of **one's potential**. It may also help with **anger, depression, headaches** (especially when flying), **hemorrhoids, circulation**, and **lowering high blood pressure**.

Single Oils Contained In This Blend:

Geranium—may help with **hormonal balance, liver** and **kidney functions** and the **discharge** of **toxins** from the **liver** that hold us back from having balance. Geranium **opens** the **liver chakra** (Solar Plexus). It may help **dilate** the **biliary ducts** for **liver detoxification**, which may help one let go of **anger** and **negative emotions**.

Spruce—**grounds** the **body**, creating the **balance** and the **opening** necessary to **receive** and to **give**. It also helps one release **emotional blocks**.

Myrrh—is part of the formula the Lord gave Moses (Exodus 30:22-27). It promotes **spiritual awareness** and is a **true gift** (one of the gifts that was brought for the Christ child). When we **open** our **hearts** and **minds** to receive the gifts, they will be given.

Ylang Ylang—may help **balance** the **male-female energies** so one can move closer towards being in spiritual attunement and allow them to focus their thoughts together, filtering out the ever-present garbage. It brings back the feeling of **self-love, confidence, joy** and **peace**.

Hyssop—was used by Moses during the Lord's Passover in Egypt (Exodus 12). It has **anti-inflammatory** and **anti-viral** properties. It may have the ability to **open** up the **respiratory system** and **discharge toxins** and **mucus**. It may also stimulate **meditation** and promote **centering**.

Bergamot—is **soothing** to the **endocrine system** and the **hormones** of the body. It may **uplift** and **calm** the **emotions** to help relieve **anxiety, stress**, and **tension**.

Melissa—is an oil that is powerful as an **anti-viral** agent, yet it is very gentle and very delicate because of the nature of the plant. It has the ability to work with and enhance the gentle aspects of the human body. It is **calming** and **uplifting** and may help to **balance** the **emotions**. It may also help to remove **emotional blocks** and **instill** a **positive outlook** on **life**.

Sandalwood—also, like frankincense, is high in sesquiterpenes, which were discovered to **increase** the amount of **oxygen** around the **pineal** and **pituitary glands**, thus helping to **improve** one's **attitude**. It **alleviates depression** and assists in the removal of **negative programming** from the cells of the body.

Rose—contains the highest frequency of the oils. It may help **enhance** the **frequency** of every cell, which could help bring **balance** and **harmony** to the body. It is thought by some to produce a magnetic energy that attracts **love** and enhances the frequency of **self-love**, bringing **joy** to the heart.

Rosewood—may help bring a synergism to all the oils. It is **soothing** to the **skin, appeasing** to the **mind, relaxing** to the **body**, and creates a feeling of **peace** and **gentleness**.

Carrier Oil Contained In This Blend: Almond Oil.

Body System(s) Affected: The oils in this blend may help it be effective for dealing with various problems related to **Emotional Balance**.

Aromatic Influence: The aroma of this blend of oils may be a tremendous aid in times of **meditation**.

Application: Apply on **shoulders, crown, chest**, behind the **ears, neck, forehead**, and **wrists**. Add to **bath** water. Wear as **perfume** or **cologne**.

Safety Data: *Avoid exposure to direct **sunlight** for 3 to 6 hours after use.*

Companion Oils: Balance with <u>Valor</u> and **protect** with <u>White Angelica</u>. Use with <u>Inspiration</u>, <u>Awaken</u>, and <u>Sacred Mountain</u> to create a feeling of wholeness in the realm of one's own spirituality and oneness with the **creator**. When the heart is stressed, use <u>Joy</u> and <u>Aroma Life</u> with <u>White Angelica</u>.

Frequency: Physical and Emotional; approximately 89 MHz.

Oil Blends

A Great Help for Alzheimer's Disease

When my mother who has Alzheimer's came to live with us, she didn't sleep at night but was up cleaning out drawers, slamming doors and being generally noisy all night. We were introduced to Young Living Oils and started putting Peace & Calming in a cool mist vaporizer 3-4 times during the day in the living area where she spent her time. In two weeks, she began sleeping ALL NIGHT!!! We've continued using a variety of oils (Lavender, Brain Power, Lemon, Clarity) and she is now in better health than she's been in 20 years. She still has Alzheimer's but her mood is mostly stabilized.

-Submitted by E. Pinar (July 2004)

Personal Care Products

These product names are all trademarks of Young Living Essential Oils and although these product names appear throughout other sections of this book without the trademark symbol, they still refer to these same trademarked products.

A·R·T™ Skin Care System
(Age Refining Technology)

This revolutionary set of three synergistic skin care products (Day Activator, Gentle Foaming Cleanser, and Night Reconstructor) provides a complete system for unprecedented protection and restoration of the skin. These products utilize the following ingredients/technologies to provide a superior skin care system: 1) Two innovative enzymes (Photolyase and Endonuclease) for advanced DNA repair; 2) A revolutionary peptide complex to enhance the production of collagen I, III, IV, and fibroconectin for softening the skin and smoothing wrinkles; 3) Wolfberry seed oil which contains essential fatty acids like linoleic acid, gamma-linoleic acid (GLA), and oleic acid for intense moisturizing and conditioning of the skin; and 4) Advanced delivery technologies like Laminar Phase Technology (for a highly efficient application and protective barrier) and Liposome Technology (to more quickly deliver greater amounts of ingredients to lower levels of the skin). Then add to all of that the cleansing, stimulating, and regenerative properties of therapeutic-grade essential oils, and these products have no equals currently on the market.

A·R·T™ Day Activator

This unique light-bodied, water-based, anti-aging day cream utilizes the innovative Photolyase enzyme. This enzyme, powered by visible light, repairs DNA segments in cells that have been damaged by UV radiation. It is quickly absorbed and perfect for wearing underneath makeup and sunscreen to help protect, repair, and build healthy, vibrant skin.

Ingredients: Deionized water, pentylene glycol, glycerin, glyceryl stearate, betaine, cetearyl alcohol, caprylic/capric triglycerides, lycium barbarum (Ningxia wolfberry) seed oil, meadowfoam seed oil and shea butter, aloe barbadensis leaf juice, phenoxyethanol, chlorphenesin, xanthan gum, sodium stearoyl lactylate, carbomer, tetrahexyldecyl ascorbate, tocopheryl acetate, polysorbate 20, squalane, dimethicone, benzoic acid, dipotassium glycyrrhizinate, sodium hyaluronate, camellia oleifera extract, chamomilla recutita (German chamomile) oil, retinyl palmitate, sodium PCA, chlorella vulgaris extract, algae extract and mugwort (artemisia vulgaris) extract, plankton extract, micrococcus lysate, palmitoyl oligopeptide, palmitoyl tetrapeptide-3, lecithin, grape (vitis vinifera) seed extract, santalum album (sandalwood) oil, and boswellia carterii (frankincense) oil as shown below. May also contain sodium hydroxide.

Essential Oils:

> **German Chamomile**—has been found to help open the liver, increase liver function and secretion, and support the pancreas. It neutralizes allergies and increases the ability of the skin to regenerate.

> **Sandalwood**—helps strengthen the lymphatic systems; revitalizes the skin; shown to increase blood oxygenation for increased skin cell regeneration.

> **Frankincense**—is high in sesquiterpenes; helps deliver oxygen to the pineal and pituitary glands; improves hGH production; increases leukocyte production; shown to inhibit elastase (the enzyme that breaks down elastin); also shown to increase lipid synthesis for higher cell volume.

Suggested Use: Apply in the morning after cleansing. Using fingertips, massage a generous amount of Day Activator over face and neck regions as needed. Suitable for all skin types.

Body System(s) Affected: Skin

Caution: As with any cosmetic, if you are currently being treated for any skin condition, consult your medical professional before using. For external use only. Keep out of reach of children. Store in a cool, dry place.

A·R·T™ GENTLE FOAMING CLEANSER

A unique foaming cleanser that gently removes dirt, oil, and makeup from the skin and, unlike so many other commercial products, leaves the skin feeling clean, fresh, hydrated, and soft.

Ingredients: Deionized water, sodium cocoyl glutamate, sodium methyl cocoyl taurate, sodium lauroamphoacetate, decyl glucoside, therapeutic-grade essential oils as shown below, aloe barbadensis leaf juice, tocopheryl acetate, glycerin, cetyl hydroxyethylcellulose, benzoic acid, sorbic acid, sodium hydroxide, ginkgo biloba leaf extract, camellia oleifera leaf extract, retinyl palmitate, citric acid, phenoxyethanol, chlorphenesin. May also contain sodium hydroxide.

Essential Oils:

> **Frankincense**—is high in sesquiterpenes; helps deliver oxygen to the pineal and pituitary glands; improves hGH production; increases leukocyte production; shown to inhibit elastase (the enzyme that breaks down elastin); also shown to increase lipid synthesis for higher cell volume.

> **Sandalwood**—helps strengthen the lymphatic systems; revitalizes the skin; shown to increase blood oxygenation for increased skin cell regeneration.

> **Lavender**—balancing and calming; works wherever there is a need; useful for any type of skin condition.

> **Lemon**—helps promote leukocyte formation; antiseptic.

Melissa—is a powerful anti-viral agent, yet is very gentle and very delicate because of the nature of the plant; has the ability to work with and enhance the gentle aspects of the human body; anti-inflammatory and energizing.

Suggested Use: With wet hands, massage gently over face. Rinse thoroughly. To be used twice daily, for a refreshing cleanse in the morning, and for a thorough cleanse at night. Suitable for all skin types. Store in a cool, dry place.

Body System(s) Affected: Skin

Caution: As with any cosmetic, if you are currently being treated for any skin condition, consult your medical professional before using.

A·R·T™ NIGHT RECONSTRUCTOR

This unique medium-bodied, water-based, anti-aging night moisturizer utilizes the innovative Endonuclease enzyme. This critical enzyme is powered by the energy in your body to cut out damaged DNA segments, reproduce the correct segments from the complimentary strands, and re-insert the new segments into the cell's DNA structure. With therapeutic-grade essential oils and superior moisturizing agents, it also provides maximum hydration to the skin during sleep.

Ingredients: Deionized water, pentylene glycol, glycerin, glyceryl stearate, betaine, lycium barbarum (Ningxia wolfberry) seed oil, cetearyl alcohol, meadowfoam seed oil and shea butter, aloe barbadensis leaf juice, phenoxyethanol, chlorphenesin, xanthan gum, sodium stearoyl lactylate, carbomer, tetrahexyldecyl ascorbate, tocopheryl acetate, polysorbate 20, squalane, dimethicone, benzoic acid, dipotassium glycyrrhizinate, sodium hyaluronate, camellia oleifera extract, chamomile recutita (German chamomile) oil, retinyl palmitate, sodium PCA, chlorella vulgaris extract, algae extract and mugwort (artemisia vulgaris) extract, micrococcus lysate, palmitoyl oligopeptide, palmitoyl tetrapeptide-3, lecithin, grape (vitis vinifera) seed extract, santalum album (sandalwood) oil, and boswellia carterii (frankincense) oil as shown below. May also contain sodium hydroxide.

Essential Oils:

German Chamomile—has been found to help open the liver, increase liver function and secretion, and support the pancreas. It neutralizes allergies and increases the ability of the skin to regenerate.

Sandalwood—helps strengthen the lymphatic systems; revitalizes the skin; shown to increase blood oxygenation for increased skin cell regeneration.

Frankincense—is high in sesquiterpenes; helps deliver oxygen to the pineal and pituitary glands; improves hGH production; increases leukocyte production; shown to inhibit elastase (the enzyme that breaks down elastin); also shown to increase lipid synthesis for higher cell volume.

Suggested Use: Apply in the evening after cleansing. Using fingertips, massage a generous amount of Night Reconstructor over face and neck regions as needed. Suitable for all skin types.

Body System(s) Affected: Skin

Caution: As with any cosmetic, if you are currently being treated for any skin condition, consult your medical professional before using. For external use only. Keep out of reach of children. Store in a cool, dry place.

A·R·T™ Purifying Toner

Although the Purifying Toner is not packaged with the other three products as part of the A·R·T Skin Care System, this remarkable formulation of ingredients is a necessary addition to any skin care regimen and the results are greatest when all four products are used together. The Purifying Toner not only cleanses the skin by removing any unwanted oil, dirt, and impurities that tend to accumulate there, but it also energizes and refreshes the skin's surface, thereby working to restore or maintain a firm, healthy-looking complexion. The added essential oils of frankincense, sandalwood, lemon, and peppermint, along with the plant extracts of lavender and melissa, help to smooth and soften skin, enhance pH balance, minimize oily shine, and reduce the appearance of pores.

Ingredients: Deionized water, SD alcohol 38-B (denatured with peppermint oil), pentylene glycol (derived from coconut and palm for moisture retention), hamamelis virginiana (Witch Hazel) distillate extract, glycerin (from coconut and vegetable sources), 100% pure essential oils as shown below, camellia oleifera leaf extract, vitis vinifera (grape) seed oil, lavandula angustifolia (lavender) extract, melissa officinalis leaf extract, aloe barbadensis leaf juice, retinyl palmitate, allantoin, and polysorbate-20.

Essential Oils:

Frankincense—is high in sesquiterpenes; helps deliver oxygen to the pineal and pituitary glands; improves hGH production; increases leukocyte production; shown to inhibit elastase (the enzyme that breaks down elastin); also shown to increase lipid synthesis for higher cell volume.

Sandalwood—helps strengthen the lymphatic systems; revitalizes the skin; shown to increase blood oxygenation for increased skin cell regeneration.

Lemon—helps promote leukocyte formation; antiseptic.

Peppermint—enhances the effect of the other oils; cooling and soothing sensations; invigorates the skin and helps with nerve regeneration.

Suggested Use: After cleansing, sweep Purifying Toner over face with a cotton ball. Can be used in the morning and again in the evening. For best results, apply the A·R·T Day Activator or Night Reconstructor cream over the Purifying Toner.

Body System(s) Affected: Skin (suitable for all skin types)

Caution: As with any cosmetic, if you are currently being treated for any skin condition, consult your medical professional before using. For external use only. Keep out of reach of children. Store in a cool, dry place.

ANIMAL SCENTS™ PET OINTMENT

Instead of the harmful chemicals and antibiotics, give your pet the same natural ingredients and powerful germ fighting essential oils that you've come to rely on. This products is wonderful blend of wholesome herbs and essential oils designed for helping your pet heal from minor skin irritations, cuts, and scrapes. It sure seems to work great on humans as well.

Ingredients: Mink oil, lecithin, beeswax, lanolin, sesame seed oil, wheat germ oil, and essential oils as shown below.

Essential Oils:

> **Rosewood**—antiseptic and antibacterial; tissue regenerative; soothing to the skin and increases elasticity.
>
> **Palmarosa**—stimulates new cell growth, regulates oil production, moisturizes and speeds healing.
>
> **Patchouli**—helps digest toxic material; tones / tightens skin; helps prevent wrinkles.
>
> **Myrrh**—is soothing to the skin; used for chapped and cracked skin and wrinkles.
>
> **Carrot seed**—a natural phytonutrient that is rich in beta carotene; helps to reduce wrinkles and dryness.
>
> *Melaleuca alternifolia*—tissue regenerative; helps promote the healing of wounds.
>
> **Rosehip seed**—helps reduce scarring and prevent premature aging of the skin.
>
> **Geranium**—improves blood flow, regenerates tissue and nerves, cleans oily skin, and may even liven up pale skin.
>
> **Balsam Fir**—is a rich source of the antioxidant limonene which has been shown to help relieve overworked and tired muscles and joints.

Suggested Use: Clean the affected area. Apply as needed. If using additional essential oils, apply oils prior to application of Animal Scents Pet Ointment.

Body System(s) Affected: Skin

ANIMAL SCENTS™ PET SHAMPOO

Stop bathing your pet in chemical-laden products. This product gives you natural ingredients, mixed with essential oils, to pamper your pet. Not only will it keep your pet clean, it will also assist in cleansing and healing their cuts and scratches.

Ingredients: Demineralized water; saponified oils of coconut and olive, essential oils (as shown below), vegetable gum, aloe vera, and rosemary extract.

Essential Oils:

> **Citronella**—deodorant; insect repellent; also good for oily skin.
>
> **Lavandin**—is an anti-fungal, an anti-bacterial, a strong antiseptic, and a tissue regenerator.
>
> **Lemon**—helps promote leukocyte formation; antiseptic.
>
> **Geranium**—improves blood flow, regenerates tissue and nerves, cleans oily skin, and may even liven up pale skin.
>
> **Spikenard**—anti-bacterial and anti-fungal; helps with staph infections.

Suggested Use: Pour a small amount of Animal Scents' Shampoo into palm and rub gently between hands. Massage thoroughly into pet's wet coat. Lather. Rinse thoroughly. Repeat if necessary.

Body System(s) Affected: Skin

Precautions: Animal Scents' Shampoo is highly concentrated. If necessary, dilute with water.

AROMAGUARD® DEODORANTS

This is one of the most unique deodorant products on the market today. Made with natural ingredients (no toxic aluminum salts or propylene glycol) and bacteria fighting essential oils, these deodorants will help keep your skin clean and fresh while not interfering with the body's natural cooling system. The formulation is also clean and evaporative, with no sticky residue.

Ingredients: Coconut oil, white beeswax, pure vegetable esters (34 and 40 from palm kernel and coconut oils), zinc oxide, natural mixed tocopherols (vitamin E), and essential oils as follows:

Mountain Mint Essential Oils:

Lemon—helps promote leukocyte formation; antiseptic.

Rosemary cineol—highly anti-infectious; anti-fungal and anti-bacterial; good for various skin conditions.

Clove—is anti-bacterial, anti-fungal, anti-infectious, anti-parasitic, a strong antiseptic, anti-viral, and an immune stimulant. It may influence healing and help create a feeling of protection and courage.

Cedarwood—rejuvenating and refreshing; antiseptic and beneficial to the skin.

Blue Cypress (*Callitris intratropica*)—is an abundant source of sesquiterpenes. It is grounding and stabilizing with a fragrance that uplifts and inspires.

May also contain peppermint, eucalyptus, and/or white fir.

Meadow Mist Essential Oils:

Lemon—helps promote leukocyte formation; antiseptic.

Geranium—can be used on almost any kind of skin; cleansing, refreshing, astringent, and a mild skin tonic; used to balance hyposecretion of androgens or estrogens which frequently occurs during menopause.

Rosewood—antiseptic and antibacterial; tissue regenerative; soothing to the skin and increases elasticity.

Rosemary cineol—highly anti-infectious; anti-fungal and anti-bacterial; good for various skin conditions.

Lavender—balancing and calming; works wherever there is a need; useful for any type of skin condition.

Melaleuca alternifolia—tissue regenerative; helps promote the healing of wounds.

Melaleuca quinquenervia—is powerfully anti-fungal, anti-viral, anti-bacterial; may help protect against radiation and is a strong tissue regenerator.

Clove—is anti-bacterial, anti-fungal, anti-infectious, anti-parasitic, a strong antiseptic, anti-viral, and an immune stimulant. It may influence healing and help create a feeling of protection and courage.

May also contain peppermint, eucalyptus, and/or white fir.

Suggested Use: After bath or shower, apply 3-4 light strokes of AromaGuard to underarms.

Body System(s) Affected: Skin

Precautions: Skin test first for sensitivity. Note: The authors of this book use these deodorants, and when first beginning to use them, the Mountain Mint deodorant would produce an itchy rash under the arms. The Meadow Mist would not produce the rash. After a few weeks of using the Meadow Mist product, the application of Mountain Mint would not produce the rash and has not since. It seems, therefore, that when switching from chemical-laden commercial products to these deodorants, a cleansing process is required and the Meadow Mist product is recommended for the first while.

BOSWELLIA™ WRINKLE CREME

Ingredients: Deionized water, calendula extract, chamomile extract, rosebud extract, orange blossom extract, St. John's wort extract, aloe vera gel, kelp extract, *Ginkgo biloba* extract, grapeseed extract, ASC 111, goat's cream, glyceryl stearate, caprylic/capric triglyceride, shea butter, essential oils (as shown below), wolfberry seed oil, stearic acid, stearyl alcohol, sodium PCA, sodium hyaluronate, allantoin, panthenol, retinyl palmitate (vitamin A), and tocopheryl acetate (vitamin E).

Essential Oils:

Frankincense—is high in sesquiterpenes; helps deliver oxygen to the pineal and pituitary glands; improves hGH production; increases leukocyte production,

Sandalwood—helps strengthen the lymphatic systems; revitalizes the skin.

Myrrh—is soothing to the skin; used for chapped and cracked skin and wrinkles.

Geranium—improves blood flow, regenerates tissue and nerves, cleans oily skin, and may even liven up pale skin.

Ylang Ylang—balances secretion of sebum (a waxy oil produced by the skin); energizing and uplifting.

Instructions: Apply directly to skin. Boswellia Wrinkle Creme is a collagen builder. Used daily, it will help minimize and prevent wrinkles. Put small amount in hand, emulsify, and apply to face and neck using upward strokes.

Body System(s) Affected: Skin.

CINNAMINT™ LIP BALM

Ingredients: Sweet almond oil, beeswax, MSM, wolfberry (*Lycium barbarum*) seed oil, essential oils (as shown below), hemp seed oil, orange wax, orange oil, tocopheryl palmitate (vitamin E), ascorbyl palmitate (vitamin A), ascorbic acid (vitamin C), and citric acid.

Essential Oils:

> **Peppermint**—enhances the effect of the other oils; cooling and soothing sensations; invigorates the skin and helps with nerve regeneration. It also enhances digestion and increases endurance.
> **Spearmint**—brings soothing relief to dry skin.
> **Cinnamon Bark**—is a powerful purifier and a powerful oxygenator; it enhances the action and the activity of the other oils while its warming action balances the cooling effect of the mint oils to bring comfortable relief to dry, chapped lips.

Instructions: To soften and moisturize lips, apply Cinnamint Lip Balm as often as needed.
Body System(s) Affected: Skin.

CLARADERM™

This product, packaged in a spray bottle, is a blend of essential oils that are most soothing and nourishing to the skin. Designed to be used topically on skin that is stressed before and after childbirth, these oils help to relieve skin irritation and itching, and may also improve skin elasticity.

Essential Oils:

> **Myrrh**—is soothing to the skin; used for chapped and cracked skin and wrinkles.
> *Melaleuca alternifolia*—tissue regenerative; helps promote the healing of wounds.
> **Lavender**—balancing and calming; works wherever there is a need; useful for any type of skin condition.
> **Frankincense**—is high in sesquiterpenes; helps deliver oxygen to the pineal and pituitary glands; improves hGH production; increases leukocyte production,
> **Roman Chamomile**—helps increase the regenerative ability of the skin; blood cleanser.
> **Helichrysum**—may help cleanse the blood and improve circulatory functions. It is anti-catarrhal in structure and nature.

Ingredients: Essential oils come in a base of fractionated coconut oil.
Suggested Use: Spray topically on location.
Body System(s) Affected: Skin

DENTAROME™/DENTAROME PLUS™ TOOTHPASTE

A revolutionary antimicrobial essential-oil-fortified toothpaste. It is an all-natural toothpaste that includes a highly antimicrobial blend of pure plant-derived essential oils. It contains no sugar, saccharine, sodium lauryl sulfate, or synthetic chemicals, colors, or preservatives of any kind. This formula was tested at Weber State University and found to have potent antimicrobial properties against a wide range of oral microbes including *streptococcus oralis, streptococcus pneumoniae, bramunella catarrhalis, and candida albicans*. Other studies confirm the plaque-fighting and antimicrobial attributes of the essential oils included in Dentarome and Dentarome Plus, including one study published in the International Journal of Food Microbiology that found the essential oils of thyme, clove, and cinnamon to exhibit antimicrobial effects. Another study listed peppermint as one of the most potent essential oils against plaque-causing elements. **The added thymol and eugenol in Dentarome Plus are derived from pure thyme (*Thymus vulgaris*) and clove (*Eugenia caryophyllata*) oils and enhance its antimicrobial potency**.

Ingredients:

Baking Soda—a mild abrasive and fast-acting cleansing agent.

Deionized Water—added for consistency.

Vegetable Glycerin—used as a moistener.

Xanthum Gum—a natural thickener.

Ionic Minerals—added as a nutritional supplement and together with the essential oil of wintergreen, help to strengthen teeth.

Thymol & Eugenol—added to Dentarome Plus for more powerful antiseptic and antimicrobial effects. Thymol is derived from thyme oil (*thymus vulgaris*) and eugenol is derived from clove oil (*eugenia caryophyllata*).

Stevioside—a natural, intensely sweet extract from a tropical plant native to South America.

Essential Oils:

Wintergreen—used here to help strengthen teeth. Also antimicrobial in nature.

Peppermint—used as a natural flavoring, breath-freshening agent.

Thieves—a proprietary blend of clove, lemon, cinnamon bark, *Eucalyptus radiata,* and rosemary essential oils which has been documented to be highly antibacterial and antimicrobial in nature.

DENTAROME ULTRA™ TOOTHPASTE

This product contains a revolutionary formula of all-natural, edible ingredients. Created to be gentle on teeth enamel, the calcium carbonate and zinc oxide in this toothpaste are substantially smaller in particle size than other popular commercial toothpastes. Add to that the germ and cavity fighting power of the essential oils and other ingredients, and this toothpaste is ultimate in dental care.

Ingredients: Calcium carbonate, essential oil concentrate containing peppermint essential oil, Thieves essential oil blend, zinc oxide, deionized water with papain, xylitol, vegetable glycerine, essential oil base (thymol from *Thymus vulgaris*, *Eucalyptus globulus*, and methyl salicylate from wintergreen), xanthum gum, zinc citrate, and stevioside.

Essential Oils:

Peppermint—used as a natural flavoring, breath-freshening agent.

Thieves—a proprietary blend of clove, lemon, cinnamon bark, *Eucalyptus radiata*, and rosemary essential oils which has been documented to be highly antibacterial and antimicrobial in nature.

Thyme—contains 46% thymol–one of the most potent antimicrobial substances known. It has been studied in Europe for its effects against bronchitis, laryngitis, and tonsillitis.

Eucalyptus—contains eucalyptol, also known as 1,8-cineol.

Wintergreen—used here to help strengthen teeth. Also antimicrobial in nature.

ESSENTIAL BEAUTY™ SERUMS

Since ancient times, essential oils have been used in numerous skin care treatments. Even in our modern cosmetic and skin care products, essential oils are utilized for their potent therapeutic benefits. However, these serums are unique in the cosmetic and skin care industries as they combine potent blends of pure essential oils that target specific skin care needs with a proprietary vegetable oil complex to nourish and protect the skin without overdrying or clogging the pores.

Ingredients: The following is a partial list of ingredients that are common between all three blends: Cocos nucifera (Coconut) oil, Simmondsia chinensis (Jojoba) oil, Persea gratissima (Avocado) oil (rich in vitamin E and lutein; lutein absorbs UV light to protect skin from sun damage), Rosa rubiginosa (Rosehip) seed oil (rich in omega-3 essential fats; improves texture and natural moisture balance), lecithin, tocopherol, and Lycium barbarum (Wolfberry) seed oil (protective and nourishing; rich in omega-3 and omega-6 essential fats; helps moisturize outer dermal layers). In addition to these ingredients are the specific essential oils listed under each blend.

How to Use: For best results, incorporate the use of the A·R·T skin care products in the following three steps.

Step 1: Thoroughly clean the skin with A·R·T Gentle Foaming Cleanser.

Step 2: Sweep the A·R·T Purifying Toner over the face with a cotton ball.

Step 3: Spot apply the desired Essential Beauty Serum to the problem areas on the face and neck regions before moisturizer, sun block, or makeup is applied. If preferred, add 3-5 drops of the serum to the A·R·T Day Activator or Night Reconstructor creams, mix well, and spread evenly over the face. Serums should be applied in the morning and again in the evening.

Body System(s) Affected: Skin.

Warning: For external use only. Store in a cool, dark place.

ESSENTIAL BEAUTY™ SERUM – ACNE-PRONE SKIN BLEND

This particular serum contains essential oils specifically blended together to help remove compacted keratin and sebum from pores and follicles that can contribute to breakouts. Then the unique vegetable oil complex, listed above in the common description under ingredients, creates a protective lipid layer that hydrates and moisturizes the skin. Some of the essential oils also remain to help provide continued antioxidant activity and cell protection.

Essential Oils:

Eucalyptus staigeriana—is anti-inflammatory, analgesic, and a powerful anti-spasmodic; it is soothing and relaxing to skin and muscles.

Melaleuca alternifolia—has powerful anti-inflammatory and antimicrobial effects; research has shown it to be very effective in combating acne.

Cedarwood—rejuvenating and refreshing; antiseptic and beneficial to the skin.

Manuka (*Leptospermum scoparium*)—is powerfully antimicrobial, and anti-fungal; studies show that it has more antioxidant activity than *Melaleuca alternifolia*; it relaxes the nerves, activates skin cells and helps to regenerate outer skin layers.

Thyme—contains 46% thymol–one of the most potently antimicrobial natural substances known; it is also anti-fungal and antiseptic; has been used medicinally in France for dermatitis, psoriasis, and candida.

ESSENTIAL BEAUTY™ SERUM – DRY SKIN BLEND

This particular serum contains essential oils specifically blended together to help remove compacted keratin and sebum from pores and follicles that can contribute to poor skin clarity. Then the unique vegetable oil complex, listed above in the common description under ingredients, creates a protective lipid layer that hydrates and moisturizes the skin. Some of the essential oils also remain to help provide continued antioxidant activity and cell protection.

Essential Oils:

Cedarwood—rejuvenating and refreshing; antiseptic and beneficial to the skin.
Blue Cypress (*Callitris intratropica*)—is an abundant source of sesquiterpenes.
Lavender—works wherever there is a need; useful for any type of skin condition.
Myrrh—is soothing to the skin; used for chapped and cracked skin and wrinkles.
Clove—is anti-bacterial, anti-fungal, anti-infectious, and a strong antiseptic
Sandalwood—revitalizes the skin; helps to repair DNA and reverse the signs of sun damage.

ESSENTIAL BEAUTY™ SERUM – OILY SKIN BLEND

This particular serum contains essential oils specifically blended together to help remove compacted keratin and sebum from pores and follicles that can contribute to excessive oil. Then the unique vegetable oil complex, listed above in the common description under ingredients, creates a protective lipid layer that hydrates and moisturizes the skin. Some of the essential oils also remain to help provide continued antioxidant activity and cell protection.

Essential Oils:

Orange—contains over 91% d-limonene (which helps to promote normal cell life cycles); rich in stress-reducing compounds.
Spearmint—is antiseptic and antispasmodic; it is soothing and relaxing to skin, nerves, and muscle tissue.
Davana—is anti-bacterial and anti-fungal; it is soothing and relaxing to skin and nerves.
Pink Pepper (*Schinus molle*)—is anti-bacterial, anti-fungal (especially against candida), anti-microbial, anti-viral, and recent research has shown it to have anti-cancer and anti-tumor properties; further research studies have demonstrated its pain-relieving, anti-spasmodic, and anti-inflammatory properties.
Nutmeg—is anti-inflammatory, antiseptic, and a circulatory stimulant; it is soothing and relaxing to skin, nerves, and muscles.

FRESH ESSENCE PLUS™ MOUTHWASH

The ultimate oral rinse, formulated with antimicrobial therapeutic-grade essential oils that naturally contain compounds which have been clinically proven to kill microbes that can cause bad breath, plaque, and periodontal diseases like gingivitis. It is formulated with a patented liposome technology (using soy-derived lecithin), which binds the essential oils to the mucus membrane inside the mouth to provide long-lasting germ-killing and breath-freshening protection. As an all-natural mouth and gum care product, Fresh Essence Plus Mouthwash contains absolutely **no dyes, no alcohol, no saccharin, and no synthetic flavors or preservatives**.

Unlike some commercially available products which contain just the active constituents of eucalyptol and menthol, Fresh Essence Plus Mouthwash uses the entire essential oil. The complete oil exhibits far stronger antimicrobial power than its active constituents alone. From his research on the essential oil of eucalyptus, Jean Valnet, M.D. made the following statement. "The antiseptic properties of the essences of eucalyptus were much more powerful than those of its principle constituent, eucalyptol." The whole oil is also safer because it contains a natural balance of elements that make it relatively harmless to human tissue.

Essential Oils:
> **Peppermint**—contains natural menthol.
> **Thieves**—is a proprietary blend of clove, lemon, cinnamon bark, *Eucalyptus radiata*, and rosemary essential oils which has been documented to be highly antibacterial and antimicrobial in nature.
> **Spearmint**—used as a natural flavoring, breath-freshening agent.
> **Vetiver**—is high in sesquiterpenes; fixative; helps stabilize essential oils.

Ingredients: Other ingredients include deionized water, peppermint floral water, melissa floral water, colloidal silver, lecithin, polysorbate 80, steviocide (a naturally sweet plant extract), and tocopherol (vitamin E).

Instructions: Rinse mouth with one tablespoon or capful of Fresh Essence Plus for 30-60 seconds or as needed. Store at room temperature.

GENESIS™ HAND & BODY LOTION

The essential oils in this product are beneficial for feeding, nurturing, and hydrating the skin. Excellent for rough, dry skin, wrinkles, and premature aging.

Ingredients: Deionized water, MSM, glyceryl stearate, stearic acid, glycerin, grapeseed extract, sodium hyaluronate, sorbitol, rosehip seed oil, shea butter, mango butter, wheat germ oil, kukui nut oil, lecithin, safflower oil, apricot oil, almond oil, tocopheryl acetate (vitamin E), retinyl palmitate (vitamin A), jojoba oil, sesame oil, calendula extract, orange blossom extract, St. John's wort extract, algae extract, aloe vera gel, ascorbic acid (vitamin C), ginkgo biloba extract, essential oils (as shown below), and honeysuckle and gardenia fragrance oils.

Essential Oils:

>**Bergamot**—helps to relieve anxiety, stress, and tension; helps to balance the hormones.

>**Geranium**—can be used on almost any kind of skin; cleansing, refreshing, astringent, and a mild skin tonic; used to balance hyposecretion of androgens or estrogens which frequently occurs during menopause.

>**Jasmine**—deeply penetrating effect on the skin; produces a feeling of confidence, energy, euphoria, and optimism.

>**Lemon**—helps promote leukocyte formation; antiseptic.

>**Palmarosa**—stimulates new cell growth, regulates oil production, moisturizes and speeds healing.

>**Roman Chamomile**—helps increase the regenerative ability of the skin; blood cleanser.

>**Rosewood**—antiseptic and antibacterial; tissue regenerative; soothing to the skin and increases elasticity.

>**Ylang Ylang**—stimulating; helps to balance male-female energies. May also contain patchouli.

Instructions: Dispense in hand and apply directly to skin.

Body System(s) Affected: Skin.

Warning: Avoid eye contact. If contact occurs, rinse thoroughly with water.

KIDSCENTS® LOTION

An extraordinarily gentle and safe lotion with the ideal pH for moisturizing, softening, and protecting young skin. It contains all natural ingredients and therapeutic-grade essential oils with no mineral oils, synthetic perfumes, artificial colorings, or toxic ingredients.

Ingredients: Deionized water, methylsulfonylmethane (MSM), glyceryl stearate, stearic acid, glycerin, grape (*Vitis vinifera*) seed extract, sodium hyaluronate, sorbitol, rose hip (*Rosa rubiginosa*) seed oil, shea butter, mango (*Mangifera indica*) butter, wheat germ oil, kukui (*Aleurites moluccana*) nut oil, lecithin, safflower (*Carthamus tinctorius*) oil, apricot (*Prunus armeniaca*) kernal oil, almond (*Prunus amygdalus dulcis*) oil, tocopheryl acetate (vitamin E), retinyl palmitate (vitamin A), jojoba (*Buxus chinensis*) oil, sesame (*Sesamum indicum*) oil, *Calendula officinalis* extract, chamomile (*Anthemis nobilis*) extract, orange (*Citrus aurantium dulcis*) blossom extract, St. John's Wort (*Hypericum perforatum*) extract, algae (*Gellidiela acerosa*) extract, aloe vera (*Aloe barbadensis*) gel, ascorbic acid (vitamin C), *Ginkgo biloba* extract, and pure therapeutic-grade essential oils (as listed below).

Essential Oils:

>**Cedarwood**—rejuvenating and refreshing; antiseptic and beneficial to the skin.

>**Western Red Cedar**—anti-bacterial; antiseptic; calming.

>**Rosewood**—antiseptic and antibacterial; tissue regenerative; soothing to the skin and increases elasticity.

>**Geranium**—improves blood flow, regenerates tissue and nerves, cleans oily skin, and may even liven up pale skin.

Instructions: Apply KidScents Lotion liberally to the skin.

Common Sense Caution: While KidScents products contain no harmful ingredients, store out of reach of children to prevent messy spills. Children do not like lotion in their mouth or eyes. Use with gentle care.

KidScents® Shampoo

This shampoo contains the finest natural ingredients for gently cleansing young, delicate hair. It is perfectly pH-balanced and contains all natural ingredients and therapeutic-grade essential oils with no mineral oils, synthetic perfumes, artificial colorings, or toxic ingredients.

Ingredients: Deionized water, decylpolyglucose, methylsulfonylmethane (MSM), aloe vera (*Aloe barbadensis*) gel, pure therapeutic-grade essential oils (as listed below), panthenol, tocopheryl acetate (vitamin E), chamomile (*Anthemis nobilis*) extract, purple coneflower (*Echinacea purpurea*) extract, kukui (*Aleurites moluccana*) nut oil, jojoba (*Buxus chinensis*) oil, citrus seed extract, babassu (*Orbignya oleifera*) oil, grape (*Vitis vinifera*) seed extract, dimethicone copolyol meadowfoamate, hyaluronic acid, wheat germ oil, keratin, linoleic acid, and linolenic acid.

Essential Oils:
Tangerine—calming to the nervous system; also a decongestant of the lymphatic system.
Lemon—promotes leukocyte formation; helps remove the dead skin cells.
Blue Tansy—helps cleanse the liver and promote a feeling of self-control.

Instructions: Apply a small amount of KidScents Shampoo to the hair. Lather, then rinse.

Common Sense Caution: While KidScents products contain no harmful ingredients, store out of reach of children to prevent messy spills. Children do not like shampoo in their mouth or eyes. Use with gentle care.

KidScents® Tender Tush™

This product is a mild, soothing, and gentle ointment designed to protect and nourish young skin and promote healing. It contains all natural ingredients and therapeutic-grade essential oils with no mineral oils, synthetic perfumes, artificial colorings, or toxic ingredients. It is particularly useful for diaper rash and other skin irritations.

Ingredients: Coconut (*Cocos nucifera*) oil, cocoa (*Theobroma cacao*) butter, bees wax, wheat germ oil, olive (*Olea europaea*) oil, almond (*Prunus amygdalus dulcis*) oil, and pure therapeutic-grade essential oils (as listed below).

Essential Oils:
Sandalwood—helps strengthen the lymphatic systems; revitalizes the skin.
Rosewood—antiseptic and antibacterial; tissue regenerative; soothing to the skin and increases elasticity.
Roman Chamomile—helps increase the regenerative ability of the skin; blood cleanser.

Lavender—balancing and calming; works wherever there is a need; useful for any type of skin condition.

Cistus—has anti-bacterial, anti-infectious, and anti-viral properties. Because it is high in oxygenating molecules, it may assist the auto-immune system and may help strengthen the immune system.

Blue Tansy—may help cleanse the liver and calm the lymphatic system to help rid one of anger and promote a feeling of self-control.

Frankincense—is anti-inflammatory; high in sesquiterpenes; helps deliver oxygen to the pineal and pituitary glands; improves hGH production; increases leukocyte production.

Instructions: Apply liberally to the skin on the bottom or wherever it is needed.

Common Sense Caution: While KidScents products contain no harmful ingredients, store out of reach of children to prevent messy spills. Children do not like ointments in their mouth or eyes. Use with gentle care.

Body System(s) Affected: Skin.

KIDSCENTS® TOOTHPASTE

This product is a completely safe and natural alternative to other commercial toothpastes. It is fluoride free and contains all natural ingredients and therapeutic-grade essential oils with no synthetic dyes or flavorings. It is safe to swallow with a great Bubble Gum flavor.

Ingredients: Calcium carbonate (tooth health agent), deionized water (consistency), colloidal silver (tooth health agent), strawberry flavor (natural flavor), vegetable glycerin (moistener), zinc oxide (tooth health agent), xanthum gum (natural thickener), ionic minerals (tooth and gum support), xylitol (tooth and gum support), stevioside (natural flavor), and pure therapeutic-grade essential oils (as listed below).

Essential Oils:

Peppermint—used as a natural flavoring, breath-freshening agent.

Spearmint—used as a natural flavoring, breath-freshening agent.

Orange—used as a natural flavor, it also contains over 91% d-limonene (which helps to promote normal cell life cycles); rich in stress-reducing compounds.

Lemon—used as a natural flavor, it also contains over 65% d-limonene (which helps to promote normal cell life cycles); helps promote leukocyte formation; helps to dissolve cholesterol and fats.

Thieves—is a proprietary blend of clove, lemon, cinnamon bark, *Eucalyptus radiata*, and rosemary essential oils which has been documented to be highly antibacterial and antimicrobial in nature.

Instructions: Brush teeth and gums thoroughly morning and night.

Common Sense Caution: While KidScents products contain no harmful ingredients, store out of reach of children to prevent messy spills. Use with gentle care.

LavaDerm™ Cooling Mist

This Cooling Mist provides wonderful relief to any type of burn, from the lightest sunburn to the most serious 3rd degree burn. It quickly cools and hydrates the skin and speeds healing and tissue regeneration.

Ingredients: Re-structured water, lavender floral water, aloe vera gel, and lavender essential oil.

Instructions: Mist directly on area of concern as often as needed to keep the skin cool and promote regeneration.

Body System(s) Affected: Emotional Balance, Skin.

Lavender Volume Conditioner™

This is a fabulous nourishing, volumizing rinse that utilizes vitamins, amino acids, MSM, and essential oils to support and feed fine hair.

Ingredients: Natural vegetable fatty acid base (saponified coconut oil), MSM, milk protein, phospholipids, amino acids cysteine (and) cysteine 8 methionine, glyco protein (glycogen and mucopolysaccharides), quinoa extract, rosemary extract, sage extract, horsetail extract, coltsfoot extract, hydrolyzed wheat protein, hydrolyzed soy protein, retinyl palmitate (vitamin A), ascorbic acid (vitamin C), tocopheryl acetate (vitamin E), panthenol (vitamin B5), grapeseed extract, and essential oils (as shown below).

Essential Oils:

Lavender—balancing and calming; works wherever there is a need; useful for any type of skin condition.

Clary Sage—astringent; good for cell regulation, cholesterol, and dry skin.

Lemon—helps promote leukocyte formation; antiseptic.

Jasmine—deeply penetrating effect on the skin; produces a feeling of confidence, energy, euphoria, and optimism.

Instructions: Apply Lavender Volume Conditioner through the hair. Leave on hair for a few seconds for light conditioning or for several minutes for deep conditioning. Rinse well. *For maximum benefit, leave on 2 to 5 minutes.*

Lavender Volume Shampoo™

As this shampoo is formulated for the gentle cleansing of fine hair, it makes an excellent shampoo for babies and children.

Ingredients: Coconut oil, decyl polyglucose, MSM, vegetable protein (wheat, oat, and soya), deionized water, nettle extract, mushroom extract, billberry extract, sugar cane extract, lemon extract, sugar maple extract, orange extract, essential oils (as shown below), aloe vera gel, retinyl palmitate (vitamin A), ascorbic acid (vitamin C), tocopheryl acetate (vitamin E), panthenol (vitamin B5), grapeseed extract, inositol, and niacin.

Personal Care Products

Essential Oils:

    Lavender—balancing and calming; works wherever there is a need; useful for any type of skin condition.

    Clary Sage—astringent; good for cell regulation, cholesterol, and dry skin.

    Lemon—helps promote leukocyte formation; antiseptic.

    Jasmine—deeply penetrating effect on the skin; produces a feeling of confidence, energy, euphoria, and optimism.

Instructions: Wet hair thoroughly. Apply small amount of Lavender Volume Shampoo. Massage thoroughly into hair and scalp. Rinse well. Repeat if desired. *For maximum benefit, leave on 2 to 5 minutes.*

LEMON SAGE CLARIFYING CONDITIONER™

This is a fabulous clarifying rinse that utilizes vitamins, amino acids, MSM, and essential oils to support and feed hair of all types without buildup.

Ingredients: Natural vegetable fatty acid base (saponified coconut oil), MSM, milk protein, phospholipids, Chenopodium quinoa extract, rosemary extract, sage extract, horsetail extract, coltsfoot extract, hydrolyzed wheat protein, hydrolyzed soy protein, retinyl palmitate (vitamin A), ascorbic acid (vitamin C), essential oils (as shown below), amino acids cysteine (and) cysteine 8 methionine, glyco protein (glycogen and mucopolysaccharides), grapeseed extract, tocopheryl acetate (vitamin E), and panthenol (vitamin B5).

Essential Oils:

    Lemon—helps promote leukocyte formation; antiseptic.

    Pine—was used by the American Indians to repel lice and flees; antimicrobial and anti-viral; may also be good against skin parasites.

    Lime—helps remove dead skin cells; tightens skin and connective tissue.

    Geranium—improves blood flow, regenerates tissue and nerves, cleans oily skin, and may even liven up pale skin.

    Roman Chamomile—helps increase the regenerative ability of the skin; blood cleanser.

    Ylang Ylang—has been used historically in hair preparations to promote thick, shiny, lustrous hair and to help control split ends.

    Sage—helps balance hormone levels; may also help with dandruff and hair loss.

Instructions: Apply Lemon Sage Clarifying Conditioner through the hair. Leave on hair for a few seconds for light conditioning or for several minutes for deep conditioning. Rinse well. *For maximum benefit, leave on 2 to 5 minutes.*

LEMON SAGE CLARIFYING SHAMPOO™

This shampoo is formulated with herbal extracts, vitamins, and essential oils to naturally remove buildup of styling products and return hair to its natural healthy shine.

Ingredients: Coconut oil, olive oil, decylpolyglucose, MSM, vegetable protein (wheat, oat, soya), deionized water, nettle extract, mushroom extract, billberry extract, sugar cane extract, lemon extract, sugar maple extract, orange extract, essential oils (as shown below), aloe vera gel, retinyl palmitate (vitamin A), ascorbic acid (vitamin C), tocopheryl acetate (vitamin E), panthenol (vitamin B5), grapeseed extract, inositol, and niacin.

Essential Oils:

Lemon—helps promote leukocyte formation; antiseptic.

Lime—helps remove dead skin cells; tightens skin and connective tissue.

Pine—was used by the American Indians to repel lice and flees; antimicrobial and anti-viral; may also be good against skin parasites.

Geranium—improves blood flow, regenerates tissue and nerves, cleans oily skin, and may even liven up pale skin.

Roman Chamomile—helps increase the regenerative ability of the skin; blood cleanser.

Ylang Ylang—has been used historically in hair preparations to promote thick, shiny, lustrous hair and to help control split ends.

Sage—helps balance hormone levels; may also help with dandruff and hair loss.

Instructions: Wet hair thoroughly. Apply small amount of Lemon Sage Clarifying Shampoo. Massage thoroughly into hair and scalp. Rinse well. Repeat if desired. *For maximum benefit, leave on 2 to 5 minutes.*

NEUROGEN™

Moisturizing Lotion

An excellent moisturizing lotion for deeper layers of the skin that can be damaged by excessive sun and wind exposure. By providing the proper nutrients to tissue layers beneath the surface of the skin, moisture and natural health is restored. Additionally, many of the ingredients and essential oils in this lotion contain properties that may help support and even regenerate damaged nerves.

Ingredients: Deionized water, pregnenolone, lecithin, MSM, essential oils (as shown below), caprylic/capric triglyceride, sorbitol, wolfberry seed oil, shea butter, glyceryl stearate, linseed oil, aloe barbadensis gel, sodium PCA, stearic acid, *Calendulla officinalis* extract, German chamomile extract, rosebud extract, orange flower extract, wild yam extract, algae extract, tocopheryl acetate (vitamin E), hydrolyzed wheat protein, locust bean gum, allantoin, natural progesterone (from soybean extract), kelp, retinyl palmitate (vitamin A), tocopheryl linoleate (vitamin E), and ascorbic acid (vitamin C).

Essential Oils:

Lemongrass—helps repair connective tissue; it helps stimulate the agents in the tissue to rejuvenate and reconnect; helps regulate the parasympathetic nervous system and strengthen vascular walls.

Peppermint—invigorating to the skin; soothing and relaxing to tired muscles; may also help with nerve regeneration. It also enhances digestion and increases endurance.

Personal Care Products

Douglas Fir—calming to tired and overworked joints; very soothing to sore muscles.

Juniper—antispasmodic; helps reduce muscle aches/pains; may also help nerve function and regeneration.

May also contain helichrysum, frankincense, and spearmint essential oils.

Body System(s) Affected: Hormonal and **Nervous Systems, Muscles and Bones**.

ORANGE BLOSSOM FACIAL WASH™

Ingredients: Deionized water, calendula extract, chamomile extract, rosebud extract, orange blossom extract, St. John's wort extract, algae, aloe vera gel, kelp extract, *Ginkgo biloba* extract, grapeseed extract, decyl polyglucose, MSM, wolfberry seed oil, essential oils (as shown below), multifruit acid complex, hydrolyzed wheat protein, citric acid, dimethyl lauramine oleate.

Essential Oils:

Lavender—balancing and calming; works wherever there is a need; useful for any type of skin condition.

Lemon—helps promote leukocyte formation; helps brighten a pale, dull complexion by removing the dead skin cells.

Rosemary verbenon—is milder than rosemary cineol and better suited for skin care.

Patchouli—helps digest toxic material; tones / tightens skin; helps prevent wrinkles.

Instructions: Apply warm water to the face to moisten skin. Apply wash directly to the face and gently massage in a gentle circular motion creating a lather. Rinse thoroughly and gently pat dry. For best results, use Orange Blossom Facial Wash twice daily. Follow up with Sandalwood Moisture Creme to promote younger and healthier looking skin.

Body System(s) Affected: Skin.

PRENOLONE™ /PRENOLONE+™

Moisturizing Cream

This cream utilizes natural pregnenolone (called the "Master Hormone" because it is a precursor to all the other hormones produced within the body including progesterone, estrogen, and testosterone) and a small amount of natural progesterone (derived from soy) to replenish and soften dry or irritated skin. With the help of the essential oils that are included in this formulation, the pregnenolone is quickly and efficiently transferred to the cellular level where it can be converted into the appropriate hormone that the body needs at that particular time. Unlike many natural progesterone creams, there is not the need to regulate the use of this cream as the body can eliminate what is not needed without any side effects. Also, unlike other natural hormone creams, this one can also be used by men. Similar natural hormone creams have been found to help with the following: wrinkles, libido (restores), blood sugar levels (normalizes), cell oxygen levels (restores), bone density (improves), weight control (helps use fat for energy), zinc and copper levels (normalizes), blood clotting (normalizes), thyroid action, breast cancer and fibroids (protects against), headaches, asthma, backaches, infertility, hair loss, depression, hypoglycemia, inflammation, exhaustion, insomnia, arthritis, and more. **The regular Prenolone contains all the same ingredients as Prenolone+ without the addition of DHEA.**

Ingredients: Deionized water, MSM, caprylic/capric triglyceride, sorbitol, pregnenolone, lecithin, wolfberry seed oil, shea butter, glyceryl stearate, aloe vera gel, sodium PCA, stearic acid, calendula extract, chamomile extract, rosebud extract, orange blossom extract, St. John's wort extract, *Ginkgo biloba* extract, grapeseed extract, algae extract, tocopheryl acetate (vitamin E), hydrolyzed wheat protein, locust bean gum, ionic trace minerals, flax seed oil, vitamin E (from wheat germ oil), ylang ylang essential oil (see below), allantoin, wild yam, ginseng, Clary sage essential oil (see below), blue cohosh, black cohosh, kelp, retinyl palmitate (vitamin A), tocopheryl linoleate, essential oils of bergamot, fennel, geranium, sage, and yarrow (see below), DHEA (only in Prenolone+), progesterone, and ascorbic acid (vitamin C).

Essential Oils:

Geranium—can be used on almost any kind of skin; cleansing, refreshing, astringent, and a mild skin tonic; used to balance hyposecretion of androgens or estrogens which frequently occurs during menopause.

Ylang Ylang—stimulating and helps to balance male-female energies.

Clary Sage—helps balance the hormones; tonic to the reproductive system.

Bergamot—helps to relieve anxiety, stress, and tension; helps to balance the hormones.

Fennel—helps balance the hormones.

Sage—contains estriol and has estrogen-like properties; believed to contain elements that contribute to the secretion of progesterone.

Yarrow—anti-inflammatory; antiseptic; excellent for menstrual problems.

May also contain fleabane essential oil.

Instructions: Apply ¼ to ½ tsp. one to two times daily for 21 continuous days. Discontinue use for 7 days and repeat. Massage cream thoroughly into soft tissue areas of the body (inside thigh, stomach, breasts, etc.) until absorbed. Individual needs may vary.

Body System(s) Affected: Emotional Balance, Hormonal and **Nervous Systems, Muscles and Bones, Skin.**

Warning: Application is intended for external use. If pregnant or under a doctor's care, consult your physician. Keep in a cool, dry place. Do not expose to excessive heat. Keep out of the reach of children.

Companion Products: FemiGen (an herbal complex for supporting the female reproductive system), Dragon Time oil blend, Thyromin (for thyroid support).

PROGESSENCE™ CREAM

This cream contains natural progesterone (derived from soy), MSM, and wolfberry oil to moisturize and nourish dry skin. With the help of the essential oils that are included in this formulation, the progesterone is quickly and efficiently transferred to the cellular level where it can be utilized by the body. Natural hormone creams like this one have been found to help with the following: wrinkles, libido (restores), blood sugar levels (normalizes), cell oxygen levels (restores), bone density (improves), weight control (helps use fat for energy), zinc and copper levels (normalizes), blood clotting (normalizes), thyroid action, breast cancer and fibroids (protects against), headaches, asthma, backaches, infertility, hair loss, depression, hypoglycemia, inflammation, exhaustion, insomnia, arthritis, and more.

Ingredients: Deionized water, MSM, caprylic/capric triglyceride, sorbitol, wolfberry oil, shea butter, glyceryl stearate, aloe vera gel, sodium PCA, stearic acid, calendula extract, chamomile extract, rosebud extract, orange blossom, St. John's wort extract, *Ginkgo biloba* extract, grapeseed extract, algae extract, tocopheryl acetate (vitamin E), hydrolyzed wheat protein, locus bean gum, allantoin, lecithin, kelp, retinyl palmitate (vitamin A), tocopheryl linoleate, ascorbic acid (vitamin C), progesterone (from soybean extract), eleuthero (*Eleuthero coccus senticosus*), trace minerals complex, ylang ylang essential oil (see below), Clary sage essential oil (see below), Canadian fleabane essential oil (see below), flax seed oil, wheat germ oil, wild yam extract, black cohosh, blue cohosh, and the essential oils of geranium, fennel, yarrow, and sage (see below).

Essential Oils:

Ylang Ylang—stimulating and helps to balance male-female energies.

Clary Sage—helps balance the hormones; tonic to the reproductive system.

Canadian Fleabane—is a rare essential oil studied for its ability to stimulate the pancreas and liver and counteract retarded puberty. It is a mood enhancer and promoter of hGH.

Geranium—can be used on almost any kind of skin; cleansing, refreshing, astringent, and a mild skin tonic; used to balance hyposecretion of androgens or estrogens which frequently occurs during menopause.

Fennel—helps balance the hormones.

Yarrow—anti-inflammatory; antiseptic; excellent for menstrual problems.

Sage—contains estriol and has estrogen-like properties; believed to contain elements that contribute to the secretion of progesterone.

Instructions: Apply ¼ to ½ tsp. one to two times daily for 21 continuous days. Discontinue use for 7 days and repeat. Massage cream thoroughly into soft tissue areas of the body (inside thigh, stomach, etc.) until absorbed. Individual needs may vary.

Body System(s) Affected: Emotional Balance, Hormonal and **Nervous Systems, Muscles and Bones, Skin**.

Warning: Application is intended for external use. If pregnant or under a doctor's care, consult your physician. Keep in a cool, dry place. Do not expose to excessive heat. Keep out of the reach of children.

Companion Products: FemiGen (an herbal complex for supporting the female reproductive system), Dragon Time oil blend, Thyromin (for thyroid support).

PROTEC™

Designed for topical use only, it should never be taken orally. This formula was designed to accompany the night long retention enema. It helps buffer the prostate from inflammation, enlargement, and tumor activity. Also suitable for women as a night long retention douche.

Ingredients:
Olive Oil—moisturizing agent.
Grape Seed Oil—antioxidant; rich in bioflavonoids; helps maintain pH balance.
Sweet Almond Oil—nourishes the skin will reducing friction for smoother application.
Wheat Germ Oil—high in natural vitamins E and B and lecithin; natural antioxidant; useful for reducing scar tissue and stretch marks; acts as a preservative for the other base oils.
Vitamin E Oil—natural antioxidant; protects and promotes regeneration of the skin.

Essential Oils:
Frankincense—anti-tumoral and anti-inflammatory; good for prostate problems.
Myrrh—anti-inflammatory and antiseptic; helps to decongest the prostate gland.
Sage—contains estriol and has estrogen-like properties; may help improve estrogen and progesterone-testosterone balance.
Cumin—anti-bacterial; antispasmodic; some anti-tumoral properties.

Instructions: For the retention enema or douche, use ½ to 1 oz. and hold all night long for 21 consecutive nights. If irritation occurs, discontinue use for three days before restarting.

Body System(s) Affected: Hormonal System.

REGENOLONE™

Moisturizing Cream

This cream utilizes natural pregnenolone (called the "Master Hormone" because it is a precursor to all the other hormones produced within the body including progesterone, estrogen, and testosterone) and a small amount of natural progesterone (derived from soy) to replenish and soften dry or irritated skin. With the essential oils that are included, this product may be effective in promoting the regeneration of damaged nerves and tissues.

Ingredients: Deionized water, MSM, caprylic/capric triglyceride, sorbitol, wolfberry oil, shea butter, glyceryl stearate, aloe vera gel, sodium PCA, stearic acid, calendula extract, chamomile extract, rosebud extract, orange blossom extract, St. John's wort extract, *Gingko biloba* extract, grapeseed extract, algae extract, tocopheryl acetate (vitamin E), hydrolyzed wheat protein, locust bean gum, allantoin, lecithin, kelp, retinyl palmitate, tocopheryl linoleate, ascorbic acid (vitamin C), progesterone, pregnenolone, wild yam, ginseng, flax seed, trace minerals, vitamin E (from wheat germ), blue cohosh, and essential oils (as shown below).

Essential Oils:
Wintergreen—has a cortisone-like action that helps to reduce inflammation in the tissues; contains methyl salicylate.

Douglas Fir—calming to tired and overworked joints; very soothing to sore muscles.

Peppermint—invigorating to the skin; soothing and relaxing to tired muscles; may also help with nerve regeneration.

Oregano—powerful antimicrobial; anti-inflammatory; locally warming.

May also contain spearmint essential oil.

Instructions: Apply ⅛ to ¼ tsp. on location as needed. Individual needs may vary. May be best not to use more than 5 times a day.

Body System(s) Affected: Hormonal and **Nervous Systems, Muscles and Bones, Skin**.

Warning: Application is intended for external use. If pregnant or under a doctor's care, consult your physician. Keep in a cool, dry place. Do not expose to excessive heat. Keep out of the reach of children.

Companion Oils: Oregano, thyme, <u>Dragon Time</u>, <u>Mister</u>.

Companion Products: Prenolone/Prenolone+, Thyromin (for thyroid support).

ROSE OINTMENT™

Dramatically improves the effectiveness of other essential oils that are applied for skin conditions. When applied on top of oils such as <u>PanAway</u>, lavender, helichrysum, and <u>Melrose</u>, this product seals in the volatile constituents of the essential oil, increasing their effectiveness by prolonging their contact with the skin. It also helps maintain the natural pH balance of the skin, conserve its acid mantle, and balance the drying effect that some essential oils may have on the skin.

Ingredients: Lecithin (natural dispersing agent; used in place of sodium lauryl sulfate), lanolin (taken from sheep wool; excellent for skin care), beeswax (used as the thickening and stabilizing agent), mink oil (nurture and regenerate the skin), sesame seed oil (high in linoleic acid; maintains pH balance of the skin), vitamin E oil (antioxidant; excellent for the skin and the cells of the skin), rosehip seed oil (helps reduce scarring and premature aging), and essential oils (as shown below).

Essential Oils:

Carrot seed—a natural phytonutrient that is rich in beta carotene; helps to reduce wrinkles and dryness.

Melaleuca—tissue regenerative; helps promote the healing of wounds.

Myrrh—helps to heal chapped or cracked skin and reduce inflammation.

Palmarosa—stimulates new cell growth, regulates oil production, moisturizes and speeds healing.

Patchouli—for protection against UV radiation and for tissue regeneration; helps tighten loose skin and prevent wrinkles.

Rosewood—tissue regenerative; soothing to the skin and increases elasticity.

Rose otto—brings balance and harmony by enhancing the frequency of every cell.

Instructions: Apply directly to skin.

Body System(s) Affected: Skin.

ROSEWOOD MOISTURIZING CONDITIONER™

This is a fabulous nourishing, moisturizing rinse that utilizes vitamins, amino acids, MSM, and essential oils to support and feed dry hair.

Ingredients: Natural vegetable fatty acid base, MSM, milk protein, phospholipids, amino acids cysteine (and) cysteine 8 methionine, glyco protein (glycogen and mucopolysaccharides), quinoa extract, rosemary extract, sage extract, horsetail extract, coltsfoot extract, hydrolyzed wheat protein, hydrolyzed soy protein, retinyl palmitate (vitamin A), ascorbic acid (vitamin C), tocopheryl acetate (vitamin E), panthenol (vitamin B5), grapeseed extract, and essential oils (as shown below).

Essential Oils:

Bergamot—may help with oily complexion, eczema, and psoriasis. It calms the emotions to helps relieve anxiety, stress, and tension.

Wintergreen—has a cortisone-like action that helps to reduce inflammation in the tissues.

Geranium—improves blood flow, regenerates tissue and nerves, cleans oily skin, and may even liven up pale skin.

Sandalwood—helps strengthen the lymphatic systems; revitalizes the skin.

Clary Sage—astringent; good for cell regulation, cholesterol, and dry skin.

Rosewood—skin cell regenerative; soothing to the skin and promotes elasticity; appeasing to the mind and relaxing to the body.

Instructions: Apply Rosewood Moisturizing Conditioner through the hair. Leave on hair for a few seconds for light conditioning or for several minutes for deep conditioning. Rinse well. *For maximum benefit, leave on 2 to 5 minutes.*

ROSEWOOD MOISTURIZING SHAMPOO™

This shampoo is formulated for the gentle cleansing of dry hair while nourishing and moisturizing it with herbal extracts, vitamins, and essential oils.

Ingredients: Coconut oil, olive oil, decyl polyglucose, MSM, vegetable protein (wheat, soya, and/or oat), deionized water, nettle extract, mushroom extract (*Grandoderma lucidum* and *Trametes veriscolor*), billberry extract, sugar cane extract, lemon extract, sugar maple extract, orange extract, essential oils (as shown below), aloe vera gel, retinyl palmitate (vitamin A), ascorbic acid (vitamin C), grapeseed extract, inositol, and niacin.

Essential Oils:

Bergamot—may help with oily complexion, eczema, and psoriasis. It calms the emotions to helps relieve anxiety, stress, and tension.

Wintergreen—has a cortisone-like action that helps to reduce inflammation in the tissues

Geranium—improves blood flow, regenerates tissue and nerves, cleans oily skin, and may even liven up pale skin.

Sandalwood—helps strengthen the lymphatic systems; revitalizes the skin.

Clary Sage—astringent; good for cell regulation, cholesterol, and dry skin.

Rosewood—skin cell regenerative; soothing to the skin and promotes elasticity; appeasing to the mind and relaxing to the body.

Instructions: Wet hair thoroughly. Apply small amount of Rosewood Moisturizing Shampoo. Massage thoroughly into hair and scalp. Rinse well. Repeat if desired. *For maximum benefit, leave on 2 to 5 minutes.*

SANDALWOOD MOISTURE CREME™

Ingredients: Deionized water, calendula extract, chamomile extract, rosebud extract, orange blossom extract, St. John's wort extract, aloe vera gel, kelp, *Ginkgo biloba* extract, grapeseed extract, caprylic/capric triglyceride, sorbitol, shea butter, goat's cream, glyceryl stearate, essential oils (as shown below), wolfberry seed oil, rosehip seed oil, sodium PCA, algae extract, stearic acid, allantoin, lecithin, retinyl palmitate (vitamin A), tocopheryl acetate (vitamin E), ascorbic acid (vitamin C), locust bean gum, hydrolyzed wheat protein, sodium hyaluronate, and tocopheryl linoleate.

Essential Oils:

Myrrh—is soothing to the skin; used for chapped and cracked skin and wrinkles.

Sandalwood—helps strengthen the lymphatic systems; revitalizes the skin.

Rosewood—skin cell regenerative; soothing to the skin and promotes elasticity; appeasing to the mind and relaxing to the body.

Lavender—balancing and calming; works wherever there is a need; useful for any type of skin condition.

Rosemary verbenon—is milder than rosemary cineol and better suited for skin care.

Instructions: For best results, use Sandalwood Moisture Creme after cleansing and toning the face and neck to promote younger, healthier skin. Put small amount in hand, emulsify, and apply to face and neck using upward strokes.

Body System(s) Affected: Skin.

SATIN FACIAL SCRUB™ (MINT)

As a gentle exfoliating scrub designed for **normal skin**, Mint Satin Facial Scrub gently eliminates layers of dead skin cells with a revolutionary formula of jojoba beads and other natural ingredients. It can be used as a drying face mask to draw impurities from the skin. Peppermint essential oil is added to soothe and refresh the skin.

Ingredients: Deionized water, glycerin, caprylic/capric triglyceride, jojoba (*Buxus chinensis*) wax beads, methylsulfonylmethane (MSM), sorbitol, glyceryl stearate, peppermint (*Mentha piperita*) oil, aloe vera (*Aloe barbadensis*) gel, stearic acid, algae (*Gellidiela acerosa*) extract, rosemary (*Rosmarinus officinalis*) extract, chamomile (*Anthemis nobilis*) extract, tocopheryl acetate (vitamin E), retinyl palmitate (vitamin A), sodium PCA, shea butter, grape (*Vitis vinifera*) seed extract, titanium dioxide, mango (*Mangifera indica*) butter, ascorbic acid (vitamin C), sodium hyaluronate, tocopheryl linoleate, allantoin, hydrolyzed wheat protein, and hydrolyzed soy protein.

Essential Oils:

>**Peppermint**—is invigorating to the skin; may also help with nerve regeneration.

Instructions: Apply warm water to the face to moisten the skin. Apply scrub directly to the face and gently massage in a gentle circular motion, creating a lather. Rinse thoroughly and gently pat dry. May also be mixed with Orange Blossom Facial Wash for a milder scrub. Mix ½ tsp. of both in palm of hand before applying. Use four or five times weekly, depending on need.

Body System(s) Affected: Skin.

SATIN™ HAND & BODY LOTION

Ingredients: Deionized water, MSM, glyceryl stearate (vegetable based), stearic acid, glycerin, goat's cream, sorbitol, wolfberry seed oil, essential oils (as shown below), safflower oil, apricot oil, almond oil, jojoba oil, sesame oil, calendula extract, chamomile extract, orange blossom extract, St. John's wort extract, algae extract, aloe vera gel, *Ginkgo biloba* extract, grapeseed extract, tocopheryl acetate (vitamin E), retinyl palmitate (vitamin A), ascorbic acid (vitamin C), and sodium hyaluronate.

Essential Oils:

>**Geranium**—improves blood flow, regenerates tissue and nerves, cleans oily skin, and may even liven up pale skin.

>**Rosewood**—skin cell regenerative; soothing to the skin and promotes elasticity; appeasing to the mind and relaxing to the body.

>**Ylang Ylang**—balances secretion of sebum (a waxy oil produced by the skin); energizing and uplifting.

>**Jasmine**—deeply penetrating effect on the skin; produces a feeling of confidence, energy, euphoria, and optimism.

>**Sandalwood**—helps strengthen the lymphatic systems; revitalizes the skin.

>**Peppermint**—enhances the effect of the other oils; cooling and soothing sensations; invigorates the skin and helps with nerve regeneration.

>**Roman Chamomile**—helps increase the regenerative ability of the skin; blood cleanser.

>*Melaleuca alternifolia*—tissue regenerative; helps promote the healing of wounds.

Instructions: To moisturize the skin, promote healing, and leave the skin feeling soft, silky and smooth, apply Satin Hand & Body Lotion to hands, body, and feet. Also good for scars, burns, rashes, itching, and sunburns.

Body System(s) Affected: Skin.

SENSATION™ HAND & BODY LOTION

Ingredients: Deionized water, cocoa butter, glyceryl stearate, cetyl alcohol, lanolin oil, floral water, vitamin E, and essential oils (as shown below).

Essential Oils:

>**Rosewood**—antiseptic and antibacterial; tissue regenerative; soothing to the skin and increases elasticity.

Ylang Ylang—stimulating and helps to balance male-female energies.

Jasmine—deeply penetrating effect on the skin; produces a feeling of confidence, energy, euphoria, and optimism.

Instructions: Dispense in hand and apply directly to skin.

Warning: Avoid eye contact. If contact occurs, rinse thoroughly with water. For external use only. Keep out of reach of children.

THIEVES® CLEANING PRODUCTS

These new antiseptic products utilize the documented bacteria killing power of the <u>Thieves</u> oil blend. Throw away those chemical-laden cleaning products and fight those germs with these powerful, natural products.

Ingredients:

Thieves® Household Cleaner: Proprietary suspension base of safe surfactants (wetting agents) and <u>Thieves</u> essential oil blend.

Thieves® Spray: Pure grain alcohol, deionized water, <u>Thieves</u> essential oil blend, coconut oil, and soy lecithin.

Thieves® Wipes: Pure grain alcohol, deionized water, <u>Thieves</u> essential oil blend, coconut oil and soy lecithin.

Suggested Use: Follow label directions.

Body System(s) Affected: Immune System.

Precautions: Keep out of reach of children. Not recommended for use on infants or sensitive areas of the body.

THIEVES® LOZENGES

Freshen your breath and soothe the sore throat, while fighting bacteria with these natural lozenges. This all natural lozenge is made from natural ingredients including the sweeteners of sorbitol (derived from fruit and shown not to contribute to tooth decay) and xylitol (shown to inhibit plaque growth). The essential oils of lemon, orange and peppermint provide natural flavoring and germ fighting ability, especially when combined with the essential oil blend of <u>Thieves</u>.

Ingredients:

Soft Lozenges: Xylitol, sorbitol, orange essential oil (*Citrus aurantium*), the essential oil blend of Thieves® (a blend of clove, lemon, cinnamon, *Eucalyptus radiata*, and rosemary), peppermint essential oil (*Mentha piperita*), cellulose, silicon dioxide, magnesium silicate, and vegetable-grade lubricant (sugar cane and palm oil).

Hard Lozenges: Maltitol, lemon essential oil (*Citrus limon*), Thieves® (a blend of clove, lemon, cinnamon, *Eucalyptus radiata*, and rosemary), peppermint essential oil (*Mentha piperita*), pectin, stevioside (*Stevia rebaudiana*).

Suggested Use: Dissolve 1 lozenge in mouth as needed.
Body System(s) Affected: Immune System and **Oral Hygiene**.
Precautions: Keep out of reach of children. Swallowing lozenges whole may cause choking.

WOLFBERRY EYE CREME™

Ingredients: Deionized water, aloe vera gel, caprylic/capric triglyceride, MSM, sorbitol, glycerin, glyceryl stearate, goat's cream, avocado oil, shea butter, kukui nut oil, rosehip seed oil, essential oils (as shown below), wolfberry seed oil, hydrocotyl extract, coneflower extract, sodium PCA, lecithin, dipalmitoyl hydroxyproline, phenoxyethanol, beta-sitosterol, linoleic acid, tocopheryl, sodium ascorbate, mannitol, almond oil, jojoba oil, mango butter, sodium hyaluronate, cucumber extract, green tea extract, tocopherol acetate, tocopherol palmitate (vitamin E), ascorbyl palmitate (vitamin A), ascorbic acid (vitamin C), citric acid, soy protein, wheat protein, allantoin, witch hazel extract, and horse chestnut extract.

Essential Oils:

Lavender—balancing and calming; works wherever there is a need; useful for any type of skin condition.

Rosewood—skin cell regenerative; soothing to the skin and promotes elasticity; appeasing to the mind and relaxing to the body.

Roman Chamomile—helps increase the regenerative ability of the skin; blood cleanser.

Frankincense—is high in sesquiterpenes; helps deliver oxygen to the pineal and pituitary glands; improves hGH production; increases leukocyte production.

Geranium—improves blood flow, regenerates tissue and nerves, cleans oily skin, and may even liven up pale skin.

Instructions: Apply a tiny amount of Wolfberry Eye Creme under eye area and on the eyelid before bed. Repeat in morning if desired.

Personal
Care
Products

Bath and Shower Gels

All of the following bath and shower products (gels and bar soaps) have a base that is from a unique, proprietary soap-making process. This base contains saponified oils of palm, coconut, and/or olive. Saponification is a process by which sodium hydroxide is combined with the fatty acids from the palm, coconut, and olive oils to create a soap. By altering the amounts of the different oils, different textures of this soap base are produced. It is the same process which yields the soap bases for both the bath & shower gels and the bar soaps that follow, with only slight modifications in the formulation of the soap base. The wonderful thing about this process is that the resulting soap is vegetable-based with more than 50 percent moisturizers. Add to that liquid aloe vera extract for added moisturizing effect and rosemary extract for its antioxidant properties and you have a soap that doesn't just clean but nourishes the skin. These product names are all trademarks of Young Living Essential Oils and although these product names appear throughout other sections of this book without the trademark symbol, they still refer to these same trademarked products.

AQUA ESSENCE™

Aqua Essence bath packets utilize hydro-diffusion technology to slowly and efficiently diffuse essential oils into shower or bath water.

How to Use: Just place any number of packets into your bath while filling it with warm water. After a short time, the oils begin to diffuse into the bath water. The packets can also be placed on the soap tray in the shower where the warm moist air will pick up the aroma of the oils being diffused to create the soothing and rejuvenating experience desired.

Joy—brings back memories of being loved, being held, and sharing loving times. It is uplifting and inspiring as it brings joy to the heart. The single oils contained in this blend include lemon, mandarin, bergamot, ylang ylang, rose, rosewood, geranium, palmarosa, Roman chamomile, and jasmine.

Peace & Calming—is exquisitely relaxing to the senses. It is extremely useful at the end of a stressful day to promote relaxation and peace and to help relieve insomnia. The single oils contained in this blend include tangerine, orange, ylang ylang, patchouli, and Blue tansy.

Sacred Mountain—helps to create a feeling of protection, empowerment, and grounding. It is soothing to the respiratory system and may help one find security and sacredness within oneself. The single oils contained in this blend include spruce, ylang ylang, Balsam fir, and cedarwood.

Valor—is emotionally uplifting and helps to empower the physical and spiritual bodies. It helps to build courage, confidence, and self-esteem while promoting calmness, peace, and relaxation. The single oils contained in this blend include spruce, rosewood, Blue tansy, and frankincense.

BATH GEL BASE

Add your favorite oils to create your own fragrance or therapeutic action.

Ingredients: Saponified oils of coconut and olive, guar gum, aloe vera, rosemary extract, and glycerin.

DRAGON TIME™

For the relief of those monthly aches and pains.

Ingredients: Saponified oils of coconut and olive, guar gum, aloe vera, rosemary extract, and glycerin.

Essential Oils:

Bergamot—sedative; helps to relieve anxiety, stress, and tension.

Clary Sage—helps balance the hormones; tonic to the reproductive system.

Geranium—helps balance the hormones; tissue and nerve regenerative.

Jasmine—deeply penetrating effect on the skin; produces a feeling of confidence, energy, euphoria, and optimism.

Lemon—helps promote leukocyte formation; helps brighten a pale, dull complexion by removing the dead skin cells.

Palmarosa—stimulates new cell growth, regulates oil production, moisturizes and speeds healing.

Roman Chamomile—helps increase the regenerative ability of the skin; blood cleanser.

Rosewood—antiseptic and antibacterial; tissue regenerative; soothing to the skin and increases elasticity.

Lavender—helps balance body systems.

Blue Tansy—calms the lymphatic system; promotes a feeling of self-control.

Mandarin—good for skin problems, stretch marks, nervous tension, and restlessness.

Sage—contains estriol and has estrogen-like properties; believed to contain elements that contribute to the secretion of progesterone.

Fennel—helps balance the hormones.

Ylang Ylang—stimulating and helps to balance male-female energies.

Body System(s) Affected: Emotional Balance, Hormonal System, Skin.

Bath Gels
and
Bar Soaps

EVENING PEACE™

Perfect for that evening bath or shower, to help you relax after a very stressful day.

Ingredients: Saponified oils of coconut and olive, guar gum, aloe vera, rosemary extract, and glycerin.

Essential Oils:

Bergamot—sedative; helps to relieve anxiety, stress, and tension.

Roman Chamomile—calming and relaxing; helps increase the regenerative ability of the skin; blood cleanser.

Clary Sage—helps balance the hormones; tonic to the reproductive system.

Geranium—helps balance the hormones; tissue and nerve regenerative.

Jasmine—deeply penetrating effect on the skin; produces a feeling of confidence, energy, euphoria, and optimism.

Lemon—helps promote leukocyte formation; helps brighten a pale, dull complexion by removing the dead skin cells.

Palmarosa—stimulates new cell growth, regulates oil production, moisturizes and speeds healing.

Rosewood—antiseptic and antibacterial; tissue regenerative; soothing to the skin and increases elasticity.

Blue Tansy—calms the lymphatic system; promotes a feeling of self-control.

Sandalwood—helps strengthen the lymphatic systems; revitalizes the skin.

Ylang Ylang—stimulating and helps to balance male-female energies.

Body System(s) Affected: Emotional Balance, Skin.

KIDSCENTS® BATH GEL

A shower gel with a neutral pH, perfect for young skin. It is gentle, mild, and safe. It contains all natural ingredients and therapeutic-grade essential oils with no mineral oils, synthetic perfumes, artificial colorings, or toxic ingredients.

Ingredients: Deionized water, decylpolyglucose, glycerin, sorbitol, methylsulfonylmethane (MSM), aloe vera (*Aloe barbadensis*) gel, pure therapeutic-grade essential oils (as listed below), panthenol, tocopheryl acetate (vitamin E), chamomile (*Anthemis nobilis*) extract, PG-hydroxyethylcellulose cocodimonium chloride, purple coneflower (*Echinacea purpurea*) extract, kukui (*Aleurites moluccana*) nut oil, jojoba (*Buxus chinensis*) oil, citrus seed extract, babassu oil, grape seed (*Vitis vinifera*) extract, dimethicone copolyol meadowfoamate, soap bark extract, soapwort extract, hyaluronic acid, wheat germ oil, keratin, linoleic acid, and linolenic acid.

Essential Oils:

Cedarwood—rejuvenating and refreshing; antiseptic and beneficial to the skin; astringent; diuretic; helps reduce oily secretions.

Geranium—can be used on almost any kind of skin; cleansing, refreshing, astringent, and a mild skin tonic.

Instructions: Apply a small amount of KidScents Bath Gel to a washcloth or directly to the skin. Rub gently, then rinse.

Common Sense Caution: While KidScents products contain no harmful ingredients, store out of reach of children to prevent messy spills. Children do not like soap in their mouth or eyes. Use with gentle care.

MORNING START™

For an invigorating bath or shower, to physically and emotionally prepare you for another hectic day. Due to the deep penetrating, cleansing action of the oils in this product, Morning Start may actually help dissolve and wash away oil and grease from the skin.

Ingredients: Saponified oils of coconut and olive, guar gum, aloe vera, rosemary extract, and glycerin.

Essential Oils:
Lemongrass—helps stimulate the agents in the tissue to rejuvenate and reconnect.
Rosemary cineol—highly anti-infectious; good for various skin conditions.
Juniper—evokes feelings of health and peace and elevates one's spiritual awareness
Peppermint—is invigorating to the skin; may also help with nerve regeneration.

Body System(s) Affected: Emotional Balance, Skin.

SENSATION™

The sensual fragrance of this bath gel is a wonderful addition to those romantic evenings.

Ingredients: Saponified oils of coconut and olive, guar gum, aloe vera, rosemary extract, and glycerin.

Essential Oils:
Rosewood—antiseptic and antibacterial; tissue regenerative; soothing to the skin and increases elasticity.
Ylang Ylang—stimulating and helps to balance male-female energies.
Jasmine—deeply penetrating effect on the skin; produces a feeling of confidence, energy, euphoria, and optimism.

Body System(s) Affected: Emotional Balance, Hormonal System, Skin.

Bath Gels
and
Bar Soaps

Bar Soaps

These product names are all trademarks of Young Living Essential Oils and although these product names appear throughout other sections of this book without the trademark symbol, they still refer to these same trademarked products.

LAVENDER ROSEWOOD
MOISTURIZING SOAP™

Contains oils that nourish the skin while their fragrance is calming and relaxing.

Ingredients: Saponified oils of palm, coconut, wolfberry seed, and olive, therapeutic-grade essential oils (as listed below), liquid aloe vera extract (moisturizing agent), rosemary extract (antioxidant), and organic oatmeal (mild abrasive to stimulate pores).

Essential Oils:
>   **Lavender**—helps balance body systems.
>   **Rosewood**—antiseptic and antibacterial; tissue regenerative; soothing to the skin and increases elasticity.

LEMON SANDALWOOD
CLEANSING SOAP™

Contains oils that deep clean and revitalize the skin with an invigorating fragrance.

Ingredients: Saponified oils of palm, coconut, wolfberry seed, and olive, therapeutic-grade essential oils (as listed below), liquid aloe vera extract (moisturizing agent), rosemary extract (antioxidant), and organic oatmeal (mild abrasive to stimulate pores).

Essential Oils:
>   **Lemon**—helps promote leukocyte formation; helps brighten a pale, dull complexion by removing the dead skin cells.
>   **Sandalwood**—helps strengthen the lymphatic systems; revitalizes the skin.

MELALEUCA GERANIUM
MOISTURIZING SOAP™

Contains oils that are antiseptic and revitalizing to the skin with a calming fragrance.

Ingredients: Saponified oils of palm, coconut, wolfberry seed, and olive, therapeutic-grade essential oils (as listed below), liquid aloe vera extract (moisturizing agent), rosemary extract (antioxidant), and organic oatmeal (mild abrasive to stimulate pores).

Essential Oils:

Melaleuca—is anti-fungal, antiseptic, anti-bacterial; tissue regenerative.

Geranium—can be used on almost any kind of skin; cleansing, refreshing, astringent, and a mild skin tonic.

Melaleuca ericifolia—is very gentle and non-irritating to the skin; well suited for youth and others who may be more sensitive to the oils.

Vetiver—antispasmodic and locally warming; good for arthritis, muscular rheumatism, and sprains.

MORNING START
MOISTURIZING SOAP™

Patterned after the popular Bath and Shower Gel, this soap is uplifting and energizing.

Ingredients: Saponified oils of palm, coconut, wolfberry seed, and olive, therapeutic-grade essential oils (as listed below), liquid aloe vera extract (moisturizing agent), rosemary extract (antioxidant), and organic oatmeal (mild abrasive to stimulate pores).

Essential Oils:

Lemongrass—helps repair connective tissue; it helps stimulate the agents in the tissue to rejuvenate and reconnect; also good as an insect repellent.

Rosemary cineol—highly anti-infectious; anti-fungal and anti-bacterial; good for various skin conditions.

Peppermint—invigorating to the skin; may also help with nerve regeneration.

Juniper—evokes feelings of health, love, and peace and may help to elevate one's spiritual awareness.

PEPPERMINT CEDARWOOD
MOISTURIZING SOAP™

Contains oils that purify and invigorate the skin with a calming fragrance.

Ingredients: Saponified oils of palm, coconut, wolfberry seed, and olive, therapeutic-grade essential oils (as listed below), liquid aloe vera extract (moisturizing agent), rosemary extract (antioxidant), and organic oatmeal (mild abrasive to stimulate pores).

Essential Oils:

Peppermint—invigorates skin and enhances effects of cedarwood.

Cedarwood—rejuvenating and refreshing; antiseptic and beneficial to the skin.

Bath Gels and Bar Soaps

SACRED MOUNTAIN
MOISTURIZING SOAP™ FOR OILY SKIN

Contains extra abrasives to remove dead skin cells and oils that are antiseptic, purifying, and calming.

Ingredients: Saponified oils of palm, coconut, wolfberry seed, and olive, therapeutic-grade essential oils (as listed below), liquid aloe vera extract (moisturizing agent), rosemary extract (antioxidant), and organic oatmeal (mild abrasive to stimulate pores).

Essential Oils:

Spruce—helps to open and release emotional blocks.

Ylang Ylang—stimulating and helps to balance male-female energies.

Balsam Fir—antiseptic; helps create a feeling of grounding, anchoring, and empowerment.

Cedarwood—rejuvenating and refreshing; antiseptic and beneficial to the skin.

THIEVES®
CLEANSING SOAP™

Contains oils that are high in antiseptic properties.

Ingredients: Saponified oils of palm, coconut, wolfberry seed, and olive, therapeutic-grade essential oils (as listed below), liquid aloe vera extract (moisturizing agent), rosemary extract (antioxidant), and organic oatmeal (mild abrasive to stimulate pores).

Essential Oils:

Clove—is anti-bacterial, anti-fungal, anti-infectious, anti-parasitic, a strong antiseptic, anti-viral, and an immune stimulant. It may influence healing and help create a feeling of protection and courage.

Lemon—helps promote leukocyte formation; helps brighten a pale, dull complexion by removing the dead skin cells.

Cinnamon Bark—is anti-bacterial, anti-fungal, anti-infectious, anti-inflammatory, antimicrobial, anti-parasitic, antiseptic, antispasmodic, anti-viral, astringent, immune-stimulant, sexual stimulant, and warming.

Eucalyptus radiata—has strong anti-bacterial, anti-catarrhal, and antiseptic properties.

Rosemary cineol—may improve circulation and help stimulate the nerves. It is antiseptic and anti-infectious.

VALOR
MOISTURIZING SOAP™

Contains the oil blend of <u>Valor</u> which is soothing and nourishing for the skin with a balancing and calming fragrance.

Ingredients: Saponified oils of palm, coconut, wolfberry seed, and olive, therapeutic-grade essential oils (as listed below), liquid aloe vera extract (moisturizing agent), rosemary extract (antioxidant), and organic oatmeal (mild abrasive to stimulate pores).

Essential Oils:

Spruce—grounds the body, creating the balance and the opening necessary to receive and to give; may help dilate the bronchial tract to improve the oxygen exchange; helps one release emotional blocks.

Rosewood—is soothing to the skin, appeasing to the mind, relaxing to the body, and creates a feeling of peace and gentleness.

Blue Tansy—may help cleanse the liver and calm the lymphatic system to help rid one of anger and promote a feeling of self-control.

Frankincense—contains sesquiterpenes, which may help oxygenate the pineal and pituitary glands; may help promote a positive attitude.

Bath Gels and Bar Soaps

Tinctures

The product names displaying the trademark symbol are all trademarks of Young Living Essential Oils and although these product names appear throughout other sections of this book without the trademark symbol, they still refer to these same trademarked products.

ANTI-CANA

This unique formulation of traditional herbs was created by D. Gary Young to help support the body's defense system. When the immune system has been compromised by stress, trauma, pollutants, poor nutrition, or negative attitudes, harmful organisms can proliferate. This product is currently only available through Creer Labs at 801-418-8870.

Ingredients: Dried extracts of echinacea angustifolia, Oregon grape, red clover, burdock bark, dandelion, myrrh, and yellowdock; essential oils (as shown below); royal jelly; 50% grain alcohol by volume, necessary for herbal extraction.

Essential Oils:
    Rosemary cineol—helps balance heart function, stimulates nerves, and decongests the liver.
    Melaleuca alternifolia—anti-fungal, antiseptic, anti-bacterial; tissue regenerative.
    Cinnamon Bark—anti-fungal, anti-bacterial, and anti-viral.
    Clove—anti-infectious, anti-viral, anti-fungal, and anti-parasitic.

Suggested Use: As a dietary supplement, place 6-12 drops under the tongue or mix with juice or water. May be taken 2-3 times daily. Shake well before using. Keep out of direct sunlight.

Body System(s) Affected: Immune System.

CHELEX™

An herbal tincture synergistically formulated to help rid the body of heavy metals and other immune-damaging free radicals. Heavy metals absorbed from the air, water, food, skin care products, etc., lodge and store in the fatty layers of the body and give off toxic gases in the system, which may create allergic symptoms. Ridding our bodies of heavy metals is extremely important in order to have healthy immune function, especially if we have mercury fillings. This formula contains the essential oil of helichrysum, which may help the body in the elimination of heavy metals because of its natural chelating action.

Ingredients: Essential oils (as shown below), with extracts of astragalus, garlic, wild sarsaparilla, Siberian ginseng, red clover, and royal jelly. Extracted in a 1:4 ratio of grain alcohol and water.

Essential Oils:

> **Eucalyptus**—is highly antiseptic (eucalyptol) and antimicrobial.
>
> **Helichrysum**—may help cleanse the blood and improve circulatory functions. It is anti-catarrhal in structure and nature.
>
> **Roman Chamomile**—helps increase the regenerative ability of the skin; blood cleanser.
>
> **Rosemary cineol**—helps balance heart function, stimulates nerves, and decongests the liver.

Suggested Use: One to three droppers (25-75 drops) three times daily in distilled water or as desired.

Body System(s) Affected: Immune System.

ESTRO™

Designed with plant-derived phytoestrogens to safely help harmonize the female hormone levels. Works well with Prenolone or Prenolone+.

Ingredients: Extracts of black cohosh, blue cohosh, royal jelly, and essential oils (as shown below). Extracted in a 1:4 ratio of grain alcohol and water.

Essential Oils:

> **Fennel**—helps balance the hormones.
>
> **Lavender**—helps balance body systems.
>
> **Clary Sage**—helps balance the hormones; tonic to the reproductive system.

Suggested Use: Start with one dropper two to three times daily. Increase as needed to as much as three droppers daily. Estro may take as long as four weeks to reach maximum effectiveness.

Body System(s) Affected: Hormonal System.

FHS

This unique formulation of Native American herbs was created by D. Gary Young to help support the glandular system in women and adolescent girls who are struggling with unbalanced systems. This formula works well with FemiGen. FHS is currently only available through Creer Labs at 801-418-8870.

Ingredients: Dried extracts of black cohosh, blessed thistle, false unicorn, licorice root, sarsaparilla, Siberian ginseng, and squaw vine; essential oils (as shown below); royal jelly; 50% grain alcohol by volume, necessary for herbal extraction.

Essential Oils:

> **Clary Sage**—helps balance the hormones; tonic to the reproductive system.
>
> **Fennel**—helps balance the hormones.
>
> **Mugwort** (*Artemisia vulgaris*)—has been used to help calm nerves and balance hormones.

Suggested Use: As a dietary supplement, place 6-12 drops under the tongue or mix with juice or water. May be taken 2-3 times daily. Shake well before using. Keep out of direct sunlight.

Body System(s) Affected: Hormonal System.

Tinctures

HRT™

This formula was created out of specially selected herbs and oils to give nutritional support to help overcome deficiencies and irregularities of the heart.

Ingredients: Water, hawthorn berry juice, vegetable glycerin, blackberry brandy, lobelia extract, garlic extract, cayenne extract, and essential oils (as shown below). Extracted in a 1:4 ratio of grain alcohol and water.

Essential Oils:

Lemon—helps promote leukocyte formation; helps to dissolve cholesterol and fats.

Rosewood—antiseptic and antibacterial; tissue regenerative; helps increase elasticity.

Ylang Ylang—is a nutrient that has been found to help support heart function.

Cypress—astringent, lymphatic decongestant; strengthens connective tissue.

Suggested Use: One to three droppers (25-75 drops) three times daily in distilled water or as desired.

Body System(s) Affected: Cardiovascular System.

K & B™

The herbs contained in this supplement, combined with oils, have been traditionally used to help the kidneys and bladder in cases of irregularity, infection and bed wetting.

Ingredients: Extracts of juniper berries, parsley, uva ursi, dandelion root, German chamomile, royal jelly, and essential oils (as shown below). Extracted in a 1:4 ratio of grain alcohol and water.

Essential Oils:

Clove—anti-infectious, anti-viral, anti-fungal, and anti-parasitic.

Juniper—cleanser, detoxifier, diuretic; helps the body release fluids.

Sage—diuretic; contains estriol and has estrogen-like properties; believed to contain elements that contribute to the secretion of progesterone.

Fennel—diuretic; may break up fluids and toxins, and cleanse the tissues.

Geranium—cleansing, refreshing, astringent, diuretic; helps support the kidney and bladder functions and helps with stone removal.

Roman Chamomile—blood cleanser; helps liver discharge toxins.

Suggested Use: Take one to three droppers (25-75 drops) three times daily in distilled water or as desired.

Body System(s) Affected: Digestive System.

MALE-PRO

This formula was created by D. Gary Young to help support the normal functioning of the male glandular system. This product is currently only available through Creer Labs at 801-418-8870.

Ingredients: Dried extracts of ginger root, goldenseal root, gravel root, juniper berry, marshmallow root, parsley root, uva ursi, and cayenne; essential oils (as shown below); royal jelly; 50% grain alcohol by volume, necessary for herbal extraction.

Essential Oils:

Cardamom—is antiseptic, antispasmodic, and a tonic.

Marjoram—powerful muscle relaxant and anti-inflammatory; relaxing and soothing to the tissues.

Suggested Use: As a dietary supplement, place 6-12 drops under the tongue or mix with juice or water. May be taken 2-3 times daily. Shake well before using. Keep out of direct sunlight.

Body System(s) Affected: Hormonal System.

NERV-CAL

This formula was created by D. Gary Young with a blend of herbs that have been traditionally used to support the nervous system. This product is currently only available through Creer Labs at 801-418-8870.

Ingredients: Dried extracts of shavegrass, alfalfa, oat straw, Irish moss, and lobelia; essential oils (as shown below); royal jelly; 50% grain alcohol by volume, necessary for herbal extraction.

Essential Oils:

Ginger—is warming, uplifting, and empowering; helps reduce feelings of nausea, and motion sickness.

Peppermint—purifying and stimulating to the conscious mind; anti-inflammatory; helps with nerve regeneration. It also enhances digestion and increases endurance.

Spearmint—is antiseptic and antispasmodic; it is soothing and relaxing to skin, nerves, and muscle tissue.

Suggested Use: As a dietary supplement, place 6-12 drops under the tongue or mix with juice or water. May be taken 2-3 times daily. Shake well before using. Keep out of direct sunlight.

Body System(s) Affected: Nervous System.

NER-VUS

This formula was created by D. Gary Young with a blend of herbs that have been used relaxation and calming. This product is currently only available through Creer Labs at 801-418-8870.

Ingredients: Dried extracts of black cohosh, German chamomile, ginger root, hawthorn berry, hops, lady slipper, lobelia, scullcap, valerian root, and wood betony; essential oils (as shown below); royal jelly; 50% grain alcohol by volume, necessary for herbal extraction.

Essential Oils:

Lemon—helps promote leukocyte formation; helps to dissolve cholesterol and fats.

Ylang Ylang—is a nutrient that has been found to help support heart function.

Pine—may help improve circulation throughout the lungs. It helps soothe mental stress, relieve anxiety, and revitalize the entire body.

Spearmint—is antiseptic and antispasmodic; it is soothing and relaxing to skin, nerves, and muscle tissue.

Suggested Use: As a dietary supplement, place 6-12 drops under the tongue or mix with juice or water. May be taken 2-3 times daily. Shake well before using. Keep out of direct sunlight.

Body System(s) Affected: Nervous System.

REHEMOGEN™

This formula contains herbs that were used by Chief Sundance to clean the blood, fight free radicals and give support to the blood cells and immune system.

Ingredients: Essential oils (as shown below), extracts of red clover blossom, licorice root, poke root, peach bark, Oregon grape root, stillingia, sarsaparilla, cascara sagrada, prickly ash bark, burdock root, buckthorn bark, and royal jelly. Extracted in a 1:4 ratio of grain alcohol and water.

Essential Oils:

Roman Chamomile—blood cleanser; helps liver discharge toxins.

Rosemary cineol—helps balance heart function, stimulates nerves, and decongests the liver.

Thyme—anti-inflammatory; anti-fungal; antiseptic; anti-viral.

Melaleuca—anti-fungal, antiseptic, anti-bacterial; tissue regenerative.

Suggested Use: One to three droppers (25-75 drops) three times daily in distilled water or as desired.

Body System(s) Affected: Cardiovascular and **Digestive Systems**.

SE-6

This blend of herbal extracts and essential oils was created by D. Gary Young to help support both male and female glandular systems and promote healthy libidos. It has been reported that this tincture has helped to restore natural sexual desires. This product is currently only available through Creer Labs at 801-418-8870.

Ingredients: Dried extracts of cayenne, chickweed, damiana, echinacea angustifolia, garlic, gotukola, periwinkle sarsaparilla, saw palmetto berry, and Siberian ginseng; essential oils (as shown below); royal jelly; 50% grain alcohol by volume, necessary for herbal extraction.

Essential Oils:

Cardamom—is antiseptic, antispasmodic, and a tonic.

Fennel—diuretic; may break up fluids and toxins, and cleanse the tissues.

Ylang Ylang—may help balance the male-female energies so one can move closer towards being in spiritual attunement and allow them to focus their thoughts together, filtering out the ever-present garbage. It brings back the feeling of self-love, confidence, joy and peace.

Peppermint—purifying and stimulating to the conscious mind; anti-inflammatory; helps with nerve regeneration. It also enhances digestion and increases endurance.

Sandalwood—is high in sesquiterpenes, which were discovered to increase the amount of oxygen around the pineal and pituitary glands, thus helping to improve one's attitude. It alleviates depression and assists in the removal of negative programming from the cells of the body. It helps one accept others with an open heart while diminishing one's own egocentricity.

Suggested Use: As a dietary supplement, place 6-12 drops under the tongue or mix with juice or water. May be taken 2-3 times daily. Shake well before using. Keep out of direct sunlight.

Body System(s) Affected: Hormonal System.

SUGAR-UP

This formula, created by D. Gary Young, is a powerful blend of herbal extracts and essential oils that help support the pancreas. It can provide wonderful support for people that are fasting. This product is currently only available through Creer Labs at 801-418-8870.

Ingredients: Dried extracts of cinnamon bark, licorice, peppermint, and spearmint; essential oils (as shown below); royal jelly; 50% grain alcohol by volume, necessary for herbal extraction.

Essential Oils:

Fennel—diuretic; may break up fluids and toxins, and cleanse the tissues.

Rosemary cineol—helps balance heart function, stimulates nerves, and decongests the liver.

Basil—has been found beneficial for alleviating mental fatigue. It may also stimulate the nerves and the adrenal cortex.

Suggested Use: As a dietary supplement, place 6-12 drops under the tongue or mix with juice or water. May be taken 2-3 times daily. Shake well before using. Keep out of direct sunlight.

Body System(s) Affected: Digestive System.

Massage Oils

These product names are all trademarks of Young Living Essential Oils and although these product names appear throughout other sections of this book without the trademark symbol, they still refer to these same trademarked products.

CEL-LITE MAGIC™

Ingredients:

Fractionated Coconut Oil—is distilled from pure coconut oil to create an odorless, colorless vegetable oil. Because the oil's completely saturated fatty acid triglycerides are smaller, with no double bonds, the oil never goes rancid and is more readily absorbed by the skin. It easily washes out of clothes and sheets with no staining.

Grape Seed Oil—antioxidant; rich in bioflavonoids; helps maintain pH balance.

Wheat Germ Oil—high in natural vitamins E and B and lecithin; natural antioxidant; useful for reducing scar tissue and stretch marks; acts as a preservative for the other base oils.

Sweet Almond Oil—nourishes the skin will reducing friction for smoother application.

Olive Oil—moisturizing agent.

Vitamin E Oil—natural antioxidant; protects and promotes regeneration of the skin.

Essential Oils:

Grapefruit—excellent for fluid retention and cellulite; diuretic, detoxifier, and stimulant of the lymphatic system; important as an antidepressant.

Cypress—mucolytic, astringent, diuretic, lymphatic decongestant; reduces cellulite and strengthens connective tissue.

Cedarwood—astringent; diuretic; helps reduce oily secretions.

Juniper—cleanser, detoxifier, diuretic; helps the body release fluids.

Clary Sage—astringent; good for cell regulation, cholesterol, and dry skin.

Suggested Use: Shake well before using. Massage on location.

Warning: Avoid eye contact. If contact occurs, rinse thoroughly with water. For external use only. Keep out of reach of children.

Body System(s) Affected: Skin.

DRAGON TIME™

Ingredients:

Fractionated Coconut Oil—is distilled from pure coconut oil to create an odorless, colorless vegetable oil. Because the oil's completely saturated fatty acid triglycerides are smaller, with no double bonds, the oil never goes rancid and is more readily absorbed by the skin. It easily washes out of clothes and sheets with no staining.

Grape Seed Oil—antioxidant; rich in bioflavonoids; helps maintain pH balance.
Sweet Almond Oil—nourishes the skin will reducing friction for smoother application.
Olive Oil—moisturizing agent.
Wheat Germ Oil—high in natural vitamins E and B and lecithin; natural antioxidant; useful for reducing scar tissue and stretch marks; acts as a preservative.
Vitamin E Oil—natural antioxidant; protects and promotes regeneration of the skin.

Essential Oils:

Clary Sage—helps balance the hormones; tonic to the reproductive system.
Fennel—helps balance the hormones.
Lavender—helps balance body systems.
Jasmine—helps relieve menstrual pains; good for uterine disorders.
Sage—contains estriol and has estrogen-like properties; believed to contain elements that contribute to the secretion of progesterone.
Ylang Ylang—stimulates adrenal glands; helps balance male/female energies.
Yarrow—anti-inflammatory; antiseptic; excellent for menstrual problems.

Warning: Shake well before using. Avoid eye contact. If contact occurs, rinse thoroughly with water. For external use only. Keep out of reach of children.

Body System(s) Affected: Emotional Balance, Hormonal System, Skin.

ORTHO EASE™

Ingredients:

Fractionated Coconut Oil—is distilled from pure coconut oil to create an odorless, colorless vegetable oil. Because the oil's completely saturated fatty acid triglycerides are smaller, with no double bonds, the oil never goes rancid and is more readily absorbed by the skin. It easily washes out of clothes and sheets with no staining.
Grape Seed Oil—antioxidant; rich in bioflavonoids; helps maintain pH balance.
Wheat Germ Oil—high in natural vitamins E and B and lecithin; natural antioxidant; useful for reducing scar tissue and stretch marks; acts as a preservative.
Sweet Almond Oil—nourishes the skin will reducing friction for smoother application.
Olive Oil—moisturizing agent.

Essential Oils:

Wintergreen—locally warming; contains methyl salicylate; has a cortisone-like action that helps to reduce inflammation in the joints and tissue.
Juniper—antispasmodic; helps reduce muscle aches/pains.
Peppermint—enhances the effect of the other oils; high in natural menthol, for a wonderful mentholatum-type of sensation.
Eucalyptus australiana—wonderful as an anti-inflammatory.
Lemongrass—helps repair connective tissue; when combined with marjoram, it helps stimulate the agents in the tissue to rejuvenate and reconnect.
Marjoram—powerful muscle relaxant and anti-inflammatory; relaxing and soothing to cartilage tissue.

Thyme—anti-inflammatory; anti-fungal; antiseptic; anti-viral.

Vetiver—antispasmodic and locally warming; good for arthritis, rheumatism, and sprains.

Warning: Avoid eye contact. If contact occurs, rinse thoroughly with water. For external use only. Keep out of reach of children.

Body System(s) Affected: Muscles and Bones, Skin.

ORTHO SPORT™

This massage oil is an enhanced version of Ortho Ease, super-charged for the more demanding athlete or sportsman.

Ingredients:

Fractionated Coconut Oil—is distilled from pure coconut oil to create an odorless, colorless vegetable oil. Because the oil's completely saturated fatty acid triglycerides are smaller, with no double bonds, the oil never goes rancid and is more readily absorbed by the skin. It easily washes out of clothes and sheets with no staining.

Grape Seed Oil—antioxidant; rich in bioflavonoids; helps maintain pH balance.

Sweet Almond Oil—nourishes the skin will reducing friction for smoother application.

Olive Oil—moisturizing agent.

Essential Oils:

Wintergreen—locally warming; contains methyl salicylate; has a cortisone-like action that helps to reduce inflammation in the joints and tissue.

Peppermint—enhances the effect of the other oils; high in natural menthol, for a wonderful mentholatum-type of sensation.

Oregano—powerful antimicrobial; anti-inflammatory; locally warming.

Eucalyptus globulus—wonderful as an anti-inflammatory.

Elemi—very powerful anti-inflammatory; similar to helichrysum as a topical anesthetic.

Vetiver—antispasmodic and locally warming; good for arthritis, rheumatism, and sprains.

Lemongrass—helps repair connective tissue; when combined with marjoram, it helps stimulate the agents in the tissue to rejuvenate and reconnect.

Thyme—anti-inflammatory; anti-fungal; antiseptic; anti-viral.

Warning: Avoid eye contact. If contact occurs, rinse thoroughly with water. For external use only. Keep out of reach of children.

Body System(s) Affected: Muscles and Bones.

RELAXATION™

Ingredients:

Fractionated Coconut Oil—is distilled from pure coconut oil to create an odorless, colorless vegetable oil. Because the oil's completely saturated fatty acid triglycerides are smaller, with no double bonds, the oil never goes rancid and is more readily absorbed by the skin. It washes out of clothes and sheets with no staining.

Grape Seed Oil—antioxidant; rich in bioflavonoids; helps maintain pH balance.

Wheat Germ Oil—high in natural vitamins E and B; natural antioxidant; useful for reducing scar tissue and stretch marks; acts as a preservative for other base oils.

Sweet Almond Oil—nourishes the skin will reducing friction for smoother application.

Olive Oil—moisturizing agent.

Essential Oils:

Tangerine—sedating and calming to the nervous system; also a diuretic and a decongestant of the lymphatic system.

Lavender—sedative; balances body systems and promotes a general sense of well being.

Peppermint—purifying and stimulating to the conscious mind; anti-inflammatory; helps with nerve regeneration.

Spearmint—acts as an anti-depressant by relieving mental strain and fatigue, and by lifting one's spirits.

Rosewood—appeasing to the mind and relaxing to the body.

Ylang Ylang—anti-depressant; calming and relaxing; balances male/female energies.

Warning: Shake well before using. Avoid eye contact. If contact occurs, rinse thoroughly with water. For external use only. Keep out of reach of children.

Body System(s) Affected: Emotional Balance, Skin.

SENSATION™

Ingredients:

Fractionated Coconut Oil—is distilled from pure coconut oil to create an odorless, colorless vegetable oil. Because the oil's completely saturated fatty acid triglycerides are smaller, with no double bonds, the oil never goes rancid and is more readily absorbed by the skin. It easily washes out of clothes and sheets with no staining.

Grape Seed Oil—antioxidant; rich in bioflavonoids; helps maintain pH balance.

Wheat Germ Oil—high in natural vitamins E and B and lecithin; natural antioxidant; useful for reducing scar tissue and stretch marks; acts as a preservative for the other base oils.

Sweet Almond Oil—nourishes the skin will reducing friction for smoother application.

Olive Oil—moisturizing agent.

Essential Oils:

Rosewood—skin cell regenerative; soothing to the skin and promotes elasticity; appeasing to the mind and relaxing to the body.

Ylang Ylang—balances secretion of sebum (a waxy oil produced by the skin); energizing and uplifting.

Jasmine—deeply penetrating effect on the skin; produces a feeling of confidence, energy, euphoria, and optimism.

Warning: Shake well before using. Avoid eye contact. If contact occurs, rinse thoroughly with water. For external use only. Keep out of reach of children.

Body System(s) Affected: Emotional Balance, Hormonal System.

V-6™
ADVANCED VEGETABLE OIL COMPLEX

This new formulation of mixing oil contains the same nourishing oils but with an increased shelf life and virtually no color or odor. Food Grade.

Ingredients:

Fractionated Coconut Oil—is distilled from pure coconut oil to create an odorless, colorless vegetable oil. Because the oil's completely saturated fatty acid triglycerides are smaller, with no double bonds, the oil never goes rancid and is more readily absorbed by the skin. It easily washes out of clothes and sheets with no staining.

Sesame Seed Oil (certified organic)—is high in linoleic acid; contains vitamins, minerals, amino acids, lecithin, and natural vegetable proteins; moisturizing; easily absorbs into the skin.

Grapeseed Oil (kosher)—nourishes the skin; antioxidant; rich in bioflavonoids; helps maintain pH balance.

Almond Oil (certified organic)—contains natural vitamin D; well suited for massage.

Wheatgerm Oil (non GMO)—high in lecithin and natural E and B vitamins; natural antioxidant; useful for reducing scar tissue and stretch marks; acts as a preservative for the other base oils.

Sunflower Seed Oil (certified organic)—contains natural vitamin E; antioxidant; suitable for a variety of skin types.

Olive Oil (Extra Virgin & certified organic)—is a moisturizing agent.

Directions: Suggested blending is 15-30 drops of essential oil to 1 oz. mixing oil. V-6 Mixing Oil is good for mixing massage oils, creating your own blends and formulas, for cooking and making salad dressings, etc.

Supplements and Vitamins

This section contains product information about the authors' favorite food supplements. Most of this information was obtained from the product labels. We chose to review these supplements because they are the only products, known to the authors, that contain both herbs and essential oils. The essential oils in these products act as catalysts to deliver oxygen and nutrients through the cell walls while assisting the body in the removal of toxic waste.

When taking supplements, it is important to give the body a rest one or two days a week. Taking supplements only five or six days out of the week gives the body time to regain its own balance and allow its own healing powers to operate rather than rely solely on the supplements being taken. These supplements are usually dissolved and assimilated by the body within a couple hours so the effectiveness of the supplements can be increased by taking them throughout the day instead of all at once.

An approximate frequency is indicated for some of the supplements. However, please keep in mind that there are many variables involved in determining frequency. Consequently, these numbers may be difficult to duplicate.

These product names are all trademarks of Young Living Essential Oils and although these product names appear throughout other sections of this book without the trademark symbol, they still refer to these same trademarked products.

USING ESSENTIAL OIL FOOD SUPPLEMENTS

TO

CLEANSE, BUILD, AND SUPPORT THE BODY

Summary of an article written by Rita Anderson, Wellness Consultant

1. Start with the **Cleansing Trio** of Essentialzyme, ComforTone, and ICP.
   A. Begin immediately to take **Essentialzyme** before each meal. It may also be taken between meals to help lessen allergy symptoms.
   B. Take enough **ComforTone** each morning and before bedtime to allow your body to have several smooth bowel movements each day.
      Comments: If I began using **ComforTone** and actually felt clogged the first day or two, I would increase my **ComforTone** intake until I had very good movements two to three times a day. I would also increase my water intake to help my cells wash away the toxins.
   C. Once you are having several smooth bowel movements each day, begin taking **ICP** fiber beverage in juice or water. Warm water seems to help it "slide" down. Do not use citrus juices as they are too acidic.
2. Two weeks after the **Cleansing Trio** is working smoothly, start on the **Body Balancing Trio** (Bodygize, Vita Green, and Master Formula His (or Master Formula Hers)) to re-nutrient and fortify the body.
3. Two weeks after starting on the **Body Balancing Trio**, start using **Mineral Essence** and **ImmuneTune** to support the immune system.

Comments: Anyone who has not worked with a cleansing program in the past two years may want to continue on the **Cleansing Trio** for at least 90 days in a very consistent manner to rid the body of all stages of parasites. **Di-Gize** may also be used on the digestive Vita Flex points of the feet or as a hot compress over the abdominal area to help relax intestinal spasms and expel parasites. Apply full strength; if your skin is sensitive, it may be necessary to dilute with V-6 Mixing Oil. If you have a degenerative disease you will want to stay on the **Cleansing Trio** for at least a year.

NOTE: Learn to feed the body by taking supplements throughout the day.

AD&E™

This product contains Vitamins A, D, and E. These vitamins are known as powerful antioxidants. They contain the essential nutrients for supporting immune function. They may also help nourish the eyes, hair, nails, skin, and be instrumental in bone development. These vitamins are extremely important to the metabolism and elasticity of cells for increased longevity.

Ingredients: Vitamins A, D, and E, beta carotene, grapeseed oil, mixed tocopherols.
Suggested Use: Take five droppers once a day in distilled water or as desired.
Body System(s) Affected: Immune and **Nervous Systems, Skin**.

ALKALIME™

A precisely-balanced acid-neutralizing mineral formulation designed to combat yeast and fungus overgrowth and preserve the body's proper pH balance - the cornerstone of health. This specially designed alkalizing mineral powder contains an array of high-alkaline salts and other yeast/fungus-fighting elements such as citric acid and essential oils. By boosting blood alkalinity, yeast and fungus are deprived of the acidic terrain they require to flourish. The effectiveness of other Essential Oils is enhanced when the body's blood and tissues are alkaline.

Ingredients: Sodium bicarbonate, calcium carbonate, magnesium citrate, citric acid, potassium bicarbonate, sea salts, and essential oils (as shown below).
Essential Oils:
   Lemon—helps promote leukocyte formation; helps to dissolve cholesterol and fats.
   Lime—helps remove dead skin cells; tightens skin and connective tissue. Lemon and lime both become alkaline when absorbed by the body.
Suggested Use: Take one rounded teaspoon in 6 to 8 oz. of distilled or purified water. **Mix only with water.** Drink immediately. For best results, drink one hour before or after eating. To balance pH, take one to three times per day one hour before meals or before retiring. As an antacid, AlkaLime may be taken as needed. Otherwise, an ideal time to take AlkaLime would be prior to bedtime.
Body System(s) Affected: Cardiovascular and **Digestive Systems, Muscles and Bones**.
Companion Products: Essentialzyme, Mineral Essence, Royaldophilus, VitaGreen.
Companion Oils: <u>Valor</u>, <u>3 Wise Men</u>, <u>Harmony</u>, <u>Forgiveness</u>, <u>Joy</u>, <u>Present Time</u>, <u>Release</u>, <u>Inner Child</u>, <u>Grounding</u>, <u>Hope</u>, <u>SARA</u>, <u>White Angelica</u>, <u>Di-Gize</u>, <u>Purification</u>, <u>Thieves</u>, peppermint, and spearmint.

AlkaLime may help reduce the following signs of acid-based yeast and fungus dominance: Fatigue/low energy, unexplained aches and pains, overweight conditions, low resistance to illness, allergies, unbalanced blood sugar, headaches, irritability/mood swings, indigestion, colitis/ulcers, diarrhea/constipation, urinary tract infections, rectal/vaginal itch.

ALLERZYME™

A vegetable enzyme complex designed to provide some relief from occasional symptoms such as fullness, pressure, bloating, gas, pain, and/or minor cramping that occur after eating. It may also help combat allergies, fermentation, fatigue, and irritable bowel syndrome. Allerzyme contains a powerful combination of sugar-splitting and starch-splitting enzymes, as well as a small amount of fat-digesting and protein-digesting enzymes, which help to promote proper digestion for people with sensitive stomachs.

Ingredients: Amylase, bromelain, peptidase, protease, invertase, phytase, lipase, lactase, cellulase, alpha-galactosidase, maltase, plantain (sulfite-free), pure therapeutic-grade essential oils (as listed below), sucrase, vegetable cellulose, rice bran, deionized water, barley sprout powder, and silica.

Essential Oils:

Tarragon—may help reduce anorexia, dyspepsia, flatulence, intestinal spasms, nervous and sluggish digestion, and genital urinary tract infection.

Ginger—is warming, uplifting, and empowering; helps reduce feelings of nausea, and motion sickness.

Peppermint—purifying and stimulating to the conscious mind; anti-inflammatory; helps with nerve regeneration. It also enhances digestion and increases endurance.

Juniper—antispasmodic; helps reduce muscle aches/pains.

Fennel—anti-parasitic; promotes the removal of toxic wastes; may break up fluids and toxins, and cleanse the tissues.

Lemongrass—helps repair connective tissue; it helps stimulate the agents in the tissue to rejuvenate and reconnect; helps regulate the parasympathetic nervous system and strengthen vascular walls.

Patchouli—protects against UV radiation and promotes tissue regeneration; helps tighten loose skin and prevent wrinkles.

Anise—may help calm and strengthen the digestive system.

Suggested Use: Take 1-2 capsules three times daily just prior to all meals. Can also be sprinkled on food or in beverages.

Body System(s) Affected: Digestive and **Respiratory Systems**.

Companion Products: ComforTone, JuvaTone, Sulfurzyme, Royaldophilus, and Power Meal.

Companion Oils: Di-Gize and JuvaFlex.

Warning: Do not give this product to children under 12 years of age except under the supervision of a doctor. If symptoms persist, discontinue use of this product and consult your physician. Keep in a cool, dry place. Do no expose to excessive heat or direct sunlight. If pregnant or under a doctor's care, consult your physician.

BALANCE COMPLETE™

(Daily Superfood Energizer + Nutritive Cleanse)

This product is power-packed with an optimal balance of nutrients from a wide variety of superfoods. Also included is a unique blend of fibers, called V-Fiber™, that delivers 11 grams of heart-healthy fiber per serving. This cutting-edge blend of soluble and insoluble fibers provides optimal viscosity for more bulk, improved elimination of fats, more absorption of toxins, less gas and bloating, better colon health, better appetite satisfaction, and incredible blood sugar balance. Not only is it a nutritional, balanced, and complete meal, it is also delicious, naturally sweet, and low glycemic as well.

Ingredients: V-Fiber Proprietary Blend (Ningxia wolfberry (*Lycium barbarum*) fruit, brown rice bran, chicory root fiber extract FOS (also known as inulin fiber, a pre-biotic that nurtures friendly flora in the intestines), larch polysaccharide (a pre-biotic that nurtures friendly flora in the intestines), guar gum, konjac, xanthan gum, and sodium alginate), whey protein concentrate (from New Zealand; is ultra-bioactive, non-denatured and certified grass-fed, hormone-free, antibiotic-free, and chemical-free), nonfat dry milk, natural vanilla flavor, virgin coconut oil, lecithin, fructose, calcium, xylitol, Proprietary Enzyme Complex (lactase, lipase, bromelain, papain, and amylase), magnesium oxide, barley grass, cream flavor, neohesperidin derivative (flavor from natural citrus), mixed carotenoids, cinnamon powder, barley grass juice, lo han kuo extract, aloe vera, vitamin C (ascorbic acid), mixed tocopherols, selenium, vitamin B3 (niacinamide), zinc oxide, molybdenum, beta-carotene, vitamin B5 (pantothenic acid), vitamin B6 (pyridoxine HCl), chromium nicotinate, vitamin B1 (thiamine HCl), vitamin B2 (riboflavin), vitamin D3 (cholecalciferol), vitamin B12 (methylcobalamin), folic acid, orange (*Citrus sinensis*) rind essential oil, biotin, and iodine.

Suggested Use: Add two scoops (1.76 oz. or 50 g) of Balance Complete to 8 oz. cold water. May be mixed with rice, almond, or other milk. Shake, stir, or blend until smooth. For added flavor, add fruit or essential oils. For **daily health maintenance**, replace your least nutritious meal with Balance Complete. For **weight management programs**, replace two daily meals with Balance Complete

5-Day Nutritive Cleanse: Young Living recommends that the following be used to replace all three meals each day for a total of five days: Digest + Cleanse (1 softgel 30-60 minutes before the Balance Complete shake), Balance Complete (1 shake as directed on label), 3 oz. of NingXia Red (to help enhance detoxification while maintaining energy levels), and an extra 8-12 oz. of water. Continue drinking water between meals so that you consume a total number of ounces that is equal to half your body weight in ounces (i.e.: 200 lbs = 100 oz. of water each day). Note: If gas and bloating cause discomfort, add Essentialzyme to each meal. If you have a high metabolism, or if you experience excessive hunger, add a snack of raw fruits or vegetables 1-2 hours after each meal.

Body System(s) Affected: Digestive System.

Companion Products: Combine with NingXia Red, Longevity capsules, and Omega Blue (all 4 of these products make up the Core Essentials Complete program and work well together). Also Digest + Cleanse, and Essentialzyme.

BE-FIT™

A high-powered formula for enhancing strength and endurance and promoting muscle formation. Several ingredients are utilized in this product to help build muscle tissue.

Ingredients: Wolfberry powder *(Refer to the Wolfberry Crisp Bar at the end of this section for more information on the benefits of the Ningxia Wolfberry)*, HMB (beta-hydroxy beta-methylbutyrate), eleuthero *(Eleuthero ciccus senticoccus)*, ginkgo biloba extract, L-arginine, L-lysine, creatine monohydrate, cayenne, essential oils (as shown below), and gelatin.

Essential Oils:
> **Nutmeg**—supports adrenal glands; anti-inflammatory; stimulates immune function.
> **Lemongrass**—helps repair connective tissue; when combined with marjoram, it helps stimulate the agents in the tissue to rejuvenate and reconnect.
> **Rosemary cineol**—helps balance heart function, stimulates nerves, and decongests the liver.
> **Wintergreen**—locally warming; contains methyl salicylate; has a cortisone-like action that helps to reduce inflammation in the joints and tissue.

Suggested Use: Two capsules morning and evening.

Body System(s) Affected: Muscles and Bones.

Companion Products: Master Formula His/Hers, NingXia Red, Power Meal, Ultra Young, Wolfberry Crisp Bars.

Companion Oils: Brain Power, En-R-Gee, EndoFlex, Envision, Live with Passion, Valor.

BERRY YOUNG JUICE™

A powerful blend of the highest known antioxidant fruit juices with the strongest anti-aging effects. With an ORAC (Oxygen Radical Absorbence Capacity) score of 1,200, it has more powerful antioxidant properties than commercially available Mangosteen and Noni juices. The Ningxia wolfberry also contains the highest levels of immune-stimulating polysaccharides.

Ingredients: Ningxia wolfberry *(Lycium barbarum)* juice, blueberry juice, pomegranate juice, agave (as a sweetener), apricot juice, raspberry juice, natural blueberry flavor, ascorbic acid, potassium sorbate, sodium benzoate, and pure therapeutic-grade essential oils (as listed below).

Essential Oils:
> **Lemon**—contains over 65% d-limonene (which helps to promote normal cell life cycles); helps promote leukocyte formation; helps to dissolve cholesterol and fats.
> **Orange**—contains over 91% d-limonene (which helps to promote normal cell life cycles); rich in compounds noted for their stress-reducing effects.

Suggested Use: Take 1 teaspoon mixed in one cup of juice or water, twice daily or as needed between meals.

Body System(s) Affected: Immune System.

Companion Products: Ultra Young, Essential Manna, Power Meal, Wolfberry Crisp Bars.

Companion Oils: En-R-Gee, EndoFlex, Envision, JuvaFlex, Magnify Your Purpose, Longevity, and Valor.

BLM™

Protect your mobility by providing your bones and joints with the proper nutritional support. This product synergistically combines some of the most potent ingredients known. Available in both powder and capsule form.

Ingredients: Manganese citrate (catalyst to synergize ingredients), potassium chloride, and a proprietary blend of glucosamine sulfate (helps formation of cartilage), **type II collagen** (joint-supporting proteoglycans, also contains cartilage matrix glycoprotein (CMGP), which can help reduce oxidative damage to joints), **MSM** (sulfur - restores flexibility to cell membranes, slows breakdown of cartilage), and essential oils as shown below.

Essential Oils:

Balsam Fir—is a rich source of the antioxidant limonene which has been shown to help relieve **overworked** and **tired muscles** and **joints**.

Wintergreen—contains 99% methyl salicylate which gives it cortisone-like properties. It may be beneficial for **arthritis, rheumatism, tendinitis**, and any other discomfort that is related to the inflammation of **bones, muscles**, and **joints**.

Clove—as an antioxidant it has one of the highest ORAC (oxygen radical absorbent capacity) scores. It helps preserve the integrity of fatty acids and has been used as a numbing agent in dentistry.

Suggested Use:

Capsules: If you weigh **less than 120 lbs**, take 1 capsule three times a day. If you weigh **between 120 and 200 lbs**, take 1 capsule four times a day. If you weigh **more than 200 lbs**, take 1 capsule five times a day.

Powder: If you weigh **less than 120 lbs**, take 1/4 teaspoon three times a day. If you weigh **between 120 and 200 lbs**, take 1/4 teaspoon four times a day. If you weigh **more than 200 lbs**, take 1/4 teaspoon five times a day.

Body System(s) Affected: Muscles and Bones.

BLUE AGAVE

This product is an organically grown, kosher certified sweetener that is 50% sweeter than table sugar with fewer calories. Because it is scientifically proven to have a low glycemic index (currently at 39), it becomes the sweetener of choice for diabetics and hypoglycemics who need to control their blood sugar levels. It also helps to support normal intestinal function.

Ingredients: *Agave tequilana.*
Suggested Use: Can be used in beverages and food recipes as a sugar replacement. Because Agave is sweeter than table sugar, use only 3/4 the amount of Agave as table sugar. It also makes a delicious replacement for honey in sandwiches and on toast. Can also be used like honey on cereals and in beverages.
Companion Products: Essential Manna, and Power Meal.
Body System(s) Affected: Hormonal System, Muscles and Bones.

BODYGIZE™

Bodygize is a nutritional drink mix with a complete profile of essential amino acids, vitamins, and minerals for improved balance and lymphatic decongestion. The purpose of Bodygize is to help balance the body at its ideal weight. Advanced technology has made low heat glass-pack pasteurization of nonfat dry milk possible, leaving the enzymes intact. Fructose (sugar derived from fruit) is a perfect sweetener and contains a proper digestive balance. The essential oils provide its unique flavor and act as a **natural antioxidant**. European research has found that the oils in Bodygize may help dissolve hard fatty deposits and decongest the lymphatic system. The high level of protein in this product may help your body maintain a good food supply for muscle tissue.

Ingredients: Non-fat dry milk, ultra-filtered whey protein, fructose, potassium citrate, vanilla, lecithin, silicon dioxide, guar gum, sodium chloride, potassium chloride, magnesium citrate, ascorbic acid (vitamin C), zinc citrate, mixed tocopherols (vitamin E), niacinamide (vitamin B3), essential oil of grapefruit (as shown below), vitamin B5 (as calcium pantothenate), copper (as amino acid chelate), vitamin A (palmitate), folic acid, vitamin B6 (as pyridoxine HCl), riboflavin (vitamin B2), thiamin (vitamin B1), lutein, lycopene, vitamin B12, biotin, potassium iodine, essential oils of lemon, tangerine, orange, mandarin, and lime (as shown below), vitamin D3 (as cholecalciferol), selenium (as selenomethionine), and essential oil of cypress (as shown below).
Essential Oils:
Grapefruit—excellent for fluid retention and cellulite; diuretic, detoxifier, and stimulant of the lymphatic system; important as an antidepressant.
Lemon—helps promote leukocyte formation; helps to dissolve cholesterol and fats.
Tangerine—sedating and calming to the nervous system; also a diuretic and a decongestant of the lymphatic system..
Orange—is rich in compounds noted for their stress-reducing effects.
Mandarin—helps to strengthen the digestive function and the liver.
Lime—turns alkaline during digestion; helps to dissolve cholesterol and fats.
Cypress—mucolytic, astringent, diuretic, lymphatic decongestant; reduces cellulite and strengthens connective tissue.
Suggested Use: One measuring scoop to 8-10 oz. of purified water, juice or low fat milk. Blend in blender for 30 seconds. Ice cubes may be added to thicken like a shake. Bodygize works

with all juices. It is a pre-digested protein and can be taken at any time. For optimum results, take with Master Formula His or Hers, and Thyromin supplements.

1. ***For Fast Weight Loss:*** Enjoy Bodygize as a replacement for breakfast and dinner. Eat a sensible, low-fat, well-balanced lunch which includes vegetables, fruits, and whole grains. As with any weight loss program, fats, sugars, and high-calorie foods should be omitted from your diet. Raw vegetables are excellent snacks.
2. ***For Weight Gain:*** Enjoy Bodygize mixed with rice/almond milk or apple juice. Add a banana or a pear and drink after each meal.
3. ***For Good Health and Weight Maintenance:*** After you have achieved your ideal weight, enjoy a Bodygize shake as a meal replacement daily, possibly for breakfast. Bodygize can also be used as a filling and nutritious snack for the entire family.

Safety Data: ***Anyone who is pregnant or nursing, has health problems, or wants to lose more than 50 pounds or more than 20% of their body weight should consult their physician before starting this or any other weight loss program.***

Body System(s) Affected: Digestive and **Immune Systems, Muscles and Bones**.

Frequency: Approximately 87 MHz.

Companion Products: Be-Fit, Cel-Lite Magic Massage Oil, ComforTone, Master Formula His/Hers, Mineral Essence, Super B, Super Cal, Thyromin.

Companion Oils: Citrus Fresh, EndoFlex, Envision, Live with Passion, Magnify Your Purpose.

Comments: The authors of this book enjoy mixing Bodygize with a glass of Rice Dream (a brown rice beverage). May also be mixed with soy or almond beverages.

CARBOZYME™

A carbohydrate-digestive blend of active ingredients that aids digestion and enhances the absorption of nutrients. Carbozyme may provide relief of occasional symptoms such as fullness, pressure, bloating, gas, pain, and/or minor cramping that may occur after eating.

Ingredients: Amylase, bee pollen, pure therapeutic-grade essential oils (as listed below), trace minerals, rice bran, vegetable cellulose, and deionized water.

Essential Oils: Thieves **Blend, containing the following oils:**

Clove—is anti-bacterial, anti-fungal, anti-infectious, anti-parasitic, a strong antiseptic, anti-viral, and an immune stimulant; helps preserve integrity of fatty acids.

Lemon—helps to dissolve cholesterol and fats.

Cinnamon Bark—anti-fungal, anti-bacterial, and anti-viral.

Eucalyptus radiata—has strong anti-bacterial, anti-catarrhal, and antiseptic properties.

Rosemary cineol—helps balance heart function, stimulates nerves, and decongests the liver.

Suggested Use: Take 1-2 capsules three times daily just before meals containing carbohydrates or as needed.

Body System(s) Affected: Digestive System.

Companion Products: ComforTone, JuvaTone, Sulfurzyme, Royaldophilus, and Power Meal.

Companion Oils: Di-Gize and JuvaFlex.

Warning: Do not give this product to children under 12 years of age except under the supervision of a doctor. If symptoms persist, discontinue use of this product and consult your physician. Keep in a cool, dry place. Do not expose to excessive heat or direct sunlight. If pregnant or under a doctor's care, consult your physician.

CardiaCare™

Strengthens and supports the heart and cardiovascular system.

Ingredients: Wolfberry powder *(Refer to the Wolfberry Crisp Bar at the end of this section for more information on the benefits of the Ningxia Wolfberry)*, hawthorn berry (may help increase blood circulation in the heart), magnesium citrate, vitamin E (d alpha succinate, naturally derived), coenzyme Q10 (CoQ10), rhododendron caucasicum extract (contains phenylpropanoids which have been shown in clinical studies to increase the efficiency of the cardiovascular system—*refer to comment below on rhododendron caucasicum*), essential oils (as shown below), and gelatin.

Essential Oils:

> **Helichrysum**—is a natural blood thickness regulator, allowing for better passage of the blood between vessels and tissues.
>
> **Lemon**—helps to dissolve cholesterol and fats.
>
> **Marjoram**—provides support for the smooth muscles of the heart.
>
> **Ylang Ylang**—is a nutrient that has been found to help support heart function.

Suggested Use: Three capsules, twice daily.

Body System(s) Affected: Cardiovascular System.

Companion Products: AD&E tincture, HRT tincture, and Mineral Essence, NingXia Red.

Companion Oils: <u>Aroma Life</u>, <u>Forgiveness</u>, <u>Harmony</u>, <u>Joy</u>, <u>Live with Passion</u>.

Comments: *Rhododendron caucasicum* contains some powerful and highly beneficial antioxidant flavonoids and polyphenols similar to those found in pine bark extract. One study showed that Rhododendron possessed the same antioxidant activity as the powerful antioxidant, Pycnogenol. Some of the clinically researched benefits of rhododendron include significant effects on physical endurance and the cardiovascular system by increasing the blood supply to the muscles and the brain, diminished heart and chest pains, normalized blood pressure, improved heart circulation, lowered blood serum cholesterol levels, improved systolic blood pressure levels, inhibition of the enzyme hyaluronidase (which may play a role in the cause of arthritis and colon cancer), increased uric acid elimination (which may help provide relief from gout).

ComforTone™

Herbal formula with Bentonite, Apple Pectin, and herbal extracts which may relieve constipation, enhance colon function, and dispel parasites and toxins. The addition of essential oils may enhance the flavor as well as the activity of the herbs contained in this formula. This products was designed as a cleanser for any type of bowel irregularity.

Ingredients: German chamomile flowers, cascara sagrada, bentonite, diatomaceous earth, psyllium seed, fennel, burdock root, garlic, barberry, *Echinacea purpurea* root, ginger root, apple pectin, licorice root, cayenne pepper, essential oils (as shown below), and gelatin.

Essential Oils:

Rosemary cineol—helps balance heart function, stimulates nerves, and decongests the liver.

Tarragon—may help reduce anorexia, dyspepsia, flatulence, intestinal spasms, nervous and sluggish digestion, and genital urinary tract infection.

Peppermint—purifying and stimulating to the conscious mind; anti-inflammatory; helps with nerve regeneration. It also enhances digestion and increases endurance.

Ginger—is warming, uplifting, and empowering; helps reduce feelings of nausea, and motion sickness.

Anise—may help calm and strengthen the digestive system.

Mugwort (*Artemisia vulgaris*)—has been used to help calm nerves.

Tangerine—sedating and calming to the nervous system; also a diuretic and a decongestant of the lymphatic system..

German Chamomile—has been found to help open the liver, increase liver function and secretion, and support the pancreas.

Suggested Use: Start with two to five capsules first thing in the morning (½ hour before breakfast) and two to five capsules just before bed. Drink eight to ten 8 oz. glasses of *purified or distilled water per day for best results. If you get cramps, skip the next morning or day, and start up again with two capsules in the morning and two in the evening. After starting ComforTone, you may cut back, but don't stop completely because all the toxins that have been pulled out of the system will go back into the system. Take at least one in the morning and one in the evening, but don't stop once you start. ComforTone can be taken every day without becoming addictive. For maximum results, use with JuvaTone and Essentialzyme.*

Caution: *Do not take ComforTone at the same time as JuvaTone! When taken together, possible reactions include bloating, gas, diaphragm and chest pains (heartburn or acid reflux). If a reaction occurs,* <u>Di-Gize</u> *or* <u>JuvaFlex</u> *applied around the navel or center of the spine has helped.* It is best to take ComforTone and JuvaTone at least one hour apart from each other.

Safety Data: ***ComforTone can be taken during pregnancy as long as you don't get diarrhea. Diarrhea can cause cramping which could bring on labor.***

Body System(s) Affected: Digestive and **Immune Systems**.

Comments: ComforTone may be used to get rid of parasites. It breaks up the encrustation along the colon wall and relaxes spasms that may occur. Use <u>Di-Gize</u> when there is nausea. If constipation is increased with five ComforTone, increase the water intake (or a spasm in the colon may cause more constipation) and decrease or stop taking ICP. If a person has a history of chronic constipation, don't start ICP and ComforTone at the same time. Start ComforTone until the system is open, then start ICP with ten glasses of water per day. One woman was paralyzed by surgery and had to have a colonic two times a day. When she started taking ComforTone, she was able to have natural bowel movements.

Frequency: Approximately 43 MHz.

Supplements

Companion Supplements: Essentialzyme and ICP, JuvaTone, Chelex, ParaFree.
Companion Oils: <u>Di-Gize</u> (use with hot compress on abdomen or rub on feet), <u>JuvaFlex</u>, <u>Purification</u>, <u>Release</u>, <u>Thieves</u>.

CORTISTOP™
(WOMEN'S)

This product is formulated specifically for women and is designed to modulate the production of cortisol (the "Death" hormone) in the body, thereby helping to maintain the natural balance and harmony of other important substances like estrogen and progesterone. The negative effects of high amounts of cortisol are also diminished by providing nutrients that influence glandular balance.

Ingredients: Pregnenolone (promotes glandular balance, improves energy, and reduces stress), l-a-lysophosphatidyl choline (Epikuron 100E) (blocks cortisol production), l-a-phosphatidyl choline (LECI-PC 35P) (blocks cortisol production), Black cohosh (has estrogen-like functions; helps with hot flashes and other menopausal problems), DHEA (dioscorea villosa) (estrogen precursor - shown to enhance memory and increase muscle strength and lean body mass), therapeutic-grade essential oils as listed below, rice flour and gelatin.

Essential Oils:

> **Fleabane** (*Conyza canadensis*)—is a rare essential oil studied by Daniel Pénoël, M.D. for its ability to stimulate the pancreas and liver and counteract retarded puberty. It is a mood enhancer and promoter of hGH

> **Peppermint**—purifying and stimulating to the conscious mind; anti-inflammatory; helps with nerve regeneration. It also enhances digestion and increases endurance.

> **Clary Sage**—helps balance the hormones; tonic to the reproductive system.

> **Fennel**—helps balance the hormones.

> **Frankincense**—anti-tumoral and anti-inflammatory; increases activity of leukocytes. It also enhances the function of the pituitary and hypothalamus.

Suggested Use: Take one capsule before retiring. If desired, for extra benefits, take another capsule in the morning before breakfast. Use daily for 8 weeks. Discontinue use for 2-4 weeks before resuming.

Precautions: Keep in a cool, dry place. Keep out of reach of children. If pregnant or under a doctor's care, consult your physician.

Comments: The natural pro-hormone activity of this formulation has led to restriction of use by some athletic organizations.

Body System(s) Affected: Hormonal System.

Companion Products: Essential Manna, NingXia Red, PD 80/20, Power Meal, Prenolone/Prenolone+, Super C, Wolfberry Crisp Bars.

DETOXZYME™

A vegetable enzyme complex designed to promote detoxification of the body and to support and maintain a healthy intestinal environment. Because it combines essential oils with enzymes that are meant to digest starches, sugars, proteins, and fats, it may also provide relief of occasional symptoms such as fullness, pressure, bloating, gas, pain, and/or minor cramping that occur after eating. By facilitating the optimal absorption of nutrients from foods and supplements, the aging process is delayed and energy levels enhanced.

Ingredients: Amylase, glucoamylase, alpha-galactosidase, invertase, lactase, cellulase, protease, bromelain, lipase, phytase, pure therapeutic-grade essential oils (as listed below), rice bran, vegetable cellulose, deionized water, cumin seed extract, and silica.

Essential Oils:

   Cumin—anti-bacterial; antispasmodic; some anti-tumoral properties.

   Anise—may help calm and strengthen the digestive system.

   Fennel—anti-parasitic; promotes the removal of toxic wastes; may break up fluids and toxins, and cleanse the tissues.

Suggested Use: Take 2-3 capsules three times daily between meals. This product may be used in conjunction with a cleansing/detoxifying program. Can also be sprinkled on food or in beverages.

Body System(s) Affected: Digestive and **Immune Systems**.

Companion Products: ComforTone, JuvaTone, Sulfurzyme, Royaldophilus, and Power Meal.

Companion Oils: Di-Gize and JuvaFlex.

Warning: Do not give this product to children under 12 years of age except under the supervision of a doctor. If symptoms persist, discontinue use of this product and consult your physician. Keep in a cool, dry place. Do not expose to excessive heat or direct sunlight. If pregnant or under a doctor's care, consult your physician.

Comments: This formula contains trace minerals that can help to detoxify the body and assist in the reduction of cholesterol and triglycerides. It also helps to open the gallbladder duct, cleanse the liver, and regulate pH levels, thereby reducing acidification which helps to prevent candida and yeast overgrowth as well as parasite colonization and infestation. It may also help provide relief from diarrhea, constipation, heartburn, and food allergies.

DIGEST + CLEANSE™

(A "Purely Oils" supplement - oil blend in softgels)

This particular supplement is not just another coated peppermint oil supplement. It is a specifically formulated blend of therapeutic-grade essential oils, all of which have been scientifically proven to soothe gastrointestinal upset and support healthy digestion. This product is ideal for anyone who either deals with bowel discomfort and digestive upsets, or who could use such a wonderful product to assist them with their cleansing program.

Ingredients: Pure therapeutic-grade essential oils (as listed below), coconut meat oil [virgin], coconut meat oil [fractionated] (contains capric acid which has been shown to inhibit the growth of three strains of candida), lecithin (from soy), gelatin, glycerin, and aqueous coating solution (oleic acid, sodium alginate, medium-chain fatty acids, ethylcellulose, and stearic acid).

Essential Oils:

Peppermint—is antispasmodic, and anti-inflammatory; soothing, cooling, and dilating to the system. It also enhances digestion and increases endurance.

Caraway—has been clinically shown to soothe the bowel, improve elimination, and ease digestive discomfort and nausea.

Lemon—contains over 65% d-limonene (which helps to promote normal cell life cycles); helps promote leukocyte formation; helps to dissolve cholesterol and fats. It helps to promote a sense of well-being while alkalizing and cleansing the digestive and lymphatic systems.

Ginger—helps reduce/alleviate feelings of nausea, motion sickness, and vomiting. Along with fennel and anise, it helps to stimulate digestion, reduce gas and bloating, and create an unfriendly environment for parasites.

Fennel—diuretic; may break up fluids and toxins, and cleanse the tissues.

Anise—may help calm and strengthen the digestive system.

Suggested Use: Take one capsule once daily with food or as needed.

Body System(s) Affected: Digestive System.

Companion Products: Combine with NingXia Red and Balance Complete to make up Young Living's 5-day Nutritive Cleanse Program. Use daily with Omega Blue and Longevity capsules.

Companion Oils: Longevity

Precautions: Keep in a cool, dry place. Do not expose to excessive heat or direct sunlight. If pregnant or under a doctor's care, consult your physician.

ESSENTIAL MANNA™

This super food has been adapted from the diet of the Hunza people, who are one of the few groups of people that live past 100 years of age with excellent health. All of the following ingredients are in their raw form.

Ingredients: Apricots, barley, wolfberries, pineapple, buckwheat, almonds, brown rice, papaya, pumpkin seeds, apricot concentrate, walnuts, amaranth, unsweetened coconut, millet, filberts, sesame seeds, rolled oats, pecans, Brazil nuts, potassium sorbate, fructooligosaccharides (FOS), sodium ascorbate, citric acid, L-lysine, and frankincense powder. May also contain cashews and stevia.

Flavors: As of October 2006, available in Carob (additional carob chips), Carob Mint (additional carob chips and peppermint essential oil), and Spice (additional cinnamon powder).

Suggested Use: Snack on Essential Manna throughout the day whenever you feel hungry.

Body System(s) Affected: Digestive and **Immune Systems, Muscles and Bones**.
Companion Products: Essentialzyme, JuvaTone, Mineral Essence, Power Meal, Sulfurzyme.
Companion Oils: Exodus II, En-R-Gee, EndoFlex, Envision, JuvaFlex, Magnify Your Purpose,
    Valor.

ESSENTIALZYME™

    A high-quality enzyme complex which may improve and aid digestion and the elimination of toxic waste from the body. Essentialzyme was formulated to help supply the enzymes to people who have difficulty digesting or assimilating food. Helps promote and re-establish proper enzyme balance in the digestive system and throughout the body. Also helps to retard the aging process. Flavor enhanced with Essential Oils. **Natural antioxidant**.

Ingredients: Betaine HCl, pancrelipase, pancreatin 4x (porcine pancreas glands originating in the
    United States), bromelain, trypsin, thyme (*Thymus vulgaris*) leaf, carrot (*Daucus carota*) root
    powder, alfalfa (*Medicago sativa*) sprouts and leaf, papain, cumin (*Cuminum cyminum*) seeds,
    essential oils (as shown below), dicalcium phosphate, stearic acid, croscarmellose sodium,
    and magnesium stearate.
Essential Oils:
    Anise—may help calm and strengthen the digestive system.
    Fennel—diuretic; may break up fluids and toxins, and cleanse the tissues.
    Peppermint—is antispasmodic, and anti-inflammatory; soothing, cooling, and dilating to the
        system. It also enhances digestion and increases endurance.
    Tarragon—may help reduce anorexia, dyspepsia, flatulence, intestinal spasms, nervous and
        sluggish digestion, and genital urinary tract infection.
    Clove—anti-infectious, anti-viral, anti-fungal, and anti-parasitic.
Suggested Use: Take three tablets, three times daily prior to or with meals (more may be taken for
    larger meals), or as needed. Take Essentialzyme with meals, especially protein meals after
    3 p.m. as it will help lessen the burden on the digestive system. Also helps with digestive
    functions in the liver.
Body System(s) Affected: Digestive System.
Frequency: Approximately 83 MHz.
Companion Products: ComforTone, JuvaTone, Mineral Essence, Royaldophilus, Power Meal.
Companion Oils: Di-Gize, Harmony, JuvaFlex.

EXODUS™

    Exodus is the ultimate supercharged antioxidant containing a Biblical Blend of Essential Oils and other valuable herbs that provide important support for the body's defenses.

Ingredients: *Uncaria tomentosa* root (or Cat's Claw), OPC grapeseed extract (highly-praised
    antioxidant), *Echinacea purpurea* root (boosts activity of T-cells), yucca root (good for

osteoarthritis and rheumatoid arthritis), pantothenic acid, vitamin A (as mixed carotenoids), amino acid complex (includes alanine, cystine, argenine, glycine, lycine, threonine, and thorine), ionic minerals, and essential oils (as shown below).

Essential Oils:

Frankincense—anti-tumoral and anti-inflammatory; increases activity of leukocytes. It also enhances the function of the pituitary and hypothalamus.

Hyssop—helps with viral infections and expelling parasites.

Laurel (*Laurus nobilis*)—anti-fungal and antiseptic.

Spikenard—anti-bacterial and anti-fungal; helps with staph infections.

Comments: Some of the company literature states that myrrh (anti-infectious and antiseptic) may also be included.

Suggested Use: Take three capsules two to three times daily.

Body System(s) Affected: Immune System.

Companion Products: ComforTone, Essential Manna, ImmuneTune, Power Meal, Super C, VitaGreen.

Companion Oils: Exodus II, ImmuPower, Purification, Thieves.

FemiGen™

An herbal formula, with glandular substances and amino acids, which helps build and balance the reproductive system and maintain better hormonal balance for developmental years all the way through menopause. When one has experienced mood swings, PMS, and symptoms related to menopause, it is an indication that the body is nutritionally out of balance. FemiGen acts as a natural estrogen and helps balance the hormones.

Ingredients: Vitamin A, vitamin C, calcium, magnesium, damiana (blood purifier), epimedium aerial parts (detoxifies kidneys), wild yam root, dong quai root, muira-puama root (potency wood), American ginseng root, licorice root, black cohosh, L-carnitine, dimethyglycine, L-phenylalanine, cramp bark, squaw vine aerial parts, L-cystine, L-cysteine HCl, essential oils (as shown below), and gelatin.

Essential Oils:

Fennel—helps balance the hormones.

Clary Sage—helps balance the hormones; tonic to the reproductive system.

Sage—contains estriol and has estrogen-like properties; believed to contain elements that contribute to the secretion of progesterone.

Ylang Ylang—stimulates adrenal glands; helps balance male/female energies.

Suggested Use: Take two capsules with breakfast and two capsules with lunch. A maintenance dose of two capsules may be taken three times a day for ten days before a period.

Body System(s) Affected: Hormonal System.

Companion Products: Dragon Time Massage Oil.

Companion Oils: Dragon Time, Mister, PanAway, Peace & Calming, Relieve It.

H₂OILS™

H Oils packets utilize hydro-diffusion technology to slowly and efficiently diffuse essential oils into drinking water. This provides a great-tasting, natural way to add the zing of essential oils to your drinking water. Children simply love the taste.

How to Use: Just place one or more packets into the Young Living Hydro Diffusion Dispenser (or other container) and fill with water. Within a few minutes, the oils will begin to diffuse into the water. The packets are re-usable until all of the oils have diffused out of the packet.

Peppermint—is refreshing and invigorating, especially on hot days. It enhances digestion and increases endurance.

Lemon—is refreshing and purifying. It helps to promote a sense of well being while alkalizing and cleansing the digestive and lymphatic systems.

Lemon-Grapefruit—is stimulating and invigorating. It helps to detoxify the system and promotes the removal of excess fat.

Lemon-Orange—is uplifting and refreshing. It helps to calm the nerves while lowering cholesterol and reducing water retention.

ICP™

Fiber Beverage - a unique source of fiber and bulk for the diet, which helps speed the transit time of waste matter through the intestinal tract. The psyllium, oat bran, flax, and rice bran are specifically balanced to eliminate allergy symptoms that many people experience when taking psyllium alone. Essential oils enhance the flavor and may help to dispel gas and discomfort. Designed as both a cleanser and a builder, this formula is unsurpassed as an aid in enhancing normal bowel function.

Ingredients: Psyllium seed powder, oat bran (binds up fat), flax seed (roto-rooter; strong antioxidant), fennel seed (anti-parasitic), rice bran (roto-rooter), guar gum (opens colon), yucca root (anti-cancerous), plant cellulose, vegetarian protease enzyme formula (aids digestion), aloe vera extract (natural laxative), and essential oils (as shown below).

Essential Oils:
Fennel, Tarragon, Ginger, Lemongrass, and **Rosemary cineol**—all anti-parasitic by nature and promote the removal of toxic wastes.
Anise—as an anti-spasmodic and relaxant, it helps relax the muscles of the colon wall.

Suggested Use: Take five times a week for maintenance (½ cup water, ½ cup apple juice, and one heaping teaspoon (tsp.) of ICP). Take more often for cleansing (start with one heaping teaspoon (tsp.) two to three times a day with carrot juice or other vegetable juices. When things are going well, increase to three teaspoons (tsp.) three times a day). ICP dilutes better in warm water. Drink immediately as this product tends to thicken quickly when added to liquid. Sprinkle on yogurt, cereal, or other foods. Drink 8 to 16 oz. of fluid per teaspoon. ICP may be added to Bodygize or Power Meal.

Supplements

Comments: For best results, take ComforTone first then ICP morning and night. If added to Citrus Juices, it creates more acid. Best to use other juices. ICP absorbs toxins so that it can build and improve the wave-like movement of the intestinal walls.

Frequency: Approximately 56 MHz.

Body System(s) Affected: Cardiovascular and **Digestive Systems**.

Companion Products: Bodygize, ComforTone, Essentialzyme, JuvaTone, ParaFree, Power Meal.

Companion Oils: Di-Gize, JuvaFlex, Purification, Thieves.

IMMUNETUNE™

A super antioxidant and dietary supplement to support the body's immune defense system and fight against free radicals that are the primary cause of disease. The curcuminoid blend in this product has been found to be 60 percent stronger in antioxidant activity than pine bark or grape pit extract. However, synergism is the key to obtaining maximum effect. Through the combining of curcuminoids and grape pit extract, the antioxidant frequency is almost doubled. The minerals are added to maintain cell electrolyte and pH balance. Chromium supports the metabolism and selenium supports the nervous system while its antioxidant ability adds to the synergism of the formula. Yucca and echineaca lend their support to the immune system and their antioxidant and anti-infectious attributes increase the nutrient support. The essential oil of orange increases the flavonoid activity; pine and fir oils increase the anti-inflammatory action; and cistus, ravensara, and lemon oils add immune system support. **Natural antioxidant.**

Ingredients: Turmeric extract, magnesium citrate, yucca root, potassium citrate, Echinacea root, calcium citrate, wild yam, pantothenic acid, grapeseed extract, selenium, chromium, alpha lipoic acid, ginger extract, essential oils (as shown below), and gelatin.

Essential Oils:

Orange—is rich in compounds noted for their stress-reducing effects.

Pine—was used by the American Indians to repel lice and flees; antimicrobial, anti-viral, and anti-inflammatory; may also be good against skin parasites.

Ravensara—is a powerful anti-viral, anti-bacterial, anti-fungal, and anti-infectious oil. It may help dilate, open, and strengthen the respiratory system. As a cross between clove and nutmeg, it may also help support the adrenal glands.

Lemon—helps promote leukocyte formation; helps to dissolve cholesterol and fats.

Fir—antiseptic and anti-inflammatory; helps create a feeling of grounding, anchoring, and empowerment.

Cistus—has anti-bacterial, anti-infectious, and anti-viral properties. Because it is high in oxygenating molecules, it may assist the auto-immune system and may help strengthen the immune system.

Suggested Use: For slow metabolism, take two to three capsules daily. For fast metabolism, take three to six capsules daily. Best taken on an empty stomach. For stomach sensitivity, take with meals.

Body System(s) Affected: Immune System.

Frequency: Approximately 108 MHz.
Companion Products: Exodus, ParaFree, Super C.
Companion Oils: <u>ImmuPower</u> (on throat and chest), <u>Thieves</u> (on feet), <u>Envision</u>, <u>Exodus II</u>, <u>Release</u>.

IMMUPRO™

ImmuPro is a unique blend of five powerful polysaccharides—natural immune system enhancers that aid in normal immune function and support the body's ability to fight illness. This vegan formula comes in a chewable tablet with a great strawberry taste.

Ingredients: Zinc (as zinc citrate), selenium (as selenomethionine), copper (as copper chelate), Ningxia wolfberry (*Lycium barbarum*) polysaccharide), Reishi (*Ganoderma lucidum*) mycelia, Maitake (*Grifola frondosa*) mycelia, *Agaricus blazei* mycelia, arabinogalactin (larch tree extract), limonene (from orange essential oil), melatonin, organic strawberry powder, fructose, raspberry juice, pure lemon powder, and silicon dioxide.

Suggested Use: Chew one tablet before retiring. If under stress, chew 2-4 tablets before retiring or one tablet as needed.

Precautions: May cause drowsiness. Keep out of reach of children. If pregnant, lactating or under a doctor's care, consult your physician. Keep in a cool, dry place.

Body System(s) Affected: Immune System

Companion Products: ImmuneTune, Super C, Exodus, and JuvaTone.

Companion Oils: <u>ImmuPower</u>, <u>Thieves</u>, <u>Exodus II</u>, <u>JuvaFlex</u>, <u>Purification</u>, <u>Release</u>, <u>Valor</u>.

JUVAPOWER™

This new food supplement is packed with ingredients that have a dual purpose, to cleanse both the liver and the intestines simultaneously. Many of the ingredients in this supplement are some of the most powerful acid-binding foods, packed into this formulation to help support and cleanse the liver by helping to remove acids from the body. Not only does it fortify with optimum nutrition, but it also tastes great. Sprinkle some on a baked potato or some scrambled eggs and you'll be providing your body with some much needed support for proper digestion.

Ingredients: Rice seed bran, spinach leaf, tomato fruit, beet root, flax seed, oat seed bran, broccoli floret, cucumber fruit, dill seed, sprouted barley seed, ginger root and rhizome, slippery elm bark, L-taurine, psyllium seed husk, essential oils (as shown below), aloe vera inner leaf extract, and peppermint leaf.

Essential Oils:
Anise—may help calm and strengthen the digestive system.
Fennel—anti-parasitic; promotes the removal of toxic wastes; may break up fluids and toxins, and cleanse the tissues.

Suggested Use: Sprinkle 1 tablespoon on food (i.e., baked potato, salad, rice, eggs, etc.) or add to 4-8 oz. purified water or rice/almond milk and drink. Use three times daily for maximum benefits.
Body System(s) Affected: Digestive System (especially the **liver**).
Companion Products: ComforTone, JuvaTone, Mineral Essence, Royaldophilus, Power Meal.
Companion Oils: Di-Gize, Harmony, Juva Cleanse, JuvaFlex.

JUVASPICE™

Contains all the same ingredients as JuvaPower, spiced up with some potassium, RealSalt™, and cayenne pepper. Great for adding both nutritional support and flavor to your favorite dishes. Sprinkle some on a baked potato or some scrambled eggs and you'll be providing your body with some much needed support for proper digestion.

Ingredients: Rice seed bran, spinach leaf, tomato fruit, beet root, flax seed, oat seed bran, broccoli floret, cucumber fruit, potassium chloride, Redmond RealSalt™, dill leaf, sprouted barley seed, cayenne pepper fruit (*Capsicum annum*), ginger root and rhizome, slippery elm bark, L-taurine, psyllium seed husk, essential oils (as shown below), aloe vera inner leaf extract, and peppermint leaf.
Essential Oils:
    Anise—may help calm and strengthen the digestive system.
    Fennel—anti-parasitic; promotes the removal of toxic wastes; may break up fluids and toxins, and cleanse the tissues.
Suggested Use: Sprinkle ⅓ - ½ teaspoon on food (i.e., baked potato, salad, rice, eggs, etc.) or add to 4-8 oz. purified water or rice/almond milk and drink.
Body System(s) Affected: Digestive System (especially the **liver**).
Companion Products: ComforTone, JuvaTone, Mineral Essence, Royaldophilus, Power Meal.
Companion Oils: Di-Gize, Harmony, Juva Cleanse, JuvaFlex.

JUVATONE™

Amino acid herbal complex with trace minerals and essential oils for enhanced liver function, diminished addictions and skin improvement in a synergistic suspension isolation process. This product was designed specifically as a cleanser of the liver. The same essential oils that are included in this product are also included in the JuvaFlex oil blend making it the perfect topically-applied companion to JuvaTone.

Ingredients: Calcium, copper citrate, sodium, choline bitartrate, dl-methionine, beet root, inositol, raw dandelion root, L-cysteine HCl, alfalfa sprouts, Oregon grape root, parsley leaves, bee propolis 5x, sodium copper chlorophyllin, echinacea root, essentials oils (as shown below), cellulose, stearic acid, croscarmellose sodium, silicon dioxide, magnesium stearate, and cellulose film coat.

Essential Oils:

> **Lemon**—helps promote leukocyte formation; helps to dissolve cholesterol and fats.
>
> **German Chamomile**—has been found to help open the liver, increase liver function and secretion, and support the pancreas.
>
> **Geranium**—cleansing, refreshing, astringent, diuretic; helps support the kidney and bladder functions and helps with stone removal.
>
> **Rosemary cineol**—helps balance heart function, stimulates nerves, and decongests the liver.
>
> **Myrtle**—is a decongestant of the respiratory system. It may help improve oxygenation and work as an expectorant in discharging mucus.
>
> **Blue Tansy**—calms the lymphatic system; promotes a feeling of self-control.

Suggested Use: Take three capsules mid-morning and three capsules mid-afternoon. For maximum results, use with ComforTone. ***Caution****: Do not take ComforTone **at the same time** as JuvaTone! When taken together, possible reactions include bloating, gas, diaphragm and chest pains (heartburn or acid reflux). If a reaction occurs, Di-Gize or JuvaFlex applied around the navel or center of the spine has helped. **It is best to take ComforTone and JuvaTone at least one hour apart from each other***. Also apply JuvaFlex over the liver, on the spine, or on the feet.

Body System(s) Affected: Digestive and **Immune Systems**.

Frequency: Approximately 140 MHz.

Companion Products: ComforTone, Essentialzyme, ICP, ParaFree, Power Meal.

Companion Oils: JuvaFlex, Di-Gize, Forgiveness, Release, Surrender, Thieves.

Comments: JuvaTone goes through five stages of isolation when made so it won't upset an empty stomach. The liver plays a major role in helping the body to detoxify. The final products of digestion are transported through the portal vein from the colon to the liver to be cleansed. People have reported that while using JuvaTone, addictions to coffee, tea, tobacco, sugar, or alcohol are diminished.

KIDSCENTS® MIGHTY MIST™

A multi-vitamin antioxidant complex with wolfberry polysaccharides.

Ingredients: Vitamin A (solubilized), vitamin C (ascorbic acid), vitamin D (cholecalciferol), vitamin E (d-tocopheryl acetate), vitamin K (menadione), thiamin (vitamin B1), riboflavin (vitamin B2), niacin, vitamin B6 (pyridoxine HCl), folic acid, vitamin B12 (cyanocobalamin), biotin, pantothenic acid (Ca pantothenate), magnesium, zinc (zinc gluconate), selenium (selenomethionine), manganese, *Echinacea purpurea* extract, wolfberry polysaccharide, aloe vera, distilled water, vegetable glycerin, trace mineral complex, amino acid complex, phosphatidycholine, ginkgo biloba, PABA (para-amino benzoic acid), inositol, stevia extract, and natural fruit flavoring.

Suggested Use: Spray 3 mists inside cheeks, three times daily or as needed. Shake well before using.

Body System(s) Affected: Emotional Balance, Cardiovascular, Immune, and **Nervous Systems**.

KIDSCENTS® MIGHTY VITES™

A great-tasting, chewable multi-vitamin for kids. The essential oils of lime, mandarin, and orange, along with the Ningxia wolfberry and the stevia extract, give this vitamin supplement a taste that makes children ask for more.

Ingredients: Vitamin A (retinyl palmitate), vitamin C (sodium ascorbate and ascorbic acid), vitamin D3 (cholecalciferol), vitamin E (d-alpha tocopheryl acid succinate), thiamin (vitamin B1), riboflavin (vitamin B2), niacin (niacin and niacinamide), vitamin B6 (pyroxidoxine HCl), folic acid, vitamin B12 (cyanocobalamin), biotin, pantothenic acid (dicalcium pantothenate), calcium, iodine (potassium iodine), magnesium, zinc, selenium, copper, manganese, chromium, potassium (potassium citrate), fructose, sorbitol, Ningxia wolfberry (*Lycium barbarum*), bee pollen, inositol, pure therapeutic-grade essential oils (as listed below), wolfberry polysaccharides, and stevia extract.
   Note: The calcium, iron, magnesium, zinc, selenium, copper, manganese, and chromium were derived from hydrolyzed protein complex.

Essential Oils:
   Lime—helps remove dead skin cells; tightens skin and connective tissue.
   Mandarin—good for skin problems, stretch marks, nervous tension, and restlessness.
   Orange—is rich in compounds noted for their stress-reducing effects.

Suggested Use: Chew 3 tablets with breakfast daily.

Body System(s) Affected: Emotional Balance, Cardiovascular, Immune, and **Nervous Systems**.

KIDSCENTS® MIGHTYZYME™

With a special micro-encapsulation process to give the enzyme capsule a subtle peppermint flavor and sweetened with pure apple syrup, this vegetarian formula is sure to appeal to every child. It will also provide them with the natural enzymes to unlock and metabolize the vitamins, minerals and amino acids they desperately need for their growing bodies. It's **chewable** as well.

Ingredients: Calcium, folic acid, protease (3.0, 4.5, & 5.0), amylase, bromelain, cellulase, peptidase, lipase, phytase, alfalfa leaf, carrot root, peppermint (*Mentha piperita*) leaf, fructose, apple syrup, coconut oil, and silicon dioxide.

Suggested Use: Take 1 tablet, three times daily prior to or with meals.

Body System(s) Affected: Digestive System.

KIDSCENTS® ROYALDOPHILUS™

Our intestines are host to trillions of bacteria with a whole host of "friendly" bacteria that are essential to keeping harmful bacteria and viruses in check. Excessive use of antibiotics and drugs, chlorinated water, and junk and processed foods reduce the number of friendly bacteria in our intestines. Studies show that lactic acid bacterial strains help to increase immune-system activity including that of monocytes and NK cells. That is why Royaldophilus contains eleven of the most helpful bacterial strains. KidScents Royaldophilus uses the LiveBac process, a patent-pending, gastric-bypass system, to help move these tablets through the digestive system and only allow them to break down when they reach the gastrointestinal tract. This not only helps to maintain the full potency of these helpful microorganisms, but also allows the tablets to be safely stored at room temperature. These tablets are even **chewable** and they taste great!

Ingredients: *Lactobacillus acidophilus*, *L. plantarum*, *L. rhamnosus*, *L. salivarius*, *Bifidobacterium bifidum*, *B. infantis*, *B. longum*, *L. casei*, *L. brevis*, *L. keferi*, *L. helveticus*, crystalline fructose, dextrose, natural strawberry flavor, magnesium stearate, stearic acid, and citric acid.

Suggested Use: Chew two tablets daily. After taking antibiotics, it may be necessary to double the amount. Can be taken with food.

Body System(s) Affected: Digestive and **Immune Systems**.

Companion Products: Other KidScents products as show on previous pages.

Companion Oils: Di-Gize, Forgiveness, JuvaFlex, Harmony, Release, Thieves.

LIPOZYME™

A fat-digestive blend of active ingredients that aids digestion and enhances the absorption of nutrients. Lipozyme may provide relief of occasional symptoms such as fullness, pressure, bloating, gas, pain, and/or minor cramping that may occur after eating.

Ingredients: Lipase, bee pollen, pancreatin 10x, pure therapeutic-grade essential oils (as listed below), trace minerals, vegetable cellulose, and deionized water.

Essential Oils:

Tarragon—may help reduce anorexia, dyspepsia, flatulence, intestinal spasms, nervous and sluggish digestion, and genital urinary tract infection.

Ginger—is warming, uplifting, and empowering; helps reduce feelings of nausea, and motion sickness.

Peppermint—purifying and stimulating to the conscious mind; anti-inflammatory; helps with nerve regeneration. It also enhances digestion and increases endurance.

Juniper—antispasmodic; helps reduce muscle aches/pains.

Fennel—anti-parasitic; promotes the removal of toxic wastes; may break up fluids and toxins, and cleanse the tissues.

Lemongrass—helps repair connective tissue; it helps stimulate the agents in the tissue to rejuvenate and reconnect; helps regulate the parasympathetic nervous system and strengthen vascular walls.

Anise—may help calm and strengthen the digestive system.

Patchouli—protects against UV radiation and promotes tissue regeneration; helps tighten loose skin and prevent wrinkles.

Suggested Use: Take 1-2 capsules three daily just prior to meals containing fat or as needed.

Body System(s) Affected: Digestive System.
Companion Products: ComforTone, JuvaTone, Sulfurzyme, Royaldophilus, and Power Meal.
Companion Oils: Di-Gize and JuvaFlex.
Warning: Do not give this product to children under 12 years of age except under the supervision of a doctor. If symptoms persist, discontinue use of this product and consult your physician. Keep in a cool, dry place. Do not expose to excessive heat or direct sunlight. If pregnant or under a doctor's care, consult your physician.

LONGEVITY™ CAPSULES
(Longevity oil blend in gel capsules)
NEW FORMULATION!

This blend of therapeutic-grade essential oils, as measured on the ORAC (oxygen radical absorbent capacity) scale, has scored near 150,000! 220 mg of this blend of oils has been placed in gelatin capsules for easier consumption as a dietary supplement. It may help to promote longevity and prevent premature aging. For the regular oil blend, refer to Longevity in the Blends section of this book. **NOW the formulation has changed**. Frankincense essential oil was added to the blend, the amount of oil blend per softgel was increased from 100 mg to 220 mg, coconut oil (virgin and fractionated) was added (to help disperse the oils more evenly in the body, help protect against rancidity, preserve the integrity of the essential oils and extend shelf life), and an aqueous coating solution (enteric type coating produced from seaweed) was added to the outside of the softgel to help delay the breakdown of the softgel until it had reached the intestines (for optimal absorption and minimal aftertaste).

Ingredients: Pure therapeutic-grade essential oils (as listed below), coconut meat oil [virgin], coconut meat oil [fractionated], lecithin (from soy), gelatin, glycerin, aqueous coating solution (oleic acid, sodium alginate, medium-chain fatty acids, ethylcellulose, and stearic acid), and mixed tocopherols.

Essential Oils:

Thyme CT Thymol—has been shown in studies to dramatically boost glutathione levels in the heart, liver, and brain; further studies show that it helps maintain DHA (a nutrient that supports brain function and cardiovascular health) levels in the brain, liver, heart, and kidneys of aging subjects. Because it can also help to prevent the oxidation of fats in the body, it may help to slow the aging process. It is also anti-fungal and anti-viral.

Orange—is rich in compounds noted for their stress-reducing effects; lipid-soluble traits; antioxidant properties which enhance vitamin absorption.

Clove—has one of the highest ORAC (oxygen radical absorbent capacity) scores of any known substance. It is anti-bacterial, anti-fungal, anti-infectious, anti-parasitic, a strong antiseptic, anti-viral, and an immune stimulant; helps preserve integrity of fatty acids. Clove may also influence healing and help improve memory.

> **Frankincense**—anti-tumoral and anti-inflammatory; increases activity of leukocytes for healthy immune function and supports cell regeneration. It also enhances the function of the pituitary and hypothalamus.

Suggested Use: Take one capsule once daily with food or as needed.

Body System(s) Affected: Cardiovascular, Immune, and Nervous Systems, and Skin.

Companion Products: Combine with NingXia Red, Omega Blue, and Balance Complete (all 4 of these products make up the Core Essentials Complete program and work well together). Also Essential Manna, Power Meal, and Wolfberry Crisp Bars.

Companion Oils: <u>Longevity</u>

Precautions: Keep in a cool, dry place. Do not expose to excessive heat or direct sunlight. If pregnant or under a doctor's care, consult your physician.

MASTER FORMULA HERS™ AND HIS™

In addition to the following list of ingredients, each of these formulations has their own additional ingredients to customize them to the needs of either females or males.

Ingredients: Vitamin A (retinyl palmitate), vitamin C (sodium ascorbate and ascorbic acid), vitamin D3 (cholecalciferol), vitamin E (d-alpha tocopheryl acid succinate), thiamin (vitamin B1), riboflavin (vitamin B2), niacin (vitamin B3), vitamin B6, folic acid, vitamin B12, biotin, pantothenic acid, calcium, iron, iodine, magnesium, zinc, selenium, copper, manganese, chromium, potassium, choline bitartrate, PABA, betaine HCl, cellulose, maltodextrin, croscarmellose sodium, stearic acid, magnesium stearate, cellulose film coat in a Synergistic Suspension Isolation, L-cystine, L-cysteine, L-lysine, L-aspartic acid, L-glutamic acid, L-methionine, L-leucine, L-isoleucine, L-arginine, L-alanine, L-threonine, L-glutamine, L-tyrosine, L-valine, L-histadine, L-phenylalanine, L-serine, L-proline, L-hydroxyproline, L-citruline, and molybdenum.

Suggested Use: For slow metabolism, three to six tablets daily. For fast metabolism, six to eight tablets daily. Take half of the daily amount with breakfast and half with dinner. Best taken before meals.

Body System(s) Affected: Emotional Balance, Cardiovascular, Immune, and **Nervous Systems**.

Note: Free of allergens. Contains no artificial flavors, preservatives, sugar, cornstarch, corn, wheat, yeast, or soy products.

MASTER FORMULA HERS™

This high-potency, time released multi-vitamin and mineral supplement (with all the vitamins and minerals as listed previously) was formulated specifically for women with more magnesium, calcium, and B vitamins. It also contains silica (from hydrolyzed soy protein chelate), citrus flavonoid complex, and glycine. It has been found to reduce the symptoms of PMS as well as increase energy levels in general. This product was designed to help build and feed the reproductive system and because of the specific ingredients, it may also help women who have had an hysterectomy. **Natural antioxidant.**

Safety Data: If pregnant or under a doctor's care, please contact your physician.
Frequency: Approximately 88 MHz.
Companion Products: Be-Fit, Estro, FemiGen, VitaGreen.
Companion Oils: Dragon Time (contains more Clary sage and fennel), Mister (more estrogen-like oils—may be better for women who have had an hysterectomy), Abundance, Harmony, Joy, Magnify Your Purpose.

MASTER FORMULA HIS™

This high-potency, time released multi-vitamin and mineral supplement, designed specifically for men, includes all the vitamins and minerals listed previously with more zinc. It also contains citrus bioflavonoids, montmorillonite, maltodextrin, silicon dioxide, alfalfa sprouts, rutin, inositol, and L-glycine. This product was designed to build and feed the male reproductive organs. **Natural antioxidant**.

Suggested Use: Three tablets with breakfast and three with lunch (take before meals).
Frequency: Approximately 86 MHz.
Companion Products: Be-Fit, Essential Manna, Mineral Essence, NingXia Red, ProGen, Power Meal, Sulfurzyme, VitaGreen, Wolfberry Crisp Bars.
Companion Oils: Mister, Envision, Magnify Your Purpose, Sacred Mountain.

MEGACAL™

Calcium is important for proper health. 98% of the calcium in the body is found in the bones and 1% in the teeth. The other 1% supports these crucial metabolic functions: Steady heartbeat, muscle contraction, transmission of nerve impulses, and blood clotting. If this last 1% is not available from ones diet, it is pulled from the bones, creating osteoporosis. Current statistics indicate that 25 million American women and 5 million American men are affected by osteoporosis, showing just how difficult it has become to obtain enough calcium and other minerals through diet alone.

MegaCal differs from other calcium supplements (Super Cal, described in this book, and other popular Coral Calcium supplements) as shown on the following page. This particular product is formulated into a time-released mineral complex and is ideal for those who already have adequate calcium levels due to high consumption of dairy products. It may help alleviate osteoporosis and muscle cramps and support normal thyroid function.

Ingredients: Xylitol, calcium, magnesium, zinc, manganese, copper, fractionated coconut oil, and lemon (*Citrus limon*) therapeutic-grade essential oil.

Suggested Use: Take 1 tablespoon daily mixed in 1 cup of water or juice one hour after meals (or medications) or before retiring.
Body System(s) Affected: Cardiovascular System, Muscles and Bones, Nervous System.

	MegaCal™	SuperCal™	Coral Calcium
Calcium per serving	618 mg	242 mg	1300 mg
Type of calcium	Lactate pentahydrate, carbonate, glycerophosphate, ascorbate	Citrate	Carbonate
Calcium to magnesium ratio	1:1	3:1	30:1
Additional minerals/nutrients	Magnesium (carbonate, citrate, and sulfate), potassium, zinc gluconate, copper gluconate, manganese sulfate, xylitol, vitamin C	Potassium, zinc, boron	Magnesium, potassium, zinc, selenium, 60 other micronutrient minerals

MINERAL ESSENCE

Over 60 organic, ionic trace minerals perfectly blended with Royal Jelly and Essential Oils to enhance bio-availability, provide anti-microbial protection, and significantly improve oxygenation to the cells. Mineral Essence differs from other Colloidal Mineral products on the market in that the ingredients are an ionic, electrolyte solution of minerals and trace minerals. The fluids of the body are largely ionic solutions and every body process is dependent on ions. Calcium, potassium, sodium, chloride, and copper ions are some key ions that participate in the body's electrical events. Potassium is the major positive ion inside the cell. Sodium is the major positive ion found in the fluid outside the cell. Ionic chlorine is the most abundant negative ion. The minerals and trace minerals in an ionic solution like Mineral Essence are balanced and in associations such as ion pairs, which keep them from being reactive.

In contrast, colloidal minerals are a suspension of tiny non-soluble mineral and trace mineral particles in water. Most colloidal minerals are held in suspension by their tiny size and/or a static electrical charge. Colloids do not dissolve into true solutions and are not capable of passing through a semipermeable membrane (such as a cell wall). True colloidal minerals suspended in a aqueous solution are not capable of conducting electricity and are not associated with bio-electric activity in the body.

The physical opposite of a colloid is a crystalloid. The minerals from Utah's Inland Sea (the Great Salt Lake) as used in Mineral Essence are ionic and are electrolytes, thus capable of conducting electrical energy in the body. The full spectrum of minerals and trace minerals found in Mineral

Essence will form perfect crystals if all liquid was removed. When blended with essential oils, Mineral Essence becomes the most bio-available mineral product on the market.

To demonstrate how blending trace minerals with essential oils increases their bio-availability, a group of volunteers consumed a teaspoon of liquid trace minerals without any essential oils. Each volunteer experienced diarrhea within 24 hours. Within days the same volunteers were given double the dosage of the same liquid trace minerals, but this time blended with essential oils. No diarrhea symptoms were experienced. This was due to the fact that the liquid trace minerals, blended with essential oils, were delivered more efficiently and utilized by the body's cells, or in other words made more bio-available.

In the July 1996 issue of Young Living Essential Edge, an article entitled "Sunburn Relief" contained the following information. "Dr. Alex Schauss, a prominent mineral researcher, has discovered that burns are painful because certain trace minerals are depleted from the skin and surrounding tissue. If the trace minerals are replenished to the affected area, then the pain will subside almost immediately. . . . We have had many who have topically applied Mineral Essence directly on the sunburn or burn and received instant pain relief as the healing process began. . . ."

The minerals shown in the table below are in descending order according to the best testing information available. Several independent lab results for Mineral Essence were compared for this approximation.

Oxygen	Bismuth	Holmium
Hydrogen	Selenium	Lutetium
Chloride	Cesium	Rhenium
Magnesium	Molybdenum	Samarium
Sulfur	**Xenon	Terbium
Potassium	Lead	Thulium
Sodium	Arsenic	Ytterbium
Boron	Tungsten	Platinum
Lithium	Thorium	Dysprosium
Calcium	Tin	Erbium
Carbon	Thallium	Neodymium
Silicon	Mercury	Praseodymium
Phosphorus	Titanium	Yttrium
Fluorine	Hafnium	Zirconium
Nitrogen	Gold	Cerium
**Argon	Barium	Cobalt
Iron	Lanthanum	Niobium
Zinc	Cadmium	Gallium
Bromine	Uranium	Rubidium
Manganese	**Helium	Tantalum
Copper	Silver	Germanium
Chromium	Strontium	Aluminum
**Krypton	Iodine	Vanadium
Tellurium	Scandium	**Radon
Nickel	Beryllium	**Noble gases never tested for or not
**Neon	Europium	found, but are present in sea water
Antimony	Gadolinium	according to CRC Press.

Comments: Some people may wonder if it is safe to consume trace minerals that have trace elements of mercury, arsenic, lead, etc., in such a product. Dr. Alex Schauss explains that our bodies possess the same chemical makeup as sea water. In fact, sea water has been used many times for blood transfusions when plasma was not available. Products created in nature, like sea water, have many elements. Some of these elements, if separated and taken in larger quantities, can be dangerous to our health. When these same elements are synergistically blended by the Creator, we have a totally different product than the sum of the individual elements. Dr. Schauss suggests we consume sea water for its mineral content each day, for sea water provides the perfect balance of trace mineral intake that our body needs for optimum health.

Ingredients: Purified water (for diluting the minerals and liquefying the blend), ionic trace minerals (as listed in the previous chart), and essential oils (as shown below) in a base of royal jelly and honey.

Essential Oils:

Cinnamon Bark—is a powerful purifier and a powerful oxygenator; it enhances the action and the activity of the other oils; anti-fungal, anti-bacterial, and anti-viral.

Peppermint—enhances the effect of other oils; cooling and soothing; aids digestion.

Lemon—helps promote leukocyte formation; helps to dissolve cholesterol and fats.

Suggested Use: Shake well before using. Take one to two droppers morning and night or as needed as a food supplement.

Body System(s) Affected: Emotional Balance, Cardiovascular, Hormonal, Immune, and **Nervous Systems, Muscles and Bones**.

Companion Products: Bodygize, KidScents Mighty Mist/Vites, Master Formula His/Hers, Power Meal, Sulfurzyme, Wolfberry Crisp Bars.

Companion Oils: Citrus Fresh, Envision, Gathering, Harmony, Valor.

NINGXIA RED™

By employing the patented "Nutrient-Guard" technology, this antioxidant drink captures the full power of the whole wolfberry fruit in puree form. Combine that with some of the highest known antioxidant fruit juices with the strongest anti-aging effects and you have the most incredible nutritional product on the market. With an ORAC (Oxygen Radical Absorbence Capacity) score from Brunswick Laboratories of 1,500 per oz. and an S-ORAC score of 363 per oz. (specific test for scavenging activity against the powerful superoxide radical), it has the most powerful antioxidant properties than any other commercially available product including the previous leader, Berry Young Juice. In fact, on the S-ORAC test, the next closest product scored only 8.6! The Ningxia wolfberry also contains the highest levels of immune-stimulating polysaccharides and with an ultra low glycemic index score of 10.6, it won't spike blood sugar levels. *(Refer to the Wolfberry Crisp Bar at the end of this section for more information on the benefits of the Ningxia Wolfberry)*

Ingredients: Whole Ningxia wolfberry (*Lycium barbarum*) puree, blueberry (*Vaccinium corymbosum*) juice, pomegranate (*Punica granatum*) juice, apricot (*Prunus armeniaca*) juice,

Supplements

raspberry (*Rubus idaeus*) juice, organic blue agave *(A. tequilana)* nectar, dark grape (*Vitis vinifera* - seed, skin, and stem - water extracted), ascorbic acid (vitamin C), natural blueberry flavor, potassium sorbate, sodium benzoate, and pure therapeutic-grade essential oils (as listed below).

Essential Oils:
> **Lemon**—contains over 65% d-limonene (which helps to promote normal cell life cycles); helps promote leukocyte formation; helps to dissolve cholesterol and fats.
> **Orange**—contains over 91% d-limonene (which helps to promote normal cell life cycles); rich in compounds noted for their stress-reducing effects.

Suggested Use: Take 1-2 fluid ounces daily or as needed. Shake well before using and refrigerate after opening.

Body System(s) Affected: Immune System. Also targeted effects to **Liver Function**, **Eye Health**, and **Energy Levels**.

Companion Products: Essential Manna, Power Meal, Ultra Young / Ultra Young+.

Companion Oils: En-R-Gee, EndoFlex, Envision, JuvaFlex, Magnify Your Purpose, Longevity, and Valor.

OMEGA BLUE™
(Pure Fish Oil + Omega Enhance™)

This particular supplement is one of the most natural and bio-available fish oils on the market for several reasons. First is the source of the fish oil. The fish oil in this product is harvested from small fish (sardine, anchovy, and mackerel) which grow wild in pristine waters. This initially helps to reduce the amount of toxins (mercury, lead, PCBs and dioxins) that have to be removed through processing. Next is the processing itself. A unique, proprietary process that uses non-molecular distillation helps to maintain the naturally occurring balance of EPA (eicosapentaenoic acid) and DHA (docosahexaenoic acid). This is necessary to help reduce rancidity and minimize the "fishy" flavor of the oil. EPA should represent about 14-18% of the fish oil and DHA should be 8-12%. According to the labeling of this product at the time of this revision, the total amount of fish oil in this product is 1.65 grams while EPA is measured at 265 mg (about 16%) and DHA is measured at 182 mg (about 11%). Another thing that makes this product so unique is the addition of the proprietary Omega Enhance™ blend of essential oils shown below. This powerful blend of oils helps to protect the fragile Omega-3 fatty acids by increasing the stability of the fish oil by a minimum of 10 times throughout its entire lifecycle (from preparation, through storage in the softgel, all the way through metabolism within the body). Finally, a unique aqueous solution coating (enteric type coating derived from seaweed) helps to protect the fish oil from oxidation and also helps to ensure that it is released in the intestines for up to 3 times the Omega-3 absorption with no "fishy" aftertaste.

Ingredients: Fish oil, rice bran oil, pure therapeutic-grade essential oils (as listed below), gelatin, glycerin, and aqueous coating solution (oleic acid, sodium alginate, medium-chain fatty acids, ethylcellulose, and stearic acid).

Essential Oils:

Lemongrass—helps repair connective tissue; it helps stimulate the agents in the tissue to rejuvenate and reconnect; enhances Omega-3's cardiovascular protection; helps regulate the parasympathetic nervous system and strengthen vascular walls. It has also been clinically shown to help maintain normal, healthy cholesterol levels.

Myrrh—anti-inflammatory and antiseptic; has high levels of sesquiterpenes and is the second highest ranking substance on the ORAC scale behind clove essential oil.

Clove—has one of the highest ORAC (oxygen radical absorbent capacity) scores of any known substance. It is anti-bacterial, anti-fungal, anti-infectious, anti-parasitic, a strong antiseptic, anti-viral, and an immune stimulant; helps preserve integrity of fatty acids. Clove may also influence healing and help improve memory. Studies show that when it is combined with fish oil, it reduces inflammation an additional 30%.

German Chamomile—has been found to help open the liver, increase liver function and secretion, and support the pancreas. It promotes digestion and has strong antioxidant and anti-inflammatory properties.

Suggested Use: Adults, take three softgels daily or as needed.

Body System(s) Affected: Cardiovascular and Nervous Systems.

Companion Products: Use daily with Digest + Cleanse and Longevity capsules. Combine with NingXia Red, Longevity capsules, and Balance Complete (all 4 of these products make up the Core Essentials Complete program and work well together).

Precautions: Keep in a cool, dry place. Do not expose to excessive heat or direct sunlight.

ParaFree™

With virtually everyone in the world having parasites of one form or another, there is a tremendous need for a product like this that utilizes the anti-parasitic properties of essential oils to help combat this worldwide problem.

Ingredients: Base oils of sesame seed and olive.

Essential Oils:

Black Cumin (*Nigella sativa*)—anti-parasitic, antispasmodic; enhances immune function.
Thyme—anti-inflammatory; anti-fungal; antiseptic; anti-viral.
Clove—anti-parasitic.
Anise—anti-parasitic; anti-inflammatory; promoter of better digestion.
Nutmeg—supports adrenal glands; anti-inflammatory; stimulates immune function.
Fennel—anti-parasitic; supports digestive and pancreatic functions.
Vetiver—antiseptic; anti-inflammatory; calming; grounding; locally warming; muscular rheumatism; arthritis; anxiety, insomnia, depression, oily skin, acne.
Idaho Tansy—highly regarded for its worm-expelling properties.
Melaleuca—anti-fungal, antiseptic, anti-bacterial.
Laurel (*Laurus nobilis*)—antiseptic, anti-bacterial, anti-parasitic, anti-viral; diuretic; fungicide; digestive for stomach; purifier; loss of appetite.

Liquid Form:
>   **Suggested Use:** Take two to four droppers three times daily for 21 consecutive days and rest for 7 days. Cycle may be repeated three times.

Soft Gel Form:
>   **Suggested Use:** Five capsules two to three times daily. For best results take for 21 days and rest 7 days. Cycle may be repeated three times.
>
>   *** Better results may be obtained when using ParaFree with ComforTone and ICP to help break up and remove the plaque and incrustation from the system.

Body System(s) Affected: Digestive and **Immune Systems**.

Safety Data: *Do not take during pregnancy. Many of the oils contained in this product are contraindicated for pregnancy.*

Comments: Since both forms of this product are to be used orally and contraindications do exist, one would be well advised to review the safety data in the **appendix** of this book. For additional information, review the books, Essential Oil Safety—A Guide for Health Care Professionals by Robert Tisserand and Tony Balacs and Aromatherapy for Health Professionals by Shirley and Len Price.

PD 80/20™

A dietary supplement which provides the nutrients necessary to support internal health and bodily functions.

Ingredients: Pregnenolone and DHEA. Also includes rice flour and gelatin.

Body System(s) Affected: Emotional Balance, Hormonal System, Muscles and Bones.

Companion Products: Essentialzyme, Royaldophilus, Sulfurzyme (capsules or powder), and VitaGreen.

Companion Oils: Clary sage, Dragon Time, and fennel.

POLYZYME™

A protein-digestive blend of active ingredients that aids digestion and enhances absorption of nutrients. Polyzyme may provide relief of occasional symptoms such as fullness, pressure, bloating, gas, pain, and/or minor cramping that may occur after eating.

Ingredients: Protease, phytase, peptidase, papain, bromelain, lipase, pure therapeutic-grade essential oils (as listed below), vegetable cellulose, rice bran, deionized water, and silica.

Essential Oils:
>   **Anise**—may help calm and strengthen the digestive system.
>
>   **Peppermint**—is antispasmodic, and anti-inflammatory; soothing, cooling, and dilating to the system. It also enhances digestion and increases endurance.
>
>   **Rosemary cineol**—helps balance heart function, stimulates nerves, and decongests the liver.

Suggested Use: Take 2-3 capsules three times daily just prior to or with meals containing protein. Can also be sprinkled on food or in beverages.

Body System(s) Affected: Digestive System, Muscles and Bones.

Companion Products: ComforTone, JuvaTone, Sulfurzyme, Royaldophilus, and Power Meal.

Companion Oils: Di-Gize and JuvaFlex.

Warning: Do not give this product to children under 12 years of age except under the supervision of a doctor. If symptoms persist, discontinue use of this product and consult your physician. Keep in a cool, dry place. Do not expose to excessive heat or direct sunlight. If pregnant or under a doctor's care, consult your physician.

POWER MEAL™

A complete vegetarian protein drink mix containing Ningxia Wolfberry (high in protein and amino acids) and MSM with high-powered, immune-supporting, super-antioxidant properties, and Siberian ginseng. The Power Meal is designed as a high-protein, vitamin-rich meal replacement containing a large spectrum of vitamins, trace minerals, and amino acids. The Power Meal provides the body with the tools to build lean muscle tissue while providing a vital source of organic sulfur, which is an important facet of proper cellular metabolism and organ function.

Whether used as a meal replacement or a filling and nutritious snack, the Power Meal can help serve as an excellent weight management tool. Free of fats, sugars, and synthetic ingredients, Power Meal provides most of the building blocks the body requires for regeneration and maintenance.

The protein rich formula of Power Meal, when combined with exercise, can help the body build lean muscle tissue that is the foundation of a lean physique and an important element to weight control. Because muscle burns 22 times as many calories as fat, the addition of muscle tissue can significantly accelerate metabolism and contribute to a more slender body. Because muscle tissue weighs more than adipose (fat) tissue, the addition of muscle mass to the body may not always be accompanied by weight loss–even though body fat may have dropped substantially.

Ingredients: Rice protein concentrate, *Lycium barbarum* (Ningxia wolfberry), rice bran, bee pollen, fructose, guar gum, calcium carbonate powder, lecithin (food for the brain), liquid vanilla flavoring, fructooligosaccharides, choline bitartrate, multi-enzyme complex (lipase (digests fats), mixed protease (digests proteins), phytase, and peptidase), silicon dioxide, magnesium oxide, potassium chloride, Eleuthero, methylsulfonylmethane (MSM—regenerates nerve tissue; detoxifies liver), alpha lipoic acid, inositol, carotenoid complex (Lycopene 3%, astaxanthin, carocare betacarotene 7.5%, lutein 70%, zeaxanthin 50%, betain HCl), kelp extract, PABA (para-amino benzoic acid), gingko biloba extract, L-carnitine tartrate (helps convert fatty acids into energy), ascorbic acid (vitamin C), zinc citrate, wolfberry polysaccharides, boron amino acid chelate (helps in the absorption and utilization of calcium), betatene, copper amino acid chelate, manganese citrate (antioxidant; regulates blood sugar levels; increases cellular energy), biotin (helps cell growth and fatty acid production), essential oils (as listed below), d-alpha tocopheryl succinate (vitamin E), niacin, ferrous citrate, calcium pantothenate (pantothenic acid), folic acid, vitamin D3, pyridoxine HCl (vitamin B6), selenium amino acid chelate (antioxidant, supports pancreas and heart functions), riboflavin (vitamin B2), thiamine HCl (vitamin B1), chromium nicotinate (helps body build enzymes and proteins, stabilizes blood sugar; helps build lean muscle tissue, and burns fat), and vitamin B12.

Essential Oils:

Grapefruit—excellent for fluid retention and cellulite; diuretic, detoxifier, and stimulant of the lymphatic system; important as an antidepressant.

Orange—is rich in compounds noted for their stress-reducing effects.

Lemon—helps promote leukocyte formation; helps to dissolve cholesterol and fats.

Cypress—mucolytic, astringent, diuretic, lymphatic decongestant; reduces cellulite and strengthens connective tissue.

Anise—anti-parasitic; anti-inflammatory; promoter of better digestion.

Fennel—anti-parasitic; supports digestive and pancreatic functions.

Nutmeg—supports adrenal glands; anti-inflammatory; stimulates immune function.

Note: The Canadian version of Power Meal contains all the same ingredients except creatine replaces L-carnitine.

Suggested Use: Take 2 full scoops with 8 to 12 oz. of pure water or juice. Use as a meal alternative or dietary supplement. For added flavor, mix one serving (2 scoops) with rice or almond milk *(the authors enjoy mixing this with Rice Dream - a brown rice beverage)*. For children under 12, use 1 scoop (½ serving).

Body System(s) Affected: Cardiovascular, Digestive, and **Immune Systems, Muscles and Bones**.

Precautions: If pregnant or under a doctor's care, consult your physician. Keep in a cool, dry place. Do not expose to sunlight.

Companion Products: Be-Fit, Bodygize, Master Formula His/Hers, ComforTone, Essential Manna, Essentialzyme, ICP, NingXia Red, Thyromin, VitaGreen, Wolfberry Crisp Bars.

Companion Oils: Abundance, Citrus Fresh, EndoFlex, Envision, Live with Passion, Magnify Your Purpose.

PROGEN™

All-vegetable and herbal support for the male glandular system. The *Pygeum africanum* has been used for years to prevent prostate atrophy and malfunction while saw palmetto is widely used for protecting the prostate from enlargement. This formula should help protect men from prostate cancer and promote better glandular function. The oils used to flavor enhance this formula have been reported in Europe to also help support and prevent degeneration.

Ingredients: *Dioscorea villosa* root (wild yam), *Pygeum africanum* bark, saw palmetto (*Seronoa serrulata*), alpha glutaric acid, L-glutathione (sulfur-bearing antioxidant for the liver), zinc aspartate, L-carnitine (helps lower cholesterol; supports the heart), L-alanine, L-arginine, magnesium citrate, Eleuthero, blessed thistle, marshmallow, sesame oil, dimethylglycine (supports heart muscle and tissue), and essential oils (as shown below).

Essential Oils:

Sage—contains estriol and has estrogen-like properties; may help improve estrogen and progesterone-testosterone balance.

Fennel—diuretic; may break up fluids and toxins, and cleanse the tissues.

Lavender—sedative; balances body systems; promotes a general sense of well being.

Myrtle—is a Decongestant of the respiratory system. It may help improve oxygenation and work as an expectorant in discharging mucus.

Yarrow—is a powerful decongestant of the prostate and a hormone balancer.

Peppermint—purifying and stimulating to the conscious mind; anti-inflammatory; helps with nerve regeneration. It also enhances digestion and increases endurance.

Suggested Use: Take four capsules daily (two with breakfast and two with lunch).

Body System(s) Affected: Hormonal System.

Companion Products: Be-Fit, Exodus, Master Formula His, Protec tincture, Power Meal, Sulfurzyme, VitaGreen.

Companion Oils: Exodus, Live with Passion, Magnify Your Purpose, Mister, Valor.

PURE PROTEIN COMPLETE™

(Ultra-Bioactive Whey Protein)

This product is meant for those interested in a high-protein diet as part of a fitness or weight-loss program. It is unique among protein drinks that exist commercially. For one thing, it contains a proprietary blend of proteins (see ingredients below). This ultra-clean protein blend comes from New Zealand and is certified grass-fed, hormone-free, antibiotic-free, and chemical-free. It is also prepared with a gentle filtering process that does not denature amino-acids and maintains ultra-bioactivity. These different proteins all metabolize at different rates which helps to reduce muscle breakdown and provides for better protein synthesis. This sustained protein metabolism helps to maintain stable blood sugar levels, which has been shown to reduce food cravings. Each serving provides 20 grams of this proprietary protein blend which is then supported by a specialized enzyme blend, a low-glycemic carbohydrate matrix, and lots of complementary vitamins and minerals.

Ingredients: Pure Protein Complete Proprietary Protein Blend (whey protein concentrate, sweet whey, milk protein concentrate, nonfat dry milk, and whey protein isolate), Proprietary Carbohydrate Matrix (chicory root fiber extract (FOS) [inulin], natural vanilla flavor, fructose, guar gum, xanthan gum, xylitol, cellulose, lo han kuo extract, and stevia [*S. rebaudiana*] leaf extract), lecithin, Proprietary Enzyme Complex (lactase, papain, bromelain, amylase, lipase, and bioperine), magnesium oxide, tri-calcium phosphate, mixed carotenoids, vitamin C (ascorbic acid), potassium citrate, vitamin E (natural mixed tocopherols), zinc gluconate, vitamin B3 (niacin), beta carotene, vitamin B5 (calcium pantothenate), neohesperidin derivative (flavor from natural citrus), vitamin B6 (pyridoxine HCl), vitamin B2 (riboflavin), vitamin B1 (thiamine HCl), orange (*Citrus sinensis*) rind essential oil, chromium nicotinate, vitamin D3 (cholecalciferol), vitamin B12 (methylcobalamin), folic acid, biotin, potassium iodide, and sodium selenite.

Suggested Use: Add two scoops of Pure Protein Complete to 8 oz. cold water. May be mixed with rice, almond, or other milk. Shake, stir, or blend until smooth. For added flavor, add fruit or essential oils.

Body System(s) Affected: Muscles and Bones.

Companion Products: Balance Complete, Digest + Cleanse, Essentialzyme, Longevity capsules, NingXia Red, and Omega Blue.

ROYALDOPHILUS™

Our intestines are host to trillions of bacteria with a whole host of "friendly" bacteria that are essential to keeping harmful bacteria and viruses in check. Excessive use of antibiotics and drugs, chlorinated water, and junk and processed foods reduce the number of friendly bacteria in our intestines. When the "friendly" bacteria population is reduced, yeast infection (candidiasis) occurs. Currently about 70% of females and 30% of males have yeast infections. The **New England Journal of Medicine** published a research article showing that *Lactobacillus acidophilus* (just one strain of these friendly bacteria) can prevent and even cure yeast infection. Just this one strain alone has many benefits which include the following: the best natural digestive aid; corrects lactose intolerance; helps bad breath; helps acne; reduces cholesterol; inhibits candida albicans and prevents yeast infection. Studies show that other lactic acid bacterial strains help to increase immune-system activity including that of monocytes and NK cells. That is why Royaldophilus contains eleven of the most helpful bacterial strains.

However, it is extremely important for these friendly bacteria to implant on the intestinal wall for the proper flourishing of intestinal flora. That is why Royaldophilus uses the LiveBac process, a patent-pending, gastric-bypass system, to help move these tablets through the digestive system and only allow them to break down when they reach the gastrointestinal tract. This not only helps to maintain the full potency of these helpful microorganisms, but also allows the tablets to be safely stored at room temperature.

Ingredients: *Lactobacillus acidophilus, L. plantarum, L. rhamnosus, L. salivarius, Bifidobacterium bifidum, B. infantis, B. longum, L. casei, L. brevis, L. keferi, L. helveticus*, microcrystalline cellulose, hydroxypropyl methylcellulose, pectin, sodium bicarbonate, silica, stearic acid, and turmeric.

Suggested Use: Take one tablet daily. When traveling, under heavy stress, or taking antibiotics, it may be necessary to double the amount. Can be taken with food.

Body System(s) Affected: Digestive and **Immune Systems**.

Companion Products: ComforTone, Essentialzyme, ICP, VitaGreen.

Companion Oils: Di-Gize, Forgiveness, JuvaFlex, Harmony, Release, Thieves.

STEVIA EXTRACT™

This product, the whole leaf stevia extract from Paraguay, is a dietary supplement which may effectively regulate blood sugar. It is a helpful aid to people who have diabetes and hypoglycemia. After hypoglycemics ingest Stevia, blood sugar rises and their energy levels and mental activities increase rapidly. It may also lower elevated blood pressure while not affecting normal blood pressure.

It may inhibit the growth and reproduction of some bacteria and other infectious organisms, including the bacteria that causes tooth decay and periodontal (gum) disease. Individuals using Stevia have reported a lower incidence of colds and flu. Individuals who have tried using Stevia as a mouthwash or added to toothpaste have seen significant improvements in the treatment of periodontal disease.

It is a wonderful aid in weight loss and weight management because it contains no calories and research indicates that it significantly increases glucose tolerance and inhibits glucose absorption. People who ingest Stevia daily often report a decrease in their desire for sweets and fatty foods. It may also improve digestion and gastrointestinal function, soothe upset stomachs and help speed recovery from minor illnesses.

When applied to the skin, it effectively softens the skin and smooths out wrinkles while helping to heal various skin blemishes, acne, seborrhea, dermatitis, and eczema. People have reported that when Stevia is used on cuts and wounds, there is more rapid healing without scarring. **(Information obtained from United American Industries, Inc.)**

Suggested Use: Use three to six drops, or as desired, for supplementing food and/or beverages.
Body System(s) Affected: Cardiovascular, Digestive, and **Immune Systems**.
Companion Products: Essentialzyme, Mineral Essence, Thyromin, VitaGreen.
Companion Oils: JuvaFlex, Thieves.

SULFURZYME™

An unique combination of Methylsulfonylmethane (MSM), the protein-building compound found in breast milk, and Lyceum Barbarum (the Ningxia Wolfberry Powder) that together create a bold new concept in reviving the immune system, supporting almost every major body function, and forestalling an array of degenerative conditions. Of particular importance is MSM's ability to equalize water pressure inside of the cells—a considerable benefit for those plagued with bursitis, arthritis, and tendinitis. It also activates enzymes, helps the body assimilate vitamins, and metabolizes carbohydrates.

Sulfurzyme may help reduce the following signs of sulfur deficiency: Poor nail and hair growth, falling hair, eczema, dermatitis, poor muscle tone, acne/pimples, gout, rheumatism, arthritis, weakening of nervous system (MS, Parkinson's, Leu Gehrig's, and Alzheimer's disease), constipation, impairment of mental faculties, lowered libido.

Supplements

Ingredients: MSM (Methylsulfonylmethane) and wolfberry powder *(Refer to the Wolfberry Crisp Bar at the end of this section for more information on the benefits of the Ningxia Wolfberry),* and gelatin.

Comments: Sulfur metabolism requires nutritional balance. It takes calcium to metabolize sulfur, magnesium to metabolize calcium, potassium to metabolize magnesium, phosphorus to metabolize potassium, etc. The list goes on! That is why wolfberry is contained in this product; it contains all of the necessary components for sulfur to be metabolized.

Capsule Form:

> **Suggested Use:** Five capsules two to three times daily.

Powder Form:

> **Suggested Use:** Mix ½ tsp. with juice or Bodygize, two times daily, one hour before or after meals.

Body System(s) Affected: Immune and **Nervous Systems, Muscles and Bones, Skin**.

Companion Products: ComforTone, Essentialzyme, ICP, Master Formula His/Hers, Ortho Ease and Ortho Sport Massage Oils, Power Meal, Ultra Young.

Companion Oils: En-R-Gee, Envision, Magnify Your Purpose, PanAway, Valor.

SUPER B™

A B-complex is necessary for the delivery of the essential nutrients needed to support the body's cells, particularly under times of stress when assimilation is most difficult. Although research has shown that mega-doses of B vitamins are not healthy, it has been noted that the diets of many Americans do not provide the recommended amount of B vitamins, which are essential for normal functions of immune response. B vitamins included in this formula are B1, B2, B3, B6 and B12 (no essential oils are present in this formula). When all of these B vitamins are combined in the stomach it causes instant fermentation resulting in stomach upset. To alleviate this problem, this product utilizes a synergistic suspension isolation to provide the release of specific vitamins when necessary so that they can all work together in their separate stages of isolation. This product was designed to help build the body. **Natural antioxidant**.

Ingredients: Dicalcium phosphate, niacin, selenium, magnesium oxide, zinc, thiamine (vitamin B1), riboflavin (vitamin B2), vitamin B6, PABA, biotin, vitamin B12, folic acid, cellulose, magnesium stearate, and stearic acid.

Suggested Use: One half to one tablet daily, preferably with a meal and not on an empty stomach.

Body System(s) Affected: Cardiovascular and **Nervous Systems, Muscles and Bones**.

Safety Data: *If taken on an empty stomach, one may experience a niacin flush.*

Comments: If a niacin flush occurs, try one drop of peppermint in 20 drops of V-6 Mixing Oil for a full body massage. This may help the body cool down quickly.

Frequency: Approximately 63 MHz.

SUPER C™

Research has shown that physical stress, alcohol, smoking and medication can lower the blood levels of this essential vitamin. When citrus fruits are not readily available, diets may not contain enough vitamin C. Super C is properly balanced with rutin, bioflavonoids, and minerals to work synergistically, balancing the electrolytes and increasing the absorption rate of the vitamin C. Without bioflavonoids, vitamin C has a hard time getting inside the cell and without proper electrolyte balance and minerals, it will not stay there for long. The essential oils contained in this product not only enhance the flavor, but they all have high levels of bioflavonoid activity. This product was designed to help build up the body.

Ingredients: Vitamin C (ascorbic acid), cellulose, citrus bioflavonoids, calcium, potassium, stearic acid, rutin, magnesium stearate, zinc, manganese, cayenne, dicalcium phosphate, and essential oils (as listed below) in a Synergistic Suspension Isolation.

Essential Oils:
Orange—is rich in compounds noted for their stress-reducing effects.
Mandarin—good for skin problems, stretch marks, nervous tension, and restlessness.
Lemon—helps promote leukocyte formation; helps to dissolve cholesterol and fats.
Grapefruit—excellent for fluid retention and cellulite; diuretic, detoxifier, and stimulant of the lymphatic system; important as an antidepressant.
Lime—helps remove dead skin cells; tightens skin and connective tissue.

Suggested Use: For reinforcing immune strength, two tablets daily. For maintenance, one tablet daily. Best taken before meals.

Body System(s) Affected: Immune and **Respiratory Systems**.

Companion Products: Exodus, ImmuneTune, Rehemogen, VitaGreen.

Companion Oils: Citrus Fresh, Exodus II, ImmuPower, Motivation, Thieves, Valor.

Frequency: Approximately 80 MHz.

SUPER C CHEWABLE™

The vitamin C provided in this unique product is enhanced by that of the acerola cherry, a tropical fruit that contains up to 4.5% vitamin C. The addition of citrus bioflavonoids increases vitamin C's support of the immune system while increasing capillary and connective tissue strength. Now you can have one of nature's most powerful antioxidants in a natural, delicious, chewable form.

Ingredients: Vitamin C (ascorbic acid), acerola cherry (*Malphighia glabra*) fruit extract, citrus bioflavonoids from lemon (*Citrus limon*), essential oils (as shown below), fructose, silicon dioxide and vegetable-grade lubricant (sugar cane and palm oil).

Essential Oils:
Lemon—helps promote leukocyte formation; helps to dissolve cholesterol and fats.
Orange—is rich in compounds noted for their stress-reducing effects.

Suggested Use: Take 1 tablet 3 times daily as needed.

Body System(s) Affected: Muscle and Bone, Immune System.

Precautions: A study was published in 2002 suggesting that the acerola cherry can cause an allergic reaction similar to that caused by latex. If you have experienced such a reaction to latex, you may want to choose a different vitamin C supplement.

SUPER CAL™

Formulated with calcium, potassium, and magnesium citrate (which is easier for the body to utilize) specifically for proper electrolyte balance, hormonal balance, and muscle and bone development. **Natural antioxidant**. This product is ideal for those on a vegetarian diet or diets that are restricted in calories or high in carbonated beverages. It was designed to help build the body. *Refer to the chart shown under MegaCal in this same section for a comparison of SuperCal to MegaCal and to other popular coral calcium supplements.*

Ingredients: Calcium citrate, magnesium citrate, potassium citrate, zinc citrate, stearic acid, boron, essential oils (as shown below), cellulose, gelatin, and stearic acid in a Synergistic Suspension Isolation, which allows nutrients to be assimilated independently.

Essential Oils:

Marjoram—powerful muscle relaxant and anti-inflammatory; relaxing and soothing to cartilage tissue.

Lemongrass—helps repair connective tissue; when combined with marjoram, it helps stimulate the agents in the tissue to rejuvenate and reconnect.

Myrtle—is a Decongestant of the respiratory system. It may help improve oxygenation and work as an expectorant in discharging mucus. May also contain wintergreen essential oil.

Suggested Use: One to two capsules before each meal.

Body System(s) Affected: Emotional Balance, Cardiovascular and **Nervous Systems, Muscles and Bones**.

Companion Products: Essentialzyme, Ortho Ease and Ortho Sport Massage Oils, Power Meal, Sulfurzyme.

Companion Oils: Grounding, Harmony, PanAway, Valor.

Frequency: Approximately 78 MHz.

THERMABURN™

These easy-to-swallow capsules contain ingredients like HCA, chromium polynicotinate, and L-carnitine to help burn fat and build muscle while curbing the appetite. The addition of yerba maté extract helps boost energy and mental alertness.

Ingredients: Hydroxycitric acid, theobromine, L-carnitine, dl-methionine, licorice root extract, yerba maté extract, guarana seed extract, boron citrate, inositol hexaniacinate, essential oils (as shown below), and chromium polynicotinate.

Essential Oils:

>
> **Fleabane** (*Conyza canadensis*)—is a rare essential oil studied by Daniel Pénoël, M.D. for its ability to stimulate the pancreas and liver and counteract retarded puberty. It is a mood enhancer and promoter of hGH.
>
> **Myrtle**—is a Decongestant of the respiratory system. It may help improve oxygenation and work as an expectorant in discharging mucus.
>
> **Nutmeg**—supports adrenal glands; anti-inflammatory; stimulates immune function.
>
> **Peppermint**—purifying and stimulating to the conscious mind; anti-inflammatory; helps with nerve regeneration. It also enhances digestion and increases endurance.
>
> **Spearmint**—may balance and increase metabolism; helps burn up fats and toxins in the body; aids digestion.
>
> May also contain frankincense essential oil.

Suggested Use: Take 1-2 capsules two hours before or after meals. Individual needs may vary.

Body System(s) Affected: Muscles and Bones.

Companion Products: Master Formula His/Hers, Thyromin, VitaGreen.

Companion Oils: En-R-Gee.

THYROMIN™

For nourishing the thyroid, balancing metabolism, and reducing fatigue, this product is a combination of specially selected glandular nutrients, herbs, amino acids, and essential oils. All are grade A quality and are perfectly balanced to bring about the most beneficial, biological and nutritional support to the thyroid. This product was not only designed to help build up the body, but to help lay a solid foundation for the healthy functioning of the many organs, tissues, and cells which are effected by the thyroid. **Natural antioxidant**.

Ingredients: Vitamin E (d alpha tocopheryl acid succinate), iodine (derived from kelp), potassium (citrate), CoQ10, L-cysteine, L-cystine, carrageenan, bovine adrenal and pituitary extracts, parsley powder, magnesium stearate, and essential oils (as shown below).

Essential Oils:

>
> **Peppermint**—purifying and stimulating to the conscious mind; anti-inflammatory; helps with nerve regeneration. It also enhances digestion and increases endurance.
>
> **Spearmint**—may balance and increase metabolism; helps burn up fats and toxins in the body; aids digestion.
>
> **Myrtle**—is a Decongestant of the respiratory system. It may help improve oxygenation and work as an expectorant in discharging mucus.
>
> **Myrrh**—anti-inflammatory and antiseptic; helps to decongest the prostate gland.

Suggested Use: One to two capsules daily, immediately before going to sleep.

Body System(s) Affected: Hormonal System.

Companion Products: Essentialzyme, FemiGen, JuvaTone, Mineral Essence, Ultra Young, VitaGreen (enhances effect of Thyromin; take together for greater effect).

Companion Oils: EndoFlex, Clarity, En-R-Gee, JuvaFlex, Magnify Your Purpose.

Frequency: Approximately 52 MHz.

Comments: Thyromin can replace thyroid medication. If currently using thyroid medication, work with your health care professional before starting Thyromin to ensure that the thyroid medication is properly regulated/reduced. For those that are not on thyroid medication, but wonder if their thyroid is working properly, here is a simple way to find out. Take your **basal cell temperature** with a mercury thermometer upon awakening first thing in the morning, even before you go to the bathroom or get out of bed. Put the thermometer under your arm pit and rest for 10 minutes. If it reads below 97.6° F (36.5° C) then your thyroid is low (hypothyroidism) and Thyromin may help. Start out with one capsule each night at bedtime and check your temperature in a couple of days. If it is not up to 97.6° F, add one more capsule, *but take it in the morning.* Continue adding more capsules and checking your basal cell temperature until it reads 97.6° F. *Alternate the additional capsules between morning and evening so that half of the number of capsules taken each day are immediately before bed and the other half are in the morning after rising.* Follow the directions on the bottle.

ULTRA YOUNG™

This spray neutriceutical utilizes a unique nutrient delivery system through **oral mucosa absorption** (directly into the bloodstream through the dense network of blood vessels lining the mucus membrane inside the mouth). The advantages of this type of delivery system are protection from rapid first-pass metabolism by the liver and up to ten times the amount of nutrients being delivered to the system compared to the pill or capsule form of the same ingredients. Ultra Young is **not** a human growth hormone (hGH or somatotrophin) supplement. This unique product is formulated in such a way as to allow the body to use the hGH it produces naturally. Also, because low blood sugar levels are the key to hGH conversion and assimilation at the cellular level, Ultra Young contains Ningxia wolfberry extract for its insulin–like action. *(Refer to the Wolfberry Crisp Bar at the end of this section for more information on the benefits of the Ningxia Wolfberry.)*

Ingredients: Vitamin A, natural vitamin E, *Vicia faba* extract, L-arginine, niacin, zinc complex, L-ornithine, pyroglutamate, L-glutamine, L-glycine, GABA (gamma amino butyric acid), grapeseed extract, L-lysine, wolfberry extract, *Ginkgo biloba*, stevia, vitamin B6 , selenium, and essential oils (as shown below), in a base of deionized water, vegetable glycerine, alcohol, hydrolyzed vegetable protein, natural raspberry flavor, ionic trace minerals, potassium sorbate, mono-, poly-, and oligo-saccharides, and extracts of Siberian ginseng, bee pollen, inosine, ginger, and octocosanol. **Total mgs per Serving:** 405.2

Essential Oils:

    Sandalwood—helps strengthen the cardiovascular and lymphatic systems as well as increasing oxygen levels around the pineal and pituitary glands.

    Fleabane (*Conyza canadensis*)—is a rare essential oil studied by Daniel Pénoël, M.D. for its ability to stimulate the pancreas and liver and counteract retarded puberty. It is a mood enhancer and promoter of hGH.

Suggested Use: Three sprays, three times a day for six consecutive days; no sprays on the seventh day. (This gives the body the opportunity to continue to generate its own supply of hGH.) Vial contains approximately 30 servings (on average, 9 sprays per day). Shake gently before using.

Instructions On Use: Spray Ultra Young directly on inside cheeks and on roof of mouth. Avoid swallowing for one to two minutes. Spray upon waking, between meals, and just before retiring. Avoid spraying on the tongue because this generates saliva, promotes swallowing, and reduces its effectiveness. (Comment: It is most effective when given time to penetrate the mucus membranes of mouth and directly enter the blood stream.) Ultra Young is best used two to four hours before or after meals with no snacking in between because high blood sugar levels reduce its effectiveness.

Body System(s) Affected: **Hormonal** and **Immune Systems**.

Companion Supplements: AD&E, Be-Fit, Essential Manna, JuvaTone, Mineral Essence, NingXia Red, Power Meal, Sulfurzyme, Thyromin, VitaGreen, Wolfberry Crisp Bars.

Companion Oils: Frankincense, lavender, <u>Abundance</u>, <u>En-R-Gee</u>, <u>EndoFlex</u>, <u>Envision</u>, <u>Joy</u>, <u>JuvaFlex</u>, <u>Live with Passion</u>, <u>Magnify Your Purpose</u>, <u>Release</u>, <u>Valor</u>.

ULTRA YOUNG+™

This product contains the same ingredients as Ultra Young with the addition of DHEA (*dehydroepiandrosterone*). DHEA is produced in the adrenal gland and is a precursor to many important hormones. Like growth hormone, DHEA production steadily declines after the age of 20.

More Information on the Human Growth Hormone (hGH)

Benefits:
1. Reverses aging of the thymus gland, a part of our immune system.
2. Dramatically raises levels of cytokines, interleukin 1 & 2, and tumor necrosis factor, all of which play a central role in the human immune system.
3. Improves fat-to-lean ratios.
4. Reverses heart disease.
5. Boosts bone formation.
6. Firms and tightens skin by activating the production of skin proteins, collagen, and elastin.
7. Increases energy.
8. Lifts depression.
9. Restores deep sleep.

Supplementation is not enough: Taking a growth hormone (hGH) supplement is not the answer since research shows that most people continue to produce ample amounts of the human growth hormone well into their advanced years. The problem is not a lack of hGH, but the inability of the liver to convert it to IGF-1. IGF-1 is responsible for actually carrying out the actions of the chemical message sent by hGH. Without a properly functioning liver, IGF-1 conversion does not take place and hGH has a limited effect in the body. This is why Ultra Young contains ingredients that dramatically facilitate the conversion of hGH to IGF-1 in the liver; ingredients such as amino acids, the essential oil of *Conyza canadensis*, zinc, vitamin B6, Ningxia Wolfberry extract and more.

Ultra Young contains the anterior pituitary peptide isolate because it is a combination of all hormones secreted by the pituitary gland. Although hGH is the most important, the other hormones must be supplemented to help buffer and activate the effects of hGH. Without them, the body is being stimulated on only one level, a one-sided approach that is inherently abnormal.

Tips for maximizing Ultra Young's benefits:
1. Exercise. Rigorous exercises like running or weight lifting increase hGH levels.
2. Fasting. Extended periods (4 to 8 hours or more) of low blood sugar increase hGH levels and cell receptivity to hGH.
3. Thyroid, pancreas and liver support. For Ultra Young to work at its best, the liver needs to be supported and the thyroid and pancreas need to be functioning normally. For best results, take one to two Thyromin and two to four JuvaTone a day with Ultra Young.
4. Use lavender and frankincense. These oils are principle ingredients in supplements that support the pituitary. Because essential oils have the same lipid structure as the cell membrane, they have an unmatched ability to penetrate cell walls and transport hormones into the cells.

VITAGREEN™

High protein, high energy chlorophyll formula that helps the body maintain a high energy level. VitaGreen contains ingredients that may aid in cleansing the blood and supporting the immune system. Barley grass and spirulina have been reported to help balance blood sugar levels, alleviating that tired, run down feeling. High in chlorophyll, VitaGreen may support the thyroid, the digestive system, and strengthen and stimulate muscle development. According to European research, the essential oils in this formula may enhance immune function. Flavor enhanced with essential oils. **Natural antioxidant**.

Ingredients: Bee pollen, barley juice concentrate, spirulina, choline bitartrate, ginseng, alfalfa juice concentrate, Pacific kelp, L-arginine, L-cystine, L-tyrosine, essential oils (as shown below), and gelatin.
Essential Oils:
   Lemon—helps promote leukocyte formation; helps to dissolve cholesterol and fats.
   Lemongrass—helps repair connective tissue; when combined with marjoram, it helps stimulate the agents in the tissue to rejuvenate and reconnect.
   Melissa—is a powerful anti-viral agent, yet is very gentle and very delicate because of the nature of the plant; has the ability to work with and enhance the gentle aspects of the human body; anti-inflammatory and energizing.

- **Rosemary cineol**—helps balance heart function, stimulates nerves, and decongests the liver.
- **Suggested Use:** For slow metabolism, take three to six capsules daily. For fast metabolism, take four to eight capsules daily. Best taken before meals.
- **Body System(s) Affected: Cardiovascular, Digestive, Immune**, and **Nervous Systems, Muscles and Bones**.
- **Companion Products:** Be-Fit, JuvaTone, NingXia Red, Power Meal, Sulfurzyme, Thyromin, Wolfberry Crisp Bars.
- **Companion Oils:** Abundance, Awaken, En-R-Gee, Envision, JuvaFlex, Live with Passion, Magnify Your Purpose, Motivation, Release, Valor.
- **Frequency:** Approximately 76 MHz.
- **Comments:** Before putting oils in VitaGreen there was 42 percent blood absorption in 24 hours. After adding essential oils to VitaGreen, blood absorption increased to 64 percent in 30 minutes and 86 percent in an hour. The conclusion was that the cells were now receiving nutrients that they had previously not been able to assimilate. Therefore, VitaGreen is excellent for promoting pH (Alkaline/Acid) balance and for regulating blood sugar levels. (For more details, refer to page 105 of D. Gary Young's Aromatherapy—The Essential Beginning.)

WHEYFIT™

This whey-based fitness drink is formulated with ingredients that provide three sources of protein (MF/UF whey, egg whites, and non-GMO soy) for building muscle and increasing strength. These high-quality sources of protein are combined with a digestion-promoting enzyme to ensure proper absorption. Blueberry and strawberry powders were added to provide natural antioxidants and FOS (fructooligosaccharides) was added as a sweetener and also for its ability to improve the absorption of calcium and magnesium.

- **Ingredients:** MF/UF whey protein, egg whites, and non-GMO soy protein (none of which contain lactose); lecithin, fructooligosaccharides (FOS - low-glycemic sweetener; improves blood sugar control), stevia, blueberry powder (strong antioxidant compounds), strawberry powder (antioxidant; contains ellagic acid which slows growth of abnormal cells), blueberry flavor (liquid), natural flavors, vanilla extract, zinc citrate, sodium selenate, magnesium citrate, citric acid, essential oil (as shown below), and an enzyme complex blend, which includes amylase, cellulase, lactase, lipase, and neutral protease.
- **Essential Oils:**
  - **Lemon**—helps promote leukocyte formation; helps to dissolve cholesterol and fats; contains antioxidant compounds which helps strengthen immune function.
- **Suggested Use:** Take one heaping scoop daily. Mix with water or, for added flavor, mix with rice milk or almond milk.
- **Body System(s) Affected: Muscles and Bones**.
- **Companion Products:** Be-Fit, NingXia Red, Power Meal, Sulfurzyme, ThermaBurn, Wolfberry Crisp Bars.

WOLFBERRY CRISP™ BAR

A delicious, nutritious whole-food bar, made with the Ningxia Wolfberry and other nutrient packed, natural ingredients. With over 15 grams of protein per serving, this bar makes an ideal meal replacement.

Ingredients: Soy/whey protein, almond butter, agave nectar (*Agave salmiana/angustifolia*), Ningxia wolfberry, pumpkin seeds (*Curcubita pepo*), xylitol, cashews (*Anacardium occidentale*), walnuts (*Juglans regia*), vanilla bean extract (*Vanilla planifolia*), and a natural banana flavor.

Suggested Use: Take 1 bar a day or as a meal alternative or a high-energy snack.

Body System(s) Affected: Digestive and **Immune Systems, Muscles and Bones**.

Companion Products: Be-Fit, Berry Young Juice, ComforTone, Essential Manna, Essentialzyme, ICP, JuvaPower, JuvaSpice, KidScents Mighty Mist/Vites, Master Formula His/Hers, NingXia Red, Thyromin, VitaGreen.

Companion Oils: Abundance, Citrus Fresh, EndoFlex, Envision, Juva Cleanse, Live with Passion, Magnify Your Purpose.

Benefits of the Ningxia Wolfberry

A group of research scientists from Natural Science University in Beijing, China discovered a village in Inner Mongolia. Some of the people of the village were 120 or 130 years old and had no signs of cancer, arthritis, AIDS, or lupus. They lived predominately on the wolfberry and the vegetables from their gardens. This prompted research into the amazing benefits of the wolfberry. The wolfberry is over 12% protein by weight, has 18 amino acids (6 times higher in proportion than bee pollen), 21 trace minerals, 6 essential fatty acids, vitamins B1, B2, B6, C, and E, calcium, betaine, polyphenols (including a range of carotenoids), and fiber. *(For more information on the amazing research and powerful benefits of the Ningxia wolfberry, refer to the book, Discovery of the Ultimate Superfood)* The following is a sample of some of the amazing benefits of the Ningxia wolfberry.

Possibly Support the Immune System: According to scientific research in China, the Wolfberry contains compounds known as *lycium polysaccharides*, which have been studied for their effects on immune function. One study involving cancer patients found that the Wolfberry triggered an increase in both *lymphocyte transformation rate* and *white blood cell count* (measures of immune function). In another study, it was shown to increase *phagocytosis* (another index of immune function). Yet another study showed that the consumption of Wolfberry led to a strengthening of immunoglobulin A levels (a part of our immunity).

A Powerful Antioxidant: One clinical study of individuals who consumed Wolfberry, *superoxide dismutase (SOD)* levels in the blood increased 48% while *hemoglobin* increased 12%. Even better, *lipid peroxide* levels dropped 65%.

Possibly Inhibit Tumor Growth: From July 1982 to January 1984, the Ningxia Institute of Drug Inspection conducted a clinical experiment using multi-index screening. They concluded: The fruits and pedicels of the wolfberry were effective in increasing white blood cells, protecting the liver, and relieving hypertension. The alcoholic extract of wolfberry fruits inhibited tumor growth in mice by 58%, and the protein of wolfberry displayed an insulin-like action that was effective in promoting fat decomposition and reducing blood sugar.

Possibly Reverse Aging: A clinical experiment by the Ningxia Institute of Drug Inspection (Register No. 870306, from October 1982 to May 1985) studied the effects of Wolfberry on the blood of aged volunteers. The results were published by the State Scientific and Technological Commission of China, and the authors concluded that the wolfberry caused the blood of older people to **noticeably revert to a younger state**.

Great Potential for High Performance Gains: Wolfberry has a high concentration of the branched-chain amino acid *L-leucine*. Inside the body, L-leucine is converted into a powerful compound called HMB (beta-hydroxy beta-methylbutyrate). According to Richard Passwater, Ph.D., a noted researcher in the field of health-maintenance, "HMB showed that it lowered total and LDL cholesterol levels in blood and helped strengthen the immune system while building muscles and burning body fat. This news is certainly of interest to body builders and other athletes, but it may also become of interest to cancer, AIDS, and muscular dystrophy patients.

Supplements

$\mathscr{P}$ersonal $\mathscr{G}$uide

APPLICATION NOTES AND EXPLANATIONS

1. *Aromatic* means diffuse, breathe, or inhale.
2. A superscripted "F" (i.e. ^{F}Clary sage) means the oil has been used medicinally in France.
3. *Neat* means to apply the oil without diluting it with a pure vegetable oil.
4. If essential oils get into your eyes by accident or they burn a little, do not try to remove the oils with water. This will only drive the oils deeper into the tissue. It is best to dilute the essential oils with a pure vegetable oil.
5. The FDA has approved some essential oils for internal use and given them the following designations: GRAS (Generally Regarded As Safe for internal consumption), FA (Food Additive), or FL (FLavoring agent). *These designations are listed in the Single Oil Summary Information chart in the Appendix of this book under Safety Data.*
6. Using some oils such as lemon, orange, grapefruit, mandarin, bergamot, angelica, etc. before or during exposure to direct sunlight or UV rays (tanning beds, etc.) may cause a rash, pigmentation, or even severe burns. These oils are designated as photosensitive (PH) or extremely photosensitive (PH*) in the Single Oil or Blend Summary Information in the Appendix of this book. It is best to check the safety data for the oils to be used, then either dilute and test a small area or avoid their use altogether.
7. Caution should be used with oils such as Clary sage, sage, and fennel during pregnancy. These oils contain active constituents with hormone-like activity and could possibly stimulate adverse reactions in the mother, although there are no recorded cases in humans.
8. Particular care should be taken when using cinnamon bark, lemongrass, oregano, and thyme as they are some of the strongest and most caustic oils. It is best to dilute them with a pure vegetable oil.
9. Essential oils are not listed in a specific order (an attempt was made to list them alphabetically) so you will have to be intuitive on which one(s) to use. It is not necessary to use all of the oils listed. Try one oil at a time. If you do not see a change soon, try a different one. What one person needs may be different than another person. (Hint: Use Kinesiology to test yourself on the oils that are right for you.)
10. In this document, several homemade blends are suggested. However, it is done with great hesitancy. Some of the blends listed come from individuals who may not be experts in the field of essential oils and aromatherapy. Rather than mix the oils together, it may be better to **layer the oils**; that is, apply a drop or two of one oil, rub it in, and then apply another oil. If dilution is necessary, a pure vegetable oil can be applied on top.

11. When someone is out of electrical balance, try the following:
     A. Place a drop or two of <u>Harmony</u> into one hand, then rub the palms of both hands together in a clockwise motion.
     B. Place one hand over the thymus (heart chakra) and the other hand over the navel.
     C. Take three deep breaths and switch hands, then take three more deep breaths. *(Refer to **Allergies** in this section for more information).*

12. Less is often better; use one to three drops of oil and no more than six drops at a time. Stir and rub on in a clockwise direction.

13. When applying oils to **infants** and **small children**, dilute one to two drops pure essential oil with ½-1 teaspoon (tsp.) of a pure vegetable oil (V-6 Mixing Oil). If the oils are used in the bath, always use a bath gel base as a dispersing agent for the oils. See Babies/Children for more information about the recommended list of oils for babies and children.

14. The body absorbs oils the fastest through inhalation (breathing) and second fastest through application to the feet or ears. Testing on the thyroid, heart, and pancreas showed that the oils reached these organs in three seconds. Layering oils can increase the rate of **absorption**.

15. When an oil causes **discomfort** it is because it is pulling toxins, heavy metals, chemicals, poisons, parasites, and mucus from the system. Either stop applying the oils for a short time, to make sure your body isn't eliminating (detoxifying) too fast, or dilute the oils until the body catches up with the releasing. Toxins go back into the system if they cannot be released.

16. When the cell wall thickens, oxygen cannot get in. The life expectancy of a cell is 120 days (4 months). Cells also divide, making duplicate cells. If the cell is diseased, new diseased cells will be made. When we stop the **mutation** of the diseased cells (create healthy cells), we stop the disease. Essential oils have the ability to penetrate and carry nutrients through the cell wall to the nucleus and improve the health of the cell.

17. Each oil has a **frequency**, and each of our organs and body parts have a frequency. The frequency of an oil is attracted by a like frequency within the body. Lower oil frequencies become a sponge for negative energy. The frequency is what stays in the body to maintain the longer-lasting effects of the oil.
     Low frequencies can make **physical** changes in the body.
     Middle frequencies can make **emotional** changes in the body.
     High frequencies can make **spiritual** changes in the body.
     A. Average frequency of the human body during the day time is between 62 and 68 Megahertz (MHz). 1) Bone frequency is 38 to 43 MHz. 2) Frequencies from the neck down vary between 62 and 68 MHz.
     B. Spiritual frequencies range from 92 to 360 MHz.

18. *Use extreme caution when diffusing cinnamon bark* because it may burn the nostrils if you put your nose directly next to the nebulizer of the diffuser.

19. When traveling by air, you should always have your oils hand-checked. X-ray machines may interfere with the frequency of the oils. ***See COMMENTS under Asthma for a discussion on plastic nasal inhalers for using oils on the airplane instead of taking the bottles of oil.***

20. Keep oils away from the light and heat, although they seem to do fine in temperatures up to 90 degrees. If stored properly, they can maintain their maximum potency for many years.

The following information will be useful to those who are familiar with the art and technique of blending. (*See the Science and Application section of Reference Guide for Essential Oils for more information.*)

    1st—The **Personifier** (1-5% of blend) oils have very sharp, strong and long-lasting fragrances. They also have dominant properties with strong therapeutic action.

    Oils in this classification may include: Angelica, birch, cardamom, German chamomile, cinnamon, cistus, Clary sage, clove, coriander, ginger, helichrysum, mandarin, neroli, nutmeg, orange, patchouli, peppermint, petitgrain, rose, spearmint, tangerine, tarragon, wintergreen, ylang ylang

    2nd—The **Enhancer** (50-80% of blend) oil should be the predominant oil as it serves to enhance the properties of the other oils in the blend. Its fragrance is not as sharp as the personifiers and is usually of a shorter duration.

    Oils in this classification may include: Basil, bergamot, birch, Roman chamomile, Black cumin, cajeput, cedarwood, dill, eucalyptus, frankincense, galbanum, geranium, grapefruit, hyssop, jasmine, lavender, lemon, lemongrass, lime, marjoram, melaleuca (Tea Tree), melissa, myrtle, orange, oregano, palmarosa, patchouli, petitgrain, ravensara, rose, rosemary, sage, spruce, thyme, wintergreen

    3rd—The **Equalizer** (10-15% of blend) oils create balance and synergy among the oils contained in the blend. Their fragrance is also not as sharp as the personifier and is of a shorter duration.

    Oils in this classification may include: Basil, bergamot, cedarwood, Roman chamomile, cypress, fennel, fir, frankincense, geranium, ginger, hyssop, jasmine, juniper, lavender, lemongrass, lime, marjoram, melaleuca (Tea Tree), melissa, myrrh, myrtle, neroli, oregano, pine, rose, rosewood, sandalwood, spruce, tarragon, thyme.

    4th—The **Modifier** (5-8% of blend) oils have a mild and short fragrance. These oils add harmony to the blend.

    Oils in this classification may include: Angelica, bergamot, cardamom, coriander, eucalyptus, fennel, grapefruit, hyssop, jasmine, lavender, lemon, mandarin, melissa, myrrh, neroli, petitgrain, rose, rosewood, sandalwood, tangerine, ylang ylang.

The Science and Application section of Reference Guide for Essential Oils contains more information on the art of blending. In that same section, another method of blending explains how to use "notes (top, middle, and base notes)" to help determine how different single oils are to be blended together. It also includes an odor intensity chart that further assists in the blending process. Refer to that section for more details and instructions on blending.

There are some tools that make blending much easier and much more enjoyable. Abundant Health offers dispensing syringes with corresponding caps called, "adapt-a-caps" that fit on your 15 ml bottles (caps for other size bottles as well), and allow for accurate, measured dispensing of the oils. There are even 1 ml syringes with drop markings for easy blend creations. Look for these dispensing tools at www.abundanthealth4u.com under Glass and Plastic Products.

Abandoned: *See Emotions.* <u>Acceptance</u>, <u>Forgiveness</u>, <u>Valor</u>**.**

Abscess: *See Anti-fungal, Anti-bacterial, Fungus: FUNGAL INFECTION, or Infection.* Bergamot, birch, elemi, frankincense, galbanum, lavender, melaleuca (Tea Tree), <u>Melrose</u>, myrrh, <u>Purification</u>, Roman chamomile, <u>Thieves</u>, thyme, wintergreen. To reduce swelling, pain, inflammation, and to draw out toxins, it may help to apply the oil(s) with a hot compress.
> **BLEND #1**—Roman chamomile, lavender, and melaleuca (Tea Tree).
> *SUPPLEMENTS*—Royaldophilus, Super B. Put <u>Thieves</u> on a rolled up gauze and place over abscess to pull out the infection.
> **DENTAL**—Helichrysum, <u>Purification</u>, Roman chamomile. Apply using a hot compress on face. It may also help to apply one drop of oil to a cotton ball and apply directly to the abscess. Put <u>Thieves</u> on a rolled-up gauze and place over abscess to pull out the infection.

> *I had an abscess tooth. The dentist and the specialist he referred me to insisted I have a root canal. I used 3 to 4 drops of Thieves in a glass of water to gargle with. Then I used a mixture of half Thieves and half olive oil and rubbed this on both sides of my gums on the infected area. I then used the Dentarome Plus toothpaste. It has been 2 months and my mouth is fine.*
> **-Submitted by K. Ernst (July 2004)**

> **BLEND #2**—Use clove, birch/wintergreen, myrrh, and helichrysum to help with infection.
> **MOUTH**— ᶠLavender.
> ****COMMENTS—Some sources recommend a non-toxic diet and an increase in liquid intake.*

Absent Minded: *See Memory.* Basil, <u>Brain Power</u>, cardamom, <u>Clarity</u>, frankincense, lemongrass, <u>M-Grain</u>, peppermint, rosemary, sandalwood.
> *SUPPLEMENTS*—Mineral Essence, Omega Blue, Power Meal, Sulfurzyme, Ultra Young, VitaGreen.

Abundance: <u>Abundance</u>, <u>Acceptance</u>, bergamot, cinnamon bark, cypress, <u>Harmony</u>, <u>Gathering</u>.
> **ATTRACTS**—<u>Abundance</u>, cinnamon bark.
> **MONEY**—Ginger, patchouli.
> ****COMMENTS—One waitress demonstrated her luck when she wore <u>Abundance</u> and <u>Harmony</u> together; she received a whopping $120.00 tip! Who knows, it may work for you too!*

Abuse: <u>Acceptance</u>, <u>Brain Power</u>, <u>Citrus Fresh</u>, <u>Christmas Spirit</u>, geranium, <u>Forgiveness</u>, <u>Grounding</u>, <u>Harmony</u>, <u>Hope</u>, <u>Humility</u>, <u>Inner Child</u>, <u>Joy</u>, lavender, melissa, <u>Peace & Calming</u>, <u>Release</u>, 3 Wise Men, sandalwood, <u>SARA</u> (releases memory and trauma of sexual or ritual abuse), <u>Surrender</u>, <u>Trauma Life</u>, <u>Valor</u>, ylang ylang. Apply 1 drop of the desired oils on each chakra to allow blocked emotions to come out.
> *SUPPLEMENTS*—Power Meal, Super B, Super C / Super C Chewable.
> **BY FATHER**—<u>Forgiveness</u>, lavender, <u>Sacred Mountain</u> (empowers self).
> **BY MOTHER**—<u>Forgiveness</u>, geranium, lavender.

***COMMENTS**—*Refer to the page on Auricular Emotional Therapy in the Basic Information section of this book for the points where oils can be applied.*

FEELINGS OF REVENGE—<u>Forgiveness</u> (around navel), <u>Present Time</u> (on thymus), <u>Surrender</u> (on sternum over heart).

PROTECTION OR BALANCE—<u>Harmony</u> (over thymus; on energy centers/chakras), <u>White Angelica</u> (on shoulders).

SEXUAL/RITUAL—<u>Forgiveness</u> (around navel), <u>Harmony</u>, <u>Joy</u>, <u>Present Time</u>, <u>Release</u> (liver Vita Flex point on feet; under nose), sage, <u>SARA</u> (over area of abuse), <u>3 Wise Men</u>, <u>Trauma Life</u>, <u>Valor</u>, and <u>White Angelica</u>.

ESPOUSAL—<u>Acceptance</u>, <u>Envision</u>, <u>Forgiveness</u>, <u>Joy</u>, <u>Release</u>, <u>Trauma Life</u>, <u>Valor</u>.

SUICIDAL—<u>Brain Power</u>, <u>Hope</u> (on rim of ears), melissa, <u>Present Time</u>.

Accidents: *See Emotions.* <u>Trauma Life</u>.

Aches/Pains: Blue cypress, Balsam fir, <u>PanAway</u>, <u>Relieve It</u>, sage lavender. Vetiver & valerian together make a powerful pain killer as do palo santo and frankincense.

MASSAGE OILS—Ortho Ease or Ortho Sport (stronger). *These massage oils help seal in and enhance the effectiveness of the single oils or oil blends.*

SUPPLEMENTS—Sulfurzyme contains MSM which has been shown to be very effective in controlling pain, especially in the joints and tissues.

BLEND #1—20 valerian, 5 vetiver, 2 helichrysum, 1 clove, 1 peppermint. Combine this ratio (in drops) in a 5 ml bottle and then apply 3-6 drops of this blend on the back of the neck (up the cervical vertebrae - top of shoulders to base of skull) and work in with Vita Flex. *Working this into the brain stem helps stop pain and reduces the production of noradrenalin and cortisol.*

BONE—All the tree oils; **birch**, cedarwood, cypress, fir, helichrysum, juniper, <u>PanAway</u>, peppermint, sandalwood, spruce, **wintergreen**.

SUPPLEMENTS—Super Cal.

CHRONIC—Basil, birch, clove, cypress, cedarwood, elemi, fir, helichrysum, Idaho tansy, ginger, juniper, <u>PanAway</u> (add 1-2 drops birch for extra strength), peppermint, rosemary cineol, <u>Relieve It</u>, sandalwood, spruce, valerian, wintergreen.

BLEND #2—Equal parts of birch/wintergreen, elemi, and Idaho tansy.

MASSAGE OILS—Ortho Ease or Ortho Sport (stronger).

SUPPLEMENTS—Super Cal.

GENERAL—<u>Aroma Siez</u>, birch, Blue cypress, Balsam fir, frankincense, ginger, helichrysum, lavender, marjoram, <u>PanAway</u>, <u>Relieve It</u>, Roman chamomile, rosemary, sage lavender, **White fir** (pain from inflammation), wintergreen.

GROWING—Massage with birch/wintergreen, cypress, peppermint, wait 5 minutes and apply <u>PanAway</u>, then seal with Ortho Ease.

MASSAGE OILS—Ortho Ease.

SUPPLEMENTS—Sulfurzyme, Super Cal.

JOINTS—Birch (discomfort), Balsam fir, nutmeg, Roman chamomile (inflamed), spruce, wintergreen.

MUSCLE—<u>Aroma Siez</u>, ᶠbirch, basil, ᶠclove, Balsam fir, ginger, helichrysum, lavender, lemongrass (especially good for ligaments), marjoram, nutmeg, oregano, palo santo, <u>PanAway</u>, peppermint, <u>Relieve It</u>, Roman chamomile, rosemary verbenon, sage lavender, spearmint, spruce (torn muscles), thyme, vetiver, **White fir** (pain from inflammation), wintergreen.

SURGICAL—Valerian, vetiver, helichrysum, clove, and peppermint. Balsam fir and frankincense (equal parts); up to 3 droppers full in water 4 times daily. Also <u>GLF</u>, topically and internally 3-4 times daily.

    BLEND #3—20 valerian, 5 vetiver, 2 helichrysum, 1 clove, 1 peppermint. Combine this ratio of oils (in milliliters) in a 1 oz. dropper bottle. In post-surgical experiments, 3 droppers full of this blend have been taken in water (internally) up to 6 times daily for effective pain control.

TISSUE—Helichrysum, <u>PanAway</u>, <u>Relieve It</u> or Balsam fir (good for deep tissue pain).

Acidosis: *See Alkaline and pH Balance.*

Lemon, myrrh, peppermint, <u>Thieves</u> (dissolves and digests acid in the interstitial tissues).

SUPPLEMENTS—AlkaLime (acid neutralizing mineral), Balance Complete, Bodygize, Exodus (may increase oxygen), JuvaPower (loaded with acid-binding foods), Mineral Essence, Power Meal, Royaldophilus, VitaGreen (for alkaline/acid balance).

***COMMENTS**—Cancer and candida need an acid condition in order to thrive and spread. In acidic conditions, the oils will neutralize the acid, but are consumed in the process and are not able to perform their physiological functions. Increase your use of the oils and take other measures to reduce acid levels in the body.* **The body can only heal in an alkaline state**.

ACID-FORMING FOODS—Avoid meat, dairy products, whole wheat or rye bread, coffee, tea, wine, beer, root beer, cider, yeast products, soy sauce, cold cereals, potato chips, etc.

> *Acidosis is a condition of over-acidity in the blood and body tissues. When the body loses its alkaline reserve, pleomorphic virus, bacteria, yeast, and fungus take over and cause degenerative diseases such as, diabetes, cancer, AIDS, arteriosclerosis, arthritis, osteoporosis, chronic fatigue, etc.*
>
> ***Symptoms of acidosis** may include: frequent sighing, insomnia, water retention, recessed eyes, rheumatoid arthritis, migraine headaches, abnormally low blood pressure, and alternating constipation and diarrhea.*
>
> ***Causes of acidosis** may include: improper diet, kidney, liver, and adrenal disorders, emotional disturbances, fever, and an excess of niacin, vitamin C, and aspirin.*
>
> ***Oxygen** reduces the acidity of the blood. All essential oils contain oxygen. We like to flavor our water with 1-2 drops of lemon or peppermint oil. Lemon has the ability to counteract acidity in the body. The citric acid found in lemons is neutralized during digestion, giving off carbonates and bicarbonates of potassium and calcium, which helps maintain the alkalinity of the system.*

NEUTRALIZING FOODS—Raw apple cider vinegar is an acid neutralizer. Add a few drops of <u>Thieves</u> to 2 oz. of raw apple cider vinegar and drink in the morning and evening to help reduce acid levels in the body.

Acne: *See Hormonal Imbalance, Scarring, Skin, and Stress.* Bergamot, cedarwood, <u>Clarity</u> (on temples), Clary sage, clove, eucalyptus, *Eucalyptus radiata*, frankincense, <u>Gentle Baby</u>, geranium, ᶠGerman chamomile, ᶠjuniper, ᶠlavender, lemon, lemongrass, marjoram, melaleuca (Tea Tree), <u>Melrose</u>, myrtle, patchouli, petitgrain, <u>Purification</u>, <u>Raven</u>, ravensara, <u>RC</u>, rosemary, ᶠrosewood, sage, sage lavender, sandalwood, <u>Sensation</u>, spearmint, thyme, vetiver, yarrow. Apply one of the above oils on location or try putting about 10 drops of an oil into a small

PERSONAL CARE—A·R·T Skin Care System, Essential Beauty Serum - Acne-Prone Skin Blend, Prenolone/Prenolone+, Progessence, Rose Ointment, Sensation Massage Oil.

SUPPLEMENTS—ComforTone, Digest + Cleanse, ICP, Essentialzyme, JuvaTone, and Sulfurzyme. Cleansing the colon may help (*see Cleansing*).

ADULT ONSET—Prenolone/Prenolone+, Progessence if the acne stems from a hormonal imbalance.

CELLULAR REGENERATIVE—Palmarosa, rosewood.

HEALING—Use anti-bacterial and anti-inflammatory oils like geranium, melaleuca (Tea Tree), <u>Melrose</u>, and rosewood.

INFECTIOUS—Clove.

MENSTRUAL—Premenstrual or mid-menstrual cycle acne may be helped by balancing the hormones.

PERSONAL CARE—Prenolone/Prenolone+, Progessence.

SUPPLEMENTS—CortiStop (Women's), FemiGen, Super B.

TOXIN RELEASE—Use sudorific oils like chamomile, hyssop, juniper, lavender, rosemary, and thyme to help promote sweating.

> *Acne* is often a result of seborrhea (an overproduction of fat from the sebaceous glands), which can oftentimes be traced back to a hormonal imbalance. Stress is another reason for increased sebum production. Consequently, it may be of help to use oils that balance the hormones and reduce stress.
>
> Essential oil treatments combined with a good diet (lots of vegetables and lots of water), exercise, and increased lymphatic and circulatory flow, will allow the toxic wastes to leave the body as the oxygen and nutrients reach the skin in greater proportions.
>
> One of the best ways to release toxins through the skin is to sweat. Chamomile, hyssop, juniper, lavender, rosemary, and thyme contain sudorific properties and may facilitate the sweating process. The anti-bacterial and anti-inflammatory oils may assist in the healing process.

Acne Rosacea: *See Rosacea.*

ADD: *See Attention Deficit Disorder.*

Addictions: <u>Acceptance</u>, bergamot (helps with over indulgences), calamus (tobacco), <u>GLF</u>, <u>JuvaFlex</u>, <u>Peace & Calming</u>, <u>Purification</u>.

> *SUPPLEMENTS*—Digest + Cleanse, JuvaTone, Mineral Essence, Super C / Super C Chewable.

The following recipe has worked for individuals who are trying to break addictions:

> **RECIPE #1**—Use JuvaPower, JuvaTone, ComforTone, <u>JuvaFlex</u> and <u>Acceptance</u> together.

ALCOHOL—(to stop drinking) <u>Purification</u>, <u>Peace & Calming</u>. Do not use Clary sage and alcohol together; it may result in nightmares. *For professional assistance, contact the local chapter of Alcoholics Anonymous.*

COFFEE/TOBACCO—Bergamot, calamus. Apply to stomach, abdomen, liver area, and feet.

DRUGS—Basil, bergamot, birch, eucalyptus, fennel, grapefruit (withdrawal), lavender, marjoram, nutmeg, orange, <u>Peace & Calming</u>, <u>Purification</u>, Roman chamomile, sandalwood, wintergreen. Apply to Vita Flex points on feet.

> *SUPPLEMENTS*—Super C / Super C Chewable (at least 250 mg per day).

SMOKING—Use the above recipe. Applying either clove or <u>Thieves</u> to the tongue before lighting up helps remove the desire to smoke. Calamus may also help.

> ****COMMENTS**—*One individual used JuvaTone to break a habit of smoking 2 ½ packs of cigarettes a day for 20 years. It only took him three to five days!*

SUGAR—Dill, <u>Purification</u>, <u>Peace & Calming</u>. Apply to Vita Flex points on feet. Place dill on wrists to help remove addiction to sweets.

> *SUPPLEMENTS*—Allerzyme (aids the digestion of sugars, starches, fats, and proteins), Cleansing Trio (ComforTone, Essentialzyme, and ICP).

WITHDRAWAL—Dill, grapefruit, lavender, marjoram, nutmeg, orange, sandalwood. Apply to temples and diffuse. Applying dill to the wrists helps reduce the sweating that often accompanies withdrawal.

Addison's Disease: *See Adrenal Glands.*
<u>En-R-Gee</u>, <u>EndoFlex</u>, <u>Joy</u>, nutmeg (increases energy; supports adrenal glands), sage (combine with nutmeg).

> *Addison's Disease is an autoimmune disease where the body's own immune cells attack the adrenal glands and either severely limit or completely shut down the production of the adrenal cortex hormones. Extreme fluid and mineral loss are the life-threatening results.*

> *SUPPLEMENTS*—ImmuPro, Master Formula His/Hers, Mineral Essence (help supplement mineral loss), **Sulfurzyme** (shown to slow or reverse autoimmune diseases), Super B, VitaGreen.

Adenitis: *See Lymphatic System.* Garlic, onion, pine, rosemary, sage.

> *Adenitis is an acute or chronic inflammation of the lymph glands or nodes. Drink a lot of water to help remove the toxins from the body.*

Adrenal Glands: *See Endocrine System, Lupus, Thyroid.* <u>EndoFlex</u>, <u>En-R-Gee</u>, <u>Forgiveness</u>, <u>Joy</u>, nutmeg (increases energy; supports adrenal glands).

> *BLEND*—Add 3 drops clove, 4 nutmeg, and 6 rosemary to 1 tsp. V-6 Mixing Oil. Apply 4-5 drops of this mixture to kidney areas and cover with hot compress. Also apply 1-2 drops of mixture to Vita Flex kidney points on the feet and work

STIMULANT— [F]Basil, clove, geranium, pine, rosemary, [F]sage.

STRENGTHEN—Spruce (Black), peppermint.

UNDERACTIVE ADRENALS—*See Addison's Disease.*

    SUPPLEMENTS—Thyromin (1-4 tablets daily. *See Suggested Use under Thyromin in the Supplements section of the Reference Guide for Essential Oils*.) Also Master Formula His/Hers, Mineral Essence, Super B, and VitaGreen.

> *The **adrenal glands** are made up of an inner part (medulla) and an outer part (cortex). The outer portion (or cortex) produces critical steroid hormones, including glucocorticoids and aldosterone. These hormones directly affect blood pressure and mineral content. They also help regulate the conversion of carbohydrates into energy. Nutmeg displays similar properties and is contained in EndoFlex.*
>
> *When the adrenal glands are working properly, it is easier to correct low thyroid function.*

Aftershave: *See Skin.* Valor. Awaken can be used instead of aftershave lotion. Try adding Awaken to Sandalwood Moisture Creme, Satin Hand & Body Lotion, Sensation Hand & Body Lotion, or Genesis Hand & Body Lotion as an aftershave.

    PERSONAL CARE—Genesis Hand & Body Lotion, KidScents Lotion (soothes and rehydrates the skin–smells great too), Prenolone/Prenolone+, Rose Ointment, Sandalwood Moisture Creme, Satin Hand & Body Lotion, Sensation Hand & Body Lotion.

Agent Orange Poisoning: GLF or JuvaFlex (over liver with hot compress), EndoFlex (over adrenal glands/kidneys).

> *Agent Orange is a toxic herbicide that was used to defoliate areas of the forest during the Vietnam War.*

    BATH—in 1 cup Epsom salts and 4 oz. of food grade hydrogen peroxide.

    SUPPLEMENTS—Balance Complete, ComforTone, Digest + Cleanse, Essentialzyme, ICP, ImmuneTune, ImmuPro, Thyromin.

    RECIPE #1—3 drops EndoFlex on throat, feet (under big toes and kidney Vita Flex point). Also across the back over the kidneys. After 90 days, start the Cleansing Trio (ComforTone, Essentialzyme, and ICP) and continue for one year.

    RECIPE #2—3 ImmuneTune four times a day, 2 Thyromin at bedtime. After 90 days, start on Cleansing Trio (ComforTone, Essentialzyme, and ICP) and continue for one year.

Aging: *See Wrinkles.* Carrot, frankincense, Longevity (take as a dietary supplement to help prevent premature aging), rosehip, rosewood, sandalwood.

    SUPPLEMENTS—Berry Young Juice, Longevity Capsules, **NingXia Red**.

MOISTURIZERS—

    PERSONAL CARE—A·R·T Skin Care System (builds collagen, repairs DNA damage, and smooths wrinkles), Boswellia Wrinkle Creme, Essential Beauty Serums (Dry, Oily & Acne-Prone Skin Blends), Satin Facial Scrub - Mint, Prenolone/Prenolone+, Progessence, Rose Ointment, Sandalwood Moisture Creme, Sensation Hand & Body Lotion, Wolfberry Eye Creme.

SUPPLEMENTS—Essentialzyme, Mineral Essence (antioxidant), Wolfberry Crisp Bars
(Refer to the Wolfberry Crisp Bar in the Supplements section of the <u>Reference Guide for Essential Oils</u> for more information on the benefits of the Ningxia Wolfberry).

Agitation: ^FBergamot, cedarwood, <u>Chivalry</u>, Clary sage, <u>Forgiveness</u>, frankincense, geranium, <u>Harmony</u>, <u>Joy</u>, juniper, lavender, marjoram, myrrh, <u>Peace & Calming</u>, rose, rosewood, sandalwood, <u>Transformation</u>, <u>Trauma Life</u> (calms), <u>Valor</u>, ylang ylang.

AIDS: <u>Brain Power</u>, cistus, cumin (supports immune system; inhibits HIV virus), <u>Exodus II</u>, helichrysum, <u>ImmuPower</u>, lemon, nutmeg, <u>Thieves</u>, <u>Valor</u>. Apply to Thymus and bottom of feet.
SUPPLEMENTS—Balance Complete, Cleansing Trio (ComforTone, Essentialzyme, and ICP), Digest + Cleanse, Exodus, ImmuneTune, ImmuPro, Mineral Essence, NingXia Red, Power Meal (contains wolfberry which is an immune stimulator), Super B, Super C / Super C Chewable, Thyromin, Ultra Young, VitaGreen.
***COMMENTS—*Refer to the chapter entitled "How to Use - The Personal Usage Reference" in the <u>Essential Oils Desk Reference</u> under "AIDS" for specific oil blend and supplement recommendations.*

Airborne Bacteria: Cinnamon bark, fir, Balsam fir, Mountain savory, oregano, <u>Purification</u>, and <u>Thieves</u>.

> *Diffusing essential oils in the home or work place is one of the best ways to purify our environment. The anti-viral, anti-bacterial, and antiseptic properties of the oils, along with the negative ions and oxygenating molecules that are released when essential oils are diffused, all help to reduce chemicals, bacteria, and metallics in the air.*
>
> *Cinnamon bark, Mountain savory, oregano, and <u>Thieves</u> were all tested by Weber State University and were shown to kill 100% of the airborne bacteria present. This was all done by diffusing the oils into the atmosphere.*
>
> *(KID-Radio with Lance Richardson and Dr. Gary Young, N.D., Aromatologist, March 5, 1996)*

Air Pollution: <u>Abundance</u>, <u>Christmas Spirit</u>, cypress, eucalyptus, fir, grapefruit, <u>ImmuPower</u>, lavender, lemon (sterilize air), lime, <u>Purification</u>, rosemary, <u>Thieves</u>.
DISINFECTANTS—Birch, citronella, clove, eucalyptus, grapefruit, ^Flemon, peppermint, <u>Purification</u>, sage, spruce, wintergreen.

Alcoholism: *See Addictions.* Fennel, juniper, and rosemary (<u>Alternative Medicine—A Definitive Guide</u>, p. 492). Can also use <u>Acceptance</u>, elemi, <u>Forgiveness</u>, <u>GLF</u>, helichrysum, <u>Joy</u>, <u>JuvaFlex</u>, lavender, <u>Motivation</u>, orange, Roman chamomile, rosemary verbenon, <u>Transformation</u>, <u>Surrender</u>.
SUPPLEMENTS—Mineral Essence, Power Meal, Thyromin. Work on cleaning out the colon and liver with Balance Complete or the Cleansing Trio, Digest + Cleanse, JuvaPower/JuvaSpice, and JuvaTone or the Master Cleanser (*see Cleansing*).

Alertness: Basil, <u>Citrus Fresh</u>, <u>Clarity</u>, lemon, peppermint, rosemary. Apply to temples and bottom of feet.

Alkaline: *See Acidosis, pH Balance.*

> *Alkaline refers to a substance or solution that has a pH of 7.0 or above. The optimum pH for our blood and body tissues is about 7.2 (The use of saliva and urine test strips will show a much lower pH level due to the protein present in the solution. Saliva and urine tests from a healthy body should be about 6.6 to 6.8).*
>
> *The body heals best when it is slightly alkaline. To keep the blood and body tissue at an optimum pH, avoid acid-forming food. See Acidosis. Make sure your food intake is 80 percent alkaline and drink plenty of water.*

ALKALI-FORMING FOODS—Dark green and yellow vegetables, sprouted grains, legumes, seeds, nuts, essential fats (omega 3 and 6), and low sugar fruits like avocados and lemons.

PERSONAL CARE—Genesis Hand & Body Lotion balances pH on the skin.

SUPPLEMENTS—AlkaLime, JuvaPower (contains many acid-binding foods), Mineral Essence, Omega Blue (loaded with omega-3 fatty acids of EPA and DHA), Power Meal (pre-digested protein), Royaldophilus (replaces intestinal flora), VitaGreen (helps normalize blood pH levels).

Alkalosis: *See pH Balance.* Anise, <u>Di-Gize</u>, ginger, tarragon.

> *Alkalosis refers to a condition where the blood and intestinal tract becomes excessively alkaline. Slight alkalinity is important for a healthy body but excessive alkalinity can cause depression, fatigue, and sickness.*

SUPPLEMENTS—Bodygize, Digest + Cleanse, Essentialzyme, Mineral Essence, Power Meal (pre-digested protein), Royaldophilus (replaces intestinal flora), Sulfurzyme, VitaGreen (helps normalize blood pH levels).

Allergies: Elemi (rashes), eucalyptus, Harmony, [F]lavender, ledum, *Melaleuca ericifolia, Melaleuca quinquenervia*, melissa (skin and respiratory), [F]patchouli, peppermint, <u>ImmuPower</u>, <u>Raven</u>, <u>RC</u>, Roman chamomile, spikenard. Apply to sinuses, bottom of feet, and diffuse.

> *If you have a reaction to the oils, it is only a reaction to all of the chemicals you have been dumping into your body throughout the years. The oils are merely reacting with the toxins in the sub-dermal tissues and beginning their removal. **Cleanse the body!***

***COMMENTS—*According to the <u>Essential Oils Desk Reference</u>, ". . . rub three drops [<u>Harmony</u>] on sternum, breathing deeply." (EDR-June 2002)*

SUPPLEMENTS—AlkaLime, ComforTone, ICP fiber beverage (beneficial when there is an allergy to psyllium), ImmuneTune, ImmuPro, Mineral Essence, Super C / Super C Chewable, Super Cal.

COUGHING—<u>Purification</u> (diffuse).

HAY FEVER—*See Hay Fever.*

PSYCHOLOGICAL ALLERGIES (IN THE MIND)—Put <u>Harmony</u> on feet, neck, navel, or in your shoes for one to five days.

To Oils—Put one drop of the oil, to which there is an allergy reaction, on a cotton ball and place it in a shoe. Add a drop each day until the allergy to that particular oil is gone. Since allergies often indicate an electrical imbalance, try the following:

    A. Place a drop or two of <u>Harmony</u> into one hand, then rub the palms of both hands together in a clockwise motion.

    B. Place one hand over the thymus (heart chakra) and the other hand over the navel.

    C. Take three deep breaths and switch hands, then take three more deep breaths. <u>Harmony</u> helps open the energy meridians and balance the bio-electric field of the body.

The following recipes have been used for allergies:

    Recipe #1—Apply 1 drop of peppermint on the base of the neck two times a day. Tap the thymus (located just below the notch in the neck) with pointer and index fingers (energy fingers). Diffuse peppermint. For some individuals, the use of peppermint oil has resulted in no more allergy shots!

    Recipe #2—Apply 1 drop of <u>RC</u> and <u>Raven</u> on the base of the neck two times a day. Tap on thymus, massage chest and back with 5 <u>Raven</u>, 5 <u>RC</u>, and 2 tsp. V-6 Mixing Oil. Diffuse <u>RC</u> and <u>Raven</u>.

    Recipe #3—For allergy rashes and skin sensitivity, Dr. Gary Young applies 3 lavender, 6 Roman chamomile, 2 myrrh, and 1 peppermint on location.

Alone (feeling): *See Emotions.* <u>Acceptance</u>, <u>Valor</u>.

Alopecia Areata: (Inflammatory hair-loss disease) *See Hair: Loss.*

Aluminum Toxicity: *See Attention Deficit Disorder.* <u>Juva Cleanse</u>.
    SUPPLEMENTS—Chelex helps remove aluminum from the body.

> *Aluminum toxicity may contribute to the cause of colic, rickets, kidney and liver dysfunction, speech and memory problems, osteoporosis, and Alzheimer's disease.*

Alzheimer's Disease: *See Brain, Memory, Pineal Gland, Pituitary Gland.*
    SUPPLEMENTS—Chelex, Cleansing Trio (ComforTone, Essentialzyme, and ICP), Digest + Cleanse, JuvaTone, Omega Blue, Power Meal, Sulfurzyme.
    ***COMMENTS—*The gingko biloba that is found in Power Meal has been shown to help improve memory loss, brain function, depression, cerebral and peripheral circulation, oxygenation, and blood flow.*

> *Autopsies have revealed that victims of **Alzheimer's disease** have four times the normal amount of aluminum in the nerve cells of their brain.*
>
> ***Prevention:*** *Use glass, iron, or stainless steel cookware. Avoid products containing aluminum, bentonite, or dihydroxyaluminum. Some of these products are: aluminum cookware, foil, antacids, baking powders, buffered aspirin, most city water, antiperspirants, deodorants, beer, bleached flour, table salt, tobacco smoke, cream of tartar, Parmesan and grated cheeses, aluminum salts, douches, and canned goods.*

BLOOD-BRAIN BARRIER—Studies have shown that sesquiterpenes can pass the blood-brain barrier. Oils that are high in sesquiterpenes include cedarwood, vetiver, sandalwood, Black pepper, patchouli, myrrh, ginger, German chamomile, spikenard, galbanum, and frankincense. Some essential oil blends containing some of these oils include: 3 Wise Men, Acceptance, Brain Power, Forgiveness, Gathering, Harmony, Inspiration, Into the Future, Transformation, and Trauma Life. Apply to temples, bottom of feet, and diffuse.

   ***COMMENTS—*Oils that pass through the blood-brain barrier cannot carry unwanted substances with them.*

BRAIN FUNCTION—Clarity, Omega Blue.

EMOTIONS—Acceptance, cypress, Peace & Calming, 3 Wise Men (crown).

Amino Acids: Lavender.

   SUPPLEMENTS—Bodygize, Cleansing Trio (ComforTone, Essentialzyme, and ICP), Exodus, FemiGen, JuvaTone, KidScents Mighty Mist/Vites, Master Formula His/Hers, Mineral Essence, NingXia Red (18 amino acids in whole food form), Power Meal, Pure Protein Complete (has a complete array of ultra-bioactive amino acids), Thyromin.

> *Amino acids have the ability to neutralize and help eliminate free radicals in the system.*

Amnesia: *See Memory.* Basil, clove, rosemary.

Analgesic: Bergamot, birch, clove, eucalyptus, geranium, helichrysum, lavender, lemongrass, marjoram, melaleuca, oregano, PanAway, peppermint, Roman chamomile, rosemary, wintergreen.

   ***COMMENTS—*See the "Single Oil Property Chart" in the Appendix of this book for additional analgesic oils and their strengths.*

Anemia: Carrot, ImmuPower, Juva Cleanse, lavender, ᶠlemon. Apply to bottom of feet and stomach.

   FOOD—Flavor water with a drop of lemon. Can also use an H2Oils packet of lemon to infuse the drinking water with lemon oil.

   SUPPLEMENTS—Rehemogen tincture (10 drops twice a day) and JuvaTone together help raise blood cell count.

Anesthesia: *See Analgesic.* Clove, helichrysum, PanAway.

   ***COMMENTS—*One individual applied helichrysum every 15 minutes during gum surgery and there was no bleeding and no pain. No other anesthetic was used.*

Aneurysm: *See Blood.* Aroma Life (chelates plaque), cypress (strengthens the capillary walls and increases circulation), frankincense, helichrysum, Idaho tansy. Apply to temples, heart, Vita Flex heart points, and diffuse.

BLEND—5 frankincense, 1 helichrysum, and 1 cypress. **Diffuse**.
HERBS—Cayenne pepper, Garlic, Hawthorn Berry.
MASSAGE OIL—Cel-Lite Magic dilates blood vessels for better circulation.
SUPPLEMENTS—Cleansing Trio (ComforTone, Essentialzyme, and ICP), Sulfurzyme,
    Super C / Super C Chewable.
TINCTURES—HRT.

Anger: *See Liver*. Australian Blue, Bergamot, cedarwood, cypress, Forgiveness, frankincense,
    geranium, German chamomile, Grounding, Joy, Harmony, helichrysum, Hope,
    Humility, Inspiration, lavender, lemon, mandarin, marjoram, melissa, myrrh
    (soothes), myrtle, orange, Peace & Calming, petitgrain, Present Time, Release,
    Roman chamomile, rose, Sacred Mountain, sandalwood, Surrender, Trauma Life,
    Valor, ylang ylang.
***COMMENTS—*Refer to the Emotional Release part of the Science and Application section of
    the* Reference Guide for Essential Oils.
CALMS ANGER—Australian Blue, Inspiration, Peace & Calming, spruce, Trauma Life.
CLEANSING AFTER ARGUMENT AND PHYSICAL FIGHTING—Eucalyptus.
CLEANSE THE LIVER—(Anger is stored in the liver) JuvaFlex, ᶠgeranium (cleanses and detoxifies
    the liver), GLF, grapefruit (liver disorders).
DISPELS ANGER—Ylang ylang.
FOR COMMUNICATION WITHOUT ANGER—Roman chamomile.
LESSENS ANGER—Myrrh.
OVERCOME—Bergamot, ᶠcedarwood, Release, Roman chamomile.
RELEASES LOCKED UP ANGER AND FRUSTRATION—Roman or German chamomile, Release (together
    with JuvaFlex), Sacred Mountain, sandalwood, Surrender, Transformation, Valor.
SUPPLEMENTS—JuvaTone, Thyromin, Super B.
BLEND—4 drops lavender, 3 geranium, 3 rosewood, 3 rosemary, 2 tangerine, 1 spearmint,
    2 Idaho tansy, 1 German chamomile, and 1 oz. V-6 Mixing Oil. Apply to back of
    neck, wrist, and heart.

Angina: Aroma Life, ᶠginger, laurel, ᶠorange
    (for false angina). Apply to heart
    and Vita Flex heart point.
TINCTURES—HRT.

Angina pectoris is a severe spasmodic pain in the chest that is due to an insufficient supply of blood to the heart.

Animals: Only a 1-2 drops of oil is all that is necessary on animals as they respond much more
    quickly to the oils than do humans. V-6 Mixing Oil can be added to extend oil
    over larger areas and to heavily dilute the essential oil for use on smaller animals,
    especially cats.
PERSONAL CARE—Animal Scents Pet Shampoo, Animal Scents Pet Ointment. Other
    alkaline shampoos without chemicals are good for animals.

SUPPLEMENTS—BLM (added to their food, can help speed the healing of bones), Power Meal and Sulfurzyme.

BLEEDING—Geranium, helichrysum.

BONES (PAIN)—Birch/wintergreen, lemongrass, <u>PanAway</u> , spruce.

MASSAGE OILS—Ortho Ease or Ortho Sport.

SUPPLEMENTS—BLM (added to their food, can help speed the healing of bones), Power Meal and Sulfurzyme.

CALM—<u>Citrus Fresh</u>, lavender, <u>Peace & Calming</u>, Roman chamomile (for horses, add to feed), <u>Trauma Life</u>. Dilute well for cats.

CANCER—

SKIN—Frankincense and cumin.

CATS—Valerie Worwood says that you can treat a cat like you would a child (*see Babies*). Dilute oils heavily with V-6 Mixing Oil. Avoid melaleuca.

***COMMENTS—*Cat physiology is so different from other animals and from humans that oils should be used with extreme caution on cats. In fact, melaleuca (or Tea Tree oil) should never be used on a cat as death can result. Some cases exist where a blend of oils containing melaleuca have killed cats.*

COLDS AND COUGHS—Eucalyptus, melaleuca (not for cats). Apply on fur or stomach.

COWS—For scours, use 5 drops <u>Di-Gize</u> on stomach (can mix with V-6 Mixing Oil to cover larger area) and repeat 2 hours later.

I have a large brown tabby cat that was limping bad so I took him to the vet. The vet said he had a knee injury (he compared it to a football player's injured knee–"Cruciate Ligament Rupture") and said it would need surgery. He wanted me to bring my cat back in a week to see his son (who is also a vet) to make arrangements for the surgery. Later, using V-6 as my carrier oil and a couple drops of lavender oil, I rubbed my cat from the bottom of the paw up to his hip area. The next day I could see an improvement, and by the time I took him back to the vet he was walking on his leg with only a slight limp. The vet said he would heal nicely on his own and there would be no need for surgery. Today he walks, runs and is even now jumping with no problems.

-Submitted by M. Rynicki (July 2004)

One Saturday in February, my husband woke me up by yelling from the living room for me to bring my oils and any oil books I had at hand to him immediately. Our dog, Buddy, (a mutt from the pound, age approx. 7+ years) was lying on the floor and all of his muscles were completely seized up and tensed to the point where we couldn't move any part of his body. I had most of my oils in my large case and the Higley reference guide at my side. I put 4 or 5 drops of lavender oil in my husband's hand and he put that on Buddy's paws, ears and all over his back and legs, anywhere he was tense that we could reach. We followed the lavender with Peace & Calming, Valor and frankincense applied the same way. Those four were the oils I was drawn to by instinct. We massaged him and continued to stroke and pet him during and after the application of oils and after about 10 minutes he was able to get up and go to the door to go outside and run around. In between applying oils I looked up the info on animals as well as the info on seizures and strokes (we weren't sure what kind of episode he was having), just to make sure my instincts were near to on target (which they were). We had plans to travel about an hour out of town to visit with family, and kept Buddy with us the whole day just to be sure he was ok. When I tell this story to other people they tell me about how their dog(s) had seizures and had to be put on steroids and eventually put down because of the seizures. I am very thankful for Young Living and the oils that allowed me to go the natural route for the care of our dog.

-Submitted by A. Cornn
Machesney Park, Illinois (July 2004)

CUTS AND SORES—<u>Melrose</u> (not on cats). 1 drop on location. Work in with finger.

DOGS—There was a dog that walked with its head down and its tail between its legs. <u>Valor</u> was put on its feet and <u>3 Wise Men</u> and <u>Joy</u> on its crown. The next day its head was up and it was happy.

ANXIETY/NERVOUSNESS— Lavender, <u>Peace & Calming</u>, valerian, <u>Valor</u>. Rub 1-2 drops between hands and apply to muzzle, between toes, on top of feet to smell when nose is down, and on edge of ears.

ARTHRITIS—A blend of rosemary, lavender, and ginger diluted with V-6 Mixing Oil. Ortho Ease Massage Oil can also be applied to arthritic areas. Add Sulfurzyme (powder) or Vitamin C to their food.

BONE INJURY—Birch/wintergreen and Ortho Ease Massage Oil on injury. Sulfurzyme and BLM in food.

CHEWING ON FURNITURE—Mineral Essence (helps satisfy mineral deficiency).

DIGESTION—Essentialzyme.

HEART PROBLEMS—Myrtle, ravensara, and <u>Thieves</u> on back using Raindrop Technique with warm wet pack. Peppermint on paws. HRT Tincture can be added to food.

LIMPING—Sulfurzyme (powder with food).

PAIN AND STRESS—Do Raindrop Technique (*the video "Essential Tips for Happy, Healthy Pets" demonstrates this technique on a dog and a horse*). This technique helps relieve stress on the back, shoulders, and legs as well as raise immune function and protect against illness.

SLEEP—Lavender (on paws), <u>Peace & Calming</u> (on stomach).

STROKE—<u>Brain Power</u> (on head), frankincense (on brain stem/back of neck), <u>Valor</u> (on each paw).

TICKS AND BUG BITES— <u>Purification</u>. 1 drop directly on live tick. Can also be applied to untreated tick wound and worked in with finger.

> I went to visit my son in Ft. Lauderdale, FL... and was also happy to see his dog, Luna, who I've known for 7 years since she was a puppy. I could tell she was in pain, as she was not as active as usual and was limping. My son, Jason, told me that she is part German Shepherd-a breed that is prone to hip dysplasia. It broke my heart to see her in such pain. Jason had been giving her various vitamins and other supplements for several months, without much success. I myself have had success with Sulfurzyme for an arthritic knee, and asked if he would like to try that for Luna. We began to give her 1/4 tsp. twice a day with her meals. Within two days, we began to see a change. My son was amazed! As the two weeks passed while I was visiting, we saw a huge change. She was running like her old self, and you could sense that the pain was almost (if not totally) gone. Within a month, Jason told me that she was now even jumping up on furniture, which she was unable to do when we started with the Sulfurzyme. That was 18 months ago, and Luna is still taking Sulfurzyme... and still doing great!
>
> *-Submitted by Linda Griffith Dixon, New Mexico (July 2004)*

TRAVEL SICKNESS—Peppermint. Dilute with V-6 Mixing Oil and rub on stomach. Also helps calm stomachaches.

TRAUMATIZED—<u>Trauma Life</u>. Rub 1-2 drops between hands and cup over nose and mouth for dog to inhale.

EARACHE—1 drop <u>Melrose</u> or a blend of 1 drop melaleuca (Tea Tree), 1 lavender, and 1 Roman chamomile diluted in V-6 Mixing oil. Put in ear and rub around the ear.

EAR INFECTIONS—<u>ImmuPower</u>, <u>Purification</u> (helps ward off insects too). Dip cotton swab in oil and apply to inside and front of ear.

FLEAS—Citronella, eucalyptus, lemongrass, <u>Melrose</u>, pine. Add 1-2 drops of oil to shampoo.
> *BLEND*—Combine eucalyptus, orange, citronella, and cedarwood. Add blend to distilled water in a spray bottle, shake well, and mist over entire animal.

HORSES—
> ANXIETY/NERVOUSNESS—<u>Peace & Calming</u>. Rub 1-2 drops between hands and apply to nose, on front of chest, knees, and tongue.
>
> FLIES—Idaho Tansy Floral Water. Spray over animal to keep flies away.
>
> HOOF ROT—Blend of Roman chamomile, thyme, and melissa in V-6 Mixing Oil.
>
> INFECTION—<u>Melrose</u>, <u>Thieves</u>.
>
> INJURIES—Do Raindrop Technique (*the video "Essential Tips for Happy, Healthy Pets" demonstrates this technique on a dog and a horse*). When a frisky race horse took a fall and was unable to walk, application of the oils using the Raindrop Technique brought the horse out of it in a matter of days.
>
> LEG FRACTURES—Ginger and V-6 Mixing Oil. Wrap the leg with a hot compress. Massage leg after the fracture is healed with a blend of rosemary and thyme with V-6 Mixing Oil. This may strengthen the ligaments and prevent calcification.
>
> MUSCLE TISSUE/LIGAMENTS—Equal parts lemongrass and lavender on location and wrap to help regenerate torn muscle tissue.

WOUNDS—Helichrysum, <u>Melrose</u>, and Rose Ointment.

I have a 21 year old gelding who was diagnosed with "kidney colic" back in January. He would be down one day, up the next, down the next, up for several days, down again, etc. He would show all the general signs of colic but was also wanting to urinate frequently, passing little or nothing. This went on for about four weeks, and the vet thought he probably was trying to pass kidney stones. Since it was happening so often, I was wanting something to give him for the pain instead of using Banamine so much. I had used marjoram, clary sage and lavender successfully on an intestinal colic, so I tried them, but they just didn't work as well on the kidneys. So I tried Juva-Flex, and the results were dramatic! Four drops over each kidney, with or without a warm compress, would get him up and back to eating and drinking in 10-20 minutes. The pain-killing effects would last from 2-4 hours and seemed to be cumulative. After I had done this for two separate "episodes," the symptoms went away completely. I don't know if the stones dissolved or he passed them, but he's been pain free for six months.

-Submitted by Jan Early
Tallahassee, Florida (July 2004)

One couple had a horse that got kicked in the flank, creating a large wound. The Vet treated the wound and gave her some medication. Unfortunately, the wound became reinfected and worsened to the point that the horse almost died. The Vet came over and reopened the wound and flushed out nearly two gallons of blood clots. However, the Vet had no medication with him and would not be able to deliver any more for a couple of days. So, the wife put 15 drops of <u>Thieves</u> *in about ¼ cup of olive oil and while the husband held open the horse's mouth, she poured the oil down its throat. This was repeated three or four times and within just a few days, the horse was fully recovered.*

SADDLE SORES—<u>Melrose</u> and Rose Ointment.

INFECTION—<u>Di-Gize</u> and <u>ImmuPower</u> on the paws.

PARASITES—Cedarwood, lavender, <u>Di-Gize</u>. Rub on paws to release parasites.

SUPPLEMENTS—ParaFree.

SNAKE BITES (VENOMOUS WOUNDS)—Do Raindrop Technique (*the video "Essential Tips for Happy, Healthy Pets" demonstrates this technique on a dog and a horse*).

Anorexia: Angelica, <u>Christmas Spirt</u>, <u>Citrus Fresh</u>, coriander, grapefruit, <u>Purification</u>, <u>Melrose</u>, [F]tarragon, <u>Valor</u>. Apply to stomach and bottom of feet. It may also help to diffuse anti-depressant oils.

***COMMENTS—*Some studies have shown that people suffering from anorexia have a tendency to have lower levels of zinc.*

SUPPLEMENTS—Mineral Essence.

ANTI-DEPRESSANTS—<u>Acceptance</u>, basil, bergamot, Clary sage, lavender, neroli, Roman chamomile, ylang ylang.

Anthrax: [F]Thyme.

> *Anthrax is an infectious, fatal animal disease found in cows and sheep. It can be transmitted to human beings through contact with contaminated animal substances, such as hair, feces, or hides. It may also be used in biological warfare and is transmitted as spores through the air. It is characterized by ulcerative skin lesions.*

Anti-bacterial: Oils high in thymol (a phenol), such as [F]thyme and Mountain savory, tend to be highly anti-bacterial. Other effective, though less potent, anti-bacterial oils include [F]Basil, bergamot, cassia, cedarwood, citronella, <u>Christmas Spirit</u>, <u>Citrus Fresh</u>, [F]cinnamon bark, Clary sage, [F]clove, [F]cypress, <u>Egyptian Gold</u>, eucalyptus, <u>Evergreen Essence</u>, fir, geranium, grapefruit, Idaho tansy, juniper, lavender, lemon, marjoram, melaleuca, *Melaleuca ericifolia*, neroli, [F]oregano, palmarosa, petitgrain, pine, <u>Purification</u>, ravensara, <u>RC</u>, Roman chamomile, [F]rosemary, [F]rosewood, <u>Sacred Mountain</u>, [F]spearmint, tarragon, <u>Thieves</u> (annihilates bacteria), valerian, Western Red cedar.

***COMMENTS—*All oils are anti-bacterial; see the "Single Oil Property Chart" in the Appendix of this book for additional anti-bacterial oils and their strengths.*

AIRBORNE—*See Airborne Bacteria.*

Cinnamon bark, fir, Mountain savory, oregano, <u>Purification</u>, <u>Thieves</u>.

CLEANSING—<u>Purification</u>.

INFECTION—Nutmeg (fights).

PREVENTS GROWTH OF—Melrose.

> *Research at Weber State University has shown that out of 67 oils tested, 66 of them were powerful anti-bacterial agents. Oregano, cinnamon bark, Mountain savory, ravensara, and peppermint were all more powerful as anti-bacterial agents than Penicillin or Ampicillin. Thieves was shown to be 60 percent higher in activity against bacteria, germs, and anti-microbial action than either Ampicillin or Penicillin!*
>
> *(KID-Radio with Lance Richardson and Dr. Gary Young, N.D., Aromatologist, March 5, 1996)*

Anti-cancerous: Clove, frankincense, <u>ImmuPower</u>, ledum (may be more powerful than frankincense). Also, oils high in limonene (like grapefruit, tangerine, orange, palo santo, mandarin, fleabane, and lemon) have been shown to be effective in fighting cancer.

SUPPLEMENTS—Exodus, Power Meal, Sulfurzyme.

Anti-catarrhal: Black pepper, ^Fcypress, elemi, eucalyptus, ^Ffir, frankincense, ginger, ^Fhelichrysum (discharges mucus), hyssop (opens respiratory system and discharges toxins and mucous), jasmine, onycha (benzoin), RC, Raven, ravensara, rosemary, Thieves (dissolves excess mucus). Apply on lung area, feet, around nose, Vita Flex lung points, and diffuse.

***COMMENTS—See the "Single Oil Property Chart" in the Appendix of this book for additional anti-catarrhal oils and their strengths.*

Anti-coagulant: Angelica, cassia, ^Fhelichrysum, lavender, tangerine, tarragon. Apply on location, bottom of feet, and diffuse.

Anti-depressant: *See Depression.* Elemi, ^Ffrankincense, lavender, onycha (combine with rose for massage). Apply to bottom of feet, heart, and diffuse.

SUPPLEMENTS—Omega Blue

***COMMENTS—See the "Single Oil Property Chart" in the Appendix of this book for additional anti-depressant oils and their strengths.*

RECOVERY FROM COMMERCIAL ANTI-DEPRESSANTS LIKE PROZAC— Brain Power, Clarity, Joy, Peace & Calming, and Valor all help repair brain damage from the commercial drugs that inhibit serotonin metabolism. They also stimulate the pineal gland which normally metabolizes 50% of the serotonin in the body. The liver and pancreas are extremely toxic. Cleanse with GLF, JuvaPower, Juva Cleanse, and/or JuvaFlex. Coriander, dill and Thieves help regulate the blood sugar. Frankincense helps prevent cancer (risk of breast cancer increases by 7x with use of Paxil). Balsam fir helps to decrease the cortisol levels. Also focus on strengthening the smooth muscle tissues (especially heart and intestines) as they are contracted by the drugs.

SUPPLEMENTS—Carbozyme (to help control blood sugar levels), CortiStop (Women's), Digest + Cleanse, JuvaPower/JuvaSpice, Omega Blue, Power Meal.

Anti-fungal: Abundance, ^Fcinnamon bark, ^Fclove, Egyptian Gold, geranium, ImmuPower, juniper, lavender, lemon, lemongrass, mandarin, ^Fmelaleuca, *Melaleuca ericifolia*, Mountain savory, ^Foregano, palmarosa, ^Frosewood, sage, ^Fspearmint, ^Fthyme. Apply to bottom of feet, on location, and diffuse.

***COMMENTS—See the "Single Oil Property Chart" in the Appendix of this book for additional anti-fungal oils and their strengths.*

BLEND—2 myrrh and 2 lavender. Rub on location.

SUPPLEMENTS—AlkaLime, Essentialzyme, ICP.

Anti-hemorrhaging: *See Hemorrhaging.* Helichrysum, rose.

Anti-infectious: ^FBasil, cassia, ^Fcinnamon bark, clove, ^Fcypress, davana, elemi, eucalyptus, hyssop, Idaho tansy, ^Flavender, marjoram, melaleuca, *Melaleuca ericifolia*, **myrrh** (with oregano), ^Fpatchouli, petitgrain, ^Fpine, ^Fravensara, rose, ^Frosemary, ^Frosewood, Purification, Roman chamomile, spearmint, spikenard, ^Fspruce, tarragon, ^Fthyme. Apply on location and bottom of feet.

   ***COMMENTS—*See the "Single Oil Property Chart" in the Appendix of this book for additional anti-infectious oils and their strengths.*
   SUPPLEMENTS—Super C / Super C Chewable.

Anti-inflammatory: Oils high in carvacrol (a phenol), like oregano, Mountain savory, and thyme, are very effective as anti-inflammatory agents. Other effective oils include Balsam fir, ^Fbirch, Black pepper, Blue cypress, Blue tansy, calamus (gastrointestinal), citronella, coriander, cypress, eucalyptus, frankincense, ^FGerman chamomile, helichrysum, hyssop (of the pulmonary), ^Flavender, lemongrass, melaleuca, ^Fmyrrh, onycha (benzoin), palo santo, ^Fpatchouli, peppermint, petitgrain, ravensara, ^FRoman chamomile, spearmint, spikenard, ^Fspruce, tangerine, ^Ftarragon, and wintergreen. **Apply on location and to brain stem**. One study showed that oils which inhibit the production of nitric oxide (NO) could greatly reduce the resulting inflammation and tissue damage. The six oils which showed the greatest percentage of NO inhibition were oregano, nutmeg, lemongrass, *Melaleuca ericifolia*, dill and peppermint.

   ***COMMENTS—*See the "Single Oil Property Chart" in the Appendix of this book for additional anti-inflammatory oils and their strengths.*

Anti-parasitic: ^FCinnamon bark, clove, Di-Gize, fennel, ginger, hyssop, lemon, lemongrass, melaleuca, Mountain savory, oregano, ^FRoman chamomile, rosemary, rosewood, spearmint, spikenard, tarragon. Apply to stomach, liver, intestines, and Vita Flex points on feet.

   ***COMMENTS—*See the "Single Oil Property Chart" in the Appendix of this book for additional anti-parasitic oils and their strengths.*
   SUPPLEMENTS—Cleansing Trio (ComforTone, Essentialzyme, and ICP), Digest + Cleanse (contains oils that create an unfriendly environment for parasites), ImmuneTune, ParaFree.

Anti-rheumatic: Birch, eucalyptus, juniper, onycha (benzoin), oregano, rosemary, thyme, wintergreen.

   ***COMMENTS—*See the "Single Oil Property Chart" in the Appendix of this book for additional anti-rheumatic oils and their strengths.*

Anti-sexual: ^FMarjoram (helps balance sexual desires).

Anti-tumoral: Clove, [F]frankincense, ImmuPower, ledum (may be more powerful than frankincense).

Anti-viral: Melissa oil has shown some of the strongest anti-viral activity. Oils high in limonene (a monoterpene), like grapefruit, orange, tangerine, palo santo, mandarin, and lemon, are very effective anti-viral agents. Other effective anti-viral oils include Abundance, bergamot, [F]cinnamon bark, Clary sage, [F]clove, Egyptian Gold, *Eucalyptus radiata*, galbanum, geranium, hyssop, Idaho tansy, ImmuPower, juniper, lavender, [F]melaleuca, Mountain savory, myrrh, [F]oregano, palmarosa, pine, RC, [F]ravensara, [F]rosewood, sandalwood, tarragon, Thieves, and [F]thyme.

   ***COMMENTS—*See the "Single Oil Property Chart" in the Appendix of this book for additional anti-viral oils and their strengths. Dr. J. C. Lapraz found that viruses cannot live in the presence of cinnamon oil. However, because of its high phenol content, it must be diluted before being applied to the skin.*
   *SUPPLEMENTS—*ParaFree.

Antibiotic: Bergamot, cinnamon bark, clove, eucalyptus, frankincense, hyssop, lavender, lemon, melaleuca, Melrose, myrtle, nutmeg, oregano, patchouli, Purification, ravensara, Roman chamomile, Thieves, thyme. Apply on location, liver area, bottom of feet, and diffuse.

> *Dr. Terry Friedmann, MD would often recommend the following **Essential Oil Antibiotic Regimen**:*
>
> *In a "00" capsule put 12 drops of Thieves, 6 drops of oregano, and 2 drops of frankincense. Ingest one capsule every 4 hours for 3 days, then every 8 hours for 4 days.*

Antihistamine: Lavender, Roman chamomile. Apply to sinuses, Vita Flex points, and diffuse.

Antimicrobial: Abundance, cinnamon bark, cypress, helichrysum, jasmine, lavender, lemongrass, *Melaleuca ericifolia* (powerful), melissa (shown in lab tests to be effective against *Streptococcus haemolytica*), myrrh, palmarosa, pine, rosemary, rosewood, sage, thyme.

   ***COMMENTS—*See the "Single Oil Property Chart" in the Appendix of this book for additional antimicrobial oils and their strengths.*

Antioxidants: Cinnamon bark, Di-Gize, Exodus II, frankincense, helichrysum, hyssop, ImmuPower, JuvaFlex, melaleuca, Longevity (take as a dietary supplement to promote longevity), melaleuca, Melrose, onycha (benzoin), oregano, PanAway, Purification, ravensara, RC, Relieve It, Roman chamomile, Thieves, thyme.

> ***Antioxidants** create an unfriendly environment for free radicals. They prevent all mutations, work as free radical scavengers, prevent fungus, prevent oxidation in the cells, and help to oxygenate the cells.*

SUPPLEMENTS—Berry Young Juice, Essentialzyme, Exodus, ImmuneTune, JuvaTone, CardiaCare (with *Rhododendron caucasicum*), Longevity Capsules (contains clove oil, which has the highest known ORAC score, and thyme oil, which increases antioxidant levels in heart, liver, & kidneys and doubles antioxidant activity in the entire body), Master Formula His/Hers, Mineral Essence, NingXia Red (tested at Brunswick Laboratories with S-ORAC score of 363 per oz. The next closest "functional drink" competitor was tested at 8.6), Super C / Super C Chewable, Super B, VitaGreen, Wolfberry Crisp Bars (*Refer to the Wolfberry Crisp Bar in the Supplements section of the Reference Guide for Essential Oils for more information on the benefits of the Ningxia Wolfberry*).

TINCTURES—AD&E

Antiseptic: Bergamot, ᶠcedarwood, cinnamon bark, citronella, clove, cumin, Di-Gize (all oils in this blend are antiseptic), elemi, eucalyptus, Evergreen Essence, fennel, ᶠfir, Balsam fir, frankincense, lavender, lemon, mandarin, marjoram, melaleuca, Melrose, Mountain savory, mugwort, ᶠmyrtle (skin), ᶠnutmeg (intestinal), orange, onycha (benzoin), ᶠoregano, ᶠpatchouli, ᶠpeppermint, ᶠpine (pulmonary, urinary, hepatic), Purification, ravensara, Roman chamomile, rosemary cineol, rosemary verbenon, ᶠsage, ᶠsandalwood, ᶠspearmint, ᶠthyme, thyme linalol, Western Red cedar, ylang ylang. Apply on location.

   ***COMMENTS—*Most oils can be used as antiseptics. See the "Single Oil Property Chart" in the Appendix of this book for additional antiseptic oils and their strengths.*

PERSONAL CARE—Rose Ointment (apply over oils to increase antiseptic properties and extend effectiveness).

SUPPLEMENTS—Super C / Super C Chewable.

TINCTURES—AD&E.

Antispasmodic: Anise, ᶠ**basil**, calamus, citronella, cumin, fennel, ᶠGerman chamomile, helichrysum, ᶠlavender, mandarin, ᶠmarjoram, mugwort ᶠpeppermint, petitgrain, ᶠRoman chamomile (relaxes spastic muscles of the colon wall), ᶠrosemary, ᶠsage, spearmint, spikenard, ᶠspruce, tarragon, valerian, ylang ylang.

   ***COMMENTS—*See the "Single Oil Property Chart" in the Appendix of this book for additional antispasmodic oils.*

Anxiety: Basil, bergamot, cedarwood, Clary sage, cypress, Evergreen Essence, frankincense, geranium, hyssop, jasmine, juniper, lavender, lemon, lime, marjoram, melissa, onycha (combine with rose for massage), patchouli, pine, Release, Roman chamomile, rose, sandalwood, Surrender, tangerine, tsuga (grounding), ᶠylang ylang.

Apathy: Frankincense, geranium, <u>Harmony</u>, <u>Highest Potential</u>, <u>Hope</u>, jasmine, <u>Joy</u>, marjoram, orange, peppermint, rose, rosemary, rosewood, sandalwood, <u>3 Wise Men</u>, <u>Transformation</u>, thyme, <u>Valor</u>, <u>White Angelica</u>, ylang ylang.

Aphrodisiac: Cinnamon bark, Clary sage, ginger, jasmine, <u>Lady Sclareol</u>, patchouli, rose, ᶠsandalwood, <u>Sensation</u>, neroli, ylang ylang.
>   *BATH & SHOWER GELS*— Sensation Bath & Shower Gel.
>   *MASSAGE OILS*—Sensation Massage Oil.
>   *PERSONAL CARE*—Sensation Hand & Body Lotion.

> *Many books of aromatherapy tout the **aphrodisiac** qualities of a number of oils. Perhaps an aphrodisiac to one individual may not be to another. The most important factor is to find an oil that brings balance to the mind and body. A balanced individual is more likely to extend love.*

Apnea: <u>Brain Power</u>, <u>Clarity</u> (diffuse), <u>Raven</u>, RC, <u>Valor</u> (on feet).
>   *SUPPLEMENTS*—Super B, Thyromin, VitaGreen.
>   **RECIPE #1**—Try 3 VitaGreen twice per day, 1 Super B three times per day with meals, and 1 Thyromin before bed.

> ***Apnea*** *is the cessation of breathing. During sleep, periods of apnea can occur for a few seconds before breathing resumes. May be due to irregular heartbeats, high blood pressure, obesity, or damage to the area of the brain responsible for controlling respiration.*

Appetite-loss of: ᶠBergamot, calamus, cardamom, ginger, hyssop, lemon, myrrh, ᶠnutmeg, orange, spearmint. Apply to stomach, bottom of feet, and diffuse.
>   *SUPPLEMENTS*—ComforTone, Essentialzyme.

Appetite Suppressant:
>   *SUPPLEMENTS*—ThermaBurn (tablets).

Argumentative: <u>Acceptance</u>, cedarwood, <u>Chivalry</u>, eucalyptus, frankincense, <u>Harmony</u>, <u>Hope</u>, <u>Humility</u>, jasmine, <u>Joy</u>, orange, <u>Peace & Calming</u>, Roman chamomile, thyme, <u>Transformation</u>, <u>Trauma Life</u>, <u>Valor</u>, ylang ylang.

Arms-flabby: Cypress, fennel, juniper, lavender.

Arterial Vasodilator: <u>Aroma Life</u>, ᶠmarjoram. Apply to carotid arteries in neck, over heart, Vita Flex points on feet.

Arterial Walls: <u>Aroma Life</u> (strengthens).

Arteries: (blocked after surgery), <u>Aroma Life</u>, lavender, <u>Melrose</u>.
>   *MASSAGE OIL*—Cel-Lite Magic and drink Chamomile Tea.
>   *SUPPLEMENTS*—Cleansing Trio (ComforTone, Essentialzyme, and ICP).

Arteriosclerosis: *See Blood.* <u>Aroma Life</u>, birch, ^Fcedarwood, ginger, juniper, lemon (increase white and red blood cells), rosemary, thyme, wintergreen. Apply to heart and Vita Flex points on feet.

BLOOD CLOTS—(*See Blood*) Balsam fir, grapefruit, helichrysum.

SUPPLEMENTS—In addition to Vitamins E and C, all supplements containing essential oils should help increase the supply of oxygen in the blood stream. Rehemogen (tincture) together with JuvaTone may help build blood and hemoglobin platelets (raise cell count). ImmuneTune is good for building white blood cells.

Arthritis: *See Acidosis.* <u>Aroma Life</u>, <u>Aroma Siez</u>, basil, birch (drains toxins that cause pain), cedarwood, clove, ^Fcypress, eucalyptus, fir (has cortisone-like action), Balsam fir, ginger, <u>Harmony</u> (with <u>Valor</u>), helichrysum, hyssop, Idaho tansy, <u>ImmuPower</u>, lavender, ^Fmarjoram, <u>Melrose</u>, nutmeg, onycha (benzoin), palo santo, <u>PanAway</u>, <u>Peace & Calming</u>, peppermint, pine, <u>Purification</u>, Roman chamomile, ^Frosemary, sage lavender, ^Fspruce, <u>Valor</u>, white fir (has cortisone-like action), wintergreen (drains toxins that cause pain). Apply oils on location and diffuse.

BLEND #1—Combine 1 oz. Ortho Ease with 25 drops birch/wintergreen, 12 cypress, 9 Roman chamomile, and 3 juniper. Massage on location.

BLEND #2—Combine Ortho Ease with birch/wintergreen alone and apply on location.

BLEND #3—Birch/wintergreen with <u>PanAway</u>.

MASSAGE OILS—Ortho Ease.

PERSONAL CARE—Prenolone/Prenolone+, Progessence, Regenolone.

SUPPLEMENTS—AlkaLime, BLM, CardiaCare (with *Rhododendron caucasicum* which inhibits the enzyme hyaluronidase), Mineral Essence, NingXia Red, Power Meal (contains wolfberry), Sulfurzyme (contains wolfberry), Super C / Super C Chewable, Super Cal, Thyromin (improves thyroid function and energy levels), VitaGreen.

ARTHRITIC PAIN—Birch, ginger, palo santo, <u>PanAway</u>, spruce, wintergreen.

OSTEOARTHRITIS—Basil, birch, eucalyptus, lavender, lemon, marjoram, thyme, wintergreen.

> *Detoxify with cypress, fennel, and lemon. Massage affected joints with rosemary, chamomile, juniper and lavender (Alternative Medicine—A Definitive Guide, p. 537).*

RHEUMATOID—Angelica, ^Fbirch, ^Fbergamot, Black pepper, cajeput, cinnamon bark, coriander, ^Fcypress, eucalyptus, fennel, fir, Balsam fir, galbanum, geranium, ^Fginger, hyssop, juniper, lavender, ^Flemon, ^Fmarjoram, ^Fnutmeg, oregano (chronic), palo santo, <u>PanAway</u>, <u>Peace & Calming</u>, peppermint, ^Fpine, Roman chamomile, rosemary, ^Fspruce, tarragon, thyme, wintergreen.

PERSONAL CARE—Prenolone/Prenolone+, Progessence, Regenolone.

BLEND #4—Combine 2 oz. of Ortho Ease with 7 drops birch/wintergreen, 6 ginger, 19 eucalyptus, 6 juniper, 8 marjoram, and 3 peppermint. Rub on location.

Ashamed: *See Emotions.* <u>Acceptance</u>, <u>Forgiveness</u>, <u>Valor</u>.

Assault: *See Emotions.* Trauma Life.

Assimilating Food:

> *SUPPLEMENTS*—Enzyme products: Allerzyme (aids the digestion of sugars, starches, fats, and proteins), Carbozyme (aids in the digestion of carbohydrates), Detoxzyme (helps maintain and support a healthy intestinal environment), Essentialzyme, Lipozyme (aids the digestion of fats) and Polyzyme (aids the digestion of protein and helps reduce swelling and discomfort). Also Balance Complete, Digest + Cleanse, Power Meal (pre-digested protein) and Super B.

Asthma: *See Respiratory System.* Cajeput, calamus, Clary sage, cypress, ᶠeucalyptus, Evergreen Essence, fir, ᶠfrankincense (on crown), hyssop, laurel, lavender, ᶠlemon, ᶠmarjoram, myrrh, myrtle, onycha (benzoin), ᶠoregano, ᶠpeppermint, ᶠpine, Raven (diffuse), ravensara, RC (some people use RC or Raven instead of inhaler), rose, rosemary, ᶠsage, sage lavender, ᶠthyme, tsuga (opens respiratory tract). Avoid steam inhalation. Apply topically over lungs and throat. Drop on pillow or diffuse. May insert RC and Raven with 1 tsp. V-6 Mixing Oil in rectum, **or** Raven rectally with RC on chest and back; reverse each night, **or** *Eucalyptus radiata* and frankincense in rectum.

> ***COMMENTS—**Plastic nasal inhalers** *work very well for this purpose. Nasal inhaler blanks (empty inhalers) are available from Abundant Health to fill with your choice of oil. Just saturate an absorbent wick with the essential oil or blend, insert into the inhaler blank and plug the end. Then, just unscrew the cap, place inhaler next to or inside each nostril and breathe deeply. Replace the cap to prevent evaporation.* ***These are great to take on airplanes instead of the messy, bulky oil bottles.***

> BLEND #1—Combine 10 drops cedarwood, 10 eucalyptus, 2 Roman chamomile, and 2 oz. water. Put on hanky and inhale. Can also be used to gargle.

> BLEND #2—Combine 10 drops Raven, 5 hyssop, and 2 tsp. V-6 Mixing Oil. Massage on spine and chest.

> *PERSONAL CARE*—Prenolone/Prenolone+.

> *SUPPLEMENTS*—ImmuneTune (drainage), Super C / Super C Chewable, Thyromin.

> ***COMMENTS—*Do a colon and liver cleanse with either the* **master cleanser** *(see Cleansing) or the Cleansing Trio supplements (ComforTone, ICP, Essentialzyme) and JuvaTone.*

> ATTACK—RC or Raven. Just smelling from bottle has stopped attacks.

> RECIPE #1—3 Wise Men on crown, Raven on throat, RC on lungs, Thieves on feet, ImmuPower on spine. May insert RC and Raven with V-6 Mixing Oil in rectum, **or** Raven rectally with RC on chest and back; reverse each night.

> RECIPE #2—Inhale or diffuse bergamot, eucalyptus, hyssop, lavender, or marjoram. Try frankincense for calming. (Alternative Medicine—The Definitive Guide, p. 824).

> RECIPE #3—Apply frankincense to the crown, RC on the throat and chest and Raven on the back. Then, inhale the aroma of the oils from your hands.

Astringent: Lemon, onycha (benzoin).

Athletes Foot: Cajeput, cypress, *Eucalyptus citriodora*, geranium, lavender, ᶠmelaleuca, myrrh, thyme.
> *BLEND*—Combine 2 oz. of Genesis Hand & Body Lotion with 10 drops thyme, 10 lavender, and 10 melaleuca. Rub on feet.

Attention Deficit Disorder (ADD): *See Hyperactivity.* Ledum.
> *BLEND*—Lavender with basil (on crown), Harmony, or Peace & Calming; Basil with Clarity; Frankincense with Valor. Apply 1-3 drops of any of these blends on the bottom of the feet and on the spine; Diffuse.
> *MASSAGE, BATH, DIFFUSE*—Citrus Fresh, lavender.
> *SUPPLEMENTS*—Allerzyme (aids the digestion of sugars, starches, fats, and proteins), Chelex, Digest + Cleanse, Mineral Essence, NingXia Red (provides a full range of vitamins, trace minerals, amino acids, and essential fatty acids), Omega Blue (absolutely necessary).
> CHELATING AGENT—Helichrysum.
> SLEEPING—Diffuse either Peace & Calming or Gentle Baby.
> ****COMMENTS*—Avoid sweeteners such as sugar and corn syrup. Eliminate caffeine and food additives from diet. Individuals who have ADD often have high aluminum toxicity. Chelex may help remove aluminum from the body.*

Aura: Awaken, Joy, Sacred Mountain, White Angelica.
> INCREASE AURA AROUND BODY—White Angelica (use with Awaken and Sacred Mountain).
> PROTECTION OF—White Angelica.
> STRENGTHEN—White Angelica.

Autism:
> REDUCE ANXIETY/FEAR—Bergamot, geranium, and Clary sage. Layer or dilute in V-6 Mixing Oil for a massage.
> STIMULATE THE SENSES—Basil, lemon, peppermint, and rosemary. Layer or dilute in V-6 Mixing Oil for a massage.
> ****COMMENTS*—Make sure that no negativity exists when the oils are used because the autistic child will make those associations when the oil is used again.*

Auto-immune System: *For diseases, see Grave's Disease, Hashimoto's Disease, and Lupus.* Cistus, ImmuPower.
> *SUPPLEMENTS*—ImmuPro, NingXia Red, Sulfurzyme (helps mitigate effects of autoimmune diseases), Thyromin, VitaGreen.

Avoidance: *See Emotions.* Magnify Your Purpose, Motivation.

Awake:

JET LAG—Eucalyptus, geranium, grapefruit, lavender, lemongrass, peppermint.
STAYING AWAKE WHILE DRIVING—Clarity and En-R-Gee together.

Awaken the Mind, Spirit: Awaken, myrrh.

Awaken the Past: Cypress.

Awareness:

GREATER AWARENESS OF ONES POTENTIAL—Believe, Into the Future, White Angelica.
INCREASES SENSORY SYSTEM—Awaken, birch, wintergreen.
OPENS SENSORY SYSTEM—Birch, peppermint, wintergreen.
REVITALIZES—Lemongrass.
SELF—Acceptance, Believe.
SPIRITUAL—Believe, Frankincense, Inspiration (enhances spiritual mood), myrrh, 3 Wise Men.

Babies/Children:

FORMULA—Bodygize. Mix 1/3 scoop in 10 oz. distilled water or Rice Dream.
PERSONAL CARE— KidScents Bath Gel, KidScents Lotion, KidScents Shampoo, KidScents
  Tender Tush, KidScents Toothpaste, Rose Ointment.
SUPPLEMENTS—KidScents Mighty Mist (vitamin spray), KidScents Mighty Vites
  (chewable tablets), KidScents MightyZyme (chewable enzymes).
BONDING—Gentle Baby (one drop gently rubbed on baby's feet and another drop or two
  brushed over mom's hair and aura–open palms skimming body surface, head to foot).
COLIC— [F]Bergamot, ginger, mandarin, [F]marjoram, Roman chamomile, rosemary, or ylang
  ylang.
  BLEND #1—Combine 2 Tbs. Almond oil with 1 drop Roman chamomile, 1 drop lavender,
  and 1 drop geranium. Mix and apply to stomach and back.
  ***COMMENTS—*Burping the baby, and keeping the abdomen warm with a warm water
  bottle will often bring relief.*
COMMON COLD—Cedarwood, lemon, *Melaleuca ericifolia*, rosemary, rose, sandalwood, or
  thyme.
  BLEND #2—Combine 2 Tbs. V-6 Mixing Oil with 2 drops melaleuca (Tea Tree), 1 lemon,
  and 1 rose otto. Massage a little of the blend on neck and chest.
CONSTIPATION—Ginger, mandarin, orange, or rosemary. Dilute one of the oils and massage
  stomach and feet.
CRADLE CAP REMEDY—
  BLEND #3—Combine 2 Tbs. Almond oil with 1 drop lemon and 1 geranium or with 1 drop
  cedarwood and 1 sandalwood. Mix and apply a small amount on head.
CROUP—Marjoram, ravensara, rosewood, sandalwood, or thyme. Dilute for massage; diffuse.
  Bundle the baby up and take outside to breathe cold air.

CRYING—Cypress, frankincense, geranium, lavender, Roman chamomile, rose otto, or ylang ylang. Dilute for massage or diffuse.

DIAPER RASH—Lavender (dilute and apply).

BLEND #4—Combine 1 drop Roman chamomile and 1 lavender with V-6 Mixing Oil or Genesis Hand & Body Lotion. Apply.

PERSONAL CARE—KidScents Tender Tush (formulated specifically for diaper rash), Rose Ointment.

DIGESTION (sluggish)—Lemon or orange. Dilute and massage feet and stomach.

DRY SKIN—Rosewood or sandalwood. Dilute and apply.

EARACHE—Lavender, melaleuca (Tea Tree), *Melaleuca ericifolia*, Roman chamomile, or thyme (sweet). Put a diluted drop of oil on a cotton ball and place in the ear; rub a little bit of diluted oil behind the ear.

BLEND #5—Combine 2 Tbs. V-6 Mixing Oil with 2 drops lavender, 1 Roman chamomile, and 1 melaleuca (Tea Tree). Put a drop on a cotton ball and put in ear, rub behind the ear and on the ear Vita Flex feet points.

OTHER—Garlic oil works great too, but it is stinky!

FEVER—Lavender. Dilute in V-6 Mixing Oil and massage baby (back of neck, feet, behind ears, etc.). Peppermint (diffuse only).

FLU—Cypress, lemon, *Melaleuca ericifolia*. Dilute 1 drop of each in 1 Tbs. Bath Gel Base for a bath; diffuse.

When using essential oils on babies and children, it is always best to **dilute 1-2 drops of pure essential oil with ½-1 tsp. V-6 Mixing Oil**. If the oils are used in the bath, always use a bath gel base as a dispersing agent for the oils.

Keep the oils out of children's reach. If an oil is ever ingested, give the child an oil-soluble liquid such as milk, cream, or half & half. Then call your local poison control center or seek emergency medical attention. A few drops of pure essential oil shouldn't be life-threatening, but for your protection, it is best to take these precautions.

In Shirley Price's book, <u>Aromatherapy for Babies and Children</u>, she mentions **twenty oils that are safe for children**. Nineteen of them are oils with the same botanical names as those mentioned in this book. These oils are:

Bergamot (Citrus bergamia)*
Cedarwood (Cedrus atlantica)**
Chamomile, Roman (Chamaemelum nobile),
Cypress (Cupressus sempervirens)
Frankincense (Boswellia carterii)
Geranium (Pelargonium graveolens)
Ginger (Zingiber officinale)
Lavender (Lavandula angustifolia)
Lemon (Citrus limon)*
Mandarin (Citrus reticulata)*
Marjoram (Origanum marjorana)
Melaleuca-Tea Tree (Melaleuca alternifolia)
Orange (Citrus aurantium)*
Rose Otto (Rosa damascena)
Rosemary (Rosmarinus officinalis)**
Rosewood (Aniba rosaeodora)
Sandalwood (Santalum album)
Thyme (Thymus vulgaris CT linalol)
Ylang Ylang (Cananga odorata)

*These oils are photosensitive; always dilute. To prevent a rash or pigmentation of the skin, do not use citrus oils when exposed to direct sunlight.

**These oils should never be used undiluted on babies and children.

Caution: Do not use synthetic or adulterated oils. Do not use oils with different botanical names until the safety data has been thoroughly reviewed.

Hiccoughs—Mandarin. **Diffuse**.

Jaundice—Geranium, lemon, lime, mandarin, or rosemary. Dilute and apply on the liver area and on the liver Vita Flex feet points.

Premature—Since premature babies have very thin and sensitive skin, it is best to avoid the use of essential oils.

Rashes—Lavender, Roman chamomile, rose, or sandalwood. Dilute and apply.

Teeth Grinding—Lavender (rub on feet), Peace & Calming (on feet or diffuse).

Teething—German chamomile, ginger, lavender, marjoram, or melaleuca (Tea Tree). Dilute and apply.

Tonsillitis—Ginger, lavender, lemon, or melaleuca (Tea Tree), Roman chamomile. Dilute and apply.

Thrush—Geranium, lavender, lemon, melaleuca (Tea Tree), *Melaleuca ericifolia*, rosewood, or thyme. Dilute and apply.

>   Blend—2 Tbs. garlic oil, 8 drops lavender, 8 drops *Melaleuca ericifolia*, 1 ml. (1 softgel) Vitamin E oil. Apply to nipples just before nursing, or with a clean finger into baby's mouth. Also try Animal Scents Pet Ointment.

***Comments—Besides Gentle Baby listed under bonding, no other commercial blends are listed in this section because many of them contain oils that are not recommended for babies. *The author's admit that they have used many of the commercial blends mentioned in this book on their babies and children with great success and no side effects. We are careful, however, to use only a couple drops at a time, diluted in V-6 Mixing Oil, and only for external application. Also, we do not continue applications for any extended period of time.*

Back: Basil, birch, Black pepper, cypress, EndoFlex, eucalyptus, geranium, ginger, juniper, lavender, oregano, peppermint, PanAway, Relieve It, Roman chamomile, rosemary, sage, tangerine, thyme (for virus in spine), Valor (aligns; a chiropractor in a bottle), wintergreen.

I was about 8½ hours into a 10 hour round trip drive and my back started to seize up. I have an old muscle injury and I knew I was in trouble. I had my oils on the seat next to me and grabbed my PanAway at a stoplight and poured it in my hand. I was in a hurry. I had planned on putting on about 5 drops, but the oil was warm and I think I ended up with about 20 in my hand. Rather than waste it, I put it all on my lower back and sat back in my seat. Within a few minutes my spine did a complete correction starting at the base and going up to the back of my head. I felt each click as it ran up my spine. Needless to say, my back no longer hurt and I had no stiffness when I finally got out of the car!
-Submitted by Andrea Safford Warrenton, Virginia (July 2004)

Supplements—BLM

Calcified (spine)—Geranium, PanAway, rosemary.

Massage Oils—Ortho Ease and PanAway (on spine).

Deteriorating Discs—Do **raindrop therapy** with just the application of the oils, none of the working along the spine.

Herniated Discs—Cypress (strengthens blood capillary walls, improves circulation, powerful anti-inflammatory), PanAway, Relieve It, (massage up disc area three times to help with pain), pepper, peppermint (a compress is good too). <u>Valor</u> (3 drops) on location may help relieve pressure. Do **raindrop therapy** with just the application of the oils, none of the working along the spine.

BLEND—Lemongrass with Idaho tansy, then marjoram with Balsam fir or frankincense to help repair the damage.

MASSAGE OILS—Ortho Ease.

SUPPLEMENTS—BLM, Super C / Super C Chewable.

LOW BACK PAINS—

RECIPE #1—Rub <u>Valor</u> on top and bottom of feet, <u>Di-Gize</u> on colon, Ortho Ease up the back. Massage cypress up the disc area three times. Cypress strengthens blood capillary walls, improves circulation, and is a powerful anti-inflammatory. Use helichrysum to increase circulation, decongest, and reduce inflammation and pain. Use peppermint to stimulate the nerves (may need to dilute with Ortho Ease). Layer basil, <u>Aroma Siez</u>, <u>Relieve It</u>, and spruce.

SUPPLEMENTS—BLM

MUSCULAR FATIGUE—Clary sage, lavender, marjoram, rosemary.

PAIN—

BLEND #1—5 to 10 drops each rosemary, marjoram, sage **or**

BLEND #2—5 to 10 drops each of lavender, eucalyptus, ginger **or**

BLEND #3—5 to 10 drops each of peppermint, rosemary, basil.

RECIPE #2—Apply <u>PanAway</u> and <u>Valor</u> on the shoulders. If the individual being worked on is laying on their stomach, the person applying the oils to the shoulders should cross their arms so the electrical frequency is not broken (right to right etc.). Apply the following oils **up** the spine, one at a time, using a probe on each vertebra if possible, stroke with fingers, feathering gently in 4" strokes three times for each oil: Peppermint (excites the back), cypress (anti-inflammatory), <u>Aroma Siez</u>, <u>Relieve It</u>, and spruce. Follow the procedure with a hot compress. The blends above have also been used with success. Follow the same stroking procedure and dilute the blends with a little V-6 Mixing Oil for a massage.

SUPPLEMENTS—BLM.

Bacteria: *See Anti-bacterial.*

Balance: <u>Acceptance</u>, <u>Aroma Siez</u>, <u>Awaken</u>, cedarwood, frankincense (balances electrical field), <u>Harmony</u>, <u>Mister</u>, palo santo, Roman chamomile, <u>Valor</u>, ylang ylang. Vetiver is also shown to have a balancing effect on the whole body when applied to the brain stem.

BALANCE MALE/FEMALE ENERGIES—<u>Acceptance</u>, ylang ylang.

CHAKRAS—<u>Harmony</u>, <u>Valor</u>.

EMOTIONAL—<u>Envision</u>.

ELECTRICAL ENERGIES—Frankincense, <u>Harmony</u>, <u>Valor</u>. Start by applying 3-6 drops <u>Valor</u> on the bottom of each foot. Some may be applied to the neck and shoulders if desired.

When working on someone else, place the palms of the hands on the bottom of each foot (left hand to left foot and right hand to right foot) and hold for 5 to 15 minutes. If working on yourself, perform the Cook's Hookup by lifting the right foot and placing the right ankle on top of the left knee in cross-legged fashion. Next place the left hand on the right ankle and cup the front of the ankle with the fingers. Then cross the right hand over the left and with the right hand grasp the heel of the right foot (with thumb around the back and fingers cupping the bottom of the heel). Hold this for 5 to 15 minutes. The balancing of the electrical energies can be felt by either a pulse in the hands and feet or a warming sensation.

FEELING OF—Envision, spruce.

HARMONIC BALANCE TO ENERGY CENTER—Acceptance, Harmony.

SUPPLEMENTS—Bodygize, Master Formula His/Hers.

Baldness: *See Hair.* Cedarwood, lavender, rosemary, sage. Apply 2-3 drops of each oil on location and on bottom of feet before bedtime and/or in the morning after washing with Lavender Volume products shown below.

PERSONAL CARE—Lavender Volume Shampoo and Lavender Volume Conditioner together.

SUPPLEMENTS—Sulfurzyme may help if the hair is falling due to a sulfur deficiency.

Bath: While tub is filling, add oils to the water; oils will be drawn to your skin quickly from the top of the water, so use gentle oils like: Lavender, Roman chamomile, rosewood, sage, ylang ylang, etc. For the most benefit, add 5-10 drops of your favorite essential oil to one-half ounce Bath and Shower Gel Base.

BATH & SHOWER GELS—Evening Peace, Relaxation, and Sensation Bath and Shower Gels as well as Lavender Rosewood, Sacred Mountain, and Peppermint Cedarwood Moisturizing Soaps are all wonderfully soothing in the evening. Morning Start Bath and Shower Gel as well as Lemon Sandalwood and Thieves Cleansing Soaps are all terrific ways to jump-start your day.

AQUA ESSENCE BATH PACKS—Finally, some of the most popular essential oil blends have been combined with the latest hydro-diffusion technology to create the perfect solution for adding oils to your bath water. Just place a packet in the tub while hot water is being added and the oils are perfectly dispersed into the water. The packets contain 10 ml of oil and are reusable. Packets can be ordered with either Joy, Valor, Peace & Calming, or Sacred Mountain.

Bed Wetting: *See Bladder.* Before bedtime, rub the abdomen with a couple drops of cypress mixed with V-6 Mixing Oil.

Belching: Di-Gize. Apply to stomach and on Vita Flex points.

Bereavement: Basil, cypress.

B

Betrayed (Feeling): *See Emotions.* Acceptance, Forgiveness, Transformation, Valor.

Birthing: *See Pregnancy.*

Bites: *See Insect.* Basil, cinnamon bark, garlic, lavender, lemon, sage, thyme (all have antitoxic and anti-venomous properties).

ALLERGIC—Purification.

BEES AND HORNETS—Remove the stinger, apply a cold compress of Roman chamomile to area for several hours or as long as possible. Then, apply 1 drop of Roman chamomile three times a day for two days. Idaho tansy may also work.

GNATS AND MIDGES—Lavender, or 3 drops thyme in 1 tsp. cider vinegar or lemon juice. Apply to bites to stop irritation.

INSECT—Cajeput, patchouli.

MOSQUITO—Helichrysum, lavender.

SNAKE—Basil, patchouli.

SPIDERS, BROWN RECLUSE, BEE STINGS, ANTS, FIRE ANTS—**Basil** (neutralizes), cinnamon bark, lavender, lemon, lemongrass, peppermint, Purification, thyme.

SPIDERS—3 drops lavender and 2 drops Roman chamomile in 1 tsp. alcohol. Mix well in clockwise motion and apply to area three times a day.

TICKS—After getting the tick out, apply 1 drop lavender every 5 minutes for 30 minutes. How to remove:
- Do not apply mineral oil, Vaseline, or anything else to remove the tick as this may cause it to inject the spirochetes into the wound.
- Be sure to remove the entire tick. Get as close to the mouth as possible and firmly tug on the tick until it releases its grip. Don't twist. If available, use a magnifying glass to make sure that you have removed the entire tick.
- Save the tick in a jar and label it with the date, where you were bitten on your body, and the location or address where you were bitten for proper identification by your doctor, especially if you develop any symptoms.
- Do not handle the tick.
- Wash hands immediately.
- Check the site of the bite occasionally to see if any rash develops. If it does, seek medical advice promptly.

WASPS (are alkaline)—1 drop basil, 2 Roman chamomile, 2 lavender, and 1 tsp. cider vinegar. Mix in clockwise motion and put on area three times a day.

Bitterness: *See Emotions.* Acceptance, Forgiveness, Roman chamomile, Valor.

Bladder: Apply EndoFlex over kidneys as a hot compress.

BED WETTING AND INCONTINENCE—Before bed, rub cypress on abdomen.

TINCTURES—Take K&B morning, noon, and night.

INFECTION—*See Cystitis.* Cedarwood, Inspiration, onycha (benzoin), and sandalwood (for 1st stages of bladder infection), ᶠlemongrass, or 1 drop Thieves in 8 oz. juice or water and drink three times a day.

SUPPLEMENTS—K&B Tincture, NingXia Red.

***COMMENTS—*One individual who had bladder infection took 1 oz. NingXia Red (followed by 6-8 oz. water) every four hours. They were over the infection in two days.*

HANGING DOWN—Valor on feet, 3 drops ravensara and 1 drop lavender on calves, (bladder should pull up).

Blame: *See Emotions.* Acceptance, Forgiveness, Valor.

Blister: (on lips from sun): Lavender (Apply as often as needed. It should take fever out and return lip to normal).

Bloating: Di-Gize. Apply to stomach, Vita Flex points, and diffuse.

SUPPLEMENTS—ComforTone.

Blocked (Emotionally): *See Emotions.*

Blood: Red blood cells carry oxygen throughout the body.

BLOOD TYPES—Different blood types have different dominating glands.

TYPE A: more prone to be alkaline pH balanced. Natural vegetarians. Type A child living in a home of type O parent is affected by parents' programing or conditioning or visa versa. They have problems with their thyroid, may have tendency to gain weight, and need exercise.

TYPE AB: may want to be a vegetarian some days, but not on others. Can go either way like A or O types. They may be affected by either the A or O parent. AB types haven't decided whether to be an A or B type. They may even need more protein than O types.

TYPE B: down the middle, more balanced. Takes them about 3 years to convert to being a vegetarian.

TYPE O: more prone to acidic condition in blood. AlkaLime is an acid-neutralizing mineral formulation and may help preserve the body's proper pH balance. Big eaters may need to take more supplements because they are not assimilating the nutrients. If they are not assimilating their food, they eat and get full quick and one hour later they are hungry again. They get more gas because they lack enzyme secretion. They may need **Essentialzyme** for the enzymes, and **Digest + Cleanse** to improve digestion and assimilation of nutrients. They eat more, digest less, but don't gain weight. May take 8 years to totally convert to vegetarian diet. Need more protein; **Bodygize, Pure Protein Complete, Vitagreen** and **Power Meal** are mainstays for O types as they are high protein and high energy formulas; nuts and seeds are good too. Nutrients in purest form reduces the need to eat. They have a harder time structuring their diet and they get cold because of poor circulation. If an O type is slender, has high energy, is compulsive in behavior, and/or is a hard worker, they may need as many as 16 VitaGreen and 10 Master Formula His/Hers per day.

BLOOD PRESSURE—

HIGH (hypertension)—<u>Aroma Life</u>, Fbirch, Clary sage, clove, Balsam fir (lowers), goldenrod, Flavender, lemon, Fmarjoram (regulates), nutmeg, Fspearmint, wintergreen, Fylang ylang (arterial; put in hand, rub palms together, cup over nose, and

> ### *OILS TO AVOID IF HYPERTENSIVE*
>
> **Single oils:** *Hyssop, rosemary, sage, thyme, and possibly peppermint.*
>
> **This list is a compilation of the safety data contained in aromatherapy books written by the following authors: Ann Berwick, Julia Lawless, Shirley & Len Price, Jeanne Rose, Robert Tisserand, and Tony Balacs.*

breathe deeply for 5 minutes and/or put on feet). Place oils on heart points on left arm, hand, foot, and over heart. Can also smell from palms of hands, diffuse, or place a few drops on a cotton ball and put in a vent. *See COMMENTS under Asthma for a discussion on using* **plastic nasal inhalers**.

***COMMENTS—*Refer to the chapter entitled "How to Use - The Personal Usage Reference" in the <u>Essential Oils Desk Reference</u> under "Blood Pressure, High" for specific product recommendations.*

BATH—3 ylang ylang and 3 marjoram in bath water. Bathe in the evening twice a week.

BLEND #1—5 geranium, 8 lemongrass, 3 lavender, and 1 oz. V-6 Mixing Oil. Rub over heart and heart Vita Flex points on left foot and hand.

BLEND #2—10 ylang ylang, 5 marjoram, 5 cypress, and 1 oz. V-6 Mixing Oil. Rub over heart and heart Vita Flex points on left foot and hand.

TINCTURES—HRT (1-2 droppers two to three times per day).

LOW—<u>Aroma Life</u>, hyssop (raises), pine, Frosemary, ylang ylang.

SUPPLEMENTS—CardiaCare (with *Rhododendron caucasicum* which helps to normalize blood pressure).

BLOOD PROTEIN—Bodygize, VitaGreen.

BLEEDING (STOPS)—<u>Aroma Life</u>, cistus, geranium (will increase bleeding first to eliminate toxins, then stop it), helichrysum, onycha (benzoin), Cayenne pepper, rose.

***COMMENTS—*Some have found that taking 14 capsules of helichrysum internally over a 24 hour period, right before surgery, can help prep the blood so that bleeding is reduced. Can also topically apply helichrysum to the surgical location before surgery.*

BROKEN BLOOD VESSELS—Grapefruit, helichrysum.

***COMMENTS—*One woman had some blood vessels break in her brain which effected her short-term memory, concentration, focus, and emotions. She used the oils of <u>Clarity</u>, basil, rosemary, peppermint, and cardamom. Not only did her blood vessels heal, but her concentration, awareness, focus, and self-esteem increased.*

BUILD—Rehemogen (tincture) together with JuvaTone and Juva Cleanse may help build blood and hemoglobin platelets (raise cell count). ImmuneTune is good for building white blood cells.

CHOLESTEROL—Helichrysum (regulates).

CLEANSING— ᶠHelichrysum, Juva Cleanse, Roman chamomile. Apply on bottom of feet.
   SUPPLEMENTS—VitaGreen.
   TINCTURES—Rehemogen (purifier).

CLOTS—Balsam fir (reduces pressure), grapefruit, helichrysum. Balsam fir, helichrysum, and cistus together (both topically and internally 3-4 times per day) help to dissolve blood clots.

HEMORRHAGING—*See Female Problems*. Cistus, helichrysum, rose, Cayenne pepper.

LOW BLOOD SUGAR—Cinnamon bark, clove, Thieves (balances blood sugar), thyme.
   SUPPLEMENTS—AlkaLime, VitaGreen (balances blood sugar), Mineral Essence.
   TINCTURES—Sugar-Up (balances blood sugar; available through Creer Labs 801-418-8870).

STICKY—Clove, thyme (inhibits blood platelet aggregation)
   SUPPLEMENTS—Longevity Capsules (contains both clove and thyme oils)

STIMULATES—ᶠLemon (helps with the formation of red and white blood cells).

VESSELS—Aroma Life, cypress (strengthens the capillary walls, and increases circulation), lemongrass (vasodilator).
   SUPPLEMENTS—Cel-Lite Magic dilates blood vessels for better circulation.

Body Systems:

CARDIOVASCULAR SYSTEM: *See Cardiovascular System*. Aroma Life, clove, cypress, goldenrod, helichrysum, marjoram, onycha (benzoin), rosemary, tsuga (opens and dilates for better oxygen exchange), ylang ylang.
   SUPPLEMENTS—CardiaCare (contains ingredients that have been scientifically tested for their abilities to support and strengthen the cardiovascular system), ICP, Mineral Essence, Omega Blue, Super B, Super Cal.
   TINCTURE—HRT.

DIGESTIVE SYSTEM: *See Digestive System*. Clove, Di-Gize (acid stomach; aids secretion of digestive enzymes), ᶠfennel (sluggish), ginger, laurel, myrtle, ᶠpeppermint, rosemary, spearmint, tarragon (nervous and sluggish). Add the oil(s) to your food, rub on stomach, or apply as a compress over abdomen.
   SUPPLEMENTS—Balance Complete, Digest + Cleanse, Essential Manna, Essentialzyme (digestive enzymes; take before meals for acid stomach), KidScents Royaldophilus, ParaFree, Royaldophilus.

EMOTIONAL BALANCE: *See Emotions*. Australian Blue, Balsam fir, Forgiveness, frankincense, geranium, Grounding, Harmony, Hope, Inner Child, Joy, juniper, lavender, onycha (combine with rose for massage), orange, Present Time, Release, Roman chamomile, sage lavender, sandalwood, SARA, 3 Wise Men, Transformation, Trauma Life, Valor, vetiver, White Angelica.

HORMONAL SYSTEM: *See Hormonal System.* Clary sage, EndoFlex, fennel, goldenrod, Mister, myrrh, myrtle, peppermint, sage, sage lavender, ylang ylang. The most common places to apply oils for hormonal balance are the Vita Flex points on ankles, lower back, thyroid, liver, kidneys, gland areas, the center of the body, along both sides of the spine, and on the clavicle area. Diffusing may also help.

> *MASSAGE OILS*—Dragon Time.
> *PERSONAL CARE*—Prenolone/Prenolone+, Progessence.
> *SUPPLEMENTS*—CortiStop (Women's), FemiGen (female), ProGen (male), Thyromin, Ultra Young+.
> *TINCTURES*—Estro.

IMMUNE SYSTEM: *See Immune System.* Clove, Exodus II, frankincense, ImmuPower, ledum (supports), lemon, Mountain savory, rosemary (supports), Thieves (enhances; massage on feet and body), thyme (supports immunological functions).

> *SUPPLEMENTS*—Essential Manna, Exodus, ImmuneTune, ImmuPro, NingXia Red, Super B, Super C / Super C Chewable, Ultra Young (may help raise levels of cytokines, interleukin 1 & 2, and tumor necrosis factor).

MUSCLES AND BONES: *See individual listings for Bones and Muscles.* Aroma Siez, basil, birch, cypress, Balsam fir, lavender, lemongrass, marjoram, oregano, palo santo, peppermint, sage lavender, thyme, Valor, wintergreen.

> *MASSAGE OILS*—Ortho Ease or Ortho Sport Massage Oils.
> *SUPPLEMENTS*—Be-Fit, BLM, Essential Manna, Mineral Essence, Power Meal, Pure Protein Complete, Sulfurzyme, Super C Chewable, Super Cal, WheyFit.

NERVOUS SYSTEM: *See Nervous System.* Brain Power, cedarwood (nervous tension), Balsam fir, ginger, lavender, Peace & Calming, **peppermint** (soothes and strengthens), rosemary, sage lavender, vetiver.

> *PERSONAL CARE*—NeuroGen, Regenolone (nerve regeneration).
> *SUPPLEMENTS*—Mineral Essence, Omega Blue, Sulfurzyme, Super B.

RESPIRATORY SYSTEM: *See Respiratory System.* FEucalyptus (general stimulant and strengthens), *Eucalyptus radiata*, ledum (supports), melaleuca, Fmyrtle, Fpeppermint (aids), pine (dilates and opens bronchial tract), RC, Raven (all respiratory problems), ravensara, rosemary verbenon, sage lavender, tsuga (dilates and opens respiratory tract).

> *SUPPLEMENTS*—Super C / Super C Chewable.

SKIN: *See Skin.* Frankincense, Gentle Baby (youthful skin), geranium, German chamomile (inflamed skin), lavender, ledum (all types of problems), Melrose, myrrh (chapped and cracked), onycha (chapped and cracked), patchouli (chapped; tightens loose skin and prevents wrinkles), rosewood (elasticity and candida), sage lavender, Valor, vetiver, Western Red cedar.

BAR SOAPS—Lavender Rosewood Moisturizing Soap, Lemon Sandalwood Cleansing Soap, Peppermint Cedarwood Moisturizing Soap, Sacred Mountain Moisturizing Soap for oily skin, Thieves Cleansing Soap.

PERSONAL CARE—A·R·T Skin Care System, AromaGuard Deodorants, Boswellia Wrinkle Creme, ClaraDerm, Essential Beauty Serums (Dry, Oily & Acne-Prone Skin Blends), Genesis Hand & Body Lotion (hydrates, heals, and nurtures the skin), Satin Facial Scrub - Mint (eliminates layers of dead skin cells and slows down premature aging of the skin), Orange Blossom Facial Wash combined with Sandalwood Moisture Creme (cleans and moisturizes dry or prematurely aging skin), Prenolone , Progessence, Regenolone (helps moisturize and regenerate tissues), Rose Ointment (for skin conditions and chapped skin), Satin Hand & Body Lotion (moisturizes skin leaving it feeling soft, silky, and smooth).

SUPPLEMENTS FOR SKIN—Sulfurzyme.

TINCTURES—AD&E.

BALANCE—Harmony, Joy, lavender, spruce, Valor.

CONTROL—Cedarwood.

ODORS—Purification (obnoxious odors), sage.

STRENGTHEN VITAL CENTERS—Oregano.

SUPPORT—Fir, ledum, Valor.

Boils: Bergamot, Clary sage, frankincense, galbanum, Gentle Baby, lavender, lemon, lemongrass, melaleuca, Melrose, Purification, Raven, ravensara, RC, Roman chamomile.

PERSONAL CARE—Rose Ointment.

***COMMENTS*—*One individual put lemon oil on a sore that looked like a boil. The next day it turned black, puss came out and it got smaller and finally disappeared.*

> *I have suffered large boils on the tops of my legs for about 30 years and nobody could help me get rid of them. Last fall I counted 12 boils. I started using Lavender and did the Master Cleanser, lemonade cleanse. On the third day, my boils opened and ran freely. This was in January of this year. Now I only occasionally get them and they are many times smaller than before. I know if I continue the regimen, they will eventually leave altogether.*
> **-Submitted by K. Ernst (July 2004)**

Bonding: *See Emotions.* Gentle Baby.

***COMMENTS*—*Use Release or other oils listed under Emotional Release in the Science and Application section of the Reference Guide for Essential Oils to help release emotional connections to one who has passed on. Also, to help children create good bonds with others, tell them about the person when working with the oils.*

Bones: All the tree oils, **birch**, cedarwood, cypress, fir, juniper, lavender, lemongrass, marjoram, PanAway (bone pain), peppermint, Relieve It, sandalwood, spruce, wintergreen.

SUPPLEMENTS—Be-Fit, BLM, Essential Manna, Mineral Essence, Power Meal, Sulfurzyme, Super Cal.

BONE SPURS—Birch/wintergreen, cypress, marjoram, <u>RC</u> (dissolves). Rub on location.

> One lady had a heel spur flare up one evening, so she took a bath with birch and cypress before retiring. The next morning, the pain was a little better. She then put 6 drops birch, 6 drops cypress, and on top of that, 5 drops RC on a cotton pad and applied it to her heel. In 10 minutes all pain was gone and even after four days, the pain had not returned.

BROKEN HEAL—Birch/wintergreen and cypress (before bed), helichrysum, oregano and <u>Valor</u> (in morning). Frankincense and Balsam fir can also be used internally and externally.

> BLEND #1—9 drops birch/wintergreen, 8 drops each of spruce, White fir, and helichrysum, 7 drops clove (good when inflammation is causing the pain).
>
> BLEND #2—Equal parts lemongrass, clove, *Eucalyptus radiata*, and *Melaleuca alternifolia* (Tea Tree). Has been used to heal an infected bone fracture in as little as 3 months.
>
> *MASSAGE OILS*—3 droppers full of Ortho Ease mixed with lavender, lemongrass, and <u>PanAway</u>. Ortho Sport with juniper, lemongrass, and marjoram (apply over broken bones).
>
> *SUPPLEMENTS*—BLM and Super Cal.

BRUISED—Helichrysum, <u>Relieve It</u>, and <u>PanAway</u>.

CARTILAGE—Sandalwood (regenerates), White fir (pain from inflammation).

DEGENERATION—Ortho Ease then peppermint.

> *SUPPLEMENTS*—Super C / Super C Chewable.

DEVELOPMENT—

> *SUPPLEMENTS*—Super C / Super C Chewable, Ultra Young (may help boost bone formation).

PAIN—**Birch**, <u>PanAway</u>, White fir, wintergreen.

ROTATOR CUFF (sore)—*See Shoulder*. **Birch/wintergreen** (bone), lemongrass (torn or pulled ligaments), <u>PanAway</u>, peppermint (nerves), <u>Relieve It</u>, spruce, White fir (inflammation).

Boredom: <u>Awaken</u>, <u>Believe</u>, cedarwood, cypress, <u>Dream Catcher</u>, fir, frankincense, <u>Gathering</u>, juniper, lavender, <u>Motivation</u>, pepper, Roman chamomile, rosemary, sandalwood, spruce, thyme, <u>Valor</u>, ylang ylang.

Bowel:

IRRITABLE BOWEL SYNDROME—<u>Di-Gize</u> and peppermint. Take 2 drops of each in distilled water 1-2 times per day. Idaho tansy and <u>Juva Cleanse</u> (as a dietary supplement) may also help. Dilute 1-2 drops with V-6 Mixing Oil and apply over abdomen with a hot compress.

> BLEND—10-15 drops <u>Di-Gize</u>, 5-6 drops ledum, and 1 drop peppermint in a capsule and take internally. *Abundant Health offers capsules that work well with the oils.*
>
> *SUPPLEMENTS*—Balance Complete, ComforTone, Digest + Cleanse, ICP (fiber beverage), JuvaPower/JuvaSpice, JuvaTone, NingXia Red, Royaldophilus.

NORMAL FUNCTION OF—
>   SUPPLEMENTS—Balance Complete (utilizes five different fibers for optimal cleansing power), ComforTone, Digest + Cleanse, ICP (fiber beverage for normal function of bowels).
>   PARALYSIS—ComforTone, Digest + Cleanse.
>   ***COMMENTS—One women was paralyzed by surgery and had to have 2 colonics a day. She took ComforTone and then she was able to have natural bowel movements.*

Boxed in (Feeling): Peace & Calming, Valor.

Brain: Aroma Life, Blue cypress (improves circulation), Clary sage (opens brain, euphoria), cypress, geranium, lemongrass, spearmint, Transformation.

> *The **blood-brain barrier** is the barrier membrane between the circulating blood and the brain that prevents certain damaging substances from reaching brain tissue and cerebrospinal fluid. The American Medical Association (AMA) determined that if they could find an agent that would pass the blood-brain barrier, they would be able to heal **Alzheimer's, Lou Gehrig's, Multiple Sclerosis, and Parkinson's disease.** In June of 1994, it was documented by the Medical University of Berlin, Germany and Vienna, Austria that **sesquiterpenes have the ability to go beyond the blood-brain barrier. High levels of sesquiterpenes** are found in the essential oils of cedarwood, vetiver, sandalwood, Black pepper, patchouli, myrrh, ginger, vitex, German chamomile, spikenard, galbanum, and frankincense. Some blends containing these oils include: 3 Wise Men, Acceptance, Brain Power Forgiveness, Gathering, Harmony, Inspiration, Into the Future, and Trauma Life (refer to Single Oil Chart in the Appendix for other blends that contain these oils).*

>   SUPPLEMENTS—Longevity Capsules (contains thyme oil, which helps preserve omega-3s in the brain, and clove oil, which helps to protect the neurons), Omega Blue (contains pure fish oil with naturally occurring ratios of EPA and DHA)

ACTIVATES RIGHT BRAIN— Bergamot, birch, geranium, grapefruit, helichrysum, Roman chamomile, wintergreen.
BROKEN BLOOD VESSELS—*See Blood.*
CEREBRAL (BRAIN)— ᶠNutmeg.
INJURY—Frankincense, Valor. Massage on brain stem and diffuse.
INTEGRATION—Clary sage, cypress, geranium, helichrysum (increases neurotransmitter activity), lemongrass, spearmint, Valor.
NEUROLOGICAL INJURY (break down of Myelin Sheath)—Peppermint, lemongrass, frankincense, Valor. Massage on brain stem and spine; diffuse.
>   FOOD—Omega 3 fatty acids found in Flax Seed Oil and Sesame Oil (taken internally).
OXYGENATE—3 drops each of helichrysum and sandalwood once or twice a day on the back of neck, temples, and behind ears down to jaw. Also Blue cypress.
TUMOR—*See Cancer.* Frankincense, Valor. Massage on brain stem and diffuse.

Breast: Clary sage, cypress, elemi (inflammation), fennel, geranium, lemongrass, sage, spearmint, vetiver.
>   PERSONAL CARE—ClaraDerm, Prenolone/Prenolone+/Progessence (for tenderness and swelling).

ENLARGE AND FIRM—Clary sage, fennel, sage, <u>SclarEssence</u>.
>   *BLEND*—Equal parts vetiver, geranium, and ylang ylang.
>   *PERSONAL CARE*—A·R·T Purifying Toner (to tone and tighten skin)

LACTATION—*See Pregnancy*.

MASTITIS (breast infection)—<u>Citrus Fresh</u> (with lavender), <u>Exodus II</u>, lavender, tangerine.
>   *BLEND*—Equal amounts of lavender and tangerine. Dilute with some V-6 Mixing Oil and apply to breasts and under arms twice a day.
>   *SUPPLEMENTS*—Exodus.

MILK PRODUCTION—*See Pregnancy*.

SORE NIPPLES—Roman chamomile.
>   *PERSONAL CARE*—Animal Scents Pet Ointment

STRETCH MARKS—<u>Gentle Baby</u>.

Breath(ing): Cinnamon bark, <u>Exodus II</u>, frankincense, ginger, hyssop, juniper, marjoram, nutmeg, Roman chamomile, rosemary, thyme. <u>Raven</u> or <u>RC</u> may work instead of an inhaler. (*See* COMMENTS *under Asthma for a discussion on using* **plastic nasal inhalers**.)

HYPERPNEA (Abnormal rapid breathing)— [F]Ylang ylang.

OXYGEN—Cedarwood, frankincense, sandalwood, all essential oils.
>   *PERSONAL CARE*—Satin Facial Scrub - Mint (deep cleansing that dispenses nutrients and oxygen). Mix with Orange Blossom Facial Wash for a milder cleanse.
>   *SUPPLEMENTS*—Exodus.

SHORTNESS OF—<u>Aroma Life</u>. (*See* COMMENTS *under Asthma for a discussion on using* **plastic nasal inhalers**.)
>   BLEND #1—For shortness of breath due to overexertion (lots of work, no sleep, etc.) add 10 drops each of eucalyptus and peppermint to a basin of lukewarm water. Soak some cloths in this water and wring them out leaving them fairly moist. Then wrap the joints (ankles, knees, wrists, elbows, and neck) with the cloths. While relaxing and allowing the compresses to cool the joints, have another person do Vita Flex on the Pineal Gland and Adrenal Gland points on the feet.

Bronchitis: *See Respiratory System*. <u>Abundance</u>, basil, bergamot, birch, cajeput, [F]cedarwood, [F]Clary sage, clove, [F]cypress, elemi, *Eucalyptus radiata*, [F]fir (obstructions of Bronchi), frankincense, ginger, <u>ImmuPower</u>, lavender, ledum, lemon, [F]marjoram, [F]melaleuca, *Melaleuca ericifolia*, [F]myrtle, myrrh, nutmeg, onycha (benzoin), [F]peppermint, [F]pine, <u>RC</u>, <u>Raven</u>, ravensara, Roman chamomile, rose, [F]rosemary, sage lavender, sandalwood, [F]spearmint, <u>Thieves</u> (drops in drinking water, also put on chest & feet, may need to dilute with V-6 Mixing Oil), [F]thyme, tsuga (opens respiratory tract), wintergreen. Diffuse the oils or rub on chest (dilute with V-6 Mixing Oil if necessary). *See* COMMENTS *under Asthma for a discussion on using* **plastic nasal inhalers**.

BLEND #1—10 cedarwood, 10 eucalyptus, 2 Roman chamomile, and 2 oz. water. Put on hanky and inhale. Blend can also be added to water for gargle.

BLEND #2—Clove, cinnamon bark, melissa, and lavender (Alternative Medicine—The Definitive Guide, p. 55).

***COMMENTS—*Refer to the chapter entitled "How to Use - The Personal Usage Reference" in the Essential Oils Desk Reference under "Bronchitis" for specific oil blend and supplement recommendations.*

CHRONIC—Elemi, eucalyptus, laurel, ᶠravensara, ᶠsage, ᶠsandalwood, ᶠoregano.

CHILDREN—Eucalyptus, lavender, melaleuca, *Melaleuca ericifolia*, Roman chamomile, rosemary, thyme (CT linalol).

SUPPLEMENTS—ImmuneTune.

CLEAR MUCUS—Bergamot, sandalwood, and thyme (Alternative Medicine—The Definitive Guide, p. 824). Onycha (benzoin) and Thieves may also help.

***COMMENTS—*Diffusing the oils is a great way to handle a respiratory problem.*

According to Dr. Daniel Pénoël, bronchitis can be broken down into three separate areas, each of which should be considered separately. Following are the three areas and specific blends recommended by Dr. Pénoël:

Inflammation—Mix equal portions of *Eucalyptus citriodora* and lemongrass. Apply 36 drops per foot to the sinus and lung Vita Flex points. Add to V-6 Mixing Oil and apply over the chest.

Infection—Mix 1 tsp. melaleuca, 25 drops palmarosa or geranium, 3 drops peppermint, 1 drop thyme. Apply 3-6 drops per foot to the sinus and lung Vita Flex points. Add to V-6 Mixing Oil and apply over the chest.

Accumulation of Fluids (mucus)—Mix 25 drops each of *Eucalyptus dives*, peppermint, dill. Apply 3-6 drops per foot to the sinus and lung Vita Flex points.

Bruises: Angelica, fennel, geranium, helichrysum, hyssop, lavender, Melrose, PanAway, Thieves. Apply on location.

***COMMENTS—*Refer to the chapter entitled "How to Use - The Personal Usage Reference" in the Essential Oils Desk Reference under "Bruising" for some excellent blend recipes and supplement recommendations.*

Bugged (Feeling): *See Emotions.* Acceptance, Forgiveness, Peace & Calming, Valor.

Bugs (Repel): *See Bites and Insect.* Lemon (kills bugs), Purification. Diffuse.

BITES (All spiders, Brown Recluse, bee stings, ants, fire ants)—Basil, cinnamon bark, lavender, lemon, lemongrass, peppermint, Purification, thyme.

INSECT—Patchouli.

REPELLENT—Idaho tansy may work as a mosquito repellent. Also, Idaho Tansy Floral Water (used to keep flies away from horses while shoeing).

SNAKE—Patchouli.

Bulimia: Grapefruit. Apply to stomach and bottom of feet.

Bumps: Frankincense, Melrose, PanAway, Peace & Calming.

Bunions: *See Bursitis.* <u>Aroma Siez</u>, carrot, cypress, German chamomile, juniper, <u>M-Grain</u>.

> **Bunions** *are from bursitis located at the base of a toe.*

      BLEND—6 drops eucalyptus, 3 lemon, 4 ravensara, and 1 birch/wintergreen in 1 oz. V-6 Mixing Oil. Apply a couple drops of this blend directly on area of concern as often as desired.

Burdens: *See Emotions.* <u>Acceptance</u>, <u>Hope</u>, <u>Release</u>, <u>Transformation</u>, <u>Valor</u>.

Burns: Eucalyptus, geranium, helichrysum, Idaho tansy, [F]lavender (cell renewal), melaleuca (Tea Tree), peppermint, ravensara (healing), Roman chamomile, rosehip, tamanu (mix with helichrysum).

> *Dr. Alex Schauss, a prominent mineral researcher, has discovered that **burns** are painful because certain trace minerals are depleted from the skin and surrounding tissue. If the trace minerals are replenished to the affected area, then the pain will subside almost immediately. Many people have received instant pain relief when Mineral Essence was either taken internally or topically applied on the sunburn or burn.*

    PERSONAL CARE—LavaDerm Cooling Mist (soothing and cooling for all burns), Satin Hand & Body Lotion (moisturizes and promotes healing).

    SUPPLEMENTS—Mineral Essence (can be taken internally and applied topically).

    BLEND #1—Put 3 drops of lavender in some Satin Hand & Body Lotion and apply. This is effective for pain, healing, peeling, and sunburns.

    BLEND #2—10 German chamomile, 5 Roman chamomile, and 10 lavender. Mix together and add 1 drop to each square inch of burn after it has been soaked in ice water. If you don't have the chamomile, lavender will do great. Can top with LavaDerm Cooling Mist to keep skin cool and moist.

    CLEANSING—<u>Melrose</u>.

    INFECTED—<u>Purification</u>.

    PAIN—Blend #1 (above), Mineral Essence (apply topically).

    HEALING—*See Scarring.* Rosehip. Blend #1 (above), ravensara or geranium mixed with helichrysum.

> *René Maurice Gattefossé, Ph.D., a French cosmetic chemist who coined the phrase "Aromatherapy," severely burned his hand in a laboratory accident. The continual application of lavender oil soothed the pain, nullified the effects of gas gangrene, and healed his hand without a scar.*

    PEELING—Blend #1, Blend #2 (both shown above).

    SUNBURN—*See Sunburn.* <u>Australian Blue</u>, [F]Melaleuca (Tea Tree), tamanu (mix with helichrysum), Mineral Essence (applied topically), Blend #1 (above).

PERSONAL CARE—A·R·T Skin Care System, LavaDerm Cooling Mist, Satin Hand & Body Lotion.

BLEND #3—Put 10 drops of lavender in 4 oz. glass or plastic spray bottle full of distilled water. Shake well then spray on location. This is effective for pain and healing.

SUN SCREEN— ᶠHelichrysum, tamanu.

Bursitis: Aroma Siez, cajeput, cypress, ginger, hyssop, juniper, onycha (benzoin), PanAway, Roman chamomile.

> *Bursitis is a chronic inflammation of the fluid-filled sac that is located close to the joints. It is caused by infection, injury, or diseases like arthritis and gout. Since it can be very tender and painful, it may restrict the ability to move freely.*

BLEND—Apply 6 drops of marjoram on shoulders and arms; wait 6 minutes. Then apply 3 drops of birch/wintergreen; wait 6 minutes. Then apply 3 drops of cypress.

MASSAGE OILS—Ortho Ease, Ortho Sport.

SUPPLEMENTS—BLM

Calcium: *See Hormonal Imbalance.*

SUPPLEMENTS—Allerzyme (aids the digestion of sugars, starches, fats, and proteins), Digest + Cleanse, Super Cal, Mineral Essence, Polyzyme (aids the digestion of protein and helps reduce swelling and discomfort).

> *According to Dr. John R. Lee, processed foods, carbonated soft drinks, caffeine, and high protein, sugar and salt consumption all contribute to increased calcium deficiency in the human body (Burton Goldberg Group, Alt. Med., The Definitive Guide, pp 773-4). Sulfur cannot be metabolized if there is a calcium deficiency. This can cause poor nail and hair growth, falling hair, eczema, dermatitis, poor muscle tone, acne, pimples, gout, rheumatism, arthritis, and a weakening of the nervous system.*

Callouses: Carrot, Melrose and oregano (callouses on feet), peppermint, Roman chamomile.

Calming: Bergamot, ᶠcedarwood, Citrus Fresh, Clary sage (aromatic), Gentle Baby, jasmine, lavender, *Melaleuca ericifolia*, myrrh, onycha (benzoin), Peace & Calming, Release, Surrender, tangerine, Trauma Life, Western Red cedar, ylang ylang.

Cancer: *See Chemicals, Tumors, Radiation.* All conifer oils have great value in fighting cancers, while Balsam fir and White fir have more specific actions. Di-Gize (rub on feet and stomach), ImmuPower (put on throat and all over feet, three times a day), Melrose (cancer sores, fights infection), clove, frankincense (diffuse; combine with ledum and take internally), Juva Cleanse, rose, sage, ᶠtarragon (anti-cancerous). Since it is very important to maintain a positive attitude while healing, it may be helpful

> *When the cell wall thickens, oxygen cannot get in. The life expectancy of a cell is 120 days (4 months). Cells also divide, making duplicate cells. If the cell is diseased, new diseased cells will be made. When we stop the mutation of the diseased cells (create healthy cells), we stop the disease. Essential oils have the ability to penetrate and carry nutrients through the cell wall to the nucleus and improve the health of the cell.*

to address the emotions using <u>Acceptance</u>, <u>Believe</u>, <u>Envision</u>, <u>Forgiveness</u>, <u>Gathering</u>, <u>Gratitude</u>, <u>Hope</u>, <u>Joy</u>, <u>Live with Passion</u>, and/or ravensara (*refer to the emotional therapies in the Science and Application section of the <u>Reference Guide for Essential Oils</u>*). One of the most common emotions cancer patients have to deal with is anger or a pattern of resentment. Others are fear, judgement, and doubt. Doubt limits God and restricts His ability to work miracles in our lives. Praying for all those with cancer can help release these emotions. Also, work on recognizing why cancer was chosen.

***COMMENTS—*Refer to the chapter entitled "How to Use - The Personal Usage Reference" in the <u>Essential Oils Desk Reference</u> under "Cancer" for some excellent blend recipes, supplement recommendations, and cleansing and maintenance programs for many different kinds of cancer.*

***Important Notice: Health care professionals are emphatic about avoiding heavy massage when working with cancer patients. Light massage may be used, but never over the trauma area. Also, the information in this section should not be perceived as a cure for cancer. Always consult with your health care professional.**

SUPPLEMENTS—AlkaLime (acid-neutralizing mineral formulation), Balance Complete, Bodygize (especially good for cancer), Cleansing Trio (ComforTone, Essentialzyme, and ICP), Digest + Cleanse, ImmuneTune, ImmuPro, NingXia Red (nutrient powerhouse), Power Meal, Super C / Super C Chewable, VitaGreen, Wolfberry Crisp Bars (*Refer to the Wolfberry Crisp Bar in the Supplements section of the <u>Reference Guide for Essential Oils</u> for more information on the benefits of the Ningxia Wolfberry*).

***COMMENTS—*One lady, who was receiving Chemo treatments for cancer of the spleen, used <u>Di-Gize</u> to promote elimination through the colon. Her doctors wondered why her Chemo treatments had not made her*

> *There must be an acid condition in the body for cancer to thrive and spread. See pH Balance. VitaGreen and Power Meal contain predigested proteins and help the body move towards an alkaline balance. AlkaLime combats yeast and fungus overgrowth and helps preserve the body's proper pH balance.*
>
> *Cancer cells also have a very low frequency.*

sick. When she felt any discomfort (light nausea or cramps in descending colon), she rubbed four to six drops of <u>Di-Gize</u> on her abdomen and within 10 minutes, all discomfort stopped.

The following are recipes that some individuals have used successfully:

RECIPE #1—For the first month, supplement with the following: 6 VitaGreen three times a day, 6 Super C / Super C Chewable three times a day, and 4 ImmuneTune three times a day. After remission, apply <u>ImmuPower</u> on the spine three times a day. Do a *light* full body massage with 6 clove and 15 frankincense in 1 oz. V-6 Mixing Oil.

RECIPE #2—Supplement with the following: Cleansing Trio (ComforTone, Essentialzyme, and ICP), 12 Super C / Super C Chewable, 15 ImmuneTune, and 9 VitaGreen.

Drink ½ gallon of carrot juice each day. Eliminate white flour, white sugar and red meat from the diet. Rub <u>Thieves</u> on the feet and do a *light* full body massage with frankincense.

RECIPE #3—Supplement with the following: 1 Master Formula His/Hers, 2 VitaGreen, 6 Super C / Super C Chewable, and 1 ImmuneTune. Do a *light* full body massage with frankincense, clove, and V-6 Mixing Oil. Apply <u>ImmuPower</u> to the spine and feet twice a day.

BONE—Frankincense on neat, all supplements. The following is a recipe that has been used on some individuals with bone cancer:

RECIPE #1—ImmuneTune (antioxidant) and Cleansing Trio (ComforTone, Essentialzyme, and ICP) for a week, then JuvaTone was added for six days, then Super B was added morning and evening. Other vitamin supplements included Super C / Super C Chewable, MegaCal, and Super Cal. All processed foods were eliminated and a strict Vegetarian Diet was followed, including 8 glasses of water each day. Birch was applied on location for pain. Frankincense and lavender were applied on the feet.

BRAIN TUMOR—The following are recipes that some individuals have used successfully:

RECIPE #1—*Light* massage daily on spine with 1 oz. V-6 Mixing Oil, 15 drops frankincense, and 6 drops clove. Rub brain stem with <u>ImmuPower</u>. Diffuse 15 drops frankincense and 6 drops clove for ½ hour three times a day.

> *Frankincense contains sesquiterpenes which allow it to go beyond the blood brain barrier. Sesquiterpenes are also found in many of the emotional blends. ImmuPower builds the immune system. Clove is anti-parasitic and anti-tumoral.*

RECIPE #2—Diffuse frankincense 24 hours a day and massage the brain stem with frankincense.

BREAST—Frankincense and clove. Often, there is an emotional issue of self-worth that must be dealt with as well.

CERVICAL—Clove, cypress, frankincense, geranium, lavender, lemon.

COLON—

SUPPLEMENTS—ICP (fiber beverage that helps prevent), CardiaCare (with *Rhododendron caucasicum* which inhibits the enzyme hyaluronidase), Super Cal (studies have shown that taking calcium supplements at night helps protect the colon from polyps and cancer).

DIET—fast 21 days (*See Fasting or Cleansing*) then have soup. *See Diet.*

HEART—HRT

LIVER—Frankincense (hot compress over liver), <u>GLF</u>, <u>JuvaFlex</u>, <u>Juva Cleanse</u>, and/or myrrh may help with liver congestion and function.

> *One woman had **cancer of the heart** which literally ate a hole in the heart. She took the tincture HRT and the tissue of her heart regenerated and the cancer disappeared!*
>
> ***JuvaTone** and **Rehemogen** build blood and hemoglobin platelets One individual had total **liver regeneration** by using JuvaTone, Rehemogen, and <u>JuvaFlex</u>.*

SUPPLEMENTS—JuvaTone was formulated to fight cancer in the liver.

C

LUNG—Frankincense (rub on chest or add 15 drops to 1 tsp. V-6 Mixing Oil for nightly retention enema), lavender.

> *BLEND #1*—15 drops frankincense, 5 drops clove, 6 drops ravensara, 4 drops myrrh, and 2 drops sage. This blend can be mixed with 1 tsp. V-6 Mixing Oil if it is too strong. It is best when inserted into rectum.

LYMPHOMA—(nodes or small tumors) in neck and groin. Cleanse liver.

> *BLEND #2*—10 drops frankincense, 5 drops myrrh, and 3 drops sage. Mix with small amount of V-6 Mixing Oil and apply daily over nodes or tumor areas and rectally. Every other day apply frankincense neat.

LYMPHOMA STAGE 4 (bone marrow)—extreme fatigue; eat vegetables and fruits, **"no meat"**. ImmuPower on the spine.

> *SUPPLEMENTS*— Royaldophilus, Bodygize morning and night, Cleansing Trio (ComforTone, Essentialzyme, and ICP), 4 ImmuneTune three times a day (for one month or until remission), 6 Super C / Super C Chewable three times a day, 6 VitaGreen three times a day. After remission, continue one more month then reduce amounts for maintenance.

MELANOMA (skin cancer)—*See Corns, Warts*. Frankincense and lavender.

OVARIAN—ImmuPower on spine three times a day.

> BLEND #3—15 drops frankincense, 6 geranium, and 5 myrrh in ½ tsp. V-6 Mixing Oil; alternate one night in vagina (tampon to retain), next in rectum.

> *SUPPLEMENTS*—Bodygize three times a day, ImmuneTune six times a day, 6 FemiGen a day, 8 Super C / Super C Chewable a day. Those with "A" type blood should take 8 VitaGreen a day while those with "O" type blood should take 12 or more a day; VitaGreen is a mainstay, it is a predigested protein and helps maintain an alkaline balance.

> *Aloha! I have been using essential oil for many years, resulting in many amazingly wonderful results. One of the best took place when a dear friend was being consumed by cancer. She was in stage 4 for 4 years- amazing in itself. RC and frankincense were used the most. When she was put into the hospice, with only days left, the oils were still used and she remained in the hospice for another year and a half. Others at the hospice got sick with colds and flu, including the workers, but my friend never got any of the passing bugs... amazing to say the least but a true testimonial to the anti-viral and antibiotic effects of the oils.*
> **-Submitted by Yvonne Vnuk-Nielsen**
> **Kailua, Hawaii (July 2004)**

PROSTATE—Anise (blend with frankincense, fennel, ImmuPower, Mister, sage, and/or yarrow). Apply to posterior scrotum, ankles, lower back, and bottom of feet. Juva Cleanse taken as a dietary supplement can also help.

> *PERSONAL CARE*—Protec was designed to accompany the night long retention enema. It helps buffer the prostate from inflammation, enlargement, and tumor activity.

> *TINCTURES*—3 droppers full of Male-Pro four times a day (available through Creer Labs 801-418-8870).

The following is a recipe that has been used on Prostate Cancer:

> **RECIPE #1**—Diffuse ImmuPower. Do a spinal massage and Vita Flex on the feet with ImmuPower. Blend 5 drops frankincense, 15 Mister, and 2 tsp. V-6 Mixing Oil

together OR 15 drops <u>ImmuPower</u> with 2 tsp. V-6 Mixing Oil; insert and retain in the rectum throughout the night.

CASE HISTORY #1—71 year old man had prostate cancer and bone metastasis. After three weeks of using frankincense, sage, myrrh, and cumin in rectal implants, he was free of cancer.

THROAT—Frankincense, lavender.

UTERINE—Geranium, <u>ImmuPower</u>.

BLEND #4—2 to 5 drops cedarwood **or** 2 to 5 drops lemon **or** 2 to 5 drops myrrh in 1 tsp. V-6 Mixing Oil.

Candida: *See Acidosis, Alkaline, Blood, Diet, Food, Thyroid, pH Balance.* <u>Di-Gize</u>, cinnamon bark, clove, <u>EndoFlex</u>, [F]eucalyptus, <u>ImmuPower</u>, melaleuca (dilute with V-6 Mixing Oil for body massage), *Melaleuca quinquenervia*, <u>Melrose</u> (+ rosemary), Mountain savory (dilute with V-6 Mixing Oil; can be hot), oregano, palmarosa (skin), peppermint (aromatic), rosemary, [F]rosewood, [F]spearmint, [F]spruce, tarragon (prevents fermentation), <u>Thieves</u>. Rub on stomach area and feet or over abdomen with a hot compress.

> *Candida is caused by the fermentation of yeast and sugar, antibiotics, thyroid shut down, stress, chlorinated water, etc. When there is candida there is usually hypoglycemia and hypothyroidism. It is usually a digestive problem; putrefaction in the system causes candida overgrowth. Candida is a natural fungus in the stomach; we need some, but it becomes a problem when there is an overgrowth. Yeast is not the problem but the fermentation of it. The fermentation exists because of a mineral imbalance and an enzyme imbalance in the digestive system. The enzymes needed for digestion are secreted by the thyroid, so it is necessary to support both the thyroid and the digestive system. Also, maintaining a slightly alkaline state in the blood and body can help to slow the overgrowth of candida.*

SUPPLEMENTS—Allerzyme (aids the digestion of sugars, starches, fats, proteins), AlkaLime (combats yeast and fungus overgrowth and preserves the body's proper pH balance), Balance Complete, Bodygize, ComforTone, Detoxzyme (helps maintain and support a healthy intestinal environment), Digest + Cleanse, Essentialzyme (increases digestion), ICP, Mineral Essence, ParaFree, Polyzyme (aids the digestion of protein and helps reduce swelling and discomfort), Power Meal (vegetable protein), Royaldophilus (prevents overgrowth), Super C / Super C Chewable, Thyromin (to help the thyroid), VitaGreen (balances the alkaline/acid condition in the body, and provides chlorophyll and oxygen).

TINCTURES—Anti-Cana (creates unfriendly environment for the candida; available through Creer Labs 801-418-8870).

DIGESTIVE CANDIDA—<u>Di-Gize</u> (hot compresses over abdomen; in a retention enema at night), <u>ImmuPower</u>, <u>Thieves</u>.

VAGINAL CANDIDA— [F]Bergamot, [F]melaleuca, [F]myrrh.

BLEND—2 Tbs. garlic oil, 8 drops lavender, 8 drops melaleuca, 1 ml. (1 softgel) Vitamin E oil. Apply to irritated area.

Cankers: *See Acidosis.* Australian Blue, Chamomile (both German and Roman), Envision, hyssop, laurel, melaleuca, Melrose, myrrh, oregano, sage lavender, Thieves.

> BLEND #1—Sage with clove and lavender.
> BLEND #2—Sage with Thieves.
> SUPPLEMENTS—AlkaLime (combats yeast and fungus overgrowth and preserves the body's proper pH balance), ImmuneTune, ImmuPro, Mineral Essence, VitaGreen.

Canker sores are occasionally associated with Crohn's disease, which affects the bowels. Deficiencies of iron, vitamin B12, and folic acid have been linked to this disease in some people. Stress and allergies are usually the cause of open sores in the mouth. To avoid getting canker sores, it is important to have a body chemistry that is balanced in minerals, acidity, and alkalinity (Prescription for Nutritional Healing, p. 126).

Capillaries:

> BROKEN—Cypress, geranium, hyssop, lime (soothes), Roman chamomile.
> BLEND—Apply 1 drop lavender and 1 Roman chamomile.

Carbuncles: Melaleuca.

Cardiotonic: *See Heart.*

Cardiovascular System: *See Heart.* Anise, Aroma Life, clove, cypress, fleabane (dilates), goldenrod, helichrysum, marjoram, onycha (benzoin), rosemary, tsuga (opens and dilates for better oxygen exchange), ylang ylang.

> SUPPLEMENTS—CardiaCare (contains ingredients that have been scientifically tested for their abilities to support and strengthen the cardiovascular system), ICP, Mineral Essence, Omega Blue, Super B, Super Cal.
> TINCTURE—HRT

Carpal Tunnel Syndrome: Basil, cypress, eucalyptus, lavender, lemongrass, marjoram, oregano. Apply oils on location and either use massage or Vita Flex to work them in. First start with basil and marjoram on the shoulder to help release any energy blockages. Then lemongrass on the wrist and oregano on the rotator cup in the shoulder. Next apply marjoram and cypress on the wrist and then cypress on the neck and down to the shoulder. Lastly, apply peppermint from the shoulder down the arm to the wrist then out to the tips of each finger.

Carpal Tunnel Syndrome is a condition where inflamed carpal ligaments at the wrist press upon the median nerve. Indications include tingling or numbness in the palm or thumb and first three fingers of the hand, weak grip, or impaired finger movement.

> ***COMMENTS—*Make sure it is carpal tunnel syndrome because many people who think they have carpal tunnel syndrome (one report says up to 90%) really have problems with muscles in the neck and shoulder that create similar symptoms.*

BLEND—Layer geranium, Balsam fir, juniper, peppermint, and sandalwood on the wrist. Apply several times per day for an extended period to give the nerves time to heal.

MASSAGE OILS—Ortho Ease or Ortho Sport. Massage into neck, shoulder, and wrist.

PERSONAL CARE—Prenolone/Prenolone+ / Progessence (on shoulder and wrist).

SUPPLEMENTS—BLM, Mineral Essence, Sulfurzyme, Super Cal.

Cataracts: *See Eyes.*

Catarrh (Mucus): *See Anti-catarrhal.* Cajeput, cistus, dill, ginger, hyssop (opens respiratory system to discharge mucus), jasmine, myrrh, onycha (benzoin), Thieves.

Cavities: *See Teeth.*

Celibacy (vow not to marry): Marjoram (aromatic).

Cells: All essential oils restore cells to original state. Need to change the RNA and DNA to change the habit.

SUPPLEMENTS—**NingXia Red** (nutrients promote cellular health).

DNA—cell chemistry.

SUPPLEMENTS—Super B, Thyromin, Body Balancing Trio (Bodygize, Master Formula His/Hers, VitaGreen).

FREQUENCY—Rose (enhances frequency of every cell, which brings balance and harmony to body).

LIVER—Helichrysum (stimulates cell function).

OXYGENATION—Black pepper.

REGULATING—Clary sage (removes negative programming).

RNA—cell memory.

STIMULATES—Abundance.

Cellulite: *See Weight.* Basil, Fcedarwood, cumin, cypress, fennel, geranium, Fgrapefruit, juniper, lavender, lemon, lime, orange, oregano, patchouli, Frosemary, rosewood, sage, spikenard (increases metabolism to burn fat), tangerine (dissolves), thyme. *Refer to the chapter entitled "How to Use - The Personal Usage Reference" in the Essential Oils Desk Reference under "Cellulite" for some excellent blend recipes and recommendations.*

> *Try flavoring 1 gallon of water with 5 drops grapefruit and 5 drops lemon. Adjust to taste and drink. This may also improve energy levels. The H2Oils packets can be used to more easily and effectively flavor drinking water with lemon and grapefruit oils.*

SUPPLEMENTS—Allerzyme (aids the digestion of sugars, starches, fats, and proteins), Digest + Cleanse, Lipozyme (aids the digestion of fats), Power Meal (eat for breakfast).

ATTACKS FAT AND CELLULITE—Basil, grapefruit, lavender, lemongrass, rosemary, sage, thyme.

MASSAGE OILS—Cel-Lite Magic (add grapefruit to increase activity and dissolve cellulite even faster).

Chakras (Energy Centers): (*Refer to the chart at the end of the Science and Application section of the <u>Reference Guide for Essential Oils</u>.*) <u>Harmony</u> (apply 1 drop on each chakra to open the energy centers and balance the electrical field of the chakras, starting at the base chakra located on the coccyx at the end of the spinal column and working up), lavender (brings harmony to chakras), rosemary (opens chakras), sandalwood (affects each chakra differently).

UNITES HEAD AND HEART—Helichrysum.

ANGELIC CHAKRA (#8)—Located above the crown of the head. Angelica, neroli.

CROWN CHAKRA (#7)—<u>3 Wise Men</u> (to replace void with good/positives), angelica (links 7-8, 7-1), basil, cistus, frankincense (links 1-7), lavender, myrrh, onycha, ravensara, rose, rosemary, rosewood (links 7-1), sandalwood (links 7-1), spikenard, spruce.

    BALANCE—<u>Highest Potential</u>

    OPEN—<u>Forgiveness</u>, <u>Harmony</u>.

BROW CHAKRA (3RD EYE -#6)—<u>Acceptance</u>, <u>Awaken</u>, and <u>Dream Catcher</u> (rub on lobe of ear to increase vision and spiritual vision); cedar leaf (Western Red), cedarwood, Clary sage, frankincense, <u>Harmony</u>, helichrysum, juniper, mugwort, palo santo, peppermint, pine, rose, rosemary, spruce, thymes, <u>Transformation</u>, tsuga.

    OPEN—Frankincense, <u>Harmony</u>.

THROAT CHAKRA (#5)—Carrot seed, chamomile (Roman and German), cypress, frankincense, geranium, lavender, rose geranium, sandalwood, spearmint, spruce.

    OPEN—<u>Harmony</u>.

HEART CHAKRA (#4)—Bergamot, carrot seed, cinnamon bark, frankincense, helichrysum, hyssop, inula, laurel, lavandin, lavender, marjoram, melissa, neroli, onycha, oregano, pepper (Black), rose, sage, sandalwood, spikenard, tansy.

    OPENS A CLOSED HEART—Bergamot, <u>Harmony</u>.

SOLAR PLEXUS CHAKRA (#3)—Calamus, cardamom, carrot seed, cedarwood, cinnamon bark, citronella, fennel, ginger, juniper, lemon, lemongrass, melissa, pepper (Black), peppermint, rosemary, spikenard, thymes (all), valerian, vetiver, ylang ylang.

    OPEN—<u>Harmony</u>.

SACRAL CHAKRA (SEX/NAVEL -#2)—Cassia, cinnamon bark, Clary sage, coriander, cypress, geranium, rose geranium, jasmine, myrrh, niaouli, patchouli, petitgrain, pine, rose, sandalwood, tangerine, vetiver, ylang ylang.

    BALANCE—<u>Acceptance</u> (balances Sacral Chakra which stores denial and sexual abuse), sage.

    OPEN—<u>Harmony</u>.

BASE CHAKRA (ROOT -#1)—cardamom, carrot seed, cedar leaf (Western Red), cedarwood, clove, frankincense, ginger, laurel, myrrh, onycha, patchouli, pepper (Black), peppermint, sandalwood, vetiver.

    OPEN—<u>Harmony</u>.

Change (Personal): *See Emotions.* Forgiveness, Into the Future, Joy, Magnify Your Purpose, Sacred Mountain, 3 Wise Men, Transformation.

Charley Horse: *See Muscles: SPASMS.* Aroma Siez, basil.
    PERSONAL CARE—Prenolone/Prenolone+, Progessence.

Cheeks: Jasmine.
    BLEND—5 Aroma Siez, 3 birch/wintergreen, and 3 spruce. Work oils between hands in a clockwise motion and pat on cheeks. Cup hands over nose and inhale.
    PERSONAL CARE—A·R·T Skin Care System, A·R·T Purifying Toner.

Chelation: *See Metals.* Aroma Life, cardamom, helichrysum (powerful chelator and anti-coagulant). Drink lots of distilled water.
    MASSAGE OILS—Cel-Lite Magic.
    SUPPLEMENTS—Cleansing Trio (ComforTone, Essentialzyme, and ICP), VitaGreen (use with cardamom to enhance effects of Chelex tincture).

> *Traditional intravenous chelation therapy can cause scar tissue on the vascular walls. These oils, supplements, and tinctures provide a more natural approach to chelation. They may take longer to achieve the same results, but with minimal side effects.*

    ***COMMENTS**—The apple pectin that is contained in ICP helps remove unwanted metals and toxins from the body.*
    TINCTURES—AD&E, Chelex, and Rehemogen for natural cleansing.

Chemicals: *See Metals.* [F]Helichrysum.
    SUPPLEMENTS—Chelex.

Chicken Pox: *See Childhood Diseases.*

Chiggers: *See Insect.* Lavender.

Childbirth: *See Pregnancy.*

Childhood Diseases:
    CHICKEN POX (2 WEEKS)—(shingles) sleep is very good. *See Shingles.* Australian Blue, Bergamot, eucalyptus, lavender, melaleuca (Tea Tree), Roman chamomile, sage lavender.
    BATH—(relieves the itching) 2 drops lavender, 1 cup bicarbonate of soda, and 1 cup soda in bath and soak.
    BLEND #1—5 to 10 drops each of German chamomile and lavender to one ounce Calamine lotion. Mix and apply twice a day all over body.
    BLEND #2—10 drops lavender, 10 Roman chamomile, and 4 oz. Calamine lotion. Mix and apply twice a day all over body.

C

> *BLEND #3*—Add enough ravensara to some Green clay (from health food store) to form a paste that can be dabbed on the pox to relieve itching.
>
> *DIFFUSE*—an anti-viral oil (such as lemon) and apply the same oil all over the body twice a day. *See Babies/Children.*
>
> MEASLES— ᶠEucalyptus, German chamomile, lavender, melaleuca. Spray or vaporize the room.
>
> GERMAN (3 DAY)—use anti-viral oils. *See Anti-viral.*
>
> RUBELLA—sponge down with one of these oils: Chamomile (Roman or German), lavender, melaleuca.
>
> MUMPS—Lavender, lemon, melaleuca.
>
> WHOOPING COUGH—Basil, cinnamon bark (diffuse or dilute well; avoid for children), Clary sage, cypress, grapefruit, hyssop, lavender, ᶠoregano, thyme.

Children: *See Babies/Children, Hyperactive, Childhood Diseases.*

> *PERSONAL CARE*—KidScents Bath Gel, KidScents Lotion, KidScents Shampoo, KidScents Tender Tush, KidScents Toothpaste.
>
> *SUPPLEMENTS*—KidScents Mighty Mist (vitamin spray), KidScents Mighty Vites (chewable vitamin tablets), KidScents MightyZyme (chewable enzymes), KidScents Royaldophilus, NingXia Red.
>
> HYPERACTIVE—Citrus Fresh, Peace & Calming, Trauma Life. **Diffuse**.

Chills: Ginger, onycha (benzoin), sage lavender. Apply on bottom of feet and on solar plexus.

Chlorophyll:

> *SUPPLEMENTS*—VitaGreen.

Cholera: Clove, ᶠravensara, ᶠrosemary.

Cholesterol: ᶠClary sage, ᶠhelichrysum (regulates), lemongrass (internally - clinically shown to help lower). Apply on Vita Flex points, over heart, and along arms.

Chorea: *See Saint Vitus Dance.*

Chronic Fatigue: *See Acidosis, Hormonal Imbalance.* Basil, Clarity, Di-Gize, ImmuPower, lavender, lemongrass, peppermint, rosemary, Thieves, Transformation. (Note: Basil and peppermint are a good combination together). *Combine any of these with the Raindrop Technique.*

> *Chronic Fatigue is often caused by the Epstein Barr virus. It may also be a result of chemical and metal toxicity, or conditions of high acidity.*
>
> *Women who are pregnant seldom have Chronic Fatigue Syndrome because of the higher amounts of natural progesterone being produced.*

SUPPLEMENTS—AlkaLime (acid neutralizing mineral), Balance Complete (*refer to the 5-Day Nutritive Cleanse program listed under Balance Complete in the Supplements section of the <u>Reference Guide for Essential Oils</u>. This program also uses Digest + Cleanse and NingXia Red to help enhance detoxification while maintaining/increasing energy levels*), Body Balancing Trio (Bodygize, Master Formula His/Hers, VitaGreen), Cleansing Trio (ComforTone, Essentialzyme, and ICP), Digest + Cleanse, ImmuneTune, ImmuPro, Longevity Capsules, Mineral Essence, **NingXia Red**, Power Meal, Royaldophilus, and Super Cal.

PERSONAL CARE—Prenolone/Prenolone+, Progessence.

Dr. Friedmann uses the following recipe on his patients:

RECIPE #1—1) Use the Cleansing Trio (ComforTone, Essentialzyme, and ICP) to detoxify. 2) Build the body and tissues with Mineral Essence and Master Formula His/Hers. 3) Build the immune system with <u>ImmuPower</u> and ImmuneTune or ImmuPro.

Cigarettes:

PURIFY AIR—<u>Purification</u>.

QUIT SMOKING—*See Addictions.* <u>GLF</u>, <u>Peace & Calming</u>, <u>Purification</u>.

SUPPLEMENTS—JuvaPower/JuvaSpice, JuvaTone.

Circulation: <u>Aroma Life</u>, basil, birch, cinnamon bark, <u>Citrus Fresh</u>, Clary sage, cumin, ^F**cypress**, geranium, helichrysum, hyssop, <u>Juva Cleanse</u>, nutmeg, onycha (benzoin), oregano, peppermint, <u>Peace & Calming</u>, <u>RC</u>, rosemary, sage lavender, thyme, wintergreen. Use in a bath, massage, or a compress.

CAPILLARY—**Cypress** (strengthens the capillary walls, and increases circulation), oregano, thyme.

PROMOTES HEALTHY—Onycha (benzoin), <u>PanAway</u>.

MASSAGE OILS—Cel-Lite Magic dilates the blood vessels for better circulation; may add grapefruit or cypress to enhance. Also Ortho Ease and Ortho Sport.

SUPPLEMENTS—Cleansing Trio (ComforTone, ICP, Essentialzyme), JuvaTone, NingXia Red, Thyromin.

***COMMENTS—*Constipation affects circulation. Improving the circulation in the colon and liver improves the circulation in the blood.*

Circulatory System: *See also Cardiovascular System.* <u>Aroma Life</u>, Clary sage, cypress, <u>En-R-Gee</u>, helichrysum, <u>PanAway</u>.

STIMULANT— ^FNutmeg, onycha (benzoin), pine.

SUPPORT—Goldenrod.

Cirrhosis: *See Liver.*

Clarity of Thoughts: <u>Clarity</u>, rosemary, <u>Transformation</u>.

Cleansing: <u>Di-Gize</u> when cramping, fennel, hyssop, juniper, melaleuca (aromatic), <u>Melrose</u>, <u>Release</u> (over liver), <u>3 Wise Men</u> when trauma, put on liver to let emotions go.

> *Cleansing may help to prevent disease, improve immune function, and make the body stronger. It may also cause an emotional cleansing! DRINK LOTS OF WATER!! Any age child can go on a cleanse. Dr. Gary Young suggests that you spend two days cleansing for every year old you are. He recommends that you take ICP and Essentialzyme five days a week and fast once a week on distilled water and lemon juice.*

CUTS—Elemi, lavender, <u>Melrose</u>.

BODY CLEANSE—

SUPPLEMENTS—Balance Complete (*refer to the 5-Day Nutritive Cleanse program listed under Balance Complete in the Supplements section of the <u>Reference Guide for Essential Oils</u>. This program also uses Digest + Cleanse and NingXia Red to help enhance detoxification while maintaining energy levels*), Cleansing Trio (ComforTone, Essentialzyme, and ICP), Digest + Cleanse. The oils contained in the Cleansing Trio will push heavy metals into the system; use <u>Sacred Mountain</u> and <u>Peace & Calming</u> to balance the system. If colon is blocked, start with ComforTone to open it. JuvaTone is the final stage of cleansing and can be taken as often as four times a day.

TINCTURES—Rehemogen supports the body during a cleanse.

MASTER CLEANSER OR LEMONADE DIET—

2 Tbs. fresh lemon or lime juice (approx. ½ lemon), 2 Tbs. of grade B maple syrup (grade A is not as rich in nutrients but can be used if grade B is not available). 1/10 tsp. cayenne pepper or to taste (cayenne is a thermal warmer and dilates the blood vessels; also has vitamin A). Combine above ingredients in a 10 oz. glass of distilled water. No substitute sugars.

> *Lemon converts to alkaline in the body. Lemons can be harmful to teeth only when in water that is not distilled because there can be a reaction with the minerals in the water. Toxins are eliminated from the bowels and bladder. Drink 6 to 12 glasses of the lemonade drink daily. When you get hungry, just drink another glass of lemonade. No other food or vitamins should be taken; the lemonade is already a food in liquid form. An herbal laxative tea may be used to help elimination. More details can be found in the book by Stanley Burroughs, <u>Healing for the Age of Enlightenment</u>. It will take 30 days on lemon to change the chemistry in the body. We have to change the DNA and RNA (memory or belief system) to change a habit. Then, do 30 days on carrot juice.*

In the case of diabetes, use black strap molasses instead of the maple syrup. Drink between three quarts and a gallon of this lemonade each day with an herbal laxative tea first thing in the morning and just before retiring for the night. Refer to the book <u>Healing for the Age of Enlightenment</u> for more specific details including suggestions and specific instructions for how coming off the cleanse.

Closed Minded: <u>Awaken</u>, <u>Inspiration</u>.

Clothes: Western Red cedar. Place a few drops on a cotton ball and put it in a plastic sack. Leave the sack open so the odor of the oil can do its work without it staining any clothes. Place the bag in a closet or storage box.

Cockroaches:

> *BLEND*—Combine 10 peppermint and 5 cypress in ½ cup of water and spray.

Coffee (Stop Drinking): (*See case study on the body's frequency reaction to coffee in the Science and Application section of the <u>Reference Guide for Essential Oils</u>*). <u>Peace & Calming</u>, <u>Purification</u>.

> *SUPPLEMENTS*—JuvaTone.

Colds: Angelica, <u>Australian Blue</u>, basil, Blue cypress (aches and pains), cajeput, eucalyptus (in hot water, breathe deep), <u>Exodus II</u>, fir (aches and pains), ginger, Idaho tansy, lavender, ledum, [F]lemon, [F]melaleuca, myrtle, onycha (benzoin), orange, oregano, peppermint (relieves nasal congestion), pine, <u>Raven</u>, ravensara, <u>RC</u> (put a few drops

> *It seems that because we live in the South there is a lot of "stuffy noses" in the spring and fall. When I have a client in my business complaining of these types of symptoms, I offer them some oils to sniff for relief. I offer a drop of peppermint first then a drop of <u>RC</u> blend. Then, if they have used the word "infection", I offer a drop of <u>Thieves</u> blend. I offer one drop of each in the palm of their hand, one at a time. Then I show them how to stir 3 times and cup their hands over the nose and deeply inhale each oil. They are always amazed at the immediate relief.*
> **-Submitted by Pam Jones**
> **Benton, Arkansas (July 2004)**

in a box of tissue), [F]rosemary, sage lavender, <u>Thieves</u>, thyme. Apply <u>Raven</u> to the back and <u>RC</u> to the chest with <u>Thieves</u> on the feet. Next application rotate <u>Raven</u> and <u>RC</u>. Other oils can be diffused or applied to the forehead, temples, back of neck, and chest. *Refer to the chapter entitled "How to Use - The Personal Usage Reference" in the <u>Essential Oils Desk Reference</u> under "Colds and Flu" for some excellent recipes and supplement recommendations. Also, refer to COMMENTS under Asthma for a discussion on using* **plastic nasal inhalers**.

> *BLEND*—Mix 6 <u>RC</u> and 2 ravensara. Apply to the chest, neck, throat, and sinus area. Diffuse or put 4 drops in a half cup of hot water, then place nose and mouth over the opening of the cup (not in the water) and breathe deeply.

> *SUPPLEMENTS*—Exodus, Thieves Lozenges.

> ***COMMENTS*—*Dr. Pénoël recommends applying a trace of melaleuca alternifolia to the tip of the tongue and swallowing. This works best when done immediately upon noticing a sore throat. Repeat every minute until the throat feels better. Then apply it behind the ears and down under the jaw line. After repeating this a few times (every 5-10 minutes), massage a couple drops on the back of the neck to relieve any blockage.*

Cold Sores: *See Herpes Simplex.* <u>Australian Blue</u>, Bergamot, Blue cypress, geranium, lavender, lemon, melaleuca (Tea Tree), <u>Melrose</u> (fights infection), <u>RC</u>, Roman chamomile, <u>Thieves</u>.

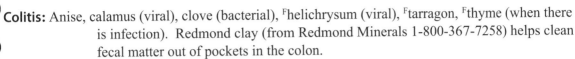

Colic: *See Babies/Children.* Angelica, bergamot, cardamom, carrot with fennel, coriander, cumin, dill, ginger, marjoram, melissa, Mountain savory, orange, pepper, peppermint, Roman chamomile, spearmint.

Colitis: Anise, calamus (viral), clove (bacterial), ᶠhelichrysum (viral), ᶠtarragon, ᶠthyme (when there is infection). Redmond clay (from Redmond Minerals 1-800-367-7258) helps clean fecal matter out of pockets in the colon.

> SUPPLEMENTS—AlkaLime, Balance Complete (uses 5 different fibers for optimal absorption and cleansing action), Cleansing Trio (ComforTone, Essentialzyme, and ICP), Digest + Cleanse.

Colon: *See Colitis and Diverticulitis.* Calamus may help reduce inflammation. <u>Di-Gize</u> and peppermint. Take 2 drops of each in distilled water 1-2 times per day. Use Redmond clay (from Redmond Minerals 1-800-367-7258) to remove fecal matter from pockets in the colon. Also <u>Release</u> topically with compress.

> SUPPLEMENTS—Balance Complete (*refer to the 5-Day Nutritive Cleanse program listed under Balance Complete in the Supplements section of the <u>Reference Guide for Essential Oils</u>. This program also uses Digest + Cleanse and NingXia Red to help enhance detoxification while maintaining energy levels.*), Cleansing Trio (ComforTone, Essentialzyme, and ICP), Digest + Cleanse, JuvaPower/JuvaSpice, Royaldophilus. *Refer to the Supplements section of the <u>Reference Guide for Essential Oils</u> for specific usages.*

> POLYPS—*See Polyps.* Cleanse the colon! Stanley Burroughs' Master Cleanse is an ideal cleansing program which affects

> > *Polyps are tumors that arise from the bowel surface and protrude into the inside of the colon. Most polyps eventually transform into malignant cancer tumors.*

> the entire body. However, if fecal matter is not being eliminated from the colon 2-3 times per day, it may be necessary to start with ComforTone first until bowel movements are more frequent. Then toxins released during the Master Cleanse can be quickly eliminated from the body. (*See MASTER CLEANSER under Cleansing*)

> > SUPPLEMENTS—Cleansing Trio (ComforTone, Essentialzyme, and ICP). *Refer to the Supplements section of the <u>Reference Guide for Essential Oils</u>.*

> PROLAPSED COLON—not assimilating; use Essentialzyme.

> > ***COMMENTS—*Stanley Burroughs recommends performing a colon lift and describes the procedure for doing so in his book <u>Healing for the Age of Enlightenment</u> on pages 55 to 59.*

> SPASTIC—*has no peristaltic action.*

> > SUPPLEMENTS—Balance Complete, ComforTone then ICP (fiber beverage).

Coma: <u>Awaken</u>, Black pepper, cypress, frankincense, <u>Hope</u>, peppermint, sandalwood, <u>Surrender</u>, <u>Trauma Life</u>, <u>Valor</u>. Massage on brain stem, mastoids (behind ears), temples, and bottom of feet.
   SUPPLEMENTS—Mineral Essence, Ultra Young.

Comforting: <u>Gentle Baby</u>.

Compassion: Helichrysum.

Complexion: *See Skin*. Apply oils to face, neck and intestines.
   PERSONAL CARE—A·R·T Skin Care System
   DULL—Jasmine, orange.
   OILY—Bergamot, orange.
   PERSONAL CARE—Essential Beauty Serum - Oily Skin Blend.

Concentration (Poor): <u>Awaken</u>, basil, <u>Brain Power</u>, cedarwood, <u>Clarity</u>, cypress, <u>Dream Catcher</u>, eucalyptus, <u>Gathering</u>, juniper, lavender, lemon, myrrh, orange, peppermint, rosemary, sandalwood, <u>3 Wise Men</u>, ylang ylang.
   SUPPLEMENTS—Omega Blue

Concussion: Cypress. Rub on brain stem and bottom of feet.
   ****COMMENTS—One woman had a concussion with headaches and hallucinations. By applying cypress over her brain stem, her headaches left for good.*

Confidence: Jasmine, <u>Live with Passion</u>, sandalwood (self), <u>Transformation</u>, <u>Valor</u>.

Confusion: <u>Awaken</u>, basil, <u>Brain Power</u>, cedarwood, <u>Clarity</u>, cypress, fir, frankincense, <u>Gathering</u>, geranium, ginger, <u>Harmony</u>, jasmine, juniper, marjoram, peppermint, <u>Present Time</u>, rose, rosemary, rosewood, sandalwood, spruce, thyme, <u>Transformation</u>, <u>Valor</u>, ylang ylang.

Congestion: <u>Di-Gize</u>, cedarwood, coriander, cypress, *Eucalyptus radiata*, <u>Exodus II</u>, fennel, ginger, myrtle (excellent for children), <u>Raven</u>, <u>RC</u>, rosemary. To help discharge mucus, rub oil(s) on chest, neck, back, feet, and diffuse.
   MASSAGE OILS—Cel-Lite Magic.
   SUPPLEMENTS—Cleansing Trio (ComforTone, ICP, Essentialzyme), Digest + Cleanse.

Conjunctivitis: *Eucalyptus radiata*, jasmine.

Consciousness: Lavender. Diffusing these oils is a great way to affect consciousness.
   OPEN—Rosemary.

Purifying—Peppermint.

Stimulating—Peppermint, Transformation.

Constipation: *See Acidosis.* Anise, Black pepper, Di-Gize, fennel, ginger, juniper, ^Fmarjoram, ^Forange,

> *Poor bowel function may be caused by enzyme deficiency, low fiber, poor bowel tone, not enough liquid in diet, stress, incorrect pH balance, and/or bad diet.*

patchouli, rose, rosemary, sandalwood, tangerine, tarragon. Massage clockwise around abdomen and on Vita Flex points (feet & shins).

SUPPLEMENTS—AlkaLime, ComforTone, Essentialzyme, ICP (fiber beverage), Sulfurzyme, and lots of water. If there is a chronic history of constipation, use ComforTone until the system is open, then start ICP.

BLEND #1—Mix together 6 drops of ^Forange, tangerine, and spearmint and rub on lower stomach and colon.

BLEND #2—15 cedarwood, 10 lemon, 5 peppermint, and 2 oz. V-6 Mixing Oil. Massage over lower abdomen three times a day clockwise and take supplements.

CHILDREN—fruit juices or lots of water. Geranium, patchouli, Roman chamomile, rosemary, tangerine.

Contagious Diseases: ^FGinger.

Control:

OF YOUR LIFE—Cedarwood, Dream Catcher, Envision.

SELF—Motivation, Roman chamomile (aromatic).

Convulsions: *See Seizure.* Brain Power, Clary sage, lavender, neroli, Roman chamomile, Valor.

SUPPLEMENTS—KidScents Mighty Mist/Vites, Mineral Essence, Ultra Young.

Cooling Oils: Angelica, Citrus oils, eucalyptus, lavender, melaleuca, Mountain savory, peppermint, Roman chamomile, spruce. Other oils that are high in aldehydes and esters can produce a cooling effect.

> *Stanley Burroughs touts clove oil as being wonderful for corns, skin cancer, and warts. He suggests using your finger to apply a small amount of clove oil directly on warts or corns. After a short time, use an emery stick to scrape off the top of the wart or corn and apply the oil again. Repeat several times daily until wart or corn disappears. The same technique can be used for skin cancer. (Healing for the Age of Enlightenment, p. 104.)*

Corns: *See Warts.* Carrot, Citrus Fresh, clove, grapefruit, lemon, myrrh, peppermint, Roman chamomile, tangerine. Apply 1 drop of oil directly on corn.

Cortisone: Birch, EndoFlex, lavender, Relieve It, Roman chamomile, ^Fspruce (is like cortisone), wintergreen.

BLEND—Combine 3 drops Roman chamomile, 3 lavender, 5 spruce, and 1 birch/wintergreen and apply as a natural cortisone.

SUPPLEMENTS—ProGen and Thyromin, together with <u>EndoFlex</u> are beneficial for both men and women. The three items together may also help the body produce its own cortisone.

Coughs: Angelica, cajeput, cardamom, **cedarwood**, elemi (unproductive), ᶠeucalyptus, fir, **frankincense**, ginger, jasmine, juniper, ᶠmelaleuca, ᶠmyrtle (helps remove mucus from lungs), myrrh, onycha (benzoin), peppermint, pine, myrrh, <u>RC</u>, ravensara, Roman chamomile, sage lavender, sandalwood, <u>Thieves</u> (dissolves excess mucus and reduces inflammation), thyme.

> *Diffusing the oils is one of the best ways to handle a cough. It may also help to rub the oils on the throat and chest area.*

    SUPPLEMENTS—Thieves Lozenges.
    ALLERGY—<u>Purification</u> (diffuse).
    SEVERE—Elemi, frankincense.
       BLEND #1—3 drops fir, 3 lemon, 2 ravensara, 1 thyme.
       BLEND #2—15 drops <u>Raven</u>, 15 <u>RC</u>, 5 lemon, and 10 <u>Peace & Calming</u>. Rub on chest, throat, and neck. Can also be diffused.
    SMOKERS—Myrtle.

Courage: Clove (aromatic), fennel (aromatic), ginger, <u>Live with Passion</u>, <u>Valor</u> (gives).

Cradle Cap: *See Babies/Children.*

Cramps: *See Digestive System, Hormonal Imbalance, Menstruation, Muscles, PMS.* <u>Aroma Siez</u>, basil, ᶠbirch, Blue cypress (abdominal), Clary sage, ᶠcypress, <u>Exodus II</u>, galbanum, ginger, ᶠlavender, rosemary, ᶠmarjoram, wintergreen.
    MASSAGE OILS—Relaxation.
    SUPPLEMENTS—Digest + Cleanse (contains oils proven to soothe gastrointestinal upset).
    LEG CRAMPS—<u>Aroma Siez</u>, basil, German chamomile, lavender, marjoram, rosemary, vetiver.
    MASSAGE OILS—Ortho Ease, Ortho Sport, Relaxation.
    PERSONAL CARE—Prenolone/Prenolone+, Progessence.
    SUPPLEMENTS—BLM, Mineral Essence, Super Cal.
    MENSTRUAL CRAMPS—*See Dysmenorrhea.* <u>Lady Flash</u>, <u>Lady Love</u> (available through Creer Labs 801-418-8870).
    PERSONAL CARE—Prenolone/Prenolone+, Progessence.
    SUPPLEMENTS—Exodus, FemiGen.
    TINCTURES—FHS (available through Creer Labs 801-418-8870). Works best when combined with FemiGen.
       RECIPE #1—Take 2 FemiGen three times a day, 10 days before period. Start again two days after cycle. May take up to 6 tablets three times a day. <u>Lady Flash</u> and <u>Lady Love</u> may be applied to the pelvis, ankles, bottom of the feet, or as a hot compress over the abdomen.
    STOMACH CRAMPS—<u>Di-Gize</u> (add 3 drops basil in capsule with <u>Di-Gize</u>).

Creates Sacred Space: Sacred Mountain.

Crohn's Disease: Basil, calamus, <u>Di-Gize</u>, peppermint. Do Raindrop Technique on spine with
   <u>ImmuPower</u>.
   SUPPLEMENTS—AlkaLime, Balance Complete, Bodygize, Cleansing Trio (ComforTone,
   ICP, and Essentialzyme), Digest + Cleanse, Mineral Essence, Power Meal,
   Royaldophilus, **Sulfurzyme**, VitaGreen.
   ****COMMENTS**—*Refer to the chapter entitled "How to Use - The Personal Usage
   Reference" in the* <u>Essential Oils Desk Reference</u> *under "Crohn's Disease" for a
   specific regimen of supplements.*

Crown Chakra: *(See Chakras for more extensive list)*
   OPEN—<u>3 Wise Men</u> (releases and fills the void).

Cushing's Disease: *See Adrenal Glands.* Basil, <u>Forgiveness</u>, <u>ImmuPower</u>, <u>Joy</u>, lemon, <u>Thieves</u>.
   SUPPLEMENTS—Exodus, ImmuneTune, ImmuPro.

Cuts: *See Tissue.* Cypress, elemi (infected), helichrysum, lavender, melaleuca, <u>Melrose </u>(rejuvenates
   tissue), onycha (benzoin), pine, ravensara, <u>Relieve It</u>, Roman chamomile (healing),
   rosewood, sage lavender, <u>Thieves</u>.

Cystic Fibrosis: Alternate with <u>Thieves</u>, <u>RC</u>, lavender, and myrtle. Apply to brain stem (back of
   neck), temples, chest, bottom of feet, and diffuse. <u>Raven</u> is stronger and can replace
   myrtle for helping to remove mucus accumulation in the lungs. <u>EndoFlex</u> and
   helichrysum can also be used with benefit.
   BLEND—(Staphylococcus) oregano, thyme, and <u>Melrose</u> (up the spine using the Raindrop
   Technique), then 10 drops lemon, 5 drops melaleuca, and 3 drops frankincense (rub
   on feet, chest, and diffuse) OR 10 <u>Raven</u> and 5 hyssop.
   SUPPLEMENTS—Essentialzyme, Master Formula His/Hers, VitaGreen, all vitamins.

Cystitis (Bladder Infection): Basil, bergamot, cajeput, cedarwood, cinnamon bark, clove, eucalyptus,
   fennel, frankincense, FGerman chamomile, hyssop, juniper, lavender, marjoram,
   oregano, pine, sage, sandalwood, Fspearmint, rosewood, Fthyme. Massage or bathe
   with one of these oils.
   SUPPLEMENTS—NingXia Red (½ cup followed by a full cup of water has brought relief
   within 10 minutes when taken at the first sign of discomfort).
   TINCTURE—K&B.

Dandruff: Cedarwood, Flavender, melaleuca (Tea Tree), patchouli, Frosemary, sage, sage lavender,
   valerian.
   PERSONAL CARE—Lavender Volume Shampoo and Lavender Volume Conditioner.

Day Dreaming: <u>Awaken</u>, cedarwood, <u>Clarity</u>, <u>Dream Catcher</u>, eucalyptus, <u>Gathering</u>, ginger, <u>Harmony</u>, helichrysum, <u>Highest Potential</u>, lavender, lemon, myrrh, peppermint, <u>Present Time</u>, rose, rosemary, rosewood, <u>Sacred Mountain</u>, sandalwood, spruce, <u>3 Wise Men</u>, thyme, <u>Valor</u>, ylang ylang.

Death (of Loved One): *See Emotions: Loss.* <u>Trauma Life</u>.

Debility: Cardamom, cumin (nervous), ᶠnutmeg sage lavender.

Decongestant: Any of the citrus oils, ᶠcypress, ᶠGerman chamomile, juniper, melaleuca, patchouli.

Defeated: *See Emotions: Defeated.*

Degenerative Disease: *See pH Balance.* <u>Citrus Fresh</u>, <u>Exodus II</u>, frankincense, lavender, lemon, orange, <u>Purification</u>, tangerine, and <u>Transformation</u> are excellent to diffuse in the room. Not only do these oils purify the air, but they help deliver needed oxygen to the starving cells. All other essential oils and supplements are beneficial for providing oxygen and nutrients to the cells of the body. See specific ailments.

    Supplements—NingXia Red (provides a full range of nutrients), Power Meal.

    ***Comments—*A lack of nutrients at the cellular level causes degenerative disease.** *The general health condition of the body will improve if the necessary nutrients are received by the body at the cellular level. Toxins change the pH of the cell wall, which significantly reduces the ability of the cell to assimilate nutrients and oxygen. This process is the beginning of cellular starvation, which leads to degenerative disease. Then, we are hosts to viral and bacterial invasions due to our weakened or compromised immune system. Essential oils are antimicrobial and help our immune system fight off the ravages of disease. They also have the ability to deliver nutrients to our nutritionally depleted cells. When essential oils are blended with the proper nutrients that the body requires, the essential oils act as the delivery system to take the nutrients directly into the cell and through the compromised cell wall, which has had the pH altered due to chemical toxins in the body. This process allows the body to rebuild and regain its healthful condition and allows the body's immune system to normalize. In addition, essential oils have the highest oxygenating molecules of any know substance. So, they deliver oxygen to the cells which helps in the regeneration process. (Young Living Essential Edge Newsletter — July 1996).*

Dehydration: ImmuneTune, Mineral Essence.

    ***Comments—**An 18 month old infant was saved from dying of dehydration when it was given ½ capsule of ImmuneTune in applesauce.*

Delivery: *See Pregnancy: Delivery.*

Denial: Roman chamomile, sage.
>   OVERCOME—<u>Abundance</u>, <u>Acceptance</u>, <u>Awaken</u>, <u>Transformation</u>.

Dental Infection: *See Blend #2 under Metals:* PULL OUT *for method to remove dental mercury.* Clove and frankincense, helichrysum, melaleuca, myrrh, <u>Thieves</u>. Apply to jaws and gums. It may be necessary to dilute <u>Thieves</u> with V-6 Mixing Oil.
>   PERSONAL CARE—Dentarome/Dentarome Plus Toothpaste (contains <u>Thieves</u>), Fresh Essence Plus Mouthwash (contains <u>Thieves</u>), KidScents Toothpaste (for children).

Deodorant: <u>Acceptance</u>, <u>Aroma Siez</u>, bergamot, citronella, cypress, <u>Dragon Time</u>, <u>Dream Catcher</u>, <u>EndoFlex</u>, eucalyptus, geranium, <u>Harmony</u>, <u>Joy</u>, lavender, melaleuca, <u>Mister</u>, myrtle, <u>Peace & Calming</u>, <u>RC</u>, <u>Release</u>, <u>White Angelica</u>. Apply oils neat to the skin or dilute with some V-6 Mixing Oil for application under the arms. Also, 2-3 drops of an oil can be added to 4 oz. of unscented talcum powder and 2 oz. of baking soda. Mix this well and apply under the arms, on the feet, or on other areas of the body.
>   BATH & SHOWER GELS—Dragon Time, Evening Peace, Morning Start.
>   MASSAGE OILS—Dragon Time, Relaxation.
>   PERSONAL CARE—AromaGuard Deodorants, Satin Hand & Body Lotion, Sandalwood Moisture Creme. Add a couple drops of one of the oils listed above for additional fragrance.

Deodorizing: Clary sage, myrrh, ^Fmyrtle, peppermint, <u>Purification</u>, sage, thyme.

Depletion: Cypress.

Depression: *See Diet.* <u>Acceptance</u>, basil, ^Fbergamot (aromatic), calamus, Clary sage, <u>EndoFlex</u> (apply often while taking Mineral Essence and Thyromin supplements), ^Ffrankincense,

> *Depression can be caused by a calcium deficiency. Stay away from carbonated soft drinks, specifically cola drinks that are high in phosphorus; they leech calcium from the body. Eating heavy protein at night does not give the body enough time to digest the food before going to sleep. The undigested food then ferments which robs the system of needed oxygen and heightens the sense of depression.*

<u>Gathering</u>, <u>Gentle Baby</u> (on solar plexus), geranium, ginger, grapefruit, <u>Harmony</u>, <u>Highest Potential</u>, <u>Hope</u> (on ears, especially for emotional clearing), <u>Inspiration</u>, jasmine, <u>Joy</u> (5 drops in palm of non-dominant hand, stir clockwise three times with dominant hand, then apply over heart and breathe in deeply), juniper (over heart), lavender (aromatic), <u>M-Grain</u>, neroli, onycha (benzoin), <u>PanAway</u>, <u>Live with Passion</u>, patchouli, <u>Peace & Calming</u> (back of neck), pepper (on crown for spirit protection), ravensara (lifts emotions), <u>Release</u>, Roman chamomile, ^Frosemary (nervous), ^Frosewood, sage (relieves depression), sandalwood, <u>Sensation</u>, tangerine, <u>Trauma Life</u>, <u>Valor</u> (helps balance energies), ^Fylang ylang. *See COMMENTS under Asthma for a discussion on using* **plastic nasal inhalers**.

BATH AND SHOWER GELS—Sensation Bath & Shower Gel, Lemon Sandalwood or Thieves Cleansing Soaps.

MASSAGE OILS—Sensation Massage Oil.

PERSONAL CARE—Prenolone/Prenolone+, Progessence.

SUPPLEMENTS—Mineral Essence, NingXia Red (helps raise energy levels), Omega Blue, Thyromin, Ultra Young (helps lift depression).

BLEND #1—Combine 1-2 drops each of frankincense, 3 Wise Men, and Hope in the palm of your hand, rub hands together clockwise, cup hands over nose and mouth, and breathe deeply.

ANTI-DEPRESSANT—Abundance, Awaken, bergamot, Christmas Spirit, Citrus Fresh, Dream Catcher, frankincense, geranium, jasmine, Joy, lavender, lemon, melissa, Motivation, neroli, orange, onycha (benzoin), Peace & Calming, ravensara, Roman chamomile, rose, Sacred Mountain, sandalwood, 3 Wise Men, Valor.

IMMUNE DEPRESSION— FSpruce.

BATH AND SHOWER GELS—Morning Start Bath & Shower Gel, Thieves Cleansing Soap.

BLEND—5 bergamot, 5 lavender, diffuse.

SUPPLEMENTS—ImmuPro.

SEDATIVES—Bergamot, cedarwood, Clary sage, cypress, frankincense, geranium, hyssop, jasmine, juniper, lavender, marjoram, *Melaleuca ericifolia*, melissa, neroli, onycha (benzoin), patchouli, Roman chamomile, rose, sandalwood, ylang ylang. Use intuition as to which one may be best for the given situation. In addition, check the safety data for each of the oils in the Appendix of this book.

SUICIDAL DEPRESSION—Put Valor then Inspiration on feet and hold feet for a few minutes until relaxed; this may start to release a past negative memory, start crying, etc. If not, rub Present Time over thymus then a drop of Inner Child on their thumb and have them suck the thumb, pushing the pad of the thumb to the roof of the mouth. Once the emotional release starts, put Grounding on the back of neck and sternum, then put Release on the crown of the head and wait for a while, allowing then to deal with the release. After the emotional release has subsided, rub Joy over the heart and Hope on the ears. After waking up the next morning, apply a couple drops of Gentle Baby on solar plexus and over the heart. Magnify Your Purpose may also be helpful to wear as a perfume/cologne.

SUPPLEMENTS—Thyromin.

CLEANSING THE FLESH AND BLOOD OF EVIL DEITIES—Cedarwood and myrrh.

BIBLE—"Breaking the lineage of iniquity," The ancient Egyptians believed that if they didn't clear the body and mind of negative influences before dying, they could not progress into the next life and return to this world to take up the body they had left in the tomb (resurrection).

Deprogramming: Forgiveness, Inner Child, Release, SARA, Trauma Life.

Dermatitis: Bergamot, chamomile (Roman and German), geranium, ^Fhelichrysum, hyssop, ^Fjuniper, lavender, *Melaleuca ericifolia*, onycha (benzoin), ^Fpatchouli, pine, sage lavender, ^Fthyme.

> SUPPLEMENTS—Essentialzyme, JuvaPower/JuvaSpice, Sulfurzyme.
> ***COMMENTS—*Dermatitis may indicate a sulfur deficiency.*

Despair: Acceptance, Believe, cedarwood, Clary sage, fir, Forgiveness, frankincense, Gathering, geranium, Gratitude, Grounding, Harmony, Hope, Joy, lavender, lemon, lemongrass, orange, peppermint, rosemary, sandalwood, spearmint, spruce, thyme, Transformation, Valor, ylang ylang.

Despondency: Bergamot, Chivalry, Clary sage, cypress, Gathering, geranium, ginger, Harmony, Hope, Inner Child, Inspiration, Joy, orange, Peace & Calming, Present Time, rose, rosewood, sandalwood, Transformation, Trauma Life, Valor, and ylang ylang.

Detoxification: GLF, ^Fhelichrysum, ^Fjuniper (detoxifier), JuvaFlex. Apply oils to liver area, intestines, and Vita Flex points on feet.

> SUPPLEMENTS—Balance Complete (*refer to the 5-Day Nutritive Cleanse program listed under Balance Complete in the Supplements section of the Reference Guide for Essential Oils. This program also uses Digest + Cleanse and NingXia Red to help enhance detoxification while maintaining energy levels*), Cleansing Trio (ComforTone, Essentialzyme, and ICP), Digest + Cleanse, JuvaTone.

Diabetes: Coriander (normalizes glucose levels), cypress, dill (helps lower glucose levels by normalizing insulin levels and supporting pancreas function), ^Feucalyptus, fennel, ^Fgeranium, ginger, hyssop, juniper, lavender, ^Fpine, ^Frosemary, Thieves, ^Fylang ylang. Apply on back, chest, feet, and over pancreas. Diffuse.

> *Caution: Diabetics should not use angelica. Watch insulin intake carefully, may have to cut down. Keep physician informed!*

> BLEND #1—8 clove, 8 cinnamon bark, 15 rosemary, 10 thyme in 2 oz. of V-6 Mixing Oil. Put on feet and over pancreas.
> BLEND #2—5 cinnamon bark and 5 cypress. Rub on feet and pancreas.
> SUPPLEMENTS—Balance Complete (contains a blend of fibers to help maintain stable blood sugar levels), Bodygize, Carbozyme (helps control blood sugar levels— can use as much as 2 capsules twice per day), Cleansing Trio (ComforTone, Essentialzyme, and ICP), Digest + Cleanse, ImmuneTune, ImmuPro, Mineral Essence, Power Meal, Pure Protein Complete (contains a blend of proteins and fibers to help reduce spikes and maintain stable blood sugar levels), Stevia, Sulfurzyme (take in morning with Vitamin C before breakfast and at bed time), VitaGreen.

***COMMENTS—*Seven-year old girl took 6 VitaGreen a day (balances blood sugar), Bodygize three times a day, and ImmuneTune.*
PANCREAS SUPPORT—Cinnamon bark, fennel, geranium.
    TINCTURES—Sugar-Up (available through Creer Labs 801-418-8870)
SORES (diabetic)—Do the Raindrop Technique and put <u>Valor</u> on Vita Flex points. Also lavender, <u>Melrose</u>.

Diaper Rash: [F]Lavender.
    PERSONAL CARE—KidScents Tender Tush (formulated specifically for diaper rash), Rose Ointment.

Diarrhea: *See Acidosis.* Cardamom, cistus, cumin, [F]geranium, [F]ginger, [F]melaleuca, [F]myrrh, myrtle, [F]peppermint, [F]sandalwood (obstinate), spearmint (not for babies).
    SUPPLEMENTS—AlkaLime, Essentialzyme, and Royaldophilus.
ANTI-SPASMODIC—Cypress, eucalyptus, Roman chamomile.
CHILDREN—Geranium, ginger, Roman chamomile, sandalwood.
    SUPPLEMENTS—KidScents Royaldophilus.
CHRONIC—Neroli, [F]nutmeg, [F]orange, <u>Di-Gize</u> (apply over stomach, colon, and VF points).
STRESS-INDUCED—Lavender.

Diet: *See Blood, Fasting, Food, and Cleansing.* Diet is extremely important when trying to correct cancer, hypoglycemia, candida, etc. First, cleanse the body, drink a lot of distilled water, stay away from sugars and meats, eat vegetable protein in the mornings, carbohydrates and starches for lunch, and fruit in the evening. Hydrochloric acid and pepsin are secreted in the morning to help digest protein.
    SUPPLEMENTS—Enzyme products: Allerzyme (aids the digestion of sugars, starches, fats, and proteins), Carbozyme (aids the digestion of carbohydrates), Detoxzyme (helps maintain and support a healthy intestinal environment), Digest + Cleanse, Polyzyme (aids the digestion of protein and helps reduce swelling and discomfort), and Lipozyme (aids the digestion of fats).
POST-DIET SAGGY SKIN—Combine 8 drops each of sage, pine, lemongrass, and 1 oz. V-6 Mixing Oil. Rub on areas.

Digestive System: *See also Intestinal Problems.*
Anise (accelerates), basil, bergamot, Black pepper, cardamom (nervous), cinnamon bark, [F]Clary sage (weak), clove, coriander (spasms), cumin

> *Digestive problems may indicate a mineral deficiency. Use Mineral Essence. Royaldophilus is necessary when you are detoxifying or on any type of prescription drug; you must feed the intestinal tract. If you have digestion problems, take Royaldophilus to stop the fermentation process.*

(spasms and indigestion), <u>Di-Gize</u> (acid stomach; aids the secretion of digestive enzymes), [F]fennel (sluggish), ginger, <u>GLF</u>, [F]grapefruit, juniper, <u>JuvaFlex</u> (supports and detoxifies), laurel, lemon (indigestion), ᶠlemongrass (purifier), mandarin (tonic), ᶠmarjoram (stimulates), myrrh, myrtle, neroli, ᶠnutmeg (for sluggish digestion; eases), orange (indigestion), ᶠpatchouli (stimulant), ᶠpeppermint, rosemary, ᶠsage (sluggish), spearmint, tangerine (nervous and sluggish), tarragon (nervous and sluggish). Add the oil(s) to your food, rub on stomach, or apply as a compress over abdomen.

DIFFUSION—See Negative Ions for oils that produce negative ions when diffused to help stimulate the digestive system.

SUPPLEMENTS—AlkaLime (combats yeast and fungus overgrowth and preserves the body's proper pH balance), Balance Complete, Berry Young Juice (helps with the reduction of free radicals), Body Balancing Trio (Bodygize, Master Formula His/Hers, VitaGreen), ComforTone, Digest + Cleanse (contains oils proven to soothe gastrointestinal upset and promote healthy digestion), Essential Manna , Essentialzyme (enzymes help build the digestive system; take before meals for acid stomach), ICP (helps speed food through digestive system; lower incidence of fermentation), KidScents Royaldophilus (chewable for kids), Mineral Essence, NingXia Red, ParaFree, Royaldophilus (supports digestive function), Sulfurzyme. Other enzyme products include: Allerzyme (aids the digestion of sugars, starches, fats, and proteins), Carbozyme (aids the digestion of carbohydrates), Detoxzyme (helps maintain and support a healthy intestinal environment), Polyzyme (aids the digestion of protein and helps reduce swelling and discomfort), and Lipozyme (aids the digestion of fats).

Diphtheria: Frankincense, goldenrod.

Disappointment: Clary sage, Dream Catcher, eucalyptus, fir, frankincense, Gathering, geranium, ginger, Grounding, Harmony, Hope, Joy, juniper, lavender, orange, Present Time, spruce, thyme, Valor, ylang ylang.

Discouragement: Bergamot, cedarwood, Dream Catcher, frankincense, geranium, Hope, Joy, juniper, lavender, lemon, orange, rosewood, Sacred Mountain, sandalwood, spruce, Valor.

Disinfectant: Grapefruit, ᶠlemon, Purification, ᶠsage.

BLEND—Add the following number of drops to a bowl of water: 10 drops lavender (2), 20 thyme (4), 5 eucalyptus (1), 5 oregano (1). If using the larger portions, add to a large bowl of water. If using the numbers in the parentheses, add the oils to a small bowl of water. Use blend to disinfect small areas.

Diuretic: Cardamom, ᶠcedarwood, cypress, EndoFlex, fennel, grapefruit (all citrus oils), juniper, ᶠlavender, lemon, ᶠlemongrass, marjoram, mugwort, onycha (benzoin), orange, oregano, ᶠrosemary, ᶠsage, **tangerine**, valerian. Apply oil(s) to kidney area on back, bottom of feet, and on location.

ALLEVIATES FLUIDS—Cypress, fennel, **tangerine**.

BLEND—1 fennel, 2 cypress, 5 tangerine, apply from the top of the foot to the knee.

Diverticulitis: Use Redmond clay (1-800-367-7258) to help remove fecal matter from the pockets. Rub abdomen with cinnamon bark and V-6 Mixing Oil. Anise or lavender may also help. Calamus may help with earlier stages of diverticulitis.

> *Diverticula, sac-like herniations through the muscular wall of the large intestine (colon), are caused by increased pressure in the bowel from constipation. The existence of these sacs that are filled with trapped fecal sludge is called* **diverticulosis***. When they become infected, the rotting feces erodes the surrounding mucosa and blood vessels and bleeding, rupturing, and infection begins. This is known as* **diverticulitis***.*

SUPPLEMENTS—Balance Complete (*refer to the 5-Day Nutritive Cleanse program listed under Balance Complete in the Supplements section of the Reference Guide for Essential Oils. This program also uses Digest + Cleanse and NingXia Red to help enhance detoxification while maintaining energy levels*), ComforTone to open blocked colon (use daily, increasing dosage by one until bowels are eliminating waste 2-4 times per day), then ICP (fiber beverage) to cleanse colon, and Essentialzyme for digestive enzyme support. Digest + Cleanse and JuvaPower/JuvaSpice may also help.

Dizziness: Tangerine.

DNA: Chamomile strengthens positive imprinting in DNA.

UNLOCK EMOTIONAL TRAUMA IN DNA—Acceptance, 3 Wise Men (instructs DNA to open for discharge of negative trauma), sandalwood (unlocks negative programing in DNA and enhances the positive programming in the DNA cell to create a feeling of security and protection).

Down Syndrome: Clarity, Valor. Apply to bottom of feet and diffuse.

SUPPLEMENTS—Master Formula His/Hers, Mineral Essence.

Dream State: Dream Catcher dissipates negative thoughts and helps one hold onto dreams until they become reality. To help enhance the vividness of dreams, try applying cedarwood and valerian to the back of the neck (from the top of the shoulders to the base of the skull) and work them in with the Vita Flex technique. For help with getting to a deep sleep, see Blend #3 under Insomnia.

INFLUENCES—Clary sage (aromatic) enhances vivid dream recall. Transformation.

PROTECTION FROM NEGATIVE DREAMS (that might steal your vision)—Dream Catcher helps one achieve dreams.

Drowning in Own Negativity: Grapefruit (prevent, aromatic), Transformation.

Drugs: *See Addictions;* DRUGS.

Dying: <u>Awaken,</u> <u>Lazarus</u> (available through Creer Labs 801-418-8870), <u>Transformation</u>. The following combinations have also been used to help individuals pass on more peacefully into the next life: Frankincense (under the nose) and rose (over the heart), **or** <u>3 Wise Men</u> (under the nose) and <u>Joy</u> (over the heart).

Dysentery: Black pepper, cajeput, cistus, clove (amoebic), cypress, eucalyptus, lemon, melissa, [F]myrrh, Roman chamomile. Apply on abdomen and bottom of feet.
SUPPLEMENTS—JuvaPower/JuvaSpice

Dyspepsia (Impaired digestion): Cardamom, coriander, cumin, tarragon, goldenrod, [F]grapefruit, laurel, myrrh, [F]orange (nervous), [F]thyme. Apply to stomach, intestines, and Vita Flex points on feet.
SUPPLEMENTS—Balance Complete, Digest + Cleanse (contains oils proven to soothe gastrointestinal upset and promote healthy digestion), Essentialzyme.

Ears: Cumin (deafness following a bad viral flu infection), elemi, eucalyptus, geranium, **helichrysum** (improves certain hearing losses), Idaho tansy, juniper, marjoram, <u>Melrose</u> (fights infection and for earache), <u>Purification</u>, valerian (combine with helichrysum for added pain relief), <u>Valor</u>, vitex.
   Instructions to increase and restore hearing—
   1. Rub <u>Valor</u> on bottom of feet, especially 2 smallest toes and smallest fingers.
   2. For each ear, layer 2 drops of **helichrysum, <u>Purification,</u> juniper,** and **peppermint** (in that order), around the inside (not deep) and back of ear, on the mastoid bone (behind ear), along the bottom of the skull around to the back of the head, and down the brain stem.
   3. Then do the following ear adjustment.
       1. Pull one ear **up** then the other ear up 10 times each side; 20 times total.
       2. Pull one ear **back** then the other, 5 times each side; 10 times total.
       3. Pull one ear **down** then the other, 5 times each side; 10 times total.
       4. Pull one ear **forward** then the other, 5 times each side; 10 times total.
       5. Then one quick pull with finger in each direction (up/back/down/forward).
   4. Rub **geranium** all around back and front of ear.
   5. (Optional) Rub 2 drops **ravensara** around base of both ears.
   EARACHE—1 drop of either basil, **<u>Melrose</u>**, or <u>ImmuPower</u>. Can also try 1 drop each of helichrysum and valerian together. Put the drop in your hand and soak a small piece of cotton (small enough to fit snugly in the ear) in the oil. Place the piece of cotton in the ear and apply the left over oil on both the front and back of the ear with a finger.
   SUPPLEMENTS—JuvaPower/JuvaSpice.
   EARACHE IN ANIMALS—(Not cats) 1 drop <u>Melrose</u> on cotton swab then around in well of ear.
   <u>**Do not put oils directly into ear canal**</u>.

HEARING IN A TUNNEL—<u>Purification</u>, ravensara.

INFECTION—<u>ImmuPower</u>, melaleuca, <u>Melrose</u> (inside well of ear, down and around ear on the outside and under chin). <u>Purification</u> inside well of ear, *Melaleuca ericifolia* and lavender all around outside of ear. Can also try myrrh and rosemary cineol together.

> ***Ear infections*** *can be caused by food allergies!*
>
> ***Caution****: When working on the ears,* <u>*do not put the oils directly into the ear canal*</u>*. Apply only 1-2 drops of oil to the ear by rubbing on the inside, outside, and on the mastoid bone directly behind the ear.*

INFLAMMATION—Eucalyptus, palo santo.

PIMPLES (in ears)—<u>ImmuPower</u>.

TINNITUS (ringing in the ears, block in eustachian tube)—**Helichrysum** (rub on inside and out of ears), juniper.

Eating Disorders:

ANOREXIA—<u>Citrus Fresh</u>, coriander, grapefruit.

BULIMIA—<u>Citrus Fresh</u>, grapefruit.

OVEREATING—Ginger, lemon, peppermint, spearmint.

Eczema: Bergamot, eucalyptus, geranium, [F]German chamomile, [F]helichrysum, [F]juniper, lavender, *Melaleuca ericifolia*, melissa, [F]patchouli, [F]rosewood, sage, sage lavender.

SUPPLEMENTS—JuvaPower/JuvaSpice, Sulfurzyme.

***COMMENTS—*Eczema may indicate a sulfur deficiency.*

DRY—Bergamot, geranium, [F]German chamomile, hyssop, rosemary.

WET—[F]German chamomile, hyssop, juniper, lavender, myrrh.

Edema: *See Hormonal Imbalance.* [F]Cypress (alleviates fluids), fennel (breaks up fluids), juniper, geranium, [F]grapefruit, ledum, [F]lemongrass, rosemary, **tangerine** (alleviates fluids). *Drink water every 3 hours.*

BLEND—1 fennel, 2 cypress, 5 tangerine. Apply from the top of the foot to the knee.

ANKLES—5 cypress, 3 juniper, and 10 tangerine or use equal parts of cypress and tangerine. Apply from ankles to knees and on Vita Flex bladder points on feet.

DIURETIC—[F]Cedarwood, cypress, <u>EndoFlex</u>, fennel, grapefruit, juniper, [F]lavender, lemon, [F]lemongrass, onycha (benzoin), orange, oregano, [F]rosemary, [F]sage.

***COMMENTS—*For water retention in the legs, Dr. Friedmann rubs tangerine, cypress, and juniper on inside of ankle(s) and leg(s) and on the kidney and heart Vita Flex points. He also has his patients inhale the oils as they are rubbed on.*

Elbow: *See Tennis Elbow.*

Electrical Problems in the Body: *See Balance* for methods of balancing the electrical energies of the body. Frankincense, <u>Harmony</u>, <u>Valor</u>.

Electrolytes:
>BALANCING—<u>Citrus Fresh</u> (increases absorption of Vitamin C).
>*SUPPLEMENTS*—Super C / Super C Chewable, Mineral Essence.

Emergency Oils: First you need the Essential 7 (lavender, peppermint, lemon, <u>Joy</u>, <u>PanAway</u>, <u>Peace & Calming</u>, and <u>Purification</u>), then add to that cistus and helichrysum (for bleeding and tissue repair), oregano, <u>Thieves</u>, frankincense, Balsam fir, and sandalwood (for DNA repair and any tissue damage).
>The following oils are recommended by Dr. Daniel Pénoël as ones that everyone should have with them for any emergency:

>**Melaleuca** (Alternifolia)—Colds, coughs, cuts, sore throat, sunburn, wounds.

>**Ravensara**—Powerful anti-viral, antiseptic. Respiratory problems, viral infections, wounds.

>**Peppermint**—Analgesic (topical pain reliever) for bumps and bruises. Also for fever, headache, indigestion, motion sickness, nausea, nerve problems, spastic colon, vomiting.

>**Basil**—Earache, fainting, headaches, spasms (can substitute fennel), poisonous insect or snake bites, malaria.

>**Lavender**—Burns (mix with melaleuca), leg cramps, herpes, heart irregularities, hives, insect bites and bee stings, sprains, sunstroke. *If in doubt, use lavender!*

>**Geranium**—Bleeding (increases to eliminate toxins, then stops; can substitute cistus), diarrhea, liver, regenerates tissue and nerves, shingles.

>**Helichrysum**—Bruises, bleeding (stops on contact), hearing, pain, reduce scarring, regenerate tissue.

>***COMMENTS**—*Dr. Pénoël also recommends including Melaleuca ericifolia because it is more suited to children then Melaleuca alternifolia, and also elemi because it has similar properties to frankincense and myrrh but is less expensive.*

Emotions: *See Emotional Release in the Science and Application section at the beginning of the <u>Reference Guide for Essential Oils</u>. Refer to the Auricular Emotional Therapy chart in the Basic Information section of this book for points on the ears where the oils can be applied.* <u>Acceptance</u>, <u>Aroma Siez</u>, <u>Awaken</u> (supports spiritual emotions), <u>Citrus Fresh</u> and spruce (on the chest and breathe in <u>Sacred Mountain</u>), cypress (aromatic, healing), <u>Envision</u> (support and

*For **Emotions**, see other topics such as: Abuse, Agitation, Anger, Apathy, Argumentative, Boredom, Confusion, Daydreaming, Despair, Despondency, Disappointment, Discouragement, Fear, Forgetfulness, Frustration, Grief/Sorrow, Guilt, Irritability, Jealously, Mood Swings, Obsessiveness, Panic, Poor Concentration, Resentment, Restlessness, and Shock.*

For more information on using essential oils to help release stored emotions, read <u>Releasing Emotional Patterns using Essential Oils</u> by Carolyn Mein.

For some exciting information about how emotions and feelings affect one's physical health, you may want to read Karol K. Truman's books, <u>Feelings Buried Alive Never Die ...</u> and <u>Healing Feeling from Your Heart</u>.

balance), Balsam fir (balancing), Gathering (to help with feelings and thoughts), geranium (women), German chamomile (stability), goldenrod (relaxing and calming), Gratitude, Humility and Forgiveness (to help with forgiveness), lavender (men), melissa (supports mind and body), Live with Passion (balancing, uplifting, strengthening, and stabilizing), palo santo, ravensara (lifts emotions), Release (soothing), rose (brings balance and harmony to the body), sage lavender (improves mood), Surrender (calming and balancing), 3 Wise Men, Transformation, Trauma Life, valerian (helps replace emotions), White Angelica (balances and protects), White lotus. *See COMMENTS under Asthma for a discussion on using* **plastic nasal inhalers**.

BLEND—Layer the oils listed below. Wait 10 minutes between each oil to allow the emotions to be released more gently. The individual releasing the emotions should shut their eyes and should have no sounds, music, or candles in the room to distract them. They need to shut down their senses to get into their subconscious deep seated emotions. Breathe synergistically with their breathing.

1. Rub Valor on feet. If there are 2 helpers, have one person hold the individual's feet (your right hand to their right foot, left to left; cross arms if necessary) during the entire procedure. Be sure not to break the energy.
2. Rub Peace & Calming on navel, feet, and on the forehead (from left to right).
3. Put Harmony on each chakra in clockwise direction, on wrists, shoulders and inside ankles.
4. Put 3 Wise Men on crown.

BATH AND SHOWER GELS—Evening Peace or Sensation Bath & Shower Gel, Sacred Mountain, Lavender Rosewood, or Peppermint Cedarwood Moisturizing Soaps.

MASSAGE OILS—Relaxation or Sensation Massage Oil.

PERSONAL CARE—Prenolone/Prenolone+, Progessence, Sensation Hand & Body Lotion.

***APPLICATION—*The oils listed here under Emotions can either be diffused, worn as perfume/cologne, applied behind ears and across forehead, applied directly on the ears as specified, or applied to locations as listed in the Emotional Release part of the Science and Application section of the* Reference Guide for Essential Oils.

ACCEPTANCE (self-acceptance)—Acceptance, Forgiveness, Joy, and Transformation. Layer oils on the specific ear point (*refer to the Auricular Emotional Therapy chart in the Basic Information section of this book for location of the Heart point to use for Acceptance*).

ANGER AND HATE—Joy (apply to pituitary Vita Flex points on feet and hands as well), Release, and Valor. Layer oils on the specific ear point (*refer to the Auricular Emotional Therapy chart in the Basic Information section of this book for location of the point to use for Anger & Hate*). Other oils that may be useful include Acceptance, Forgiveness, helichrysum (with deep-seated anger for strength to forgive), and Humility.

BALANCE—<u>Forgiveness</u>, frankincense, geranium, <u>Grounding</u>, <u>Harmony</u>, <u>Hope</u>, <u>Inner Child</u>, <u>Joy</u>, juniper, lavender, orange, <u>Present Time</u>, <u>Release</u>, Roman chamomile, sandalwood, <u>SARA</u>, <u>3 Wise Men</u>, <u>Trauma Life</u>, <u>Valor</u>, vetiver, <u>White Angelica</u>.
   PERSONAL CARE—Prenolone/Prenolone+, Progessence.

BLOCKS—Cypress, frankincense, <u>Harmony</u>, helichrysum, <u>Release</u> (over liver), sandalwood, spearmint, spikenard, spruce, <u>3 Wise Men</u>, <u>Trauma Life</u>, and <u>Valor</u> help to release emotional blocks. <u>Acceptance</u> can help one accept the change.

BURDENED (Bearing Burdens of the World)—<u>Release</u> and <u>Valor</u>. Layer oils on the specific ear point (*refer to the Auricular Emotional Therapy chart in the Basic Information section of this book for the location of the point to use for Bearing Burdens of the World*). <u>Acceptance</u> may also be good to use.

CHILDHOOD ISSUES—<u>SARA</u>. Apply to the **heart** point on the ears.
   FEAR (relating to Childhood Issues)—<u>Gentle Baby</u>, <u>Highest Potential</u>, <u>Inner Child</u>, <u>SARA</u>. Apply to the **fear** point on the ears.
   FATHER OR MOTHER—<u>Gentle Baby</u> and/or <u>Inner Child</u>. Apply to the **father** or **mother** point on the ears (*refer to the Auricular Emotional Therapy chart in the Basic Information section of this book for the location of the Heart, Fear, Father, or Mother points to use for Childhood Issues*).

CLEARING—<u>Forgiveness</u>, <u>Grounding</u>, <u>Harmony</u> (use <u>Hope</u> when emotional clearing), <u>Inner Child</u>, <u>Joy</u>, juniper, <u>Present Time</u>, <u>Release</u> (massage a couple drops on both ears for a general clearing), <u>SARA, 3 Wise Men</u>, <u>Valor, White Angelica</u>. *For some simple instructions on how to do emotional clearing, refer to the page on Emotional Release in the Science and Application section of the <u>Reference Guide for Essential Oils</u>. Another good reference for information on clearing negative emotions is the book, "Releasing Emotional Patterns" by Carolyn L. Mein, D.C.*

> *The emotions of the mind are the most elusive part of the human body. People are extremely handicapped emotionally and are continually looking for ways to clear these negative emotions. Many of the emotional blends referred to in this book were created from the research of the ancient Egyptian rituals of clearing emotions. They were created with the intent of helping people overcome the trauma of emotional and physical abuse enabling them to progress and achieve their goals and dreams. The Egyptians took three days and three nights to clear emotions. In order to create a very peaceful setting, they would put the person in a room with 10 to 12 inch thick walls of solid cement and close the door so there would be no sight or sound.*

COLDNESS (emotional)—Myrrh, ylang ylang.

CONFIDENCE—<u>Chivalry</u>, <u>Envision</u>, <u>Highest Potential</u>, jasmine (euphoria), <u>Live with Passion</u>.

DEFEATED—<u>Acceptance</u>, cypress, fir, <u>Forgiveness</u>, <u>Inspiration</u>, <u>Joy</u>, juniper, spruce, <u>3 Wise Men</u>, <u>Valor</u>.

DEPRESSION—Most of the single oils and blends help with depression as they tend to lift by raising one's frequency. Some of the best include <u>Christmas Spirit</u>, <u>Citrus Fresh</u>, <u>Gentle Baby</u>, <u>Highest Potential</u>, <u>Hope</u>, <u>Joy</u>, <u>Peace & Calming</u>, <u>Valor</u>, and <u>White Angelica</u>. Use whichever blend(s) work best for you. Layer oils on the specific ear point (*refer to the Auricular Emotional Therapy chart in the Basic Information*

E

section of this book for the location of the point to use for Depression). Other oils that may be good to use include <u>Humility</u>, <u>Inner Child</u>, lavender, <u>SARA</u>, and <u>Transformation</u>.

SUPPLEMENTS—Omega Blue.

EMOTIONAL TRAUMA—Sandalwood, <u>Trauma Life</u>.

EXPRESSION (self-expression)—<u>Motivation</u> and <u>Valor</u> (for courage to speak out). <u>Joy</u> may be added to encourage enjoying life to its fullest. Apply to the **self-expression** point on the ears. Take deep breaths to help express oneself.

    EXCESSIVE—<u>Surrender</u>. Apply to the **self-expression** point on the ears.

    FOCUSED—<u>Release</u>, then <u>Acceptance</u> or <u>Gathering</u>. Layer oils on the **self-expression** point on the ears.

    LOST IDENTITY—<u>Inner Child</u>. Apply to the **self-expression** point on the ears (*refer to the Auricular Emotional Therapy chart in the Basic Information section of this book for the location of the Self-expression point*).

EYES—*See Eyes* for oils that help with eyesight.

    VISION OF GOALS—<u>Believe</u>, <u>Dream Catcher</u>, <u>Acceptance</u>, <u>3 Wise Men</u>. Layer on the **eyes & vision** point on the ears (*refer to the Auricular Emotional Therapy chart in the Basic Information section of this book for the location of the Eyes & Vision point*). <u>Envision</u> and <u>Into the Future</u> may also help.

FATHER—Lavender. Apply to the **father** point on the ears. Another oil that may be helpful to layer on top of lavender is helichrysum, especially when deep-seated anger is present.

    CHILDHOOD ISSUES—<u>Gentle Baby</u> or <u>Inner Child</u>. Apply to the **father** point on the ears.

    MALE ABUSE—Helichrysum and lavender. Layer oils on the **father** point on the ears.

    SEXUAL ABUSE—Lavender, <u>Release</u>, and ylang ylang. Layer oils on the **father** point on the ears. <u>SARA</u> may also be helpful (*refer to the Auricular Emotional Therapy chart in the Basic Information section of this book for the location of the Father point to use for Father related issues*).

FEAR—<u>Valor</u>, <u>Release</u>, and <u>Joy</u>. Layer on the **fear** point on the ears. <u>Acceptance</u> <u>Harmony</u>, and <u>Highest Potential</u> may also be helpful.

    CHILDHOOD ISSUES—<u>Gentle Baby</u>, <u>Inner Child</u>, or <u>SARA</u>. Apply to the **fear** point on the ears.

    FUTURE—<u>Into the Future</u>. Apply to the **fear** point on the ears (*refer to the Auricular Emotional Therapy chart in the Basic Information section of this book for the location of the Fear point*).

FEMALE ISSUES—*See Mother.*

GRIEF—Bergamot. Apply to the **heart** point on the ears (*refer to the Auricular Emotional Therapy chart in the Basic Information section of this book for the location of the Heart point to use for Grief*). Another oil that may be helpful is tangerine (when diffused, increases optimism and releases emotional stress).

HEART (Broken or Heavy Heart)—*Refer to both GRIEF and LOSS as well.* <u>Acceptance</u>, <u>Forgiveness</u>, and <u>Joy</u>. Layer oils on the **heart** point on the ears (*refer to the*

Auricular Emotional Therapy chart in the Basic Information section of this book for the location of the point to use for Heart). <u>Release</u>, <u>Transformation</u>, and <u>Valor</u> may also be good to use.

LOSS (eases the feeling)—<u>Joy</u>, <u>Sensation</u>, tangerine (stability).

MALE ISSUES—*See FATHER.*

MIND (open)—<u>3 Wise Men</u>. Apply to the **open the mind** point on the ears as well as the crown of the head and the navel (*refer to the Auricular Emotional Therapy chart in the Basic Information section of this book for the location of the Open the Mind point*). <u>Acceptance</u>, <u>Believe</u>, <u>Clarity</u>, frankincense, <u>Gathering</u>, <u>Magnify Your Purpose</u>, <u>Motivation</u>, <u>Release</u>, sandalwood, and <u>Transformation</u> may also be helpful.

MOOD ELEVATION PROTOCOL—<u>Valor</u> (one drop on each wrist, hold wrists together), <u>Harmony</u> (one drop on solar plexus), <u>Joy</u> (one drop over the heart), <u>White Angelica</u> (one drop on hands–rub hands together then brush through hair, over the face, shoulders, and chest and down the legs).

MOTHER—Geranium. Apply to the **mother** point on the ears. <u>Inner Child</u> and <u>SARA</u> may also be helpful.

    ABANDONMENT—Geranium, <u>Acceptance</u>, and <u>Forgiveness</u>. Layer oils on the **mother** point on the ears.

    SEXUAL ABUSE—Geranium and ylang ylang. Layer oils on the **mother** point on the ears (*refer to the Auricular Emotional Therapy chart in the Basic Information section of this book for the location of the Mother point to use for Mother related issues*).

OVERWHELMED—<u>Acceptance</u> and <u>Hope</u>. Layer on the **overwhelmed** point on the ears (*refer to the Auricular Emotional Therapy chart in the Basic Information section of this book for the location of the Overwhelmed point*). <u>Grounding</u> and <u>Valor</u> may also be helpful.

PITY (self-pity)—<u>Acceptance</u>. Apply to the **self-pity** point on the ears. <u>Forgiveness</u> and <u>Joy</u> may also be helpful.

    COURAGE (to move beyond feeling)—<u>Release</u> then <u>Valor</u>. Layer on the **self-pity** point on the ears.

    PAINFUL—Can feel like heaviness in the chest. <u>PanAway</u>. Apply to the **self-pity** point on the ears (*refer to the Auricular Emotional Therapy chart in the Basic Information section of this book to locate the Self-pity point*).

PROTECTION FROM NEGATIVE EMOTIONS—<u>Magnify Your Purpose</u> (empowering and uplifting), grapefruit, <u>Highest Potential</u>, palo santo, <u>3 Wise Men</u> (release), <u>White Angelica</u>. Apply oils to the forehead and over the heart.

REJECTION—<u>Forgiveness</u> and <u>Acceptance</u>. Layer on the **rejection** point on the ears. <u>Grounding</u> and <u>Valor</u> may also be helpful.

    FROM FATHER—Use lavender first then <u>Forgiveness</u> and <u>Acceptance</u>. Layer on the **rejection** point on the ears.

    FROM MOTHER—Use geranium first then <u>Forgiveness</u> and <u>Acceptance</u>. Layer on the **rejection** point on the ears (*refer to the Auricular Emotional Therapy chart in the Basic Information section of this book for the location of the Rejection point*).

RELEASE—ᶠRoman chamomile.

STRESS—<u>Believe</u>, Clary sage, <u>Evergreen Essence</u>, <u>Live with Passion</u>, <u>Surrender</u>.

SUICIDAL—<u>Gathering</u>, <u>Hope</u>, <u>Joy</u>, <u>Live with Passion</u>, <u>Release</u>, <u>Trauma Life</u>.

SYMPATHY & GUILT—<u>Joy</u> and <u>Inspiration</u>. Layer on the **sympathy & guilt** point on the ears (*refer to the Auricular Emotional Therapy chart in the Basic Information section of this book for the location of the Sympathy & Guilt point*). <u>Release</u>, <u>PanAway</u>, and/or <u>Acceptance</u> may also be helpful.

UPLIFTING—<u>Valor</u> (on feet), birch, <u>Dream Catcher</u>, <u>En-R-Gee</u>, <u>Gratitude</u>, <u>Highest Potential</u>, lemon, orange, <u>Transformation</u>, wintergreen.

VISION—*See Eyes.*

Emphysema: *See Blend #5 under Respiratory System*. Eucalyptus, *Eucalyptus radiata*, <u>Exodus II</u>, <u>Raven</u> (hot compress on chest). May use <u>Raven</u> rectally, <u>RC</u> on chest and back. Reverse each night. <u>Thieves</u> on feet, <u>ImmuPower</u> on spine.

BLEND—Equal parts rosemary cineol, lemon, and peppermint. Diffuse.

SUPPLEMENTS—Exodus.

***COMMENTS—*Dr. Terry Friedmann used Exodus on a 68 year old male who had emphysema. He was on oxygen 24 hours a day. He gave him four per day for one week. When the man came back in, Dr. Friedmann used an oxymeter to test his concentration of blood oxygen. His concentration of blood oxygen, without his oxygen tank, was higher after taking Exodus than it was when he just had his oxygen tank.*

Empowerment: <u>Magnify Your Purpose</u>, <u>Sacred Mountain</u>, <u>Transformation</u>.

Endocrine System: *See Adrenal Glands, Thyroid, Pituitary Gland, Lupus, etc.* Black pepper, cinnamon bark, dill, <u>EndoFlex</u>, ᶠrosemary, sage lavender.

PERSONAL CARE—Prenolone/ Prenolone+, Progessence.

SUPPLEMENTS—Thyromin and FemiGen (women) or ProGen (men), Power Meal (pre-digested protein).

> *The adrenal glands, pituitary gland, thyroid gland, parathyroid glands, thymus gland, pineal gland, pancreas, ovaries, and testes are all a part of the **endocrine system**. The endocrine glands secrete hormones, transmitted via the bloodstream, which are responsible for regulating growth, metabolism, enzyme activity, and reproduction. Essential oils may either act as hormones or stimulate the endocrine glands to produce hormones. This production of hormones has a regulating effect on the body.*

Endometriosis: *See Hormonal Imbalance.* Clary sage, cypress, eucalyptus, geranium, <u>Melrose</u> (hot compress on abdomen), nutmeg, <u>Thieves</u> (on feet).

> ***Endometriosis** is the growth of endometrial tissue in abnormal locations as on ovaries or peritoneal (abdominal) cavity.*

PERSONAL CARE—Prenolone/ Prenolone+, Progessence, ClaraDerm (spray).

SUPPLEMENTS—Cleansing Trio (ComforTone, Essentialzyme, and ICP), Digest + Cleanse, Super C / Super C Chewable, FemiGen.

RECIPE #1—Combine bergamot, lavender, and Clary sage and use with a hot compress over the abdomen or add 2 drops of each to 1 Tbs. V-6 Mixing Oil and insert into the vagina. Use a tampon to retain overnight. This may help rebuild the normal tissue.

Endurance:

PHYSICAL—Balsam fir (inhale from hands), En-R-Gee (on feet), peppermint (cooling). *See COMMENTS under Asthma for a discussion on using* **plastic nasal inhalers**.

SUPPLEMENTS—Be-Fit, CardiaCare (with *Rhododendron caucasicum* which has been shown clinically to enhance physical endurance by increasing blood supply to the muscles and brain), Power Meal, Pure Protein Complete, WheyFit.

Energy: Abundance, Awaken, basil (when squandering energy), Black pepper, Clarity, cypress, En-R-Gee, Envision (balances), eucalyptus (builds), ^Ffir, Hope, Joy, juniper, lemon, lemongrass, Motivation, myrtle (supports adrenal glands to increase energy), nutmeg (increases), orange (aromatic), palo santo, peppermint, rosemary, thyme (aromatic; gives energy in times of physical weakness and stress), Valor (balances), White Angelica.

BATH AND SHOWER GELS—Morning Start Bath & Shower Gel or Lemon Sandalwood Cleansing Soap gives you a fresh start with a surge of energy.

SUPPLEMENTS—VitaGreen (gives energy), Master Formula His/Hers (Multi-Vitamin), Mineral Essence, **NingXia Red**, Thyromin, Super B.

ELECTRICAL ENERGY (frequency)—Forgiveness (high frequency), rose.

INCREASE—Brain Power, Clarity, En-R-Gee, eucalyptus, grapefruit, palo santo, peppermint, rosemary.

DIFFUSION—*See Positive Ions* for oils that produce positive ions when diffused to help increase energy.

SUPPLEMENTS—Ultra Young.

INTEGRATES ENERGY FOR EQUAL DISTRIBUTION—Patchouli.

MAGNETIC—Abundance, Joy (enhances and attracts magnetic energy of prosperity and joy around the body).

NEGATIVE—White Angelica (frequency protects against bombardment of), ginger, juniper (clears negative energy), palo santo (clears).

PHYSICAL—Bergamot, cinnamon bark (aromatic), lemon (aromatic), patchouli (aromatic).

SEXUAL—Lady Love (available through Creer Labs 801-418-8870), Lady Sclareol, Ylang ylang (aromatic; influences).

TINCTURES—SE-6 (available through Creer Labs 801-418-8870)

Energy Centers: *See Chakras.*

Enlightening: Helichrysum.

Enteritis: Cajeput.

Enzymes: Fresh carrot juice has one of the largest concentrations of enzymes. Drink 8 oz. per day. Add apple and lemon to help with detoxification.
S*UPPLEMENTS*—Enzyme products: Allerzyme (aids the digestion of sugars, starches, fats, and proteins), Carbozyme (aids the digestion of carbohydrates), Detoxzyme (helps maintain and support a healthy intestinal environment), Polyzyme (aids the digestion of protein and helps reduce swelling and discomfort), and Lipozyme (aids the digestion of fats). Also KidScents MightyZyme (chewable, just for kids!).

Epilepsy: *See Seizure.* Brain Power, Clary sage. Apply to back of neck and brain Vita Flex points on bottom of feet.
S*UPPLEMENTS*—Cleansing Trio (ComforTone, Essentialzyme, ICP), JuvaPower/JuvaSpice.

> **OILS TO AVOID IF EPILEPTIC**
>
> *There are several oils that should not be used if prone to epilepsy. Please see the Appendix for safety data on the oils and products mentioned in this book. For further contraindication information, please consult the following books:*
>
> *Essential Oil Safety—A Guide for Health Care Professionals by Robert Tisserand and Tony Balacs and Aromatherapy for Health Professionals by Shirley and Len Price.*

Epstein Barr: *See Chronic Fatigue, Hypoglycemia.* Eucalyptus, ImmuPower, Thieves. Do **Raindrop Technique** on spine with the addition of ImmuPower.
S*UPPLEMENTS*—AlkaLime, ComforTone, Essentialzyme, Exodus, ICP, ImmuneTune, ImmuPro, JuvaPower/JuvaSpice, JuvaTone, Mineral Essence, Super C / Super C Chewable, Thyromin, VitaGreen.

Equilibrium: Surrender (emotional), ylang ylang.
N*ERVE*—Petitgrain.

Essential Oils: Essential oils function as a **catalyst** to deliver nutrients to starving cells.
S*ENSITIVE TO* S*KIN* (caustic, high in phenols, may need to dilute)—Cinnamon bark, clove, fennel, grapefruit, lemon, nutmeg, orange, oregano, peppermint. Test the oil first in a small, sensitive area. If irritation occurs, dilute with 1 drop of above oil to 20 drops lavender or mix 20:80 with V-6 Mixing Oil.

Estrogen: Clary sage, SclarEssence, and Mister help the body produce estrogen. Anise (increases).
***C*OMMENTS*—*Some sugar sweeteners block estrogen. Honey goes into blood stream quickly, which affects the pancreas and the production of estrogen.*
P*ERSONAL* C*ARE*—Prenolone/Prenolone+ (pregnenolone is master hormone; used to balance estrogen and progesterone, whichever is needed).

SUPPLEMENTS—2 FemiGen three times a day, ten days before period. Start again two days after cycle. May take up to 6 tablets three times a day. CortiStop (Women's) can also help increase estrogen levels by lowering cortisol levels.

TINCTURE—1 dropper of Estro three times a day in water.

Euphoria: Clary sage (aromatic), jasmine.

Exhaustion: First, work with one or more of the following nervous system oils to calm and relax: Bergamot, Clary sage, coriander, cumin, elemi, frankincense, lavender, pine, sage lavender. Secondly, use basil, ginger, grapefruit, lavender, lemon, Roman chamomile, rosemary, sandalwood, or Transformation.

Expectorant: Black pepper, elemi, eucalyptus, frankincense, helichrysum, Fmarjoram, mugwort, pine, Fravensara. Apply oils to throat, lungs, and diffuse.

Expression (Self Expression): Helichrysum, Into the Future, Joy (when unable to express physically), Motivation, Raven, RC, Transformation, Valor.

Eyes: Thieves on feet (especially 2 big toes), M-Grain on thumb prints, layer Mister, Dragon Time and EndoFlex on Vita Flex points, ankles, and pelvis. Carrot is good around eye area, cypress (also helps circulation), *Eucalyptus radiata*, fennel, frankincense, German chamomile, lavender, lemon, lemongrass (improves eyesight), sandalwood.

> ### NEVER PUT OILS DIRECTLY IN THE EYES!
> *Be careful when applying oils near the eyes. Be sure to have some V-6 Mixing Oil handy for additional dilution if irritation occurs. Never use water to wash off an oil that irritates.*

BASE OILS (good blends of)—Almond or hazelnut.

SUPPLEMENTS—Essential Manna, **NingXia Red** (provides a significant amount of minerals and carotenoids that protect against eyesight deterioration. *See* COMMENTS *below*), Power Meal, Sulfurzyme, Wolfberry Crisp Bars.

TINCTURES—Add AD&E drops for all eye problems.

***COMMENTS—*According to the book, Discovery of the Ultimate Superfood, "The Ningxia wolfberry is rich in two eye-protecting carotenoids--zeaxanthin and lutein—that are absolutely essential for protecting vision from the free radical damage, protein destruction, and blindness that occurs with age."*

EYE DROP RECIPE—Combine 5 parts distilled water, 2 parts honey, and 1 part apple cider vinegar (do not use white vinegar). Mix together and store in a bottle. Does not need to be refrigerated. This special eye drop formula is found in Stanley Burroughs' book, *Healing for the Age of Enlightenment* and has proven over the years to be superior to most commercial eye drops. These drops have been successful for helping to clear glaucoma, cataracts, spots, film, and growths of various kinds. Apply drops one at a time to each eye several times a day until condition has cleared.

CATARACTS—
> **BLEND #1**—8 lemongrass, 6 cypress, and 3 eucalyptus. Apply around the eye area two times a day. Don't get in the eyes.

DRY-ITCHY—Melaleuca (in humidifier).

EYE LID DROP (OR DROOPING EYELIDS)—
> **BLEND #2**—Aroma Life, 1 helichrysum, 5 lavender.
> **BLEND #3**—Helichrysum and peppermint (don't get in the eyes).
> *MASSAGE OILS*—Cel-Lite Magic (around eyes).
> *SUPPLEMENTS*—3 VitaGreen four times a day. After massaging Vita Flex points, eat two whole oranges a day with the white still on the orange. It is very important to eat all the white you can plus Super C / Super C Chewable, ComforTone, and ICP (fiber beverage) after meals.
> *VITA FLEX POINTS*—Fingers, toes, and around the eyes.

IMPROVE VISION—Dragon Time, EndoFlex, frankincense, juniper, lemongrass, Mister, M-Grain, sandalwood, Thieves. Apply oils to feet, Vita Flex eye points, thumbs, ankles, pelvis, eye area (not in eyes), eyebrows. *According to Dr. Mercola, just about any oil can be used if it is consistently rubbed around each eye for several minutes twice a day. This must be continued for at least 3 weeks before any improvement can be seen. He recommends using **frankincense and lavender**.*

> *I have had glaucoma for several years and have had my eye drop prescription changed numerous times because of rising pressure. I used a mixture of one third clove, one third lemon, and one third olive oil and rubbed it on my face above and below my eyes. The last time I was at the doctor, my pressure was 14. It was the lowest pressure I have had since I was diagnosed.*
> **-Submitted by K. Ernst (July 2004)**

> **BLEND #4**—10 lemongrass, 5 cypress, 3 *Eucalyptus radiata*, in 1 oz. V-6 Mixing Oil. Apply around eyes morning and night to improve eyesight. Can also be applied to Vita Flex eye points on fingers and toes, and also on the ears *(refer to the Auricular Emotional Therapy chart in the Basic Information section of this book for the Eyes and Vision point on the ears)*.
> **BLEND #5**—5 lemongrass, 3 cypress, 2 eucalyptus, in 1 oz. of V-6 Mixing Oil. Apply as a blend or layer the oils on the eye area (not in eyes).
> *TINCTURES*—AD&E to take the pressure off the liver and intestines and to improve the vision.
> ****COMMENTS*—One individual, who was not able to see color and had no peripheral vision, rubbed frankincense on his eyelids and just above his eyebrows. Soon thereafter he was able to see color and his peripheral vision returned.*

IRIS, INFLAMMATION OF—Eucalyptus.

RETINA (bleeding)—
> **BLEND #6**—5 tangerine, 5 orange, and 5 grapefruit. Mix and apply 2 drops on fingers and toes. Massage Vita Flex points two times a day or more. Diffuse and let vapor mist around eye. Rub Cel-Lite Magic around the eyes too. Then, eat two whole oranges a day with the white still on the orange. Eat all of the white you can.

SUPPLEMENTS—Super C / Super C Chewable.

RETINA (strengthen)—Cypress, lavender, lemongrass, helichrysum, juniper, peppermint, sandalwood. Apply oil(s) around eye area.

BLEND #7—5 juniper, 3 lemongrass, 3 cypress. Rub on brain stem twice a day.

SPIRITUAL EYES (3rd eye, brow chakra)—<u>Acceptance</u>, <u>Awaken</u>, <u>Dream Catcher</u>. Rub oil on ear lobe to increase both physical and spiritual vision.

SWOLLEN EYES—Cypress and helichrysum. Lavender (antiseptic) is also safe around eyes. If swollen eyes are due to allergies, try putting peppermint on the back of the neck.

Facial Oils: Myrrh, patchouli, sandalwood, vetiver. *Refer to the Personal Care Products section of the <u>Reference Guide for Essential Oils</u> for many other beneficial skin care products.*

PERSONAL CARE—Essential Beauty Serums (Dry, Oily & Acne-Prone Skin Blends).

BROKEN CAPILLARIES—Cypress, geranium, hyssop, Roman chamomile.

DEHYDRATED—Geranium, lavender.

DISTURBED—Clary sage, geranium, hyssop, juniper, lavender, lemon, patchouli, Roman chamomile, sandalwood.

DRY—Geranium, German chamomile, hyssop, lemon, patchouli, rosemary, sandalwood.

ENERGIZING—Bergamot, lemon.

HYDRATING—Cypress, fennel, geranium, hyssop, lavender, lemon, patchouli, sandalwood.

NORMAL—Geranium, lavender, lemon, Roman chamomile, sandalwood.

OILY—Cypress, frankincense, geranium, jasmine, juniper, lavender, lemon, marjoram, orange, patchouli, Roman chamomile, rosemary.

REVITALIZING—Cypress, fennel, lemon.

SENSITIVE—Geranium, German chamomile, lavender.

Fainting: *See Shock.* Nutmeg. Hold one of the following under the nose: Basil, Black pepper, <u>Brain Power</u>, <u>Clarity</u>, lavender, neroli, peppermint, rosemary, spearmint, <u>Trauma Life</u>.

Faith: <u>Hope</u> (increases), <u>Transformation</u> (for anchoring and stabilizing new-found faith).

Fasting: Fasting is the avoidance of solid foods altogether, while liquid consumption ranges between nothing (complete avoidance of all liquids as well) to fresh juices with just water being somewhere in the middle. **Complete avoidance fasting (no food or liquid) should only be done when feeling good**, while fasting on fresh juices can be very healing when sick. The Master Cleanser Lemonade fast (*see Cleansing*) is one of the most beneficial juice fasts. While it takes 30 days on this cleanse to change the chemistry in the body (such as eliminating the need or desire for animal proteins), very effective health results can be achieved after only 10 days. To enhance the effectiveness of the change in body chemistry, the 30 day lemon juice fast can be followed by a carrot juice fast for another 30 days. Bodygize and VitaGreen may be taken two times a day for two weeks but should then be stopped so changes can be made at the cellular level; protein prevents this change. When a mother fasts, the breast fed baby gets the benefits as well (the mammary glands filter the toxins so they are not harmful to the baby).

Fat: *See Cellulite, Diet and Weight.*
> BATH (**attack fat**)—Add 6 drops of the following blend to the bath water and soak in tub.
> BLEND—8 grapefruit, 5 cypress, 4 lavender, 4 basil, and 3 juniper.

Ultra Young may help stimulate the pituitary for increased production of the human growth hormone. This hormone is one of the most powerful side-effect-free agents for rejuvenating the body, restoring lean body mass, and reducing fat.

> SUPPLEMENTS—Allerzyme (aids the digestion of sugars, starches, fats, and proteins), Balance Complete, Digest + Cleanse, Lipozyme (aids the digestion of fats), Power Meal (eat for breakfast as a meal replacement), Ultra Young (improves fat-to-lean ratios by stimulating production of the human growth hormone).
> ***COMMENTS—*Eat more grapefruit to dissolve fat faster. **Also, trans-fats replace essential fatty acids in the brain and are highly acidic! Remove trans-fats from diet!***

Father (Problems With): <u>Acceptance</u>, lavender, <u>Valor</u>. Apply to ears (*refer to the Auricular Emotional Therapy chart in the Basic Information section of this book*).

Fatigue: Clove, En-R-Gee, pine, Fravensara (muscle), Frosemary (nervous), Fthyme (general).
> SUPPLEMENTS—**NingXia Red**.
> MENTAL—Basil, <u>Clarity</u>, lemongrass, <u>Peace & Calming</u>. Basil and lemongrass together are a good combination. Apply on temples, back of neck, feet and diffuse.
> OVERCOMING—Thyme or <u>En-R-Gee</u> on spine, wait a few minutes, then <u>Awaken</u> all over the back and spine; OR <u>En-R-Gee</u> on feet and <u>Awaken</u> on temples and cheeks.
> PHYSICAL—*See Energy.* <u>Clarity</u>, <u>Peace & Calming</u>. Apply on liver, feet, diffuse, and as a body massage.
> SUPPLEMENTS—AlkaLime (acid-neutralizing mineral formulation), Omega Blue, Power Meal, Sulfurzyme, Thyromin, VitaGreen, Wolfberry Crisp Bars.

Fatty Deposits: *See Cellulite and Weight.*
> DISSOLVE—
> SUPPLEMENTS—Allerzyme (aids the digestion of sugars, starches, fats, and proteins), Balance Complete (contains a mix of 5 different kinds of fibers to help cleanse the digestive system), Body Balancing Trio (Bodygize, Master Formula His/Hers, VitaGreen), Digest + Cleanse, Lipozyme (aids the digestion of fats), Power Meal.

Fear: Bergamot, Clary sage, cypress, fir, geranium, <u>Highest Potential</u>, <u>Hope</u>, juniper, marjoram,

Fear causes the blood vessels to tighten, restricting the amount of oxygen and nutrients that can reach the cells.

Motivation (releases emotional and physical fears), myrrh, orange, Present Time, Roman chamomile, rose, sandalwood, spruce, Valor, White Angelica, ylang ylang.

Feet: Fennel, lavender, lemon, pine (excessive sweating), Roman chamomile.

CALLOUSES—Melrose and oregano

CLUB FOOT—Massage with one of the following: Ginger (see below), lavender, Roman chamomile, rosemary (see below).

CORNS—*See Corns.*

NOT TO BE USED ON BABIES EXCEPT FOR CLUB FOOT—Ginger, rosemary.

ODOR—Mix 1 Tbs. baking powder with 2 drops of sage and put in a plastic bag. Shake and eliminate lumps with a rolling pin and put in shoes. Rub calamus of feet.

Female Problems: *See Hormonal Imbalance, Infertility, Menopause, Menstruation, Ovaries, PMS, Pregnancy, Uterus, etc.* Anise, Mister (during time of month when you are out of sorts), Clary sage, Sacred Mountain (female balance).

SUPPLEMENTS—Body Balancing Trio Hers (Bodygize, Master Formula Hers, VitaGreen), FemiGen, Prenolone/Prenolone+, Progessence.

ABNORMAL PAP SMEARS—

RECIPE #1—Add 10 drops ImmuPower and 5 drops frankincense to 1 Tbs. V-6 Mixing Oil and insert into vagina. Use tampon to retain overnight. Take Master Formula Hers to support nutrient levels and ImmuneTune to support the body. May continue daily for as long as necessary.

BALANCE FEMALE HORMONES—Bergamot, sage lavender, ylang ylang.

BATH AND SHOWER GELS—Dragon Time Bath & Shower Gel for that time of month which leaves women with lower back pain, stress, and sleeping difficulties. Pour 1 tsp. to 1 oz. of the gel in water while filling your tub.

SUPPLEMENTS—Three times a day one week before cycle starts, take 2 droppers full of FHS Tincture (available through Creer Labs 801-418-8870) in water after starting. One week after the cycle, take Master Formula Hers four times a day and 6 VitaGreen a day. CortiStop (Women's) can also help reduce cortisol levels and balance hormones.

HEMORRHAGING—*See Hemorrhaging.*

MASSAGE OILS—Combine 10 helichrysum with 1 tsp. V-6 Mixing Oil and massage around ankles, lower back, and stomach.

INFECTION— FBergamot (general), frankincense, and Melrose (may mix and insert in vagina at night; may alternate with the blend below).

BLEND #1— 8 juniper, 8 melaleuca, and 8 Purification. Put in water and douche **or** 3 drops of each in 1 tsp. V-6 Mixing Oil and insert at night using a tampon to retain.

BLEND #2—8 juniper, 8 lavender, and 8 Melrose. Alternate with Blend #1 and follow same instructions.

INFERTILITY (FEMALE)—*See Fertility.* Clary sage, cypress, fennel, geranium, melissa, nutmeg, Roman chamomile, SclarEssence, thyme. Before the cycle, rub 10 drops Dragon

Time around ankles, lower back, and lower stomach. During the cycle, rub 4 drops basil in the same places as before.

PERSONAL CARE—Prenolone/Prenolone+, Progessence.

SUPPLEMENTS—Essential Manna, FemiGen, Master Formula Hers.

OVARIES—*See Ovaries.*

PMS—*See PMS.*

MASSAGE OILS—Dragon Time.

PERSONAL CARE—Prenolone/Prenolone+, Progessence.

SUPPLEMENTS—Body Balancing Trio Hers (Bodygize, Master Formula Hers, VitaGreen), FemiGen, Omega Blue, Wolfberry Crisp Bars.

POSTPARTUM DEPRESSION—Basil, Clary sage, Gentle Baby, Harmony, Joy, nutmeg (see the safety data in the Appendix of this book), Peace & Calming, Valor, White Angelica.

> **Natural Progesterone or Pregnenolone may help prevent postpartum depression**. *Just before a woman has a baby her body produces about 400 mg of progesterone each day to help hold the placenta in place. When the baby is born, the production of progesterone falls dramatically. The body's inability to produce high doses of progesterone can help induce postpartum depression.*

PERSONAL CARE— Prenolone/Prenolone+, Progessence.

SUPPLEMENTS—Omega Blue.

Some women have had wonderful results with the following recipe:

RECIPE #1—Valor first (2-5 drops on each foot and hold to balance energies), Harmony (use finger to dab small amount on each energy center (chakra)), Joy (apply a drop between and just above the breasts), and White Angelica (on the crown of the head and over the top of the shoulders).

REPRODUCTIVE SYSTEM—FemiGen (may help build and balance the reproductive system and maintain better hormonal balance for developmental years all the way through menopause).

Fertility: Bergamot, Clary sage, Dragon Time, fennel, geranium, melissa, Mister, sage, SclarEssence (taken as a dietary supplement to help raise estradiol and testosterone levels), Sensation, yarrow. Apply on reproductive Vita Flex areas on feet, particularly around front of ankle, in line with ankle bone, on each side of ankle under ankle bone, and up along the Achilles tendon. Women: on lower back and on lower abdomen near pubic bone. Can also dilute with V-6 Mixing Oil and use as vaginal retention implant. Men: on lower abdomen near pubic bone, on area between scrotum and rectum, and as a rectal implant (diluted with V-6 Mixing Oil).

PERSONAL CARE—Prenolone/Prenolone+, Progessence, Protec (as rectal or vaginal implant).

SUPPLEMENTS—AlkaLime, Balance Complete (*refer to the 5-Day Nutritive Cleanse program listed under Balance Complete in the Supplements section of the Reference Guide for Essential Oils. This program also uses Digest + Cleanse and NingXia Red*

to help enhance detoxification while maintaining energy levels), Digest + Cleanse, Essential Manna, Ultra Young, VitaGreen. FemiGen (women) and ProGen (men).
***COMMENTS—*An accumulation of petrochemicals in the body can cause sterility in both men and women. Do the MASTER CLEANSER (See Cleansing) for 10 to 20 days consecutively. After coming off the cleanse, focus on alkaline-ash foods. When the body is acidic, it can be hard to conceive.*

Fever: Basil, bergamot, clove (taken internally), ^Feucalyptus, fennel (breaks up), fir, ginger, ImmuPower (rub on spine), lavender, ledum, ^Flemon or lime (reduces–1 or 2 drops in rice milk or water and sip slowly), melaleuca, ^Fpeppermint (reduces–1 or 2 drops in rice milk or water and sip slowly), rosemary cineol, sage lavender, spearmint (not on babies). Peppermint can also be diffused in the room or applied to the bottom of feet.
PERSONAL CARE—Cinnamint Lip Balm.
SUPPLEMENTS—AlkaLime, Mineral Essence, Super C / Super C Chewable.
TO COOL THE SYSTEM—Bergamot, Clove (internally), *Eucalyptus radiata*, peppermint.
TO INDUCE SWEATING—Basil, cypress, fennel, lavender, melaleuca, peppermint, Roman chamomile, rosemary.

> *My daughter, Haley, at age 18 was ill one Sunday, and later in the evening was feeling quite worse. When we checked, she had a fever of 105 degrees. I filled a gel capsule with 10 drops of Clove oil and had her take it with some water. In ½ an hour I checked her temperature again and it was down to 102. I gave her 5 more drops in another capsule and in another ½ hour, her fever was totally gone!!*
>
> ***-Submitted by Sally Donahue***
> ***Wilsonville, Oregon (July 2004)***

Fiber: There are two kinds of fiber: soluble fiber is important for absorbing toxins and removing them from the body; insoluble fiber is important for scrubbing the intestines to remove any buildup of waste material. Viscosity is the balance between soluble and insoluble fiber. A blend of different fibers provides for maximum viscosity which equals optimal absorption and cleansing capabilities. Fiber also helps to slow and balance the absorption of sugars and fats, thereby balancing blood sugar levels! Research has shown that balancing blood sugar levels can extend life expectancy by up to 50%.
SUPPLEMENTS—Balance Complete (contains a blend of 5 different fibers for maximum viscosity), Cleansing Trio (ComforTone, Essentialzyme, and ICP).

Fibrocysts: *See Hormonal Imbalance.*

Fibroids: *See Hormonal Imbalance.* Cistus, EndoFlex, frankincense, helichrysum, Idaho tansy, lavender, oregano, pine, Valor. Put 3 drops of either oil in douche. Also apply to Vita Flex points of feet.
MASSAGE OILS—Cel-Lite Magic.
PERSONAL CARE—Protec.

SUPPLEMENTS—AlkaLime, Essentialzyme, Power Meal, Thyromin, Ultra Young, VitaGreen.

Fibromyalgia: *See Acidosis, Hormonal Imbalance.* May need to detoxify the liver. ImmuPower; massage with PanAway adding

> ***Fibromyalgia*** *is a condition of high acid and generalized pain all over the body; tiny movement brings on pain; extra low pain threshold. Since there are very few positive findings, it is difficult to diagnose. Some sources say that natural progesterone may be beneficial.*

birch/wintergreen & spruce for an additional cortisone response. It may be helpful to use some anti-inflammatory oils like birch, helichrysum, lavender, myrrh, patchouli, rosemary, rosewood, spruce, thyme, or wintergreen.

MASSAGE OILS—Ortho Ease or Ortho Sport (for full body), and do Raindrop Technique.

SUPPLEMENTS— Allerzyme (aids the digestion of sugars, starches, fats, and proteins), AlkaLime (combat yeast and fungus overgrowth and preserve the body's proper pH balance), Balance Complete (high in fiber to absorb toxins and clean the intestinal tract), Bodygize (for vitamins and minerals), Digest + Cleanse, Essential Manna, ImmuneTune (four days), JuvaTone, Mineral Essence, **NingXia Red**, Power Meal, Royaldophilus, **Sulfurzyme**, Super C / Super C Chewable, Super Cal (no more than 1 per day, because of the poor ability to utilize minerals), VitaGreen.

COMMENTS— *Dr. Bernard Jensen suggested that people with fibromyalgia should eliminate all refined sugars from their diet. Refer to the chapter entitled "How to Use - The Personal Usage Reference" in the* Essential Oils Desk Reference *under "Fibromyalgia" for an excellent supplement regimen.*

Fibrositis: *See Hormonal Imbalance.*

BLEND—Combine 2 cinnamon bark, 10 eucalyptus, 10 ginger, 6 nutmeg, 10 peppermint, and 3 rosemary with 2 Tbs. V-6 Mixing Oil and massage chest and back once a day.

Finger:

MASHED—Geranium (for the bruising), helichrysum (to stop the bleeding), lavender (to help for all things), lemongrass (for tissue repair), and PanAway (for the pain).

Flatulence (Gas): Angelica, anise, bergamot, cardamom, coriander, cumin, eucalyptus, fennel, [F]ginger, juniper, [F]lavender, myrrh, nutmeg, onycha (benzoin), peppermint, Roman chamomile, rosemary, spearmint (not for babies), [F]tarragon. Apply oil(s) to stomach, abdomen, and Vita Flex points of feet.

Flu: Blue cypress (aches and pains), clove, ImmuPower, RC, Raven (apply to thymus area, Vita Flex points on feet, chest, back, and on any place where the flu has settled), *Eucalyptus radiata*, Exodus II, fir (aches and pains), goldenrod, ginger, Idaho tansy (on bottom of feet), lavender, ledum, [F]melaleuca, *Melaleuca ericifolia*, [F]myrtle, onycha (benzoin), orange, oregano, [F]peppermint, pine, [F]rosemary, sage lavender, Thieves, thyme, tsuga.

***COMMENTS—According to the
Essential Oils Desk Reference,
"[Idaho] tansy should be
applied topically on stomach
and bottom of feet." (EDR-June
2002; Ch. 28; Flu) It may be
best to dilute Idaho tansy first in
one teaspoon V-6 Mixing Oil
before topical application.

BATH—2 Tbs. Evening Peace Bath
& Shower Gel with drops of
the following oils: 1 birch/
wintergreen, 20 eucalyptus,
5 frankincense, 3 helichrysum,
15 ravensara, and 6 spruce. Mix
together and put mixture under
the faucet while running HOT
bath water. SOAK until cool.
Also consider using Thieves
Cleansing Soap to wash hands with, especially during cold and flu season.

SUPPLEMENTS—Essentialzyme, Exodus, ImmuneTune, Master Formula His/Hers,
ParaFree, Super C / Super C Chewable.

> One Sunday after church a friend commented that I looked "exhausted." I thought that strange because I had gotten a good night's sleep. I walked over to a meeting for a mission trip I would be participating in, and an hour later I started getting a headache and felt something happening to my throat. About 30 minutes later I knew I was coming down with the flu as the headache and sore throat intensified and I started feeling shaky. Fortunately I had peppermint, oregano and Thieves in my truck, and as soon as I got in, I rubbed several drops of oregano on my feet, rubbed Thieves on my neck and throat, and put several drops of peppermint in my water and started drinking it. By the time I got home the headache and sore throat had lessened. That evening and for the next several days I took by capsule a combination of lemon, Mountain savory and oregano three times a day. While I could tell my body was fighting an infection (as indicated by my desire to take naps), the oils completely stopped the flu in its tracks and the headache and sore throat never returned.
> -Submitted by Kevin Dunn
> Los Angeles, California (July 2004)

Fluids: *See Edema or Diuretic.*

Focus: Believe, Brain Power (during strenuous mental activity), Clarity, Gathering (for greater
focus), Highest Potential, Surrender (balancing; clears the mind).
SUPPLEMENTS—Omega Blue, Sulfurzyme.

Food: *See pH Balance.* Use basil for soups
and stuffing. Use cinnamon
bark, clove, orange, tangerine,
and thyme for flavorings.
*** COMMENTS—According to the
Essential Oils Desk Reference,
"They are so concentrated that only 12 drops of an essential oil is equivalent to a
full 1-2 oz. bottle of dried herbs. For a recipe that serves six to ten people, add 1
to 2 drops of an oil and stir in after cooking and just before serving, so the oil does
not evaporate" (EDR-June 2002; Ch. 4; Other Uses; Cooking). Refer to that same
section in the Essential Oils Desk Reference for more ideas on cooking with essential
oils.

> The body secretes pepsin, protease and hydrochloric acid in the morning for the digestion of protein. If you eat fruit in the morning you have almost instant putrefaction (fermentation). Sub-acid fruits (like strawberries) are the only fruit that can be eaten with protein.

BREAKFAST—Proteins (meat, fish, eggs), mixed grains, sunflower seeds, nuts, Power Meal, Pure Protein Complete, and Bodygize. Fruit in the morning will cause candida overgrowth, hypoglycemia, and dysfunction of the thyroid gland. Take Essentialzyme or Polyzyme to help with the digestion, especially when animal protein has been eaten. Also, 8 oz. of carrot juice per day with apple and lemon helps detoxify the body and provides necessary enzymes.

LUNCH—Eat salads, complex carbohydrates like rice, beans, soup, steamed vegetables, bread (Jack Sprout Bread is good) that is toasted (reduces gluten content), baked potatoes, yams, squash, Bodygize.

AFTER 3:00 P.M.—Refrain from eating animal proteins. Bodygize and Power Meal are predigested proteins and can be eaten with fruit. Foods that are easier on the digestive system at night are fruit, soups, lightly steamed vegetables, and salads.

ASSIMILATION OF—

SUPPLEMENTS—Enzyme products: Allerzyme (aids the digestion of sugars, starches, fats, and proteins), Carbozyme (aids the digestion of carbohydrates), Detoxzyme (helps maintain and support a healthy intestinal environment), Digest + Cleanse, Essentialzyme (multiple enzyme product), Polyzyme (aids the digestion of protein and helps reduce swelling and discomfort), and Lipozyme (aids the digestion of fats).

> **Buttered Basil Garlic Melt**
>
> *1 loaf cheese bread or any artisan bread,*
>   *cut into 1 inch slices*
> *1/2 stick butter*
> *1/2 teaspoon garlic powder*
> *4 drops basil essential oil*
> *Sliced mozzarella cheese*
>
> *Melt butter then add garlic powder and stir well. Add basil oil, mix well. With a large unused paint brush, brush on butter mixture until saturated. Cover sliced bread with slices of cheese and bake at 350° until golden brown. Yummmmmie! Even my Baby loved it.*
>
> *-Submitted by Jill Burk*
> *Saginaw, Michigan (July 2004)*

FIBER—Balance Complete, ICP (fiber beverage).

OIL—V-6 Mixing Oil (six different vegetable oils) is excellent for cooking and making salad dressings.

SUGAR SUBSTITUTE—Stevia.

Food Poisoning: Flavor a cup of water with 6 drops <u>Di-Gize</u>, swish around in mouth, and swallow. <u>Exodus II,</u> patchouli, rosemary cineol, tarragon, <u>Thieves</u>.
SUPPLEMENTS—Detoxzyme, Essentialzyme, Exodus.

Forehead: Jasmine.

Forgetfulness: *See Memory.* <u>Acceptance</u> (over heart and liver), <u>Brain Power</u> (1 drop under tongue), cedarwood, <u>Clarity</u>, cypress, <u>Dream Catcher</u>, <u>Highest Potential</u>, <u>Hope</u>, fir, <u>Gathering</u>, geranium, juniper, marjoram, myrrh, orange, <u>Present Time</u>, Roman chamomile, rose, sandalwood, <u>3 Wise Men</u>, rose, sage lavender <u>Valor</u>, <u>White Angelica</u>, ylang ylang.

Wear as perfume/cologne or put a couple drops in hands, rub together, cup over nose and mouth, and breathe deeply. *See* COMMENTS *under Asthma for a discussion on using* **plastic nasal inhalers**.
SUPPLEMENTS—Essential Manna, Omega Blue, Ultra Young/Ultra Young+, VitaGreen.

Forgive (and Forget): Acceptance, Forgiveness, 3 Wise Men, Transformation, Valor, White Angelica.
***COMMENTS—*It has been said that, "The conscious thought to forgive quells the fear response in the amygdalla."*

Formaldehyde: Purification (removes).

F

Fortifying: Cypress.

Freckles: Idaho tansy. Mix 2-3 drops with lotion and spread over face. Can be used two or three times per week.

Free Radicals:
ELIMINATE—Longevity
SUPPLEMENTS—Berry Young Juice, Chelex, Longevity Capsules, and NingXia Red help eliminate and prevent the build up of free radicals.

Frigidity: *See Libido, Sex Stimulant.* Chivalry, FClary sage, jasmine, Lady Love (available through Creer Labs 801-418-8870), Lady Sclareol, nutmeg (overcome frigidity and impotence), rose, Fylang ylang (helps balance male/female energies).
SUPPLEMENTS—Prenolone/Prenolone+, Progessence.
TINCTURES—SE-6 (available through Creer Labs 801-418-8870)

Frustration: Acceptance, Clary sage, frankincense, Gathering, ginger, Hope, Humility, juniper, lavender, lemon, orange, peppermint, Present Time, Roman chamomile, spruce, 3 Wise Men, thyme, Valor, ylang ylang.

Fungus: Abundance, cajeput, clove, fennel, geranium, ImmuPower, lavender, lemongrass, melaleuca, Melrose, RC, Raven, Roman chamomile, rosemary verbenon, Thieves. Apply topically (dilution with V-6 Mixing Oil may be necessary depending on the oil) or add to

*I had developed a **fungus** on my big toenails. The fungus was bad enough that the white, thick toenail was making shoes painful. I went to a podiatric doctor. The doctor removed the inside edge of the left big toenail down to the nail bed. He then prescribed some medicine that was $80 a tube to get rid of the rest. It continued to get worse and was spreading all over the nails and was headed for the rest of the nail beds. I decided to use Animal Scents Ointment on my toes 3 times a day. Now my nails are normal and the thickness is gone.*
-Submitted by K. Ernst (July 2004)

bath water. Do the **raindrop technique** to help purge the body of pathogenic fungi that may exist along the spinal cord or in the lymphatic system. May also try the MASTER CLEANSER (*See Cleansing*) to clean out the intestinal tract and re-alkalinize the body.

BLEND—2 myrrh, 2 lavender. Put on location.

SUPPLEMENTS—AlkaLime (designed to combat yeast and fungus overgrowth and preserve the body's proper pH balance), Balance Complete, Digest + Cleanse (contains coconut oil with capric acid which has been shown to inhibit the growth of three different strains of candida), Essentialzyme, Royaldophilus, Super C / Super C Chewable, Thyromin, VitaGreen.

***COMMENTS—*Refer to the chapter entitled "How to Use - The Personal Usage Reference" in the* Essential Oils Desk Reference *under "Fungal Infections" for some excellent blends and tips for combating systemic fungal infections.*

FUNGAL INFECTIONS—*Eucalyptus citriodora*, geranium, melaleuca (Tea Tree), patchouli.

PREVENTS GROWTH OF—Melrose (two times a day for seven days), Purification.

Gallbladder: Forgiveness, ᶠgeranium, ᶠGerman chamomile, **GLF**, juniper, Juva Cleanse, JuvaFlex (stimulates), lavender, Release, rosemary (supports), Surrender (over liver & pancreas). Apply over gallbladder area (can use a hot compress) and Vita Flex points on feet. Also, 2 capsules JuvaFlex - AM, 2 Juva Cleanse - PM.

SUPPLEMENTS—Essentialzyme, Sulfurzyme (aids bile secretion and magnifies effects of vitamins).

INFECTION IN— ᶠHelichrysum.

STONES—Geranium, grapefruit, juniper, Juva Cleanse, lime, ᶠnutmeg, rosemary, wintergreen.

Gangrene: Cistus, elemi, Exodus II, ImmuPower, lavender (used by Dr. Gattefossé to recover from gas gangrene), Melrose, Mountain savory, ravensara, Thieves, thyme.

SUPPLEMENTS—Exodus, ImmuneTune, ImmuPro, Super C / Super C Chewable.

Gas: *See Flatulence.* ᶠLavender, nutmeg, onycha (benzoin), tarragon. Apply to large intestine Vita Flex points on the feet.

Gastritis: (Inflammation of the stomach lining). *See Anti-inflammatory.* Calamus, Di-Gize, fennel, laurel, peppermint, pine, sage, spikenard, tarragon, yarrow. Apply over stomach area with hot compress. One drop of oil in rice or almond milk taken as a dietary supplement. Can also use capsules to take oils internally (**Note**: *use only those oils approved for internal use by the FDA. Look for GRAS or FA designations in "Single Oil Summary Information" in the Appendix*).

SUPPLEMENTS—AlkaLime, Balance Complete, Cleansing Trio (ComforTone, Essentialzyme, and ICP), Digest + Cleanse, KidScents Royaldophilus, Mineral Essence, Royaldophilus.

General Tonic: Grapefruit, lemon, Mountain savory, ^Fspruce.

Genitals: ^FClary sage.

Gentleness: Rosewood (aromatic).

Germs: *See Bacteria.*
> AIRBORNE—Fir.
> GERMICIDAL— ^FLemon, <u>RC</u>.

Gingivitis: <u>Forgiveness</u>, <u>Harmony</u>, helichrysum, melaleuca, <u>Melrose</u>, myrrh, <u>Present Time</u>, rose, rosemary, ^Fsage, <u>Thieves</u>. Apply on throat and gums.
> *PERSONAL CARE*—Dentarome/Dentarome Plus Toothpaste (contains <u>Thieves</u>), Fresh Essence Plus Mouthwash (contains <u>Thieves</u>), KidScents Toothpaste (for children).

Glandular System: <u>Egyptian Gold</u>, ^FSage, spearmint, spruce. Blue cypress may help stimulate the amygdalla, pineal gland, pituitary gland, and hypothalamus.
> *SUPPLEMENTS*—ProGen (male) or FemiGen (female) for glandular nutrients.

Glaucoma: *See Eyes.*
> *SUPPLEMENTS*—Essentialzyme (to help relieve stress on the pancreas, if congested), Sulfurzyme (to help regulate the fluid pressure in the eye), Super C / Super C Chewable, Super B.

Goiter: *See Endocrine System, Lymphatic System.* Cleanse the lymphatic system. Balance the endocrine system with EndoFlex.

Gout: Basil, birch, calamus, ^Ffennel, geranium, hyssop, <u>Juva Cleanse</u>, <u>JuvaFlex</u>, ^Flemon, nutmeg, onycha (benzoin), <u>PanAway</u>, pine, thyme, wintergreen, yarrow. Cleanse with MASTER CLEANSER (*See Cleansing*) and drink lots of fluids (water, juices, etc.).
> *MASSAGE OILS*—Ortho Ease and Ortho Sport.
> *SUPPLEMENTS*—Balance Complete, CardiaCare (with *Rhododendron caucasicum* which helps increase uric acid elimination), Cleansing Trio (ComforTone, Essentialzyme, and ICP), Digest + Cleanse, Essential Manna, JuvaTone, Mineral Essence, Sulfurzyme, Super C / Super C Chewable, Super Cal, Thyromin, VitaGreen.
> ***COMMENTS*—*Refer to the chapter entitled "How to Use - The Personal Usage Reference" in the <u>Essential Oils Desk Reference</u> under "Gout" for some excellent blend recipes and supplement recommendations.*

Grave's Disease: *See Thyroid:* HYPERTHYROIDISM. Blue tansy, <u>EndoFlex</u>, lemongrass, myrrh, spruce.
> *SUPPLEMENTS*—ImmuPro, Mineral Essence, Sulfurzyme (helps mitigate effects of autoimmune diseases), Thyromin, VitaGreen.

Grief/Sorrow: Bergamot (turns grief into joy), Clary sage, eucalyptus, <u>Forgiveness</u>, <u>Gentle Baby</u> (massage whole body), <u>Hope</u>, <u>Joy</u> (over the heart), juniper, lavender, <u>Present Time</u>, <u>Release</u>, Roman chamomile, <u>Sacred Mountain</u> (back of the neck), <u>3 Wise Men</u> (rub on crown), <u>Transformation</u>, <u>Valor</u> (on the feet), <u>White Angelica</u> (on the forehead or shoulders).

Grounding: Fir, <u>Grounding</u>, <u>Hope</u>, <u>Joy</u>, patchouli, spruce, <u>3 Wise Men</u>, tsuga.
    FEELING OF—cypress (aromatic).

Guilt: <u>Acceptance</u>, <u>Awaken</u>, cypress, <u>Forgiveness</u>, frankincense, <u>Gathering</u>, geranium, <u>Harmony</u>, <u>Inner Child</u>, <u>Inspiration</u>, juniper, lemon, marjoram, <u>Peace & Calming</u>, <u>Present Time</u>, <u>Release</u>, Roman chamomile, rose, sandalwood, spruce, thyme, <u>Valor</u>, <u>White Angelica</u>.

Gulf War Syndrome: <u>Exodus II</u>.

Gum Disease: *See Gingivitis.* <u>Forgiveness</u>, <u>Harmony</u>, ᶠmelaleuca, <u>Melrose</u> (fights infection), myrrh, <u>Present Time</u>, tsuga.
    PERSONAL CARE—Dentarome/Dentarome Plus Toothpaste (contains <u>Thieves</u>), Fresh Essence Plus Mouthwash (contains <u>Thieves</u>).

Gums: *See Gingivitis.* Lavender, <u>Melrose</u> (fights infection), myrrh (infection), Roman chamomile, sage lavender (infection).
    PERSONAL CARE—Dentarome/Dentarome Plus Toothpaste (contains <u>Thieves</u>), Fresh Essence Plus Mouthwash (contains <u>Thieves</u>), KidScents Toothpaste (for children).
    SURGERY ON GUMS—For one individual, helichrysum was applied with a Q-tip every 15 minutes to kill the pain. No other pain killer was used.

Habits: *See Addictions.* <u>Acceptance</u>, lavender, <u>Transformation</u>.
    ***COMMENTS—*To break bad habits, you need to change the DNA and RNA. Sandalwood and frankincense help with this.*

Hair: *Refer to the Personal Care Products section of the* <u>Reference Guide for Essential Oils</u> *for a list of ingredients and more details on chemical-free shampoos and conditioners.*
    TINCTURES—AD&E
    ***COMMENTS—*Refer to the chapter entitled "How to Use - The Personal Usage Reference" in the* <u>Essential Oils Desk Reference</u> *under "Hair and Scalp Problems" for some excellent blend recipes.*
    BEARD—Cypress, lavender, lemon, rosemary, thyme.
    BODY—Cedarwood (gives the hair shaft more body, more strength, and more life), tamanu.
    CHILDREN—Lavender Volume Shampoo with Lavender Volume Conditioner or KidScents Shampoo.

Color—(keep light) 1 chamomile, 1 lemon, and 1 quart of water. Rinse hair.

Damaged (perms, color-treated, bleached)—Tamanu.

> *PERSONAL CARE*—Lemon Sage Clarifying Shampoo and Lemon Sage Clarifying Conditioner (leave on hair for about 10 minutes) together helps remove buildup of styling products and recondition hair. Rosewood Moisturizing Shampoo and Rosewood Moisturizing Conditioner (leave on hair for about 10 minutes) together may restore manageability and shiny, healthy look. Also KidScents Shampoo.

Dandruff—Basil, birch, cedarwood, cypress, [F]lavender, rosemary, sage, thyme, wintergreen.

> *PERSONAL CARE*—KidScents Shampoo, Lavender Volume Shampoo, Lavender Volume Conditioner.

Dry—Birch, geranium, lavender, rosemary, sandalwood, wintergreen.

> *PERSONAL CARE*—Rosewood Moisturizing Shampoo and Rosewood Moisturizing Conditioner (leave on hair for about 10 minutes) together may restore manageability and shiny, healthy look.

Estrogen Balance—Clary sage in Lavender Volume Shampoo and Lavender Volume Conditioner help promote estrogen balance in the membrane tissue around the hair follicle. This serves to balance testosterone levels and prevent the thickening of the tissue around the follicle that results in hair loss.

> **Blend #1**—1 lavender, 6 patchouli in 2-5 oz. Rosewood Moisturizing Shampoo.
>
> **Blend #2**—Mix together 2 cinnamon bark, 4 cypress, 4 geranium, 2 juniper, 5 lavender, and 3 rosemary. Then put one drop of the blend into ¼ tsp of water and rub on bald area and entire scalp. A gentle night treatment.
>
> *PERSONAL CARE*—Lavender Volume Shampoo and Lavender Volume Conditioner with Clary sage (*see ESTROGEN BALANCE above*).
>
> *SUPPLEMENTS*—ComforTone, Essentialzyme, Super B (stress), Thyromin, VitaGreen.

Fragile Hair—Birch, Clary sage, lavender, Roman chamomile, sandalwood, thyme, wintergreen.

> *PERSONAL CARE*—KidScents Shampoo, Lavender Volume Shampoo and Lavender Volume Conditioner.

Greasy—Petitgrain.

Growth (stimulate)—Basil, Western Red cedar, cedarwood, cypress, geranium, ginger, grapefruit, hyssop, lavender, lemon, rosemary, sage, thyme, ylang ylang (promotes).

> *PERSONAL CARE*—Lavender Volume Shampoo and Lavender Volume Conditioner.
>
> *SUPPLEMENTS*—Sulfurzyme. A deficiency in sulfur can result in hair loss or poor hair growth.

Itching—Lavender and [F]peppermint (skin).

Loss—Birch, [F]cedarwood, Clary sage, cypress, [F]lavender, laurel (after infection), lemon, Roman chamomile, [F]rosemary, sage, sage lavender, thyme, wintergreen, [F]ylang ylang.

> Alopecia Areata (inflammatory hair loss disease) thyme (CT thymol), rosemary (CT cineol), lavender, cedarwood. Add any or all of these oils to jojoba and grapeseed carrier oils and massage into scalp daily.
>
> *PERSONAL CARE*—Lavender Volume Shampoo and Lavender Volume Conditioner.

SUPPLEMENTS—Sulfurzyme,
Super B, Thyromin.
***COMMENTS—*Refer to the chapter
entitled "How to Use - The
Personal Usage Reference"
in the Essential Oils Desk
Reference under "Hair Loss"
for some excellent blend recipes.*
SILKY AND SHINY—Tamanu.
PERSONAL CARE—KidScents
Shampoo, Rosewood
Moisturizing Shampoo and
Rosewood Moisturizing
Conditioner (leave on hair for about 10 minutes) together may help maintain
manageability and a shiny, healthy look.
SPLIT ENDS—
PERSONAL CARE—KidScents Shampoo, Rosewood Moisturizing Shampoo and Rosewood
Moisturizing Conditioner (leave on hair for about 10 minutes) together may restore
manageability and shiny, healthy look.

In males, hair loss can often be blamed on heredity, hormones (high levels of testosterone), and aging. Other reasons for hair loss may include poor circulation, hypertension, acute illness, surgery, radiation, Scarlet Fever, Syphilis, stress, sudden weight loss, iron deficiency, diabetes, hypothyroidism, drugs, poor diet, and vitamin deficiency.

Avoid hair products that are not natural on the hair. Avoid chlorinated swimming pools or polluted seas. Chemical products may also leave a residue build-up which can cause hair loss. Correcting a hormonal imbalance or hypertension (dilate blood vessels and stimulate cell division) may help.

Halitosis: Cardamom, lavender, ᶠnutmeg,
ᶠpeppermint, Thieves.
SUPPLEMENTS—AlkaLime.
PERSONAL CARE— Dentarome/
Dentarome Plus Toothpaste
(contains Thieves), Fresh
Essence Plus Mouthwash
(contains Thieves), KidScents Toothpaste (for children).

Don't you just love the feel of clean teeth and fresh breath! Try putting a drop of Thieves on your toothbrush instead of toothpaste. At first, it is a little warm, but it sure feels refreshing. If this doesn't work for you, try putting a drop on your toothpaste or put 10 drops of Thieves in a small spray bottle full of distilled water and mist in your mouth before brushing your teeth.

Hands: Eucalyptus, geranium, lavender, lemon, patchouli, rosemary, sandalwood.
DRY—Geranium, patchouli, sandalwood.
PERSONAL CARE—Genesis Hand & Body Lotion, Rose Ointment.
NEGLECTED—Geranium, lemon, patchouli.
TINGLING IN—Lemongrass in Genesis Hand & Body Lotion.

Hangovers: Fennel, grapefruit, lavender, lemon, rose, rosemary, sandalwood.
SUPPLEMENTS—Super C / Super C Chewable.

Happiness: Christmas Spirit, Joy.

Harmony in Body Systems: <u>Acceptance</u>, clove (aromatic), geranium (harmonizing), <u>Harmony</u>, <u>Inspiration</u>, <u>Lady Sclareol</u> (women), Roman chamomile.

> *MASSAGE OILS*—Sensation Massage Oil creates an exotic arousal and increases sexual desire. The fragrance creates a peaceful and harmonious feeling that is helpful in easing relationship stress. Relaxation Massage Oil also creates a peaceful and harmonious feeling.
>
> *PERSONAL CARE*—Sensation Hand & Body Lotion.

OF MIND AND BODY—<u>Release</u>.

Harshness: Jasmine.

Hashimoto's Disease: *See Thyroid: HYPERTHYROIDISM.* Blue tansy, <u>EndoFlex</u>, lemongrass, myrrh, spruce.

> *SUPPLEMENTS*—ImmuPro, Mineral Essence, Sulfurzyme (helps mitigate effects of autoimmune diseases), Thyromin, VitaGreen.

Hate: <u>Acceptance</u>, <u>Forgiveness</u>, <u>Release</u>.

Hay Fever: Cajeput, eucalyptus, <u>Juva Cleanse</u>, lavender, Roman chamomile, rose.

Headaches: *See Migraine Headaches.* Basil, <u>Aroma Life</u> (massage on arteries in neck), <u>Aroma Siez</u>, calamus, cardamom, <u>Clarity</u>,

> *Clarity may cause headaches when chemicals or metals are in the brain. To break this blockage put <u>Aroma Life</u> or helichrysum on arteries in the neck.*

clove, cumin, eucalyptus, <u>Dragon Time</u>, frankincense, <u>Gentle Baby</u>, lavender, marjoram, <u>Mister</u>, <u>M-Grain</u>, ᶠpeppermint, <u>Relieve It</u>, ᶠrosemary, sage lavender. Apply to temples, back of neck, forehead, and diffuse.

> ***COMMENTS*—*According to the <u>Essential Oils Desk Reference</u>, "For headaches, put one drop [<u>Thieves</u>] on tongue and push tongue against the roof of the mouth." (EDR-June 2002; Ch. 8; Thieves; Application) Also, refer to the chapter entitled "How to Use - The Personal Usage Reference" in the <u>Essential Oils Desk Reference</u> under "Headaches" for some excellent blend recipes and supplement recommendations for several different types of headaches.*

COLD/FLU HEADACHES—Cumin.

EMOTIONAL HEADACHES—<u>Joy</u>.

MENSTRUAL MIGRAINES—*See Hormonal Imbalance.* Sage lavender.

CHILDREN'S MIGRAINES—

> *BLEND*—5 drops Roman chamomile, 10 grapefruit, 5 peppermint, 3 rosemary, and 4 oz. V-6 Mixing Oil for children under seven and 2 oz. V-6 Mixing Oil for children over seven.

MIGRAINE HEADACHES—(may be caused by problems in the colon. Cleanse the colon using supplements). <u>Aroma Siez</u>, Fbasil, birch, marjoram, <u>M-Grain</u>, <u>PanAway</u>, <u>Peace & Calming</u>, Fpeppermint, <u>Relieve It</u>, <u>Release</u>, Roman chamomile, spearmint, wintergreen, ylang ylang.

> *My husband has been bothered by migraine headaches for much of his adult life. Doctors have treated this condition with various medications - all with their own bag of side-effects. So one day I decided to have him try peppermint oil, a drop on each temple. To his amazement the headache was gone in seconds and the cooling feel of the peppermint gave him a feeling of energy and revitalization.*
> **-Submitted by Kathleen Mueller,**
> **Menomonee Falls, WI (July 2004)**

SUPPLEMENTS—AlkaLime (if caused from acidosis), Balance Complete, Cleansing Trio (ComforTone, Essentialzyme, and ICP), Digest + Cleanse. Do not use ComforTone and JuvaTone together (*See ComforTone in the Supplements section of the* <u>*Reference Guide for Essential Oils*</u>).

STRESS HEADACHES—<u>M-Grain</u>, Roman chamomile.

SUGAR HEADACHES—<u>Thieves</u> for low blood sugar headaches.

SUPPLEMENTS—Allerzyme (aids the digestion of sugars, starches, fats, and proteins), AlkaLime, Carbozyme, Digest + Cleanse, Mineral Essence.

Healing: <u>Acceptance</u>, Clary sage (aromatic), clove, cypress, eucalyptus (aromatic), frankincense, <u>Humility</u>, lemon (aromatic), melaleuca, <u>PanAway</u>, sage. Combinations of sandalwood, frankincense, and lavender or frankincense and balsam fir (add myrrh if dealing with infection) have been used to help heal from surgery or major injuries. Also, combine the following oils (ratio in drops) in a 5 ml bottle: 20 valerian, 5 vetiver, 2 helichrysum, 1 clove, 1 peppermint. Applying several drops of this blend to the brain stem (cervical vertebrae on back of neck) before surgery has been shown to maintain normal white blood cell counts during surgery, thereby speeding recovery by up to 30%. Any of these combinations may be used both internally and externally.

Health: <u>Abundance</u>, lavender (aromatic), lemon (aromatic).

SUPPLEMENTS—Balance Complete, Cleansing Trio (ComforTone, Essentialzyme, and ICP), Digest + Cleanse, Longevity Capsules, NingXia Red, Omega Blue (omega-3 essential fatty acids). The following is a recommended daily regimen to help maintain and promote optimal health: NingXia Red and Longevity Capsules (for optimal antioxidant support), Omega Blue (to support cell membranes and optimal brain function), and Balance Complete (to replace the least nutritional meal; for nutritional support, toxin removal, and healthy elimination).

PROMOTES—Eucalyptus, juniper (aromatic).

Hearing: *See Ears.*

Heart: Aroma Life on heart and all Vita Flex heart points, Citrus Fresh, Clarity, cypress, Dragon Time, fleabane, Forgiveness, Gentle Baby, geranium, ginger, Harmony, Hope, hyssop, Joy, lavender, Mister, M-Grain, PanAway, Relieve It, rosemary,

> **HEART PUMP FOR HEART STRESS**
>
> *Using your thumbs, apply pressure in an alternating "pumping" fashion between the following two heart points: (1) on the left hand at the lifeline under the ring finger; and (2) just inside the elbow. Also apply Aroma Life to the chest and the hand and heart points. And of course, GET HELP FAST!*

Valor on feet, White Angelica, ylang ylang (balances heart function). Apply oils to carotid arteries, heart, feet, under left ring finger, above elbow, behind ring toe on left foot, and Vita Flex points on the feet.

> *SUPPLEMENTS*—CardiaCare, Longevity Capsules (contains thyme oil to help preserve omega-3 fatty acids in the heart), Mineral Essence, NingXia Red, Power Meal, Sulfurzyme, Ultra Young (may help reverse heart disease), Wolfberry Crisp Bars.

> *TINCTURES*—HRT and Rehemogen.

ANGINA—Aroma Life, ^Fginger, laurel, ^Forange (for false angina). Apply to heart and Vita Flex heart point.

> *TINCTURES*—HRT.

ARRHYTHMIA—PanAway on heart and Relieve It on left foot Vita Flex heart point (rotate each application). Goldenrod and lavender are also good. Research done by Dr. Pénoël indicates that ylang ylang may be beneficial in preventing or correcting an irregularity in the force or rhythm of the heart.

> *TINCTURES*—HRT.

BRINGS JOY TO HEART—Christmas Spirit, Citrus Fresh, Joy.

CARDIOTONIC—Lavender, thyme.

> *SUPPLEMENTS*—CardiaCare (strengthens and supports).

CARDIOVASCULAR SYSTEMS—*See Cardiovascular System.* Aroma Life (cardiac spasms), cinnamon bark (strengthens), cypress (strengthens the capillary walls and increases circulation), fennel, fleabane (dilates), Joy, ^Forange (cardiac spasms), palmarosa (supports), sandalwood (strengthens).

> *SUPPLEMENTS*—CardiaCare (strengthens and supports), Omega Blue.

> *TINCTURES*—1-2 droppers of HRT two to three times per day.

CORONARY ARTERY—Prenolone/Prenolone+, Progessence.

> ***COMMENTS*—*Research has shown that natural progesterone protects the coronary artery from going into spasms. Provera, a synthetic progestin, offers no protection from coronary artery spasms. In fact, it promotes the spasm to the point of completely shutting off the flow of blood. This may explain the increase in heart attacks in women 5 to 10 years after menopause, many of whom are on synthetic progestin.*

> *SUPPLEMENTS*—CardiaCare (contains Hawthorne Berry which helps dilate the coronary arteries and increase blood circulation to the heart).

HEART TISSUE—Marjoram has been found to help rejuvenate the smooth muscle tissue of the heart.

TINCTURES—HRT.

***COMMENTS—*One woman had cancer of the heart which literally ate a hole in her heart. She used HRT and the heart tissue regenerated itself and the cancer disappeared. One man had a heart attack and was awaiting a heart transplant, he used Aroma Life, Valor, and lavender topically and HRT orally. After four weeks of using the oils, he was told by his doctor that he was doing too well to have a heart transplant.*

HYPERTENSION (high blood pressure)—*See Blood.*

LARGE VALVE—Aroma Life (shortness of breath).

TINCTURES—HRT.

PALPITATIONS (rapid and forceful contraction of the heart)—Aroma Life, lavender, melissa, Forange, peppermint, Fylang ylang.

SUPPLEMENTS—CardiaCare (strengthens and supports).

TINCTURES—HRT.

PROLAPSED MITRAL VALVE—Marjoram.

STIMULANT—Coriander, cumin.

STRENGTHENS HEART MUSCLE—Lavender, marjoram, peppermint, rose, rosemary (Alternative Medicine—A Definitive Guide, p. 722).

STRENGTHENING—Cinnamon bark.

SUPPLEMENTS—CardiaCare (strengthens and supports), Wolfberry Crisp Bars.

TACHYCARDIA (accelerated rhythm of the heartbeat)—Goldenrod, Flavender, orange, spikenard, ylang ylang.

SUPPLEMENTS—CardiaCare (strengthens and supports), Power Meal, Wolfberry Crisp Bars.

TINCTURES—HRT.

Heartburn: Cardamom, Di-Gize (over stomach and colon), Gentle Baby, Flemon, Fpeppermint (over thymus).

BLEND—2 lemon, 2 peppermint, 3 sandalwood, and ½ oz. V-6 Mixing Oil. Apply to breast bone. Using palm of hand, massage in a clockwise motion applying pressure. Do Vita Flex on feet.

SUPPLEMENTS—AlkaLime, Essentialzyme, JuvaPower/JuvaSpice.

Hematoma (swelling or tumor filled with diffused blood): Aroma Life, German chamomile, Fhelichrysum.

Hemorrhaging: Helichrysum, rose, ylang ylang. Massage around ankles, lower back, and stomach. Cayenne pepper may also help.

Hemorrhoids: <u>Aroma Life</u>, basil, [F]Clary sage, [F]cypress, frankincense, helichrysum, juniper, myrrh, [F]patchouli, [F]peppermint, [F]sandalwood. Put cypress and helichrysum inside on location.

Hepatitis: Cinnamon bark, cypress, eucalyptus, <u>GLF</u>, <u>JuvaFlex</u> (over the liver), <u>ImmuPower</u> (on spine and liver), melaleuca, myrrh (with ledum internally for hepatitis B & C), oregano, patchouli, <u>Release</u> (on feet and liver), Roman chamomile, rosemary, thyme.

    SUPPLEMENTS—**NingXia Red**. The following regimen has been useful: Use the Cleansing Trio (ComforTone, Essentialzyme, and ICP) for 1 week, 4 Royaldophilus a day, Master Formula His/Hers, 1 VitaGreen a day, 4 Super C / Super C Chewable three times a day. Add JuvaTone on the 3rd day.

    ***COMMENTS—*Refer to the chapter entitled "How to Use - The Personal Usage Reference" in the <u>Essential Oils Desk Reference</u> under "Liver" subcategory "Hepatitis" for a specific daily program using supplements and blends.*

    DETOXIFY LIVER—Ledum and <u>JuvaTone</u> together.

    VIRAL— <u>GLF</u>, [F]Myrrh and <u>JuvaFlex</u>, ledum, [F]ravensara, [F]rosemary. Apply to spine, compress over liver area, and Vita Flex points on feet. Alternate oils.

    SUPPLEMENTS—Super C / Super C Chewable.

Hernia: Apply oil(s) on location, lower back, and Vita Flex points on feet.

    HIATAL HERNIA—Basil, cypress, fennel, geranium, ginger, hyssop, lavender, peppermint, rosemary, vitex. Drink water. Put the first two fingers of each hand just below the sternum (under center of rib cage), press in firmly, and brush down quickly and firmly. This can also be done after raising up on toes and while dropping down on heels to more firmly emphasize the effect.

    SUPPLEMENTS—Essentialzyme before meal, ComforTone, ICP (fiber beverage) after meal.

    INCISIONAL HERNIA (usually caused by scar tissue failing to heal from an abdominal wound or incision)—Basil, geranium, ginger, helichrysum, lavender, lemon, lemongrass, melaleuca.

    INGUINAL—Lavender, lemongrass.

Herpes Simplex: <u>Australian Blue</u>, Blue cypress, bergamot with *Eucalyptus radiata*, eucalyptus, geranium, [F]lavender, lemon, melissa, [F]ravensara, rose.

> *Jean Valnet, M.D., a French physician, recommends a blend of lemon and geranium. Tisserand suggests eucalyptus and bergamot. Dr. Wabner says that a one-time application of either true rose oil or true melissa oil led to complete remission of herpes simplex lesions. Apply the oil directly on the lesions at the first sign of an outbreak. (<u>Alternative Medicine—The Definitive Guide</u>, p. 56).*

Hiccoughs: Sandalwood, [F]tarragon.

High Blood Pressure: *See Blood.*

Hives: *See Acidosis, pH Balance.* Hives may be the result of too much acid in the blood or the result of a niacin flush (vitamin B3 taken on empty stomach). Patchouli (may relieve itching), peppermint, Roman chamomile.

> *SUPPLEMENTS*—AlkaLime (combat yeast and fungus overgrowth and preserve the body's proper pH balance), Super Cal (may prevent), VitaGreen.

> ***COMMENTS—*** *One woman broke out in hives over her entire body, she used peppermint oil diluted with V-6 Mixing Oil for a body massage. Almost instantly, her body cooled off and the hives diminished until gone.*

Hodgkin's Disease: Clove. Apply to liver, kidney, and Vita Flex points on feet.

Hope: Hope (restores).

Hormonal Imbalance: Anise, Lady Love (available through Creer Labs 801-418-8870), SclarEssence, ylang ylang.

> *PERSONAL CARE*— Prenolone/Prenolone+, Progessence.

> *SUPPLEMENTS*—Exodus, FemiGen, Mineral Essence, Sulfurzyme (lowered libido).

> *TINCTURES*—FHS (available through Creer Labs 801-418-8870). Works best when combined with FemiGen for balancing female hormones.

Hormonal System: Acceptance, Aroma Life, Clarity, davana, Dragon Time, EndoFlex, fennel, goldenrod, Gentle Baby, Lady Love (available through Creer Labs 801-418-8870), Mister, M-Grain, myrrh, myrtle, peppermint, Relieve It, sandalwood, SclarEssence, [F]spearmint (hormone-like), ylang ylang. The most common places to apply oils for hormonal balance are the Vita Flex points on ankles, lower back, thyroid, liver, kidneys, gland areas, the center of the body and along both sides of the spine, and the clavicle area. It may also help to diffuse them.

> *BALANCE*—Bergamot, [F]Clary sage, clove (aromatic), EndoFlex, fennel, geranium, Legacy, Mister (creates greater balance), nutmeg, sage, ylang ylang.

> *MASSAGE OILS*—Dragon Time.

> *PERSONAL CARE*— Prenolone / Prenolone+, Progessence.

> *SUPPLEMENTS*—CortiStop (Women's), Exodus, FemiGen (female), ProGen (male), Super B, Super Cal, Thyromin, Ultra Young+, VitaGreen.

> *TINCTURES*—Estro.

> *DISTURBANCES*—

> > *SUPPLEMENTS*—ProGen (male) or FemiGen (female).

> > *TINCTURES*—FHS (female; best when combined with FemiGen), Male-Pro (male). Both these products are available through Creer Labs 801-418-8870.

> *FEMALE*—Lady Love, Lady Sclareol, Mister (for estrogen).

> > *SUPPLEMENTS*—CortiStop (Women's), FemiGen, Ultra Young+.

> > *TINCTURES*—Estro, FHS (best when combined with FemiGen), SE-6.

MALE—<u>Mister</u>.
  SUPPLEMENTS—ProGen, Ultra
    Young+.
  TINCTURES—Male-Pro, SE-6.
SEXUAL ENERGY—Goldenrod, <u>Lady Love</u>,
    <u>Lady Sclareol</u>, ylang ylang.
  TINCTURES—SE-6 (only available
    through Creer Labs 801-418-
    8870).

Hot Flashes: *See Hormonal Imbalance.*
    Bergamot (estrogen), Clary
    sage (estrogen), <u>Dragon Time</u>,
    <u>EndoFlex</u>, fennel, <u>Mister</u>
    (estrogen) works for women in
    Canada, or ᶠpeppermint. Apply
    these oils on the ankles at the
    ovary and uterus Vita Flex
    points. If hypoglycemic, use
    <u>Aroma Siez</u> with <u>M-Grain</u>. Can
    also try <u>Lady Flash</u> or <u>Lady
    Love</u> (available through Creer Labs 801-418-8870). Apply over ovaries, pelvis,
    ankles, bottom of feet.

> *A hormonal imbalance can cause many problems including, PMS, pre- and post-menopausal conditions, depression, endometriosis, fibromyalgia, fibrocysts, infertility, insomnia, irregular menstrual cycles, lowered libido, menstrual migraines, osteoporosis, ovarian cysts, unexplained first-trimester miscarriages, water retention, etc. Carbonated water can cause hormone deficiency. But, most often, it is a result of estrogen dominance; that is, not enough progesterone to balance out the amount of estrogen. Estrogen is manufactured in several places of the body, even after menopause, and is also found in much of our food, especially animal and dairy products. Progesterone is secreted by the corpus luteum, by the placenta, and in small amounts by the adrenal glands. If the ovaries are not functioning properly, have been removed, or if they have atrophied because of menopause or hysterectomy, the woman is undoubtedly estrogen dominant. Therefore, she is a candidate for the problems listed above. One successful approach for the above problems is NATURAL PROGESTERONE (obtained from the Wild Yam or SOY). Two good books to read about natural progesterone are <u>What Your Doctor May Not Tell You About Premenopause</u> and <u>What Your Doctor May Not Tell You About Menopause</u>. Both books were written by John R. Lee, MD.*

  ***COMMENTS—*Some women have had success using a drop of <u>EndoFlex</u> under their tongue three times a day. Be cautious as it contains nutmeg and an overdose could cause problems.*
  PERSONAL CARE—Prenolone/Prenolone+, Progessence.
  SUPPLEMENTS—CortiStop (Women's), FemiGen, Mineral Essence.
  TINCTURES—AD&E.

Housecleaning: Put a few drops of oil on your dust cloth or put 10 drops in a spray bottle of water
    and mist.
  BATHROOMS/KITCHENS—Fir, lemon, or spruce for cleaning and disinfecting.
  CARPETS—<u>Purification</u>, lemon (has been used to remove black shoe polish)
  DISHES—A couple of drops of <u>Melrose</u> or lemon in the " make for sparkling dishes and a great
    smelling kitchen.
  FURNITURE POLISH—Fir, lemon, or spruce work well for polishing furniture.
  GUM/GREASE—Lemon oil is terrific for dissolving gum and grease.
  LAUNDRY—Adding oils to the washer can increase the anti-bacterial benefits, provide greater
    hygiene, and the clothes come out with a fresh, clean smell.
  MOLD/FUNGUS—<u>Purification</u>, <u>Thieves</u>.

Hyperactivity: <u>Citrus Fresh</u>, lavender, <u>Peace & Calming</u> (gets them off Ritalin), Roman chamomile, <u>Trauma Life</u> (calming), <u>Valor</u> (sometimes works better than Peace & Calming). Apply to Vita Flex points on the feet and diffuse.

> *Hyperactivity may indicate a trace mineral deficiency. Get off Prozac and Ritalin and use Mineral Essence. It is interesting to note that 48 out of 49 death row inmates were tested and found to be deficient in the same trace minerals.*

SUPPLEMENTS—ComforTone, Essentialzyme, ICP, Mineral Essence, healthy diet.

Hyperpnea (Abnormal rapid breathing): ^FYlang ylang. Apply to lung area and Vita Flex points.

Hypertension (High blood pressure): *See Blood.*

Hypoglycemia: *See Protein.* Cinnamon bark, clove, ^Feucalyptus, <u>Gentle Baby</u>, <u>Gratitude</u> (over pancreas and on Vita Flex points), <u>Thieves</u>, thyme.

> *Protein deficiency causes **hypoglycemia**. Honey enters the blood stream faster than sugar and can cause hypoglycemia. When flu and virus enter the body and mix with problems of hypoglycemia, it can cause candida, Epstein barr virus, allergies, etc. There is a progressive deterioration from hypoglycemia. Signs of hypoglycemia are: headaches, fatigue, PMS, ornery, moody, weak, light headed, not hungry in the morning because body is still digesting its food from the night before.*

SUPPLEMENTS—Allerzyme (aids the digestion of sugars, starches, fats, and proteins), AlkaLime, Balance Complete, Bodygize, Digest + Cleanse, Polyzyme (aids the digestion of protein and helps reduce swelling and discomfort), Power Meal, Pure Protein Complete, Stevia, Sulfurzyme, VitaGreen, WheyFit (lactose-free protein from three sources; provides highest ranking protein for digestibility), Wolfberry Crisp Bars.

TINCTURES—Sugar-Up (available through Creer Labs 801-418-8870)

Hysteria: Lavender, melaleuca, neroli. Apply to heart, bottom of feet, and diffuse.

Immune System: <u>Abundance</u>, cistus, clove, cumin, <u>Exodus II</u>, frankincense, geranium, Idaho tansy, <u>ImmuPower</u>, lavender, ledum (supports), lemon, melaleuca, Mountain savory, <u>Raven</u>, ravensara, rosemary (supports), <u>Thieves</u> (enhances; massage on feet and body), thyme (immunological functions), White lotus.

SUPPLEMENTS—AlkaLime (designed to combat yeast and fungus overgrowth and preserve the body's proper pH balance), Body Balancing Trio (Bodygize, Master Formula His/Hers, VitaGreen), Cleansing Trio (ComforTone, Essentialzyme, and ICP), Digest + Cleanse, Essential Manna, Exodus, ImmuneTune, ImmuPro, Longevity Capsules, Mineral Essence, NingXia Red, Power Meal, Super B, Super C / Super C Chewable, Thyromin, Ultra Young (may help raise levels of cytokines, interleukin 1 & 2, and tumor necrosis factor), VitaGreen, Wolfberry Crisp Bars (*Refer to the Wolfberry Crisp Bar in the Supplements section of the <u>Reference Guide for Essential Oils</u> for more information on the benefits of the Ningxia Wolfberry*).

TINCTURES—AD&E.

STIMULATES— ᶠCinnamon bark, ᶠfrankincense, <u>ImmuPower</u>, lavender (for immune system), ᶠmelaleuca, Mountain savory, ᶠoregano, <u>Thieves</u> (diffuse with clove). Apply oil(s) to bottom of feet, along spine, under arms, dilute for massage, and diffuse for ½ hour at a time.

BOOSTING IMMUNE DEFENSE—Cumin, ledum.

Impetigo: Lavender, myrrh. Boil 4 ounces water, cool, add 5 to 10 drops lavender and wash. You may also use myrrh (cover for an hour). Do hot compress on site.

> *Impetigo is an infection of the outer layers of the skin. It is caused by an infected scratch or insect bite. It starts as tiny red spots, then it turns into blisters that can fill with pus. It is contagious to self and others. Approach the problem and handle it as it is noticed.*

Impotency: ᶠClary sage, ᶠclove, goldenrod, ᶠginger, jasmine, <u>Mister</u>, nutmeg, rose, ᶠsandalwood, <u>SclarEssence</u> (taken internally as a dietary supplement, helps to raise testosterone levels), ylang ylang. Capsules work well for internal consumption of oils.

SUPPLEMENTS—ProGen.
PERSONAL CARE—Prenolone+

Incontinence: *See Bladder.*

Indifference: Jasmine.

Indigestion: Angelica, cumin, ginger, <u>GLF</u>, <u>JuvaFlex</u>, ᶠlavender, ᶠpeppermint, nutmeg, valerian (nervous indigestion).

SUPPLEMENTS—AlkaLime, Balance Complete, Cleansing Trio (ComforTone, Essentialzyme, and ICP), Digest + Cleanse.

Infection: *See Anti-infectious.* ᶠBergamot, cajeput (urethra), ᶠcinnamon bark, clove, ᶠClary sage, cypress, elemi (chest/bronchial infections), Idaho tansy, jasmine (bacterial infection), juniper, fennel, lavender, lemongrass, *Melaleuca quinquenervia* (viral), <u>Melrose</u> (prevents growth of all infections), myrrh (with oregano), oregano, peppermint, ᶠpine (severe), <u>Raven</u>, ravensara, rosemary (with myrrh for oral infection), <u>Thieves</u>, thyme (urinary infection).

FUNGICIDAL—Cedarwood.
INFECTED WOUNDS—Frankincense, melaleuca, patchouli.

BLEND (to draw infection out)—1 thyme. Apply hot compress twice daily. Mix together 3 lavender, 2 melaleuca, and 2 thyme with 1 tsp. V-6 Mixing Oil. After the infection and pus have been expelled, apply a little of the mixture twice daily on the infected area.

SUPPLEMENTS—Bodygize, ImmuneTune, ImmuPro, Super C / Super C Chewable.

Infectious Disease: Bergamot, cinnamon bark, clove, <u>Exodus II</u>, ginger, hyssop (viral infections), <u>ImmuPower</u>, juniper (viral infections), lemon, melaleuca, myrtle, <u>Raven</u>, <u>RC</u>, and thyme (bacterial infection).

   ***COMMENTS—*Dr. Young uses <u>Raven</u>, <u>RC</u>, and <u>ImmuPower</u> together for infectious diseases.*

Inferiority:

   OVERCOMING—Peppermint, <u>Transformation</u>.

Infertility: *See Hormonal Imbalance.* Anise, bergamot, Clary sage, cypress, <u>Dragon Time </u>(place on ankles, lower abdomen, and in vagina for women), fennel, geranium, melissa, <u>Mister</u> (for men, place in rectum, across lower back, around and under ankles), nutmeg, Roman chamomile, sage, thyme, yarrow, ylang ylang. Feed the thyroid.

   SUPPLEMENTS—ProGen (male) or FemiGen (female), Prenolone/Prenolone+ / Progessence, and 1-3 VitaGreen three times a day.

Inflammation: *See Anti-inflammatory.* Birch, Blue tansy, calamus (intestines and colon), caraway, clove, cypress, elemi (breast and uterus), Balsam fir (see Balsam fir under Injuries below), frankincense, helichrysum, juniper, lavender, myrrh, oregano, palo santo, <u>PanAway</u>, <u>Peace & Calming</u>, <u>Relieve It</u>, Roman chamomile, spruce, wintergreen. **Apply on location and to brain stem** (back of neck up to base of skull). *This helps stop pain and reduces the production of noradrenalin and cortisol.*

   MASSAGE OILS—Ortho Sport.

   SUPPLEMENTS—According to Dr. David Hill, "Inflammation and Oxidation go hand-in-hand." NingXia Red and Longevity Capsules on a daily basis are a powerful combination to help fight oxidation and inflammation system-wide. Also, Omega Blue contains clove oil and fish oil, which have been shown to work together to reduce inflammation by up to 30%!

   ***COMMENTS—*Refer to the chapter entitled "How to Use - The Personal Usage Reference" in the <u>Essential Oils Desk Reference</u> under "Inflammation" for some excellent blend recipes.*

Influenza: *See Flu or Colds.*

Injuries: *See Tissue, Scarring. Also Blend #2 under Aches/Pains for pain reduction.* Balsam fir (with frankincense, sandalwood, myrrh, and helichrysum for pain and inflammation), cistus (promotes healing of scar tissue), helichrysum (reduces scarring and discoloration), <u>Melrose</u> (regenerates tissue), sandalwood (for any DNA repair).

   SPORT—Balsam fir, helichrysum, <u>Melrose</u>, <u>PanAway</u>.

   MASSAGE OILS—Ortho Ease, Ortho Sport.

Inner Knowing: <u>Inner Child</u> (reconnects you with your inner child), <u>SARA</u>.

Insanity: <u>Hope</u> (ears), <u>Release</u> (liver), <u>Relieve It</u>.

Insect:

BITES—*See Bites*. Cajeput, bergamot cajeput, Idaho tansy.

BLEND #1—Combine 3 drops Roman chamomile, 4 eucalyptus, 10 lavender, and 1 thyme with 1 Tbs. V-6 Mixing Oil.

***COMMENTS—*Refer to the chapter entitled "How to Use - The Personal Usage Reference" in the <u>Essential Oils Desk Reference</u> under "Insect Bites" for some excellent blend recipes for bites/stings from different types of insects.*

> *Dr. Jean Valnet says that basil, cinnamon, garlic, lavender, lemon, onion, sage, savory, and thyme are effective against insect bites because of their antitoxic and anti-venomous properties.*

> *My husband was bitten by a spider on his stomach. The bite swelled with a large blister and it itched terribly. I used lavender oil - about a drop - on the area. In about 4 hours my husband asked for another application of the "magic oil". My husband has an allergy and reacts to any type of a bite. In fact, he usually has to go to the Dr. and get shots and prescriptions.*
> *-Submitted by Mary Rynicki (July 2004)*

POISONS FROM BROWN RECLUSE SPIDER OR WASPS—Basil (known to neutralize poisons), <u>Purification</u> (removes poisons from the body).

INSECTICIDAL—Citronella.

ITCHING—Lavender.

PERSONAL CARE—Satin Hand & Body Lotion with lavender.

REPELLENT—Basil, bergamot, cedarwood, <u>Purification</u>.

FLORAL WATERS—Idaho Tansy (has been used with success as a fly and mosquito repellent on horses and other animals).

BLEND #2—Combine 5 lavender, 5 lemongrass, 3 peppermint, and 1 thyme and put on feet or add to cup of water and spray on.

BLEND #3—Clove, lemon, and orange.

BLEND #4—Put 5 drops lemon and 5 <u>Purification</u> in a little spray bottle of water and mist on your skin to protect yourself against insects, flies, and mosquitoes. *1 or 2 oz. glass or plastic spray bottles work very well and are small enough to take with you.*

> *My husband was stung by a wasp last year on the inside of the hand. He removed the stinger and asked me to put something on it. I put Purification on it, and the itching stopped. After his shower that evening, I put Purification on it again. The next morning, you couldn't see or even tell that he'd been stung. I've also put Purification on coworkers who have had mosquito/bug bites that itched. After the Purification went on the bites, the itching stopped.*
> *-Submitted by Christie Krajewski Batesville, Arkansas (July 2004)*

***COMMENTS—*Dr. Friedmann came in contact with a person who had bugs growing on their face and scalp. Somehow they were subjected to a fungus to which the bugs were attracted. They established their nests, laid and hatched their eggs on her skin. She had been using many products and was only able to suppress the problem but not correct it. Dr. Friedmann applied <u>Melrose</u>, helichrysum, lavender, and <u>ImmuPower</u> on her Thymus. She stopped using all other chemicals and several weeks later the bugs were almost gone.*

Insomnia: Angelica, basil, Fbergamot, <u>Citrus Fresh</u>, Clary sage, Fcypress, Flavender (best when combined with Roman chamomile and dill), lemon, Fmarjoram, *Melaleuca ericifolia*, Fmyrtle (for hormone-related insomnia), neroli, nutmeg (small amount), Forange, <u>Peace & Calming</u>, petitgrain, Fravensara, Roman chamomile (small amount), rosemary, sandalwood, <u>Surrender</u> (behind the ears), valerian, Fylang ylang.

  BLEND #1—Combine 6 <u>Citrus Fresh</u> with 6 lavender or 6 <u>Peace & Calming</u>. Apply blend to big toes, bottom of feet, 2 drops around navel, 3 drops on back of neck.

  BLEND #2—2 drops Roman chamomile, 6 geranium, 3 lemon, and 4 sandalwood. Mix together and add 6 drops in your bath at bedtime and 5 drops with 2 tsp. V-6 Mixing Oil for a massage after bath.

  BLEND #3—Combine 20 ml valerian, 5 ml vetiver, 2 ml helichrysum, 1 ml clove, and 1 ml peppermint in 1 oz. dropper bottle. Add several drops (up to 3 droppers full) to 2-3 oz. of water and drink followed by ½ tsp. AlkaLime in water.

  SUPPLEMENTS—ImmuPro.

  ***COMMENTS—*Refer to the chapter entitled "How to Use - The Personal Usage Reference" in the* <u>Essential Oils Desk Reference</u> *under "Insomnia" for some excellent blend recipes.*

  FOR CHILDREN—12 months to 5 years—lavender, Roman chamomile; 5 to 12 years—Clary sage, geranium, *Melaleuca ericifolia*, ylang ylang (infection).

Intestinal Problems: *See Acidosis, Colitis, Colon, Constipation, Digestive System, Diverticulitis, Parasites, etc.* FBasil, cajeput, calamus (reduces inflammation and detoxifies), ginger, Fmarjoram, patchouli (aids in the digestion of toxic waste), rosemary, tarragon.

  SUPPLEMENTS—AlkaLime, Balance Complete, Cleansing Trio (ComforTone, Essentialzyme, and ICP), Digest + Cleanse (helps soothe gastrointestinal upset), KidScents Royaldophilus (for children), ParaFree, JuvaTone, Royaldophilus.

 ANTISEPTIC—Nutmeg.

 CRAMPS—Blue cypress, FClary sage, <u>Di-Gize</u> (add 3 drops basil in capsule with <u>Di-Gize</u>).

 FLORA—*Take* **kefir with Royaldophilus**, *first thing in the morning on an empty stomach, to help implant good bacteria in the intestines (yogurt will help maintain good bacteria but not implant it).*

  SUPPLEMENTS—Balance Complete (contains inulin which helps build intestinal flora), KidScents Royaldophilus (for children), Royaldophilus.

 PARASITES— FBergamot, Fclove, <u>Di-Gize</u>, Ffennel, ginger (helps to create an unfriendly environment for parasites), Flemon, peppermint, ravensara, FRoman chamomile.

  SUPPLEMENTS—AlkaLime, Cleansing Trio (ComforTone, Essentialzyme, and ICP), Digest + Cleanse (contains oils that create an unfriendly environment for parasites), and ParaFree assist in cleansing the intestinal tract of toxic debris and parasites, which are hosts for many diseases.

 SOOTHE—Spearmint.

 SPASM— FTarragon, Ffennel.

Invigorating: Birch/wintergreen.

  IN SUMMER—Eucalyptus, peppermint.

Ions:

  INCREASE NEGATIVE IONS—Bergamot, citronella, lemongrass, orange.

  INCREASE POSITIVE IONS—Cajeput, frankincense, helichrysum, juniper, *Melaleuca quinquenervia*, pine, ravensara, ylang ylang.

Iron: Important for learning. Raisins are good natural source.

  SUPPLEMENTS—Master Formula His/Hers, KidScents Mighty Vites (chewable).

Irritability: Forgiveness, Hope, Humility, Inspiration, lavender, myrrh, Present Time, Surrender, Valor. All single oils **except**: Eucalyptus, pepper, peppermint, and rosemary.

  SUPPLEMENTS—AlkaLime.

Irritable Bowel Syndrome: Calamus, caraway, Di-Gize, peppermint. Take 2 drops of each in distilled water 1-2 times per day. Anise and Juva Cleanse may also help.

  SUPPLEMENTS—Balance Complete, ComforTone, Digest + Cleanse (enteric coated to release in the bowels), JuvaPower/JuvaSpice, JuvaTone, ICP, Royaldophilus.

Itching: Lavender, Peace & Calming (ears), peppermint (ears). Apply on location too.

  BLEND—6 lavender and 3 rosemary with Satin Hand & Body Lotion.

  PERSONAL CARE—Rose Ointment, Satin Hand & Body Lotion.

Jaundice (Liver disease): ᶠGeranium, Juva Cleanse, lemon, rosemary, sage lavender.

Jealousy: Bergamot, eucalyptus, Forgiveness, frankincense, Harmony, Humility, Joy, lemon, marjoram, orange, rose, rosemary, Sacred Mountain, sandalwood, thyme, Valor, White Angelica.

Jet Lag: Brain Power, Clarity, En-R-Gee, eucalyptus, geranium, grapefruit, ImmuPower (for protection), lavender, lemongrass, peppermint, Present Time, Valor. Apply to temples, thymus, and bottom of feet. It is best not to eat heavy foods and to drink as much water as possible.

  SUPPLEMENTS—Power Meal, Sulfurzyme, Super C / Super C Chewable.

Joints: Birch (discomfort), cajeput (stiff), Balsam fir (pain from exercising), Douglas fir (calming to tired and overworked joints), nutmeg, Roman chamomile (inflamed), spruce (aching), wintergreen.

  ***COMMENTS—*Refer to the chapter entitled "How to Use - The Personal Usage Reference" in the Essential Oils Desk Reference under "Joint Stiffness and Pain" for some excellent blend recipes.*

Personal Guide

Joyous: Abundance, bergamot (turns grief to joy), Christmas Spirit, Citrus Fresh (brings joy to children), Joy, orange (aromatic).

Kidneys: Aroma Life, calamus (reduces congestion after intoxication), Clary sage, EndoFlex, geranium, grapefruit, juniper (for better function of kidneys), JuvaFlex, ledum (strengthen), Flemongrass (combine with juniper for greater synergistic effect), Release. Apply over kidneys as a hot compress. Drink plenty of distilled water (3-4 quarts each day). When kidneys start producing ammonia, it can go to the brain and people have died from that alone. Do the MASTER CLEANSER (*See Cleansing*).

    SUPPLEMENTS—Longevity Capsules (contains thyme oil to help preserve omega-3 fatty acids in the kidneys), VitaGreen (turns blood back to alkaline).

    TINCTURES—K&B.

    ***COMMENTS—*Refer to the chapter entitled "How to Use - The Personal Usage Reference" in the* Essential Oils Desk Reference *under "Kidney Disorders" for some excellent blend recipes and supplement recommendations.*

    BLOCKAGE—

        MASSAGE—Release and other oils on kidney points on feet twice a day.

        SUPPLEMENTS—Cleansing Trio (ComforTone, Essentialzyme, and ICP), JuvaTone (First week: 2 tablets a day; Second week: 3 tablets a day for 90 days).

    CAPILLARIES BEING ATTACKED IN KIDNEYS—

        SUPPLEMENTS—Need to support the body and cleanse the blood with VitaGreen, Cleansing Trio (ComforTone, Essentialzyme, and ICP).

    INFECTION IN—Rosemary. Apply to kidneys and Vita Flex points.

        BLEND #1—Cypress, marjoram, and Thieves or JuvaFlex. Apply as a hot compress.

        FOOD—Drink one gallon of distilled water and 2 quarts cranberry juice in a day.

        SUPPLEMENTS—NingXia Red (1-3 oz. followed by 8-10 oz. water 3 times daily).

    INFLAMMATION (Nephritis)—Aroma Life, juniper, JuvaFlex. Do a colon cleanse (*see Cleansing*).

        FOOD—Drink one gallon of distilled water and 2 quarts cranberry juice in a day.

        SUPPLEMENTS—ImmuneTune, Power Meal, Super C / Super C Chewable, VitaGreen.

        TINCTURES—K&B, Rehemogen.

        ***COMMENTS—*Refer to the chapter entitled "How to Use - The Personal Usage Reference" in the* Essential Oils Desk Reference *under "Kidney Disorders" subcategory "Inflammation in the Kidneys (Nephritis)" for a very specific regimen of supplements and blends.*

    MUSCLES THAT WON'T WORK IN THE KIDNEYS—Aroma Siez and EndoFlex.

        BLEND #2—8 fennel and 10 juniper.

    STONES—Eucalyptus, hyssop, juniper.

        BLEND #3—10 juniper and 10 geranium. Apply as a hot compress over kidneys once a day.

        SUPPLEMENTS—After being on the Cleansing Trio (ComforTone, Essentialzyme, and ICP) for 10 days, add ImmuneTune, and Super C / Super C Chewable.

Pass (without edges)—Drink 4 oz. distilled water with juice from ½ lemon every 30 minutes for 6 hours straight. Then take 2 Tbs. extra light virgin olive oil with the juice from 1 full lemon. Repeat daily until stone passes.

Knee Cartilage Injury:
>	*Blend*—8 clove, 12 ginger, 10 nutmeg with 2 oz. V-6 Mixing Oil. Massage three times a day. Apply ice for swelling and inflammation. Wrap knee and elevate when sitting. Use the ice method three times a day and alternate with a hot compress and the oils.
>	*Massage Oils*—Ortho Ease, Ortho Sport.
>	*Personal Care*—Regenolone.
>	*Supplements*—BLM

Labor: *See Pregnancy.* Gentle Baby, jasmine (pain).

Lactation (Secretion of breast milk): *See Nursing.* ᶠFennel or basil (increase flow), peppermint with cold compress (decrease flow). Apply above the breasts on the lymph area and 2-3 drops on the spine, about breast level.
>	*Supplements*—PD 80/20, Prenolone/Prenolone+, Progessence.

Lactose Intolerance: Lemongrass (reported to help eliminate lactic acid from fermentation of lactose in milk).
>	*Supplements*—Allerzyme, Essentialzyme, KidScents MightyZyme (chewable for children), KidScents Royaldophilus (chewable for children), Power Meal, Royaldophilus, WheyFit.

Laryngitis: Jasmine, ledum, Melrose, onycha (benzoin), sage lavender, sandalwood.
>	*Diffuse*—Frankincense, lavender, sandalwood, thyme.
>	*Blend*—Add one drop each of Melrose and lemon to 1 tsp. honey. Swish around in mouth for a couple of minutes to liquefy then swallow.

Laundry: Lemon, Purification.
>	***Comments—*Adding oils to the washer can increase the anti-bacterial benefits, provide greater hygiene, and the clothes come out with a fresh, clean smell. A few drops of oil can also be placed on a washcloth and put in the dryer with laundry or added to a bottle of water, shook well, and sprayed into the dryer before drying the laundry.*

Laxative: Hyssop, jasmine, tangerine.
>	*Supplements*—Balance Complete, Cleansing Trio (ComforTone, Essentialzyme, and ICP), Digest + Cleanse.

Legs, Restless: Restless legs are caused by the body dumping acid into the system at night. The following recipe was recommended to counteract this reaction to the over-acidification of the body.

> RECIPE #1—In the evening before bed, take 1 Tbs of JuvaPower (in almond, rice or soy milk, or water), followed by ½ tsp of AlkaLime in water. Then apply 2-3 drops each of valerian, Roman chamomile, and lavender to the brain stem (back of neck from shoulders to base of skull) and work them in with the Vita Flex technique.

Lethargy: Jasmine, Transformation.

Libido (Low): *See Frigidity, Sex Stimulant.* Chivalry, Dragon Time, Joy, Mister, nutmeg, Live with Passion, rose, SclarEssence (take internally), Sensation, ylang ylang. Do the MASTER CLEANSER (*See Cleansing*).

> SUPPLEMENTS—PD 80/20, Prenolone/Prenolone+, Progessence, Sulfurzyme.
> MEN—Additional oils include Black pepper, cinnamon, ginger, myrrh, and pine. *See also Prostate.*
> PERSONAL CARE—Protec (combine with frankincense to decongest the prostate).
> TINCTURES—Male-Pro, SE-6 (both available through Creer Labs 801-418-8870).
> WOMEN—Additional oils include Clary sage, geranium, jasmine, Lady Love, and Lady Sclareol.
> TINCTURES—FHS, SE-6 (both available through Creer Labs 801-418-8870).

Lice: Eucalyptus, geranium, lavender, lemon, pine (repels), rosemary. Apply oil(s) to bottom of feet and rub over scalp three times a day.

Ligaments: *See Muscles.* **Lemongrass** (torn or pulled; combine with marjoram to stimulate torn ligaments; combine with basil if torn ligaments produce spasms), palo santo.

> SUPPLEMENTS—BLM
> TORN—Birch, clove, helichrysum, marjoram, PanAway, wintergreen.
> MASSAGE OILS—Ortho Sport.

Lipoma: *See Tumors.*

Lips: German chamomile, lavender, lemon, melaleuca.

> DRY LIPS—
> > BLEND—2 to 5 drops geranium and 2 to 5 drops lavender.

Listlessness: Jasmine.

Liver: Acceptance, cypress, dill, Di-Gize, fleabane, [F]geranium (cleanses and detoxifies the liver), [F]German chamomile, GLF, goldenrod (supports liver function), grapefruit (liver

disorders), ᶠhelichrysum, <u>JuvaFlex</u> (detoxification), <u>Juva Cleanse</u>, **ledum** (powerful
detoxifier), myrrh, <u>Peace & Calming</u>, ravensara, ᶠsage (for liver problems), sage
lavender (congestion), <u>Release</u> (apply to liver and Vita Flex points), Roman
chamomile, <u>3 Wise Men</u> (on crown).

   Supplements—Balance Complete, Digest + Cleanse, JuvaTone, Longevity Capsules
(contains thyme oil to help preserve omega-3 fatty acids in the liver). Also NingXia
Red, Omega Blue, and Power Meal.

   ***Comments*—*When the liver is toxic, it makes the mind lethargic and slows the emotions.
For those who have liver problems, be careful about the oils used and the amounts.
Ease into a liver cleanse!*

Cirrhosis of Liver—Frankincense, geranium, juniper, lavender, myrrh, Roman chamomile,
rosemary, rose.

   Supplements—Bodygize, JuvaTone, NingXia Red, Super C / Super C Chewable.

Cleansing—Carrot seed, clove (increases detoxification), helichrysum, geranium, German
chamomile, <u>GLF</u>, <u>JuvaFlex</u>, <u>Juva Cleanse</u>, ledum (with JuvaTone), myrrh, sage
lavender.

   Supplements—Longevity Capsules, NingXia Red, Sulfurzyme (may help detoxify the
liver).

Function (improve)—<u>GLF</u>, <u>JuvaFlex</u>, goldenrod, and myrrh. Do a compress over the liver
and alternate the oils on the liver Vita Flex points.

   Supplements—NingXia Red, Omega Blue, and Power Meal.

Hepatitis—*See Hepatitis.* <u>GLF</u>, <u>JuvaFlex</u>, ledum, myrrh, **ravensara** (viral).

Jaundice (liver disease)— ᶠGeranium, <u>GLF</u>, <u>Juva Cleanse</u>.

Regeneration—NingXia Red

   ***Comments*—*One individual had total liver regeneration using JuvaTone, Rehemogen,
and <u>JuvaFlex</u>.*

Spots—Idaho Tansy Floral Water, Prenolone/Prenolone+, Progessence.

Stimulant for Liver Cell Function— <u>GLF</u>, ᶠhelichrysum, ledum (combine with JuvaTone).

   Supplements—Balance Complete, Cleansing Trio (ComforTone, Essentialzyme, and
ICP), JuvaTone (helps increase digestion in the liver), NingXia Red, Omega Blue.

Longevity: Fennel (aromatic), <u>Longevity</u>.

   Supplements—Berry Young Juice, CardiaCare (with *Rhododendron caucasicum*),
Longevity Capsules (Longevity blend + frankincense in gel caps for internal
consumption), NingXia Red (whole wolfberry puree), Omega Blue (omega-3s).

Loss of Loved One: Basil, cedarwood, cypress (diffuse), fir, <u>Forgiveness</u>, jasmine, <u>Joy</u>, rose, spruce,
<u>Transformation</u>, <u>Valor</u>, ylang ylang.

   Bath & Shower Gels—Sensation Bath & Shower Gel.

   Massage Oil—Sensation Massage Oil.

   Personal Care—Sensation Hand & Body Lotion.

L

Loss of Smell: Basil.

Lou Gehrig's Disease: *See Alzheimer's Disease, Brain, Multiple Sclerosis, Parkinson's Disease, Pineal Gland, Pituitary Gland.* Use the same oils as you would if you were handling Multiple Sclerosis, Alzheimer's, and Parkinson's Disease. Drink steam distilled water. Acceptance (may help to oxygenate the pineal and pituitary glands), Clarity (for brain function), cypress (circulation), Egyptian Gold, Peace & Calming, Valor.
> SUPPLEMENTS—Cleansing Trio (ComforTone, Essentialzyme, and ICP), Digest + Cleanse, JuvaPower/JuvaSpice, JuvaTone, Omega Blue, Sulfurzyme.

Love: Forgiveness, Joy, juniper, Lady Sclareol, lavender, Sensation, ylang ylang.
> BATH & SHOWER GELS—Sensation Bath & Shower Gel contains oils used by Cleopatra to enhance love and increase the desire to be close to that someone special.
> MASSAGE OILS—Sensation Massage Oil.
> PERSONAL CARE—Sensation Hand & Body Lotion.
> ATTRACTS—Joy.
> SELF LOVE—Joy.

Lumbago: *See Back.* Sandalwood.

Lungs: *See Respiratory System.* Aroma Life, Believe, Feucalyptus, Forgiveness, frankincense (stimulates), hyssop (diffuse to clear lungs of mucus), Joy, Raven (stronger than RC), ravensara, RC (diffuse to open lungs and to send oxygen to red blood cells), Thieves. Apply on chest with hot compress or on Vita Flex lung points on the feet.
> BLEND—Equal parts *Melaleuca ericifolia* and either RC or Raven (depending on strength desired). Add to 1 oz. V-6 Mixing Oil and insert into rectum for retention (at least 15 min. if not overnight). Rectal implant is one of the quickest ways to affect the lungs.
> PULMONARY—Aroma Life, cypress, eucalyptus, pine (antiseptic), Fsage, Fsandalwood.

> *The pulmonary is the designated artery conveying blood from the right ventricle of the heart to the lungs or any of the veins conveying oxygenated blood from the lungs to the left atrium of the heart.*

Lupus: *See Adrenal Glands, Digestive System, Endocrine System, Immune System, Thyroid.* Acceptance, clove, EndoFlex, ImmuPower (alone has cleared up Lupus), Joy, Present Time (key oil for Lupus), Thieves (every 2 hours on the feet), Valor (always use first on the feet for courage to overcome fear and build self esteem).
> BATH—Put 30 drops EndoFlex in softened Bath Gel Base (to soften, put in small container and set in hot water) and shake 30 times. Bathe 30 minutes every day. Bath Gel Base cleanses pores of the skin.
> MASSAGE—Thieves (every 2 hours on feet).
> PERSONAL CARE—A·R·T Skin Care System, Regenolone (may help reverse symptoms).

SUPPLEMENTS—Balance Complete, ComforTone, Digest + Cleanse, ICP, and Essentialzyme (cleanses the body of toxins and supports the digestive function), Thyromin (is a main stay for Lupus as it feeds and regulates the thyroid), ImmuneTune (immune support), ImmuPro, NingXia Red (contains manose, an essential sugar that helps to prevent infection - lupus patients are all deficient in this), Power Meal (pre-digested protein that contains wolfberry), and VitaGreen (high in chlorophyll; contains melissa which supports the connective tissue and the immune function). Carrot juice is also very supportive.

> *Lupus is a collagen break-down that may effect the skin, joints, and other systems of the body. It occurs because of thyroid and adrenal malfunction. The immune system cells malfunction and some of the good immune cells turn and destroy other good immune cells. This attack leads to an allergic reaction. The immune cells go crazy and attack whatever is convenient for them. The endocrine systems are usually affected and may shut down. In order to heal Lupus, it is necessary to cleanse the body, reduce the toxins, increase blood circulation, and nutritionally support the endocrine functions. When this happens, the adrenal glands can secrete the cortisone that is necessary for connective tissue repair and maintenance.*
>
> *To determine whether or not the thyroid needs help, you must monitor your basal cell temperature. Place a mercury thermometer under your arm pit and leave it there for 10 minutes. If your temperature is below 97.6° you need to work on the thyroid (See RECIPE #1 below).*

***COMMENTS—*Refer to the chapter entitled "How to Use - The Personal Usage Reference" in the <u>Essential Oils Desk Reference</u> under "Lupus" for a specific daily regimen using supplements and blends.*

ADRENAL GLANDS—Nutmeg has adrenal cortex properties and is contained in <u>EndoFlex</u>. <u>EndoFlex</u> or Blend #1 can be applied over the adrenal gland area using a hot compress. Also, apply on and massage the Vita Flex points.

BLEND #1—3 drops clove (rub in), 5 drops nutmeg (rub in), 7 drops rosemary (rub in), and 20 drops V-6 Mixing Oil. Apply a hot compress.

BLEND #2—30 cypress, 30 lemongrass, and 30 <u>EndoFlex</u> in 4 oz. V-6 Mixing Oil. Massage whole body every day.

FLUID RETENTION (caused by steroids)—<u>EndoFlex</u>.

ENDOCRINE SYSTEM SUPPORT—*See Endocrine System*. <u>EndoFlex</u>.

The following is a recipe that has been used for individuals with Lupus:

RECIPE #1—If your basal cell temperature is below 97.6° F (36.5° C), you need to work on the thyroid. Take 2 Thyromin at bedtime. If your temperature doesn't come up in three days, you will need to increase the amount of Thyromin you are taking. Take 1 upon arising along with the 2 at bedtime. When your temperature gets back up to 97.6° F, stop taking the one in the morning. Gradually go off the 2 at night. Check regularly to see that your temperature continues to stay at 97.6° F. In addition, choose one of the following oils to work as tissue generators: <u>Acceptance</u>, <u>Joy</u>, <u>Present Time</u>, or <u>Valor</u>; apply to Vita Flex points and thyroid. To support the adrenal glands, use Blend #1. To determine the adrenal area, lay a yard stick across the back from elbow to elbow and go up 2". Apply ImmuPower on the spine and Vita Flex points. Finally, supplement with Super C / Super C Chewable, 2 Thyromin or more if needed, and ImmuneTune.

CASE HISTORY #1—After doing the following for two months, one individual was totally free from Lupus: Thyromin 2 caps morning, 2 evening until temperature stayed down for three days, then increased to 3 morning and 3 evening. Also, oils used included ImmuPower, and Valor among others.

CASE HISTORY #2—Nurse in a hospital in the east gave ImmuPower to a patient as she was leaving the hospital from another serious bout with Lupus. She had Lupus for 22 years. She felt better very soon after she used ImmuPower. No symptoms of Lupus were found after eight days.

CASE HISTORY #3—After suffering from systemic lupus for some time, one lady decided there was nothing left to try from the doctors. She turned to the oils and started applying ImmuPower, EndoFlex, and Joy over her thymus and on her feet over the Vita Flex points for the pineal and pituitary glands. She also began taking Thyromin supplements. After only a day and a half of applying EndoFlex to her toes, she began to have some feeling return. After a while (specific time unknown), the "butterfly" on her face disappeared and blood tests returned "just fine".

THOUGHT PATTERNS AND EMOTIONS—Feelings experienced may be those you are not aware of or patterns you brought forward from your ancestors in the DNA. A feeling of giving up. Better to die than stand up for one's self. Anger and a need to be punished. Feelings of deep grief. Laughing on the outside, but crying on the inside. Self destructive programming, an internal cannibalism, a loss of self worth. (Remember it may not have begun with you, we carry in our cells the programming of our ancestors for 4 generations back). May feel one or more of the above. Reprogram your cells by claiming your power, loving and approving of yourself in every way (no judgment). You are free and safe; speak up for yourself freely and easily. Righteous judgment is seeing only the good we do; God's judgment. Visualize your body healed or healing. Learn the reason you chose this lesson and learn from it so you can get past it and be healed. Put as little energy as possible into your affliction.

Lyme Disease: Clarity (back of ears), Joy (over heart), RC (on chest and inhale), Sacred Mountain (on back of neck), Thieves (on feet and thymus), White Angelica (on forehead).
SUPPLEMENTS—Cleansing Trio (ComforTone, Essentialzyme, and ICP).

Lymphatic System: *See Immune System.* ᶠCypress (aromatic), Di-Gize, JuvaFlex (detoxifying), ledum (inflamed lymph nodes), ᶠsage, sandalwood (supports), tangerine.
BALANCE AND LONGEVITY—Aroma Life, Mister.
BLEND—5 drops Roman chamomile, 5 lavender, and 5 orange in 2 Tbs. V-6 Mixing Oil. Apply a few drops of blend and massage.
CLEANSING—Lemon, lime.
DECONGESTANT FOR—Aroma Life, Citrus Fresh, cumin, ᶠcypress, ᶠgrapefruit, helichrysum, lemongrass, myrtle, orange, rosemary, tangerine, thyme.

> *MASSAGE OILS*—Cel-Lite Magic.
>> *SUPPLEMENTS*—Bodygize.
> DRAINAGE OF— ^FHelichrysum, ^Flemongrass.
> ELIMINATES WASTE THROUGH— ^FLavender.
> INCREASE FUNCTION OF—Lemon.
>> *MASSAGE OILS*—Cel-Lite Magic (stimulates lymph), Relaxation.
>> *SUPPLEMENTS*—Body Balancing Trio (Bodygize, Master Formula His/Hers, VitaGreen), Power Meal.

Malaria: Lemon with honey in water to prevent.

Male: *See Aftershave or Skin.* <u>Awaken</u>.
> PERSONAL CARE—PD 80/20, Prenolone/Prenolone+, Satin Hand & Body Lotion (moisturizes skin leaving it soft, silky, and smooth), Sensation Hand & Body Lotion (moisturizes and protects skin with an alluring fragrance). KidScents Lotion makes a great aftershave as it soothes and rehydrates the skin.
> GENITAL AREA—
>> INFECTION—Eucalyptus, lavender, melaleuca, oregano, patchouli.
>> INFLAMMATION—Hyssop, lavender, Roman chamomile.
>> SWELLING—Cypress, eucalyptus, hyssop, juniper, lavender, rosemary.
> HORMONAL SYSTEM (male)—<u>Mister</u> (balances), <u>SclarEssence</u> (increases testosterone levels).
> INFERTILITY (male)—Basil, cedarwood, Clary sage, sage , <u>SclarEssence</u>, thyme.
>> *SUPPLEMENTS*—Body Balancing Trio His (Bodygize, Master Formula His, VitaGreen).
> JOCK ITCH—Cypress, lavender, melaleuca, or patchouli. Put 2 drops of any one of these oils in 1 tsp. V-6 Mixing Oil and apply to area morning and night **or** put 2 drops of any one of these oils in a small bowl of water and wash and dry area well.
>> *SUPPLEMENTS*—ProGen, Body Balancing Trio His (Bodygize, Master Formula His, VitaGreen).

Massage: Any of the different Massage Oils - Ortho Ease and Ortho Sport are excellent.
> *BLEND*—5 drops Roman chamomile, 5 lavender, 5 orange with 2 Tbs. V-6 Mixing Oil. Apply as a relaxing massage.

Measles: *See Childhood Diseases.* Eucalyptus.

Medication:
> *SUPPLEMENTS*—Super C / Super C Chewable.

Meditation: Western Red cedar, <u>Dream Catcher</u> (also for sweat lodges), elemi (aromatic), <u>Gratitude</u>, <u>Humility</u>, <u>Inspiration</u>, myrrh (aromatic), Roman chamomile, sandalwood, <u>Sacred Mountain</u>, tsuga (uplifting and grounding).

Melanoma: *See Cancer.*

OF SKIN—Frankincense and lavender.

Memory: *See Amnesia.* Aroma Life, basil (for poor memory), bergamot, calamus, Clarity, clove (memory deficiency), Dragon Time, En-R-Gee, Gentle Baby, ginger, grapefruit, Joy (of love), lavender, lemon (improves), lemongrass, Mister, Mountain savory (may bring back good memories), M-Grain, Relieve It, rose, rosemary, sage lavender. Wear as a perfume, apply to temples, and diffuse. *See COMMENTS under Asthma for a discussion on using* **plastic nasal inhalers***. These work well if used while studying material that needs to be remembered (i.e. school, exams) then used again during testing to help recall studied material.*

BLEND #1—Add a drop of lemongrass to 1-3 drops of Clarity. May be best to dilute with a few drops of V-6 Mixing Oil. Apply to forehead, temples, behind ears, and on back of neck. Cup hands over nose and mouth and breathe deeply.

BLEND #2—Add a drop of rosemary to 1-3 drops of M-Grain. Apply as described in Blend #1.

IMPROVE—Clary sage (aromatic), Fclove, lime, sage lavender.

BLEND #3—5 basil, 2 peppermint, 10 rosemary, and 1 oz. V-6 Mixing Oil.

RELEASES NEGATIVE—Forgiveness (has high frequencies), geranium (aromatic), palo santo, 3 Wise Men.

RETENTION—Clarity.

STIMULATE—Calamus, rosemary (aromatic).

BLEND #4—2 drops Blue tansy, 2 Roman chamomile, 3 geranium, 4 lavender, 3 rosemary, 3 rosewood, 1 spearmint, 2 tangerine, and 1 oz. V-6 Mixing Oil. Apply a few drops of blend to back of neck, wrist, and heart.

Menopause: *See Hormonal Imbalance.* Angelica, basil, bergamot, cardamom, Clary sage, Fcypress, Dragon Time (add V-6 Mixing Oil and use in douche, enema, or in rectum), EndoFlex (on throat, parathyroid, and thyroid), Ffennel, geranium, jasmine, Flavender, Mister, neroli, nutmeg (balances hormones), Forange, Roman chamomile, rose, rosemary, Fsage, SclarEssence, thyme. Apply oil(s) to feet, ankles, lower back, groin, and pelvis.

BATH & SHOWER GELS—Add 1 tsp. - 1 oz. Dragon Time Bath & Shower Gel to bath while filling tub with water. Soaking helps relieve lower back pain, stress, and sleeping difficulties that are associated with a woman's cycle.

MASSAGE OILS—Dragon Time.

SUPPLEMENTS—CortiStop (Women's), FemiGen, PD 80/20, Prenolone/ Prenolone+, Progessence.

***COMMENTS—*The possibility for heart attacks in women increases by 5 to 10% following menopause.*

PRE-MENOPAUSE— ᶠClary sage, EndoFlex, ᶠfennel, lavender, Mister, nutmeg (balances hormones), sage lavender (helps raise hormone levels naturally), SclarEssence, tarragon.

Menstruation: *See Hormonal Imbalance and PMS.*

AMENORRHEA— ᶠBasil, carrot, cistus, Clary sage, Dragon Time, fennel, hyssop, juniper, lavender, marjoram, myrrh, peppermint, Roman chamomile, rose, rosemary, sage, sage lavender.

DYSMENORRHEA—Clary sage then basil, cypress, Dragon Time, EndoFlex, fennel, jasmine, juniper, lavender, marjoram, peppermint, Roman chamomile, rosemary, sage, sage lavender, ᶠtarragon, yarrow.

> *Amenorrhea is the absence of menstruation. The oils listed are those which induce menstrual flow (emmenagogic).*
>
> *Emmenagogue is an agent that induces or hastens menstrual flow. Many of these oils should be avoided during pregnancy. Please see Pregnancy for safety data.*
>
> *Dysmenorrhea is painful menstruation. Apply one or more of these oils to the abdomen. It may also help to use a hot compress. Each of us have different body chemistries so if one oil doesn't work, try a different one.*
>
> *Menorrhagia is abnormally heavy or extended menstrual flow. It may also refer to irregular bleeding at any time. This situation may be a sign of a more serious condition so please see your doctor.*

BATH & SHOWER GELS— Add 1 tsp. - 1 oz. Dragon Time Bath & Shower Gel to bath while filling tub with water. Soaking helps relieve lower back pain, stress, and sleeping difficulties that are associated with a woman's cycle.

GENERAL CARE—

BLEND—Before and during cycle, combine 10 drops Dragon Time with 4 basil and rub around ankles, lower back, and lower stomach.

MASSAGE OILS—Dragon Time (uncomfortable days and irregularity)

PERSONAL CARE—PD 80/20, Prenolone/Prenolone+, or Progessence may help to regulate the hormones which

> *I have been using Young Living Essential Oils for a little over a year now. Since then, my health has improved somewhat. I decided to stop using birth control pills on Labor Day of 2003, due to being sick from them most of the time and wanting to try something else. I started putting EndoFlex on the bottom of my feet on the endocrine reflex areas. I also continued receiving colonics twice a month and eating cultured vegetables. Between the EndoFlex, colonics, and cultured vegetables, my periods have become more regular and less painful. A friend of mine who's also using EndoFlex on her feet has said that her hot flashes have stopped since she's been using EndoFlex.*
>
> **-Submitted by Christie Krajewski**
> **Batesville, Arkansas (July 2004)**

should alleviate many of the problems associated with menstruation. *See Hormonal Imbalance.*

SUPPLEMENTS—Three times a day one week before cycle starts, take 2 droppers full of FHS Tincture (available through Creer Labs 801-418-8870) in water. One week after the cycle, take Master Formula Hers four times a day and 6 VitaGreen a day. Also FemiGen (for PMS), Exodus.

IRREGULAR—Clary sage, fennel, lavender, melissa, ᶠpeppermint, Roman chamomile, rose, ᶠrosemary, ᶠsage.

MENORRHAGIA—Cypress, geranium, Roman chamomile, rose.

SCANTY—Jasmine, lavender, melissa, peppermint. *See oils listed under Amenorrhea.*

Mental: Brain Power (increases capacity and clarity by dissolving petrochemicals), ᶠoregano (mental diseases), sage (strain, aromatic), vitex (unrest). *See COMMENTS under Asthma for a discussion on using* **plastic nasal inhalers**.

SUPPLEMENTS—Omega Blue (a powerful blend of EPA and DHA from fish oil plus essential oils to preserve and support delivery to the brain; critical nutrients for proper brain function).

ACCURACY—Clarity, peppermint. Diffuse or inhale.

ALERTNESS—Clarity, En-R-Gee.

***COMMENTS—*These oils are good for night driving.*

FATIGUE—Aroma Life, Awaken, ᶠbasil, cardamom, Clarity, Dragon Time, Gentle Baby, lemongrass, Mister, M-Grain, Relieve It, ᶠrosemary, sage (diffuse), ᶠylang ylang. Basil and lemongrass together are a good combination.

IMPAIRMENT—Sulfurzyme.

RETARDATION—Can be due to a mineral deficiency. Essential Manna, KidScents Mighty Mist/ Vites, Mineral Essence.

STRESS—Clary sage, Evergreen Essence, pine (aromatic), Surrender.

SUPPLEMENTS—ImmuPro.

Metabolism:

BALANCE—Clove (aromatic), EndoFlex (increases), oregano, spearmint, Valor.

INCREASE (over all)—Spearmint (add to water & freeze to emulsify throughout), spikenard.

LIPID—Hyssop (regulates).

STRENGTHEN (vital centers)—Sage.

SUPPLEMENTS—Thyromin (regulates metabolism), ThermaBurn (tablets), Power Meal.

Metals: *See Chelation.* Clove (chelates metal ions), helichrysum, Juva Cleanse (helps to remove metals from the body), Peace & Calming, Sacred Mountain, Valor.

SUPPLEMENTS—Chelex, Cleansing Trio (ComforTone, Essentialzyme, and ICP), JuvaTone, Longevity Capsules.

> *Heavy metals in the system give off toxic gases and can create allergic symptoms and hormonal imbalances. For example, cadmium can create hyperactivity and learning disabilities in children. Cigarette smoke and caffeine all contain cadmium. Ridding the body of heavy metals is extremely important for proper immune function. Cast-iron cookware leaves heavy iron deposits in the body. Aluminum cookware leaves aluminum deposits in the body. Glass or Stainless Steel cookware is best.*

PULL OUT—Drink steam distilled water. The absence of minerals in distilled water creates a vacuum-like action that pulls metals and toxins from the body.

> **Blend #1**—Combine 10 cypress, 10 juniper, 10 lemongrass with 1 oz. V-6 Mixing Oil and massage under arms, over kidneys, and on bottoms of feet.
>
> **Blend #2**—Add 2-4 drops <u>Thieves</u> and 1-3 drops helichrysum to a rolled gauze and place between cheek and gums to pull out dental mercury. Leave in one place during the night and throw away the gauze roll in the morning. Next night place a new gauze roll with oil in a different place. Continue in like manner until all areas have been affected. ***Note: Dilute with V-6 Mixing Oil for use on very sensitive gums or on children.***

Mice (Repel): <u>Purification</u>.

Migraine Headaches: *See Headaches.* <u>Aroma Siez</u>, [F]basil, cumin, [F]eucalyptus, German chamomile, grapefruit, lavender, <u>M-Grain</u>, [F]marjoram, [F]peppermint, spearmint, valerian.
> *Supplements*—Balance Complete, Cleansing Trio (ComforTone, Essentialzyme, and ICP), Digest + Cleanse.

Mildew: <u>Purification</u> (put a few drops in a squirt bottle and spray into the air or directly onto a wall to neutralize mildew).

Mind: Basil (absent minded), <u>Believe</u> (stimulates), <u>Surrender</u> (clearing), Western Red cedar (powerful effects on subconscious and unconscious mind).

Minerals (deficiency):
> *Supplements*—Cleansing Trio (ComforTone, Essentialzyme, and ICP), Mineral Essence.

Miscarriage: *See Pregnancy.*

Mold: <u>Purification</u>, <u>Thieves</u>.
> Toxic Black—<u>Thieves</u> (on feet, as rectal implant, with Raindrop Technique on back).
> ***Comments—One young boy had toxic black mold infection. Parents gave him a rectal implant of 8 ml myrrh, 2 ml oregano, 5 ml Melaleuca alternifolia, and 5 ml Eucalyptus globulus. They followed up with <u>Thieves</u> as described above to help clear him of the infection.

Moles: Frankincense, geranium, lavender, <u>Melrose</u>.

Moment:
> Being In—<u>Present Time</u>.

> *I am not sure if this is an original idea. I used a combination of lavender and frankincense on a new **mole** that grew in with a very crusty surface. By the time I was able to have an appointment with my doctor it had totally disappeared.*
>
> *-Submitted by Judi Arndt*
> *Colorado Springs, Colorado (July 2004)*

Mono (Mononucleosis): ImmuPower, RC, Thieves.
> BLEND—3 oregano, 3 <u>Thieves</u>, and 3 thyme. Rub on feet.
> INFECTIOUS— ^FRavensara.
> SUPPLEMENTS—Build immune system. Cleansing Trio (ComforTone, Essentialzyme, and ICP), ImmuneTune, ImmuPro, Power Meal, Super C / Super C Chewable.

Mood Swings: *See Hormonal Imbalance.* Can be due to a Vitamin B deficiency. <u>Acceptance</u>, bergamot, Clary sage, <u>Dragon Time</u> or <u>Mister</u>, fennel, <u>Gathering</u>, geranium, <u>Harmony</u>, jasmine, <u>Joy</u>, juniper, lavender, lemon, <u>Peace & Calming</u>, peppermint, <u>Present Time</u>, rose, rosemary, sage, sage lavender, sandalwood, spruce, <u>Trauma Life</u>, <u>Valor</u>, yarrow, ylang ylang.
> SUPPLEMENTS—AlkaLime (if due to over-acidification), Super B.

Morning Sickness: *See Pregnancy.*

Mosquitoes: *See Insect.* Frequent mosquito bites could be due to a Vitamin B deficiency.
> SUPPLEMENTS—Super B.

Mother (Problems with): <u>Acceptance</u>, geranium, <u>Valor</u>. Apply to ears (*refer to the Auricular Emotional Therapy chart in the Basic Information section of this book*).

Motion Sickness: <u>Di-Gize</u>, ginger, <u>M-Grain</u>, nutmeg, ^Fpeppermint, spearmint. Apply to feet, temples, and wrists. Can also apply a drop or two of <u>Di-Gize</u> to the hands, stir in a clockwise motion, apply behind both ears, rub hands together, cup over nose and mouth and breathe deeply. *See COMMENTS under Asthma for a discussion on using* **plastic nasal inhalers**.
> ***COMMENTS—*According to the <u>Essential Oils Desk Reference</u>, "Mix 4 drops peppermint and 4 drops ginger in 1 ounce V-6 Mixing Oil. Rub on chest and stomach before traveling." (EDR-June 2002; Ch. 28; Digestion Problems; Travel Sickness)*

Motivation:
> TO MOVE FORWARD—<u>Envision</u> (emotional support), <u>Magnify Your Purpose</u> (empowering and uplifting), <u>Motivation</u>, myrrh, <u>Live with Passion</u>.
> SUPPLEMENTS—Sulfurzyme.

MRSA (Methicillin Resistant Staphylococcus Aureus): Cinnamon bark, clove, *Eucalyptus radiata*, geranium, grapefruit, lavender, lemon myrtle, lemongrass, *Melaleuca alternifolia* (Tea Tree), Mountain savory, orange, patchouli, peppermint, spearmint, thyme.

Mucus: *See Anti-catarrhal.* ^FCypress, helichrysum (discharge), goldenrod (discharges respiratory mucus), hyssop (opens respiratory system and discharges toxins and mucus), mugwort (expels), onycha (benzoin), ^Frosemary, <u>Thieves</u> (dissolves excess mucus).

Multiple Sclerosis (M.S.): *See Myelin Sheath.* <u>Aroma Siez</u>, birch, <u>Clarity</u>, cypress, elemi, frankincense, geranium, helichrysum, Idaho tansy, juniper, oregano, <u>Peace & Calming</u>, peppermint, rosemary, sage, sandalwood, thyme, wintergreen. Do the Raindrop Technique.

PERSONAL CARE—PD 80/20, Prenolone/Prenolone+, Progessence.

SUPPLEMENTS—Bodygize, Cleansing Trio (ComforTone, Essentialzyme, and ICP), ImmuneTune, ImmuPro, JuvaPower/JuvaSpice, JuvaTone, Mineral Essence, Omega Blue (a powerful blend of EPA and DHA from fish oil plus essential oils to preserve and support delivery to the brain; critical nutrients for proper brain function), Power Meal, Sulfurzyme, Super B, Super C / Super C Chewable, VitaGreen.

The following are recipes that have been used successfully:

RECIPE #1—Supplement with VitaGreen, Cleansing Trio (ComforTone, Essentialzyme, and ICP), ImmuneTune, and Super C / Super C Chewable. Blend 10 cardamom, 10 peppermint, and 10 rosemary with 1 oz. V-6 Mixing Oil for a full body massage. Finally, diffuse <u>Acceptance</u> and <u>Awaken</u>.

> ***Multiple Sclerosis*** *is a chronic degenerative disorder of the central nervous system where the myelin sheath, which covers the nerves, is gradually destroyed throughout the brain and/or spinal cord. Eventually it causes muscular weakness, loss of coordination, speech and visual disturbances, and bladder and bowel problems. It may be caused by a virus or a defect in the immune system.*
>
> *According to D. Gary Young, progesterone is absolutely necessary in manufacturing, building, repairing, and rejuvenating the myelin sheath. Progesterone is naturally produced from pregnenolone.*

RECIPE #2—Supplement with 8 Super Cal, 2 Super B (after breakfast), 6 Super C / Super C Chewable, 6 VitaGreen four times a day, 4 ImmuneTune, and Master Formula His/Hers. Apply juniper and peppermint, one at a time, on the spine. If the M.S. is in the neck, work up the spine. If it is in the legs, work down the spine. Do a cold compress and wait for 30 minutes. Remove the compress and repeat again.

RECIPE #3—Take 2 droppers full of Mineral Essence morning and evening to conduct current to reconnect the nerve tissues. Take ½ Super B in the morning and evening with meals for the first week. Then increase the dosage. Use juniper, geranium, and peppermint on the bottom of the feet and up the legs and spine. Apply oils in the direction of the paralysis. Apply juniper and cypress on the base of the neck, then add <u>Aroma Siez</u>. Next do the Raindrop Technique on the spine using oregano and thyme. Use <u>Peace & Calming</u> and <u>Clarity</u> for brain function and cypress for circulation. Use the Cleansing Trio (ComforTone, Essentialzyme, and ICP) and JuvaTone. Also use Super C / Super C Chewable for six days. Then start on Super B morning and evening with Bodygize or a meal, 6 VitaGreen four times a day, and 4 ImmuneTune two times a day.

BLEND—6 drops juniper, 4 sandalwood, 2 peppermint, 12 geranium. Mix and massage into neck, spine, and bottom of feet.

M

***COMMENTS—*Avoid hot baths, etc. Heat is the worst thing you can do. If anything, insulate the body with ice packs. Lowering the body temperature with cold packs helps to regenerate the myelin sheath. The person can be kept in the cold packs either for as long as they can stand it or until their body temperature drops 3 degrees. The body temperature must be monitored closely to avoid lowering it to far. This process can be repeated until the person can only stand being in the cold packs for 20 minutes. It is also best to avoid diet foods, especially those that contain aspartame as it is known to cause MS, brain damage, and other problems.*

Mumps: *See Childhood Diseases.* Lavender, melaleuca.

Muscles: <u>Aroma Siez</u>, basil, birch, cypress, Balsam fir, lavender, lemongrass, **marjoram**, palo santo, peppermint, White fir, wintergreen.

    *MASSAGE OILS—*Ortho Ease, Ortho Sport, Relaxation (these oils are great for all problems associated with muscles).

    *SUPPLEMENTS—*Be-Fit (enhances strength and endurance), BLM, CardiaCare, Essential Manna, Mineral Essence, NingXia Red, Power Meal, Pure Protein Complete (the ideal blend of 5 ultra-clean, ultra-bioactive whey proteins; provides prolonged assimilation for better protein synthesis), Sulfurzyme, Super Cal, WheyFit, Wolfberry Crisp Bars (*Refer to the Wolfberry Crisp Bar in the Supplements section of the <u>Reference Guide for Essential Oils</u> for more information on the benefits of the Ningxia Wolfberry*).

    ***COMMENTS—*One professional trainer for body builders used Be-Fit, Power Meal, and Wolfberry Bars to increase muscle mass and strength beyond anything he had previously achieved!*

    ACHES AND PAINS—<u>Aroma Siez</u>, Fbirch, Blue cypress, Fclove, Balsam fir, Douglas fir, ginger, helichrysum, lavender, lemongrass (especially good for ligaments), **marjoram**, nutmeg, oregano, palo santo, <u>PanAway</u>, peppermint, <u>Relieve It</u>, Roman chamomile, rosemary, spearmint, thyme, vetiver, White fir (with inflammation), wintergreen.

> *Every fall when the weather is hot, then cold, then hot, then cold here in Florida, I get chest pains that my doctor has characterized as **charley horses** in the deep muscles of my chest. Unlike a leg or foot muscle, you can't massage these or walk to stretch them, so there was nothing to do but "endure" these annoying episodes, which sometimes lasted for two hours. One night I woke up with this chest pain, and as I lay there thinking about what I could do for it, I remembered the instant results I had had with Aroma Siez on other people's leg cramps. So I got up and rubbed a few drops of Aroma Siez on my chest, and the pain went away in about 10 minutes!*
>
> ***-Submitted by Jan Early***
> ***Tallahassee, Florida (July 2004)***

    *SUPPLEMENTS—*Sulfurzyme.

    ***COMMENTS—*Refer to the chapter entitled "How to Use - The Personal Usage Reference" in the <u>Essential Oils Desk Reference</u> under "Muscles" for some excellent blends to help sore and tight muscles.*

    ANTI-INFLAMMATORY—Basil, Balsam fir, frankincense, peppermint, White fir. *See Anti-inflammatory and Inflammation for additional oils.*

***COMMENTS**—*Refer to the chapter entitled "How to Use - The Personal Usage Reference" in the* <u>Essential Oils Desk Reference</u> *under "Muscles" for an excellent blend to help reduce inflammation.*

CARDIAC MUSCLE—Goldenrod, lavender, marjoram, neroli, peppermint, rose, rosemary verbenon (helps regulate).
  SUPPLEMENTS—CardiaCare (strengthen and support).

CRAMPS/CHARLEY HORSES—<u>Aroma Siez</u>, basil, Clary sage, coriander, cypress, grapefruit, jasmine, lavender (aromatic), **marjoram**, pine, Roman chamomile, rosemary, thyme, vetiver.
  SUPPLEMENTS—BLM, Essential Manna, Mineral Essence, Sulfurzyme, Super Cal.
  BLEND—Equal parts rosemary and <u>Aroma Siez</u>. Apply neat or mix with V-6 Mixing Oil and massage.

DEVELOPMENT—Birch/wintergreen (with spruce), <u>PanAway</u>.
  SUPPLEMENTS—Be-Fit, Power Meal, Pure Protein Complete, Super Cal, VitaGreen (stimulates and strengthens).

FATIGUE—<u>Aroma Siez</u>, cypress, Balsam fir, Douglas fir, eucalyptus, grapefruit, **marjoram**, peppermint, ravensara, rosemary, thyme.
  SUPPLEMENTS—Essential Manna (high in magnesium), Mineral Essence, Super Cal.

OVER-EXERCISED—**Balsam fir**, Douglas fir, eucalyptus, ginger, lavender, thyme, White fir (with inflammation).
  BATH—3 drops marjoram and 2 drops lemon in a tub of water. Soak.
  BLEND—Equal parts of eucalyptus, peppermint, and ginger. Mix with V-6 Mixing Oil and massage.

RHEUMATISM (Muscular)—palo santo, rosemary, thyme.

SPRAINS—Black pepper, clove, eucalyptus, ginger, helichrysum, Idaho tansy, jasmine, lavender, lemongrass, **marjoram**, nutmeg, pine, rosemary, thyme, vetiver, White fir.

SPASMS—<u>Aroma Siez</u>, **basil**, Clary sage, cypress, lavender, jasmine, marjoram, <u>PanAway</u>, peppermint, Roman chamomile.
  MASSAGE OILS—Cel-Lite Magic, Ortho Ease.
  SUPPLEMENTS—Super Cal.

STIFFNESS—<u>Aroma Siez</u>, <u>PanAway</u>.

SMOOTH MUSCLE—Bergamot, Black pepper, Clary sage, cypress, fennel, juniper, lavender, **marjoram**, melissa, neroli, peppermint, Roman chamomile, rosemary, sandalwood. Apply as a hot compress over the affected area.
  ***COMMENTS**—Essential oils with high proportions of ester compounds are especially effective.*

TENSION (especially in shoulders and neck)—<u>Aroma Siez</u>, Douglas fir, helichrysum, juniper, lavender, **marjoram**, <u>Relieve It</u>, Roman chamomile, spruce.
  BATH & SHOWER GELS—Evening Peace Bath & Shower Gel (relaxes tired, fatigued muscles and helps alleviate tension).
  MASSAGE OILS—Ortho Ease and Ortho Sport.

M

TISSUE—

> SUPPLEMENTS—Bodygize, Pure Protein Complete, and Power Meal (contain a complete amino acid and vitamin profile and have a high level of predigested protein to maintain a good food supply for muscle tissue), Be-Fit (contains ingredients necessary to build muscle mass), BLM, Ultra Young/Ultra Young+ (increase production of growth hormone which increases formation of lean muscle tissue), WheyFit.

> ***COMMENTS—*Refer to the chapter entitled "How to Use - The Personal Usage Reference" in the Essential Oils Desk Reference under "Muscles" for some excellent blends to help improve circulation in the muscles and aid in the regeneration of muscle tissue.*

TONE—Basil, birch, Black pepper, cypress, ginger, grapefruit, juniper, lavender, lime, marjoram, orange, peppermint, petitgrain, pine, rosemary, thyme, wintergreen. Apply before exercise.

> SUPPLEMENTS—Be-Fit (promotes formation of muscle tissue), Pure Protein Complete, Sulfurzyme, WheyFit.

> ***COMMENTS—*Poor muscle tone may indicate a sulfur deficiency.*

TORN MUSCLES—Helichrysum and spruce take pain away (use hot packs), ginger (circulation), **lemongrass**, Lemon myrtle.

> MASSAGE OILS—Ortho Sport.

Muscular Dystrophy: Aroma Siez, basil, eucalyptus, geranium, ginger, lavender, lemon, lemongrass, marjoram (combine with equal parts lemongrass), orange, pine, Relieve It, rosemary.

> MASSAGE OILS—Ortho Ease, Ortho Sport.

> SUPPLEMENTS—Essentialzyme, Mineral Essence, Power Meal, Sulfurzyme, Thyromin, Ultra Young, VitaGreen.

Myelin Sheath: ImmuneTune, ImmuPro, ImmuPower, and **cold** compresses using peppermint, juniper, and geranium *(remember, **no heat!**)*.

> SUPPLEMENTS—Omega Blue (contains DHA which helps support the myelin sheath).

Nails: Citrus Fresh, eucalyptus, frankincense, grapefruit, lavender, lemon (repeated use may help harden), lime, melaleuca, myrrh, oregano, patchouli, peppermint, ravensara, rosemary, thyme.

> BLEND—Equal parts frankincense, lemon, and myrrh. Mix with a couple drops of Wheat Germ oil and apply 2-3 times per week.

> SUPPLEMENTS—Mineral Essence, Sulfurzyme (helps with growth and removal of ridges and cracks), Super Cal.

> ***COMMENTS—*A deficiency in sulfur can cause poor nail growth.*

Narcolepsy: Brain Power

SUPPLEMENTS—Mineral Essence, Thyromin, Ultra Young, VitaGreen.

***COMMENTS— *Establishing a routine of strict bedtimes and daytime naps may also help reduce the number of unexpected sleep attacks.*

> ***Narcolepsy*** *is a disorder that is characterized by sudden and uncontrollable drowsiness and attacks of sleep at unexpected and irregular intervals. It is frequently misdiagnosed as hypothyroidism (insufficient thyroid hormone), hypoglycemia (insufficient blood sugar), epilepsy, or multiple sclerosis. Proper diagnosis requires overnight monitoring with a device used to detect brain waves called an electroencephalograph.*

Nasal: *See Nose.*

Nausea: Calamus, cardamom, clove, <u>Di-Gize</u> (over stomach and colon), ginger, juniper, ^Flavender, <u>M-Grain</u>, nutmeg, ^Fpeppermint (aromatic), rosewood, spearmint, tarragon. Apply behind ears and on Vita Flex points. *See COMMENTS under Asthma for a discussion on using* **plastic nasal inhalers**.

BLEND—2 lavender, 2 spearmint, and 2 drops of another oil for your type of nausea. Mix together and put a little on a cotton ball and inhale three times a day or diffuse.

Neck: Basil, Clary sage, geranium, lemon, lemongrass, orange, helichrysum.

CHRONIC PAIN—<u>PanAway</u>. Apply to base of big toe.

SUPPLEMENTS—BLM

Negative Ions: When dispersed into the air through a cool-air nebulizing diffuser, the following oils ionize negatively: Bergamot, cedarwood, citronella, *Eucalyptus citriodora*, grapefruit, lavandin, lavender, lemon,

> ***Negative ions*** *are produced naturally by wind and rain. They help stimulate the parasympathetic nervous system which controls rest, relaxation, digestion, and sleep. However, if you live in an environment with an over-abundance of negative ions, such as in the country or by the ocean, you may benefit greatly by diffusing the oils listed under* Positive Ions. *The production of more positive ions can help bring greater balance to the area and provide a more healthy environment.*

Negativity: Sandalwood (removes negative programming from the cells), <u>Transformation</u>.

BREAKS UP—<u>Dream Catcher</u>, <u>Forgiveness</u>, palo santo.

DROWNING IN OWN—Grapefruit (aromatic).

Nervous System: ^FBasil (stimulant and for nervous breakdown), bergamot, <u>Brain Power</u>, calamus, cedarwood (nervous tension), cinnamon bark, cumin (stimulant), <u>Di-Gize</u>, Balsam fir, frankincense, geranium (regenerates nerves), ginger, jasmine (nervous exhaustion), juniper (better nerve function), lavender, lemon, lemongrass (for nerve damage; activates), marjoram (soothing), *Melaleuca ericifolia* (nervous tension), nutmeg (supports), orange, palmarosa (supports), <u>Peace & Calming</u>, pepper (stimulant),

peppermint (soothes and strengthens; place on wrists or location of nerve damage), petitgrain (re-establishes nerve equilibrium), pine (stimulant), ravensara, Roman chamomile, rosemary, ^Fsage, sandalwood, spearmint, spruce (fatigue), valerian (central nervous system depressant), vetiver.

PERSONAL CARE—NeuroGen or Regenolone (both help nerve regeneration).

SUPPLEMENTS—Mineral Essence, Omega Blue, Sulfurzyme, Super B.

TINCTURES—Nerv-Cal (supplies nerve tissues with calcium), Ner-Vus (helps heal nerve damage and relax nervous conditions). *Both tinctures are available through Creer Labs 801-418-8870.*

NERVOUSNESS—Cypress, goldenrod, orange, Surrender, tangerine.

PARASYMPATHETIC NERVES—*See Parasympathetic Nerves.* ^FMarjoram (increases tone of).

VIRUS OF NERVES—Clove and frankincense.

Neuralgia (severe pain along nerve): Cajeput, cedarwood, eucalyptus, helichrysum, juniper, lavender, ^Fmarjoram, nutmeg, pine, ^FRoman chamomile, sage lavender.

Neuritis: Cedarwood, clove, eucalyptus, juniper, lavender, ^FRoman chamomile, yarrow.

Neurological Problems: Limit the use of oils with high *ketone* content.

***COMMENTS—A 4 year old child was in a car accident where she suffered severe brain damage. The surgeon removed part of her brain which sent her into a coma. After being in a coma for two months, Dr. Friedmann was asked to help her. He used oils that are commonly used for neurological problems. He put Valor on the back of her neck, skull, and feet. He also used Present Time and Awaken. She came out of the coma and started doing physical therapy.*

Neuromuscular: Roman chamomile, tarragon.

Neuropathy: Brain Power, cedarwood, cypress, eucalyptus, geranium, helichrysum, juniper, JuvaFlex, lavender, lemongrass, peppermint, Roman chamomile, Valor.

PERSONAL CARE—NeuroGen, PD 80/20, Prenolone/Prenolone+, Progessence, Regenolone.

SUPPLEMENTS—Bodygize, Essential Manna, Mineral Essence, Sulfurzyme, Super B.

***COMMENTS—Refer to the chapter entitled "How to Use - The Personal Usage Reference" in the Essential Oils Desk Reference under "Nerve Disorders" subcategory "Neuropathy" for some excellent blends.*

PAIN—Relieve It, helichrysum (best with cold compresses), PanAway. Massage with peppermint, juniper, and geranium and reapply cold compresses.

Neurotonic: Melaleuca, ^Fravensara, thyme.

Night Sweats: *See Hot Flashes and Hormonal Imbalance.* EndoFlex, ^FSage.

Nose: Melaleuca, rosemary.

> BLEEDING—Cypress, helichrysum, frankincense, lavender, lemon.
>> *BLEND*—2 cypress, 1 helichrysum, and 2 lemon in 8 oz. ice water. Soak cloth and apply to nose and back of neck.
>
> NASAL MUCUS MEMBRANE—Both eucalyptus and peppermint may help reduce inflammation.
> NASAL NASOPHARYNX—Eucalyptus.
> POLYPS—*See Polyps.* Basil, citronella, frankincense, oregano, peppermint, <u>Purification</u>, <u>RC</u> (can be applied to inside of nose with cotton swab). Apply to exterior of nose (use caution because of close proximity to eyes) or breathe in diffused mist. A colon and liver cleanse may be helpful. Birch/wintergreen or <u>Valor</u> may also be applied to bridge of nose for possible structural realignment.
>> ***COMMENTS—*** *Nasal polyps are caused by an overproduction of fluid in the mucous membranes. They are seen with asthma, hay fever, chronic sinus infections, and cystic fibrosis. In fact, one source stated that one out of four people with cystic fibrosis have nasal polyps. They may also be a result of blockages in the brain or some trauma to the nose in which structural integrity has been compromised. Diet may also be a factor.*

Nursing: Clary sage (brings in milk production), [F]fennel or basil (increases milk production), geranium. Apply above breasts on lymph area and on spine at breast level.

> INCREASE MILK PRODUCTION—
>> *BLEND*—7 to 15 drops fennel and either 7 to 15 drops geranium or 5 to 10 drops Clary sage. Dilute 1-2 drops of blend in 2 Tbs. V-6 Mixing Oil.
>> *SUPPLEMENTS*—Body Balancing Trio Hers (Bodygize, Master Formula Hers, VitaGreen).
>
> DECREASE MILK PRODUCTION—Peppermint. Apply with cold compress over breasts. *Refer to Methods of Application under the Science and Application section of the <u>Reference Guide for Essential Oils</u> for instructions on using cold compresses.*

Obesity: *See Diet, Weight.* Fennel, <u>GLF</u>, grapefruit, juniper, <u>Juva Cleanse</u>, orange, rosemary, tangerine.

> *SUPPLEMENTS*—Balance Complete, Digest + Cleanse, JuvaPower/JuvaSpice, NingXia Red, Power Meal (eat for breakfast as a meal replacement), Wolfberry Crisp Bars.
> REDUCE—<u>Juva Cleanse</u>, Orange, tangerine.

Obsessiveness: <u>Acceptance</u>, <u>Awaken</u>, Clary sage, cypress, <u>Forgiveness</u>, geranium, helichrysum, <u>Humility</u>, <u>Inner Child</u>, <u>Joy</u>, lavender, marjoram, <u>Motivation</u>, <u>Present Time</u>, rose, <u>Sacred Mountain</u>, sandalwood, <u>Valor</u>, ylang ylang.

Odors: *See Deodorant.* Bergamot, lavender, <u>Purification</u> (neutralizes and eliminates).

> *PERSONAL CARE*—AromaGuard Deodorants.
> BODY—<u>Purification</u> (obnoxious odors).
> CONTROLLING—Cedarwood.

Opening (to receive): Fir (aromatic), Transformation.

Opposition: Valor.

Oral Infections: ^FRosewood.

Osteomyelitis: *See Bones.* Equal parts lemongrass, clove, *Eucalyptus radiata*, and *Melaleuca alternifolia* (Tea Tree) either blended together, or applied individually on the direct topical location.
  ***COMMENTS—*Osteomyelitis is infection in the bones. Often, the original site of infection is elsewhere in the body, and spreads to the bone by the blood. Bacteria or fungus may sometimes be responsible for osteomyelitis.*

Osteoporosis: *See Hormonal Imbalance.* Aroma Siez, birch, chamomile (Roman and German), clove, cypress, fennel, fir (cortisone-like action), geranium, ginger, hyssop, lemon, nutmeg, oregano, PanAway, Peace & Calming, peppermint, pine, Relieve It, rosemary, spruce, thyme, wintergreen.
  *SUPPLEMENTS—*BLM, PD 80/20, Prenolone/Prenolone+, Progessence, Super Cal.

> *Studies and clinical experience by Dr. John R. Lee indicate that bone mass can be reversed (regained) by as much as 41% with the use of Natural Progesterone. For information on Dr. Lee's book, see* Hormonal Imbalance.

Ovaries: *See Hormonal Imbalance.* Di-Gize, geranium, Gratitude, ^Fmyrtle, ^Frosemary (regulates).
  *OVARIAN CYSTS—*Basil.
  *BLEND—*5 frankincense and 5 Melrose. Mix and apply to lower back and abdomen. May also consider adding this blend to 2 tsp. of olive oil and before going to bed, while lying down, insert blend into vagina and retain with a tampon throughout the night.
  *PERSONAL CARE—*PD 80/20, Prenolone/Prenolone+, Progessence, Protec.
  *SUPPLEMENTS—*FemiGen (helps feed the body), Master Formula Hers.

Overcome and Release Unpleasant, Difficult Issues in Life: Acceptance, Release, Roman chamomile, SARA, Transformation, Trauma Life.

Overeating: *See Eating Disorders.*

Overweight: *See Obesity and Weight.*

Overwhelmed: Acceptance, Hope, Release, Valor.

> *All essential oils increase the ability of the body to take oxygen to the cells and to push toxins out. The oils pick up more oxygen and take it to the site of discomfort.*

Oxygen:
  *OXYGENATING—*Fennel, fir, frankincense, oregano, sandalwood (increases oxygen around pineal and pituitary glands).

PERSONAL CARE—Satin Facial Scrub - Mint (deep cleansing that dispenses nutrients and oxygen).

OXYGEN EXCHANGE—Tsuga (increases by opening and dilating respiratory tract).

Pain: *See Aches/Pains.*

Painting: Add one 15 ml. bottle of your favorite essential oil (or oil blend) to any five gallon bucket of paint. Stir vigorously, mixing well, and then either spray paint or paint by hand. This should eliminate the paint fumes and after-smell.

Palpitations: *See Heart.*

Pancreas: Coriander, ^Fcypress (for insufficiencies), dill, fleabane, lemon, <u>Raven</u>, <u>RC</u>, rosemary, <u>Thieves</u>.

STIMULANT FOR—Fleabane, ^Fhelichrysum.

SUPPORT—Cinnamon bark, coriander, <u>EndoFlex</u>, fennel, geranium.

SUPPLEMENTS—Essentialzyme, Stevia, Thyromin, VitaGreen.

TINCTURES—Sugar-Up (available through Creer Labs 801-418-8870)

Pancreatitis:

WEAKNESS—Lemon, marjoram.

Panic: <u>Awaken</u>, bergamot, birch, fir, Balsam fir, frankincense, <u>Gathering</u>, <u>Harmony</u>, lavender, marjoram, myrrh, Roman chamomile, rosemary, sandalwood, spruce, thyme, <u>Valor</u>, <u>White Angelica</u>, wintergreen, ylang ylang.

Paralysis: <u>Awaken</u>, cypress, geranium, ginger, helichrysum, juniper, lemongrass, nutmeg, peppermint, <u>Purification</u>, <u>Valor</u>.

BLEND—Combine 6 cypress, 15 geranium, 10 helichrysum, 5 juniper, 2 peppermint and V-6 Mixing Oil. May rejuvenate nerve damage up to 60%. Put on location and feet.

SUPPLEMENTS—Support the body with Bodygize, VitaGreen, Super B, Master Formula His/Hers, Mineral Essence. When it starts to reverse there will be pain, apply <u>PanAway</u> on location and on feet.

Parasites: *See Anti-parasitic and Intestinal Problems.* Anise, clove, <u>Di-Gize</u>, ^Ffennel, hyssop, melaleuca, Mountain savory, mugwort (blend with thyme), ^Foregano, tangerine, ^Ftarragon, ^Fthyme. Apply oil on stomach and feet to help pass parasites.

ParaFree was specifically designed to help the body rid itself of parasites. The essential oils contained in this supplement are: Black cumin, anise, fennel, laurel, vetiver, nutmeg, melaleuca alternifolia, Idaho tansy, clove, and thyme.

Since this product is to be used orally and contraindications do exist, one would be well advised to review the book, <u>Essential Oil Safety—A Guide for Health Care Professionals</u> by Robert Tisserand and Tony Balacs or <u>Aromatherapy for Health Professionals</u> by Shirley and Len Price.

ANTI-PARASITIC— ᶠNutmeg.

INTESTINAL— ᶠLemon, ravensara, ᶠRoman chamomile.

> SUPPLEMENTS—Cleansing Trio (ComforTone, Essentialzyme, and ICP), Digest + Cleanse, ParaFree.

> ***COMMENTS—*Individuals have passed parasites within 12 hours using* <u>Di-Gize</u> *on stomach.*

Parasympathetic Nervous System:

ᶠLemongrass (regulates), ᶠmarjoram (increases tone of), <u>Peace & Calming</u>, <u>Valor</u>.

> *The* **Parasympathetic Nervous System** *is responsible for preparing us for feeding, digestion, and rest by slowing the heart, contracting the bronchi, dilating the arteries, and stimulating the digestive system.*

> DIFFUSION—*See* **Negative Ions** *for a list of oils that ionize negatively when diffused to help stimulate the parasympathetic nervous system.*

> ***COMMENTS—*See the Autonomic Nervous System chart in the Science and Application section of the* <u>Reference Guide for Essential Oils</u>.

Parathyroid: <u>EndoFlex</u>. Apply over the

thyroid gland at the bottom of the throat or on the parathyroid Vita Flex point on feet.

> *The* **parathyroid gland** *is responsible for secreting a hormone necessary for the metabolism of calcium and phosphorus. It is located near or within the posterior surface of the thyroid gland.*

Parkinson's Disease: *See Brain, Pineal Gland, Pituitary Gland, and Alzheimer's Disease.* <u>Acceptance</u>,

basil, bergamot, <u>Clarity</u> (brain function), cypress (circulation), frankincense, <u>Gathering</u> (high in sesquiterpenes and in frequency), geranium, helichrysum, juniper, <u>Juva Cleanse</u>, lavender, lemon, marjoram, nutmeg, orange, <u>Peace & Calming</u>, peppermint, rosemary, sandalwood, thyme, <u>Valor</u>, vitex.

> *Cedarwood, vetiver, sandalwood, Black pepper, myrrh, patchouli, ginger, German chamomile, spikenard, galbanum, and frankincense all contain sesquiterpenes which have the ability to go beyond the blood-brain barrier. See Pineal Gland and Pituitary Gland.*

> SUPPLEMENTS—BLM, Cleansing Trio (ComforTone, Essentialzyme, and ICP), JuvaPower/ JuvaSpice, JuvaTone, Omega Blue, Power Meal (contains Choline which is beneficial for Parkinson's disease), Sulfurzyme.

> TINCTURES—Chelex. The following recipe has been used by Dr. Terry Friedmann of Paradise Valley, Arizona:

> RECIPE #1—Use the Cleansing Trio (ComforTone, Essentialzyme, and ICP) for one week, then add JuvaTone and 10 VitaGreen along with it. Drink 10 glasses of distilled water daily. Take one dropper full of Chelex tincture two times a day and diffuse the oil of helichrysum and frankincense together one hour at night.

> RECIPE #2—Apply frankincense to the top of the spine (at the base of the skull) and work it in. Then apply 3-5 drops of each of the following oils, one at a time, up the back of the neck, and work each one in individually: valerian, vetiver, Balsam fir, Roman

chamomile, and Western Red cedar. This will help to suppress the override of the sympathetic system and bring about a change in their attitude and ability.

TO PREVENT—Keep liver and blood clean with Juva Cleanse, JuvaTone and the Cleansing Trio (ComforTone, Essentialzyme, and ICP). Massage with helichrysum and sandalwood to help chelate metallics out of the body.

Past: Present Time (helps to bring you into the present so you can go forward), Transformation.

Peace: Juniper (aromatic), lavender (aromatic), marjoram, Peace & Calming, Release, Trauma Life, ylang ylang.

FINDING—Tangerine (aromatic).

PROMOTE—Roman chamomile.

SUPPLEMENTS—Cleansing Trio (ComforTone, Essentialzyme, and ICP) and JuvaTone.

Pelvic Pain Syndrome: Bergamot, clove, geranium, ginger, nutmeg, thyme.

Periodontal Disease: *See Gum Disease.*

Personal Growth: Transformation.

ELIMINATING BLOCKED—Helichrysum, frankincense.

PERSONALITY (MULTIPLE)—Inner Child, SARA, and Sensation.

Perspiration: Petitgrain, Purification.

SUPPLEMENTS—Cleansing Trio (ComforTone, Essentialzyme, and ICP).

Pest Troubles: *See Insect.* Ravensara.

pH Balance: *See Acidosis and Alkalosis.*

SUPPLEMENTS—AlkaLime (combats yeast and fungus overgrowth and preserves the body's proper pH balance), Balance Complete, ComforTone (to help clean out the colon), Digest + Cleanse, Essentialzyme, JuvaTone (to clean the liver) and Mineral Essence (if body is too alkaline), VitaGreen (brings blood back to an alkaline pH).

PERSONAL CARE—Genesis Hand & Body Lotion (balances pH on skin).

> *According to Dr. Robert O. Young in his book, One Sickness, One Disease, One Treatment, "disease is an expression of pH." He believes that there is only one disease which is "the constant over-acidification of the blood and tissues which disturbs the central regulation of the human body, all of which is mainly the result of an inverted way of living and eating." All sickness and disease that leads to death begins with an over-acidification of the blood and tissues and culminates with yeast and fungus. A normal healthy body should have a pH of about 7.2. (The use of saliva and urine test strips will show a much lower pH level due to the protein present in the solution. Saliva and urine tests from a healthy body should be about 6.6 to 6.8.) To maintain this pH, our diet should consist of 80% alkaline foods to 20% acid foods. "In the healing of disease, when the individual is acidic, the higher the ratio of alkaline elements in the diet, the faster will be the recovery."*

P

Personal Guide

Pharyngitis: *See also Rhinopharyngitis.* Goldenrod.

Phlebitis: Cypress, geranium, grapefruit, ᶠhelichrysum (prevents), ᶠlavender, Roman chamomile, or Valor. Massage toward heart and wear support hose until healed, possibly two to three months. Use Aroma Life every morning and night. Do the Raindrop Technique on leg.

Pimples: Clary sage, frankincense, Gentle Baby, ImmuPower (pimples in ears), lavender, lemongrass, melaleuca, Melrose, Purification, Raven, ravensara, RC.
   PERSONAL CARE—Rose Ointment (apply over top of other oil(s) used to enhance and extend their effectiveness).

Pineal Gland:
   OPENS AND INCREASES OXYGEN—Acceptance, Brain Power, cedarwood, Forgiveness, frankincense, Gathering, Harmony, Inspiration, Into the Future, Release, sandalwood (increases oxygen), spruce, Transformation, Trauma Life, 3 Wise Men (same frequency as pineal).
   ***COMMENTS— *Just smelling the essential oils will increase the oxygen production, particularly around the pineal and pituitary glands, and will help increase the secretion of anti-bodies, endorphins, and neurotransmitters.*

> The ***pineal gland*** *synthesizes a hormone called melatonin in periods of darkness. The pineal gland and melatonin are being studied for their roles in aging, sleep, and reproduction. The pineal gland is also involved in the process of creativity and planning things to do. If the pineal gland is not open, negative emotions will be attracted back to the aura.*
>
> ***Oils containing sesquiterpenes are especially effective in oxygenating the pineal and pituitary glands****. These include cedarwood, vetiver, sandalwood, Black pepper, myrrh, patchouli, ginger, German chamomile, spikenard, galbanum, and frankincense in order of sesquiterpene content. Blends include* 3 Wise Men, Acceptance, Brain Power, Forgiveness, Gathering, Harmony, Inspiration, Into the Future, *and* Trauma Life.

Pituitary Gland: *See Endocrine System.*
   SUPPLEMENTS—Ultra Young (a new spray neutriceutical which contains ingredients that are necessary for stimulating the pituitary gland into producing the human growth hormone (hGH) and allowing the body to utilize it).
   BALANCES—Geranium, ylang ylang. Apply to forehead, back of neck, and Vita Flex points on big toes.

> The ***pituitary gland*** *is located at the base of the brain and is considered to be the master gland because its secretions stimulate the other endocrine glands. The pituitary has an anterior and a posterior lobe. The anterior lobe secretes the human growth hormone (stimulates overall body growth), adrenocorticotropic hormone (controls steroid hormone secretion by the adrenal cortex), thyrotropic hormone (stimulates the activity of the thyroid gland), and three gonadotropic hormones (control growth and reproductive activity of the ovaries and testes). The posterior lobe secretes antidiuretic hormone and oxytocin. The antidiuretic hormone causes water retention by the kidneys. Oxytocin stimulates the mammary glands to release milk and also causes uterine contractions. An overactive pituitary during childhood can cause a child to be extremely tall while an underactive pituitary can result in the opposite. (Refer to the text box for* Pineal Gland *above for a list of oils that are high in sesquiterpenes.)*

INCREASES OXYGEN—3 Wise Men, Acceptance, Brain Power, Egyptian Gold, frankincense, Forgiveness, Gathering, Harmony, Inspiration, Into the Future, sandalwood, Trauma Life. Apply to the forehead, back of neck, and Vita Flex points on big toes. Can also rub a couple drops of oil between hands, cup over nose and mouth, and breathe deeply (*see COMMENTS under Pineal above*). *Also, refer to COMMENTS under Asthma for a discussion on using **plastic nasal inhalers**.*

Plague: Abundance, ᶠclove, Thieves (annihilates bacteria).

Pleurisy: *See Lungs or Anti-bacterial.* ᶠCypress, ᶠthyme.

PMS: *See Hormonal Imbalance.* Angelica, anise, bergamot, ᶠClary sage, Exodus II, fennel, geranium, grapefruit, jasmine, lavender (aromatic), nutmeg, Peace & Calming, Roman chamomile, ᶠtarragon.

APATHETIC-TIRED-LISTLESS—Bergamot, fennel, geranium, grapefruit, Roman chamomile.
  BATH & SHOWER GELS—Dragon Time Bath & Shower Gel.
  BLEND—10 drops Dragon Time and 4 drops basil. Rub blend around ankles, lower back, and lower stomach. Use before and during cycle.

IRRITABLE—Bergamot, Clary sage, nutmeg, Roman chamomile.
  MASSAGE OILS—Before and during cycle, combine 10 drops Dragon Time with 4 basil and rub around ankles, lower back and lower stomach.
  SUPPLEMENTS—Exodus, NingXia Red, Omega Blue, PD 80/20, Prenolone/Prenolone+, Progessence, Wolfberry Crisp Bars. Three times a day one week before cycle starts, take 2 droppers full of FHS Tincture (available through Creer Labs 801-418-8870) in water. One week after the cycle, take Master Formula Hers four times a day and 6 VitaGreen a day. Also FemiGen (for PMS)—take 2 FemiGen three times a day before period, start again two days after cycle.

VIOLENT AGGRESSIVE—Bergamot, geranium, nutmeg.
  SUPPLEMENTS—Omega Blue.

WEEPING-DEPRESSION—Bergamot, Clary sage, geranium, nutmeg.
  SUPPLEMENTS—Omega Blue.

Pneumonia: *See Respiratory System (COMMENTS, RECIPE #1, and BLEND #5).* Cajeput, eucalyptus, *Eucalyptus radiata*, Exodus II, frankincense, ImmuPower (on spine), lavender, lemon, melaleuca, *Melaleuca ericifolia*, myrrh, oregano, Raven (on back and feet), ravensara, Thieves (on feet) and thyme are good to use as compresses.

SUPPLEMENTS—Exodus, Master Formula His/Hers, Ultra Young.
  One or more of the following can be used with great effect:
  1. RC on chest.
  2. Put 15 drops of RC in 2 cups of hot water in a bowl, wet towel, ring out, and put on chest with a dry towel on top.

3. Put 4 drops of <u>RC</u> or eucalyptus in ½ cup hot water, inhale steam deeply.
4. <u>Raven</u> in rectum, <u>RC</u> on chest and back (reverse each night).

***COMMENTS—*Refer to the chapter entitled "How to Use - The Personal Usage Reference" in the <u>Essential Oils Desk Reference</u> under "Pneumonia - Emphysema" for some excellent blend recipes and supplement recommendations.*

Poison Oak/Ivy: <u>Harmony</u>, <u>Joy</u>, Lavender, <u>Melrose</u>, Roman chamomile, rose, rosewood, palmarosa.
PERSONAL CARE—Rose Ointment.

Pollution: *See Purification.* <u>Purification</u>.
AIR—Lemon, peppermint, <u>Purification</u>.
CIGARETTE SMOKE—<u>Purification</u>.
WATER—Lemon, peppermint, <u>Purification</u>.

Polyps: *See also Nose: POLYPS.* <u>Di-Gize</u>, <u>Exodus II</u>, peppermint, spikenard, and others with strong anti-bacterial properties (*See Anti-bacterial*).
SUPPLEMENTS—ComforTone, Essentialzyme, Exodus, Master Formula His/Hers, Super Cal.

***COMMENTS—*In two separate articles published in 1998, bacterial infection was found to exist when polyps were present. In the case of colorectal (intestinal) polyps, E. coli and similar bacteria were found to be adhering to the walls of the large intestine, and even partially penetrating the intestinal mucosa (Gastroenterology 1998; 115: 281-286). In the case of gastric polyps (small growths in the stomach lining), the Helicobacter pylori bacteria was found, and when eradicated, the polyps disappeared in 71% of the patients within a 12 to 15 month period (Annals of Internal Medicine 1998; 129: 712-715).*

> *Recently I got **Poison Ivy/Oak** for the first time. I looked in my "Reference Guide for Essential Oils" and decided to use <u>Melrose</u> on my poison ivy. The itching would stop for about 5 minutes and start up again. I decided to put <u>Purification</u> on, which stopped the itching for maybe an hour or two and then would start up again. Getting desperate I used <u>Joy</u> and sometimes <u>Harmony</u> (since I had more <u>Harmony</u>) on the poison ivy. The itching would stop for most of the day and I would forget about having poison ivy. I didn't start the <u>Harmony</u> and <u>Joy</u> until about 3 or 4 days into the poison ivy flare up, but it's now the 6th day and I'm not itching unless I take a shower or sweat profusely. From my experience with my poison ivy, I'm convinced that the presence of Rose, Rosewood, and Palmarosa in <u>Joy</u> and <u>Harmony</u>, have all helped in the healing of our "skin conditions". I plan to stock up on <u>Harmony</u> and <u>Joy</u> for future needs.*
>
> **-Submitted by Christie Krajewski**
> **Batesville, Arkansas (July 2004)**

Positive Feelings: <u>Acceptance</u>, <u>Abundance</u>, <u>Envision</u>, <u>Forgiveness</u>, Idaho tansy, <u>Joy</u>, <u>Motivation</u>, <u>Live with Passion</u>, <u>3 Wise Men</u> (releases negative memory/trauma and reinforces positive feelings which creates greater spiritual awareness).

Positive Ions: When dispersed into the air through a cool-air nebulizing diffuser, the following oils ionize positively: Cajeput,

> **Positive ions** are produced by electronic equipment and are typically found in man-made environments. They help stimulate the sympathetic nervous system, necessary for recovering, strengthening, and energizing. However, an over-abundance of positive ions can lead to stress and agitation. The diffusion of the oils listed under Negative Ions can help balance the ions and help produce a more stress free environment.

clove, cypress, eucalyptus, frankincense, helichrysum, juniper, marjoram, *Melaleuca quinquenervia*, palmarosa, pine, ravensara, rosemary, thyme, ylang ylang.

Potassium Deficiency:
> SUPPLEMENTS—Essential Manna, Master Formula His/Hers, Mineral Essence, Thyromin.

> *Potassium is important for a healthy nervous system and a regular heart rhythm. It works with sodium to control the body's water balance and regulates the transfer of nutrients to the cells.*

Potential: Acceptance, Awaken (realize our highest potential), Believe (release our unlimited potential), Gathering, Transformation, White Angelica (greater awareness of one's potential).

Power: Sacred Mountain, Surrender (calming and relaxing to dominant personalities), Valor.

Power Surges: *See Hot Flashes.*

Prayer: Frankincense, Inspiration, Sacred Mountain.

Pregnancy: Elemi, Gentle Baby (relieves stress during pregnancy; can also be used by fathers to relieve stress during delivery), geranium, grapefruit, jasmine, lavender, Roman chamomile, tangerine, ylang ylang.
> SUPPLEMENTS—PD 80/20, Prenolone/Prenolone+, Progessence, Thyromin (use before, during, and after).
> PERSONAL CARE—ClaraDerm (Essential oil spray - apply topically to stressed skin before and after childbirth).
> ANXIETY/TENSION—Into the Future (help let go of fear and trauma), Present Time (help mother focus on giving birth).
> BLEND—Add 10 drops lavender, 10 orange, 2 marjoram, 2 cedarwood, 1 Roman chamomile to 4 oz. sweet almond oil or V-6 Mixing Oil. Use as a massage oil or in bath water.
> SUPPLEMENTS—PD 80/20, Prenolone/Prenolone+, Progessence.
> BABY (Newborn)—Frankincense (1 drop on the crown for protection), myrrh (on remaining umbilical cord and around navel to protect from infection), Valor (1 drop - divide between both feet & 1-2 drops rubbed up spine to help ensure proper alignment).
> BREASTS—Fennel (tone), Roman chamomile (sore nipples).
> CONCEPTION—Do a proper cleansing for one year before. May want to start with the Master Cleanser (*See Cleansing for more information*).
> SUPPLEMENTS—Balance Complete (*refer to the 5-Day Nutritive Cleanse program listed under Balance Complete in the Supplements section of the Reference Guide for Essential Oils. This program also uses Digest + Cleanse and NingXia Red to help enhance detoxification while maintaining energy levels*), Cleansing Trio (especially ComforTone for the colon and ICP for the intestines), Digest + Cleanse, JuvaTone (cleanses liver).

P

CONSTIPATION—ComforTone can be taken during pregnancy as long as you don't get diarrhea. Diarrhea can cause cramping which could bring on labor.

> SUPPLEMENTS—Essentialzyme, JuvaTone (helps change genetics in the colon and purge the liver).

DELIVERY—Clary sage, Forgiveness, Gentle Baby, Harmony, lavender (stimulates circulation, calming, antibiotic, anti-inflammatory, antiseptic), nutmeg (balances hormones, calms the central nervous system, alleviates anxiety, increases circulation, and good for blood supply), Valor (align mother's hips; apply along inside and bottom of each foot, then have someone hold feet–right palm to right foot and left palm to left foot–to balance energy flows; rub a couple drops along newborn's spine for alignment).

> ***CAUTION—Nutmeg is generally non-toxic, non-irritant, and non-sensitizing. However, large doses may cause nausea, stupor, and tachycardia. Use in moderation and with great care during pregnancy. See the safety data about nutmeg in the Appendix of this book.*

PREGNANCY SAFETY DATA

Avoid During Pregnancy

Single Oils: *Basil, birch, calamus, cassia, cinnamon bark, hyssop, Idaho tansy, lavandin, rosemary, sage, tarragon.*

Blends: Di-Gize, Dragon Time, Exodus II, Grounding, Mister.

Other: *Estro, Exodus, FemiGen, ParaFree, Protec,*

Use Cautiously During Pregnancy

Single Oils: *Angelica, cedarwood, chamomile (German/ Blue), cistus, citronella, Clary sage, clove bud, cumin (Black), cypress, davana, fennel, laurel, marjoram, Mountain savory, myrrh, nutmeg, peppermint, rose, spearmint, vetiver, yarrow.*

Blends: Aroma Siez, Clarity, Harmony, ImmuPower, Relieve It, Thieves.

Other: *Prenolone/Prenolone+, ComforTone, Essentialzyme, Dragon Time Massage Oil.*

It was very difficult to compile a list of oils and products to be avoided during pregnancy. Each aromatologist has a different opinion. We feel that an oil that is unsafe is an oil that has been adulterated or one that is used improperly. Oils that are diluted, applied externally and in moderation should not create a problem. This list is a compilation of the safety data contained in aromatherapy books written by the following authors: Ann Berwick, Julia Lawless, Shirley & Len Price, Jeanne Rose, Robert Tisserand, and Tony Balacs.

AVOID EPISIOTOMY—ClaraDerm Spray (spray onto and massage into perineum three times daily), Gentle Baby or geranium (neat or added to olive oil; massage perineum).

BLEND—8 drops geranium, 5 drops lavender, 1 oz. V-6 Mixing Oil. Prepare three weeks before delivery and rub on perineum three times a day. One week before delivery, prepare same blend and add 5 drops fennel. Continue applying three times daily.

DIFFUSE—Hope, Joy, Motivation, Live with Passion, Peace & Calming.

UTERUS—Tone uterus with 1-3 drops of Clary sage around ankles (one woman dilated and had her baby in 1 ½ hours), Dragon Time, fennel, Gathering, sage.

> TRANSITION—Basil.

EARLY LABOR—Lavender (rub on tummy to stop).

ENERGY—Equal portions of Roman chamomile, geranium, and lavender in V-6 Mixing Oil.

HEMORRHAGING—Helichrysum and Gentle Baby together on lower back (prevent).

HIGH BLOOD PRESSURE—<u>Aroma Life</u> (heart). Avoid using hyssop, rosemary, sage, thyme, and possibly peppermint.

KEEP BABY IN BIRTH CANAL—<u>Gentle Baby</u>.
  ***COMMENTS—*One mother would rub <u>Gentle Baby</u> on her little fingers and little toes when contracting. The she would squeeze the sides of her little fingers while someone else squeezed her little toes. This was repeated during contractions until the baby decided to stay in the birth canal.*

LABOR (during)—Clary sage (kick labor into gear; some have combined with fennel), <u>Gentle Baby</u> (apply to ankles and hands when labor starts), <u>Into the Future</u> (to help move past fear and trauma), jasmine (speed up contractions), <u>Present Time</u> (to help focus).
  BLEND—**(Use only when ready to deliver)**. 2 oz. V-6 Mixing Oil, 8 drops Clary sage, 8 drops lavender, 8 drops jasmine. May be useful when trying to induce labor or augment a slow, lazy labor.
  PAIN—<u>PanAway</u> (apply to lower back and tummy area).
  ***COMMENTS—*Refer to the chapter entitled "How to Use - The Personal Usage Reference" in the <u>Essential Oils Desk Reference</u> under "Pregnancy" for a wonderful blend to use during labor.*

LABOR (post)—Geranium, lavender.
  ***COMMENTS—*Lavender is calming and has a slight analgesic effect. It also stimulates circulation, which is great for both mother and baby, and has anti-inflammatory and antiseptic properties. Geranium is one of the best oils to stimulate circulation, which in turn facilitates easy breathing. It has a contractive effect and helps pull together dilated tissues, so it is healing for the uterus and endometrium after the birth. Geranium is also an anti-depressant and is known for its uplifting effect (<u>Alternative Medicine—A Definitive Guide</u>, pp. 806-7).*

LACTATION—*See Milk Production below.*

MASTITIS (breast infection)—<u>Citrus Fresh</u> (with lavender), <u>Exodus II</u>, lavender, tangerine.
  BLEND—Equal amounts of lavender and tangerine. Dilute with some V-6 Mixing Oil and apply to breasts and under arms twice a day.
  SUPPLEMENTS—Exodus.

MILK PRODUCTION—Clary sage (bring in milk), fennel or basil (increase), peppermint with cold compress (decrease). ***Caution: Fennel should not be used for more than 10 days as it will excessively increase flow through the urinary tract.***
  SUPPLEMENTS—Essential Manna, Power Meal, VitaGreen.

MISCARRIAGE (after)—Frankincense, geranium, grapefruit, lavender (may help prevent), Roman chamomile, spruce (2 drops on solar plexus).
  SUPPLEMENTS—JuvaTone, Cleansing Trio (ComforTone, Essentialzyme, and ICP).

MORNING SICKNESS—Calamus, <u>Di-Gize</u> (1-2 drops in water and sip or 1-2 drops around the navel), ginger, <u>M-Grain</u>, peppermint. Apply on or behind ears,

> **Caution**: *Although <u>Di-Gize</u> is recommended for morning sickness, it contains some oils which some aromatologists strongly discourage using. It may have a lot to do with purity. Use at your own risk. I did and it worked for me!*

down jaw bone, over stomach as a compress, on Vita Flex points on feet, on hands (rub together and smell), or put a drop on your pillow. Can also put 4 to 6 drops of spearmint in a bowl of boiled and cooled water and place on floor beside the bed overnight to keep stomach calm.

SUPPLEMENTS—ComforTone, Essentialzyme.

ON CHAKRAS—<u>Awaken</u> (after pregnancy).

PLACENTA—Basil (has been use to help retain), jasmine (helps expulsion).

POSTPARTUM DEPRESSION (Baby Blues)—*See Female Problems.* Bergamot, Clary sage, fennel, frankincense, geranium, <u>Gentle Baby</u>, grapefruit, <u>Harmony</u>, <u>Hope</u>, jasmine, <u>Joy</u>, lavender, myrrh, nutmeg (use in moderation), orange, and patchouli, <u>Valor</u>, vetiver, <u>White Angelica</u>.

SUPPLEMENTS—Essential Manna, ImmuPro, Omega Blue.

SELF LOVE—<u>Joy</u>.

SKIN ELASTICITY—<u>Aroma Life</u>, <u>Clarity</u>, <u>Dragon Time</u>, <u>Gentle Baby</u>, <u>Mister</u>, <u>M-Grain</u>, <u>Relieve It</u>. *Again, many of these blends contain oils that many aromatologists feel should be avoided or used with caution during pregnancy.*

PERSONAL CARE—A·R·T Skin Care System, ClaraDerm (Essential oil spray - apply topically to stressed skin before and after childbirth).

STRETCH MARKS—<u>Gentle Baby</u> (every day on tummy).

PERSONAL CARE—ClaraDerm (Essential oil spray - apply topically to stressed skin before and after childbirth).

TOXEMIA (extremely high protein in urine)—<u>Aroma Life</u>.

Pride: Peppermint (dispels).

Procrastination: <u>Acceptance</u>, <u>Envision</u> (emotional support), <u>Magnify Your Purpose</u> (empowering and uplifting), <u>Motivation</u> (easier to take action, gets you out of the mood of procrastination).

Progesterone: <u>EndoFlex</u>, <u>Grounding</u>. *Progesterone is made from cholesterol and helps to protect against cancer.*

PERSONAL CARE—PD 80/20, Prenolone/Prenolone+, Progessence.

Prosperity: Abundance, bergamot, cinnamon bark (aromatic), cypress.

Prostate: <u>Australian Blue</u>, Blue cypress, <u>EndoFlex</u>, <u>Gratitude</u>, helichrysum, juniper, <u>Juva Cleanse</u>, <u>Mister</u>, yarrow.

PERSONAL CARE—PD 80/20, Prenolone/Prenolone+, Protec (designed to accompany the night long retention enema, it helps buffer the prostate from inflammation, enlargement, and tumor activity).

SUPPLEMENTS—Master Formula HIS, ProGen (an herbal support for the male glandular system; it may prevent prostate atrophy and malfunction and protect men from prostate cancer).

DECONGESTANT—[F]Cypress, <u>Di-Gize</u>, <u>Dragon Time</u>, <u>Mister</u> (decongests prostate and balances hormones), myrrh, [F]myrtle, sage, [F]spruce, yarrow. Apply oils to inside ankle and heel. <u>ImmuPower</u> on lower spine and in rectum.

    BLEND #1—Combine 15 frankincense and 5 <u>Mister</u> with 2 tsp. V-6 Mixing Oil. Insert blend into rectum with bulb syringe or pipet and retain throughout night.

    BLEND #2—Combine 10 frankincense and 10 lavender with 2 tsp. V-6 Mixing Oil. Insert blend into rectum with bulb syringe and retain throughout night.

    BLEND #3—Combine 10 frankincense, 5 myrrh, and 3 sage with 2 tsp. V-6 Mixing Oil. Insert blend into rectum with bulb syringe or pipet and retain through night.

    ***COMMENTS—*Abundant Health offers dispensing syringes with rectal insertion tip.*

ENLARGEMENT—Mix 10 drops of <u>Mister</u> with 1 Tbs. of V-6 Mixing oil and insert in rectum and retain overnight. May also apply either sage, fennel, or yarrow to posterior, scrotum, ankles, lower back, and bottom of feet.

INFLAMED—Cypress, lavender, thyme (<u>Alternative Medicine—A Definitive Guide</u>, p. 742).

STRENGTHEN—PD 80/20, Prenolone/Prenolone+, ProGen, Protec.

    TINCTURES—Male-Pro (available through Creer Labs 801-418-8870)

THOUGHT PATTERNS AND EMOTIONS—The prostate represents the masculine principle. Men's **prostate problems** have a lot to do with self-worth and also believing that as they get older they become less of a man. Ideas may be in conflict about sex, refusing to let go of the past, fear of aging, feeling like throwing in the towel. May be feeling inadequate in sexual role, may be holding onto unpleasant memories of previous relationships, or feeling unfulfilled in love.

Prostate Cancer: *See Cancer.*

> *Prostate Cancer may be from repressed anger. Visualize the prostate healing, don't put energy into the cancer.*

Protection: (from negative influence) Clove (aromatic), cypress, fennel (protection from psychic attack), fir (aromatic), frankincense, <u>Harmony</u>, <u>Joy</u>, palo santo, <u>Sacred Mountain</u>, <u>Valor</u>, <u>White Angelica</u>.

Protein: Carbonated water prevents the absorption of protein. Protein deficiency causes Hypoglycemia.

> *A **protein deficiency**, either from the lack of protein intake or from the inability to digest it, creates an acidic pH in the blood. A high acidity level in the blood creates an environment for cell mutation and disease. See Acidosis.*

    SUPPLEMENTS—Bodygize, Digest + Cleanse, Essentialzyme, Polyzyme (provides enzymes necessary for proper breakdown and digestion of protein), Power Meal (pre-digested protein), Pure Protein Complete, Sulfurzyme (helps digest protein), VitaGreen.

Psoriasis: Bergamot, cajeput, cedarwood, [F]helichrysum, lavender, melaleuca, patchouli, Roman chamomile, [F]thyme.

    BLEND—Combine 2-3 drops each of Roman chamomile and lavender for use as ointment for pH Balance.

P

PERSONAL CARE—A·R·T Skin Care System, Rose Ointment (helps soften cracking skin), Essential Beauty Serum - Dry Skin Blend, Lavender Volume Shampoo and Lavender Volume Conditioner for psoriasis of the scalp.

SUPPLEMENTS—AlkaLime, Balance Complete, Cleansing Trio (ComforTone, Essentialzyme, and ICP), Digest + Cleanse, JuvaPower/JuvaSpice, JuvaTone, Sulfurzyme.

Psychic: Cinnamon bark (awareness), fennel (protect from attack), lemongrass. Diffuse.
   CENTERS—Elemi (balances, strengthens, fortifies).

Puberty: Fleabane (stimulates retarded puberty).

Pulmonary: *See Lungs*.

Purge: *See Cleansing*.

Purification: <u>Abundance</u>, <u>Acceptance</u>, cedarwood, <u>En-R-Gee</u>, eucalyptus (aromatic), fennel (aromatic), lemon (aromatic), lemongrass (aromatic), melaleuca (aromatic), orange (aromatic), <u>Purification</u>, sage.
   AIR—Lemon (diffuse or add to spray bottle of water to deodorize and sterilize the air).
   CIGARETTE SMOKE—<u>Purification</u>.
   DISHES—2 drops of <u>Melrose</u> or lemon in the dish water for sparkling dishes and a great smelling kitchen.
   WATER— ᶠLemon, peppermint.
   CLOTHING—Adding oils to washer or dryer decreases bacteria, improves hygiene, and clothes have a fresh, clean smell.
   FURNITURE—A few drops of fir, lemon, or spruce oil on a dust cloth, or 10 drops in a 1 oz. glass or plastic spray bottle filled with distilled water, work well for polishing, cleaning and disinfecting furniture, kitchens and bathrooms. You may also consider adding <u>Abundance</u> to increase your abundance. Lemon oil for dissolving gum and grease. <u>Purification</u> for mold and fungus. If you don't have a diffuser, you may want to add 10-12 drops of <u>Purification</u> to 8 oz of distilled water in a spray bottle and spray into the air.

Pus: *See Infection and Anti-infectious*. Melaleuca is useful in healing pus-filled wounds.

Radiation: *See Cancer. Melaleuca quinquenervia*, <u>Melrose</u>, patchouli. May apply on location, bottom of feet, kidneys, thyroid, and diffuse.
   COMPUTER, TV, MICROWAVE—Fill a wooden bowl half full of peat moss and half full of hazel nuts and 30 drops of <u>Melrose</u> then set on the appliance. Using an equipment diode may also help (*available from Abundant Health*).

***COMMENTS—<u>Melrose</u> may
help protect the body during
radiation treatments if used 10
days before, during, and 10 days
after. **Do not use on the day of
radiation treatment**. According
to Dr. Pénoël, massage with
Melaleuca quinquenervia helps
to prevent radiation side effects.
Remember to keep all massage
light and away from trauma
area.

RADIATION BURNS—Recipe #1.
SIDE-EFFECTS–Recipe #2.
TREATMENTS—Radiation treatments can
produce tremendous toxicity
within the liver. Cut down on
the use of oils with high *phenol*
content to prevent increasing the
liver toxicity.

CHEMOTHERAPY—Because of the
greater amounts of toxicity
produced, even greater care
should be taken to limit the use
of oils with high *phenol* content.

WEEPING WOUNDS FROM—Melaleuca,
oregano, thyme.

SUPPLEMENTS—The apple pectin that
is contained in ICP helps remove unwanted metals and toxins. It is also valuable in
radiation therapy.

Valerie Worwood suggests Recipe #1 below to be used at least two to three weeks before the radiation treatments begin. Don't use it during the treatment, but use it between treatments and for at least a month after your last treatment.

RECIPE #1—10 lavender, 5 German chamomile, 5 Roman chamomile, 5 tagetes, 5 yarrow, and 2 tsp. of vinca infused oil. Massage the entire torso, including the back and abdomen and the trauma area. This treatment will not conflict with the doctor's treatment. Note: Vinca is made from periwinkle which is known to contain alkaloids that in some cases can suppress the cancerous cells. (The Complete Book of Essential Oils & Aromatherapy, pp. 249-50).

The following Dr. Westlake formula utilizes Bach Flower Remedies to counteract the side-effects of cancer patients who have received radiation therapy.

RECIPE #2—"Mix 3.5 grams of sea salt with 100 mils of distilled water. Put into a 10 ml dropper bottle 2 drops of each of the following Bach Flower Remedies: Cherry Plum, Gentian, Rock Rose, Star of Bethlehem, Vine, Walnut and Wild Oat, and top up the bottle with the sea salt solution. Take 2 drops, three or four times a day, or add 10 to 15 drops to a bath. People who have been exposed to radiation sources, such as X-rays, cobalt therapy or other medical radiation therapies, or have been contaminated in an escape from a nuclear power station or who regularly use office or domestic equipment that gives out low-level radiation, such as color television sets, microwaves, and visual display units, would do well to use this formula in a bath once or twice a week." (Aromatherapy—An A to Z by Patricia Davis, p. 269)

Rashes: Elemi (allergic), lavender, ^Fmelaleuca, <u>Melrose</u>, palmarosa, <u>Release</u> (on Vita Flex points of feet), Roman chamomile. Red spots on body may indicate a Biotin deficiency; take Super C or Super C Chewable.
PERSONAL CARE—KidScents Tender Tush, Rose Ointment.
***COMMENTS—Dr. Friedmann had a patient who had a rash for

If the rash occurs from application of oils to the skin, it may be due to the oils reacting with accumulated synthetic chemicals (toxins) that are trapped in the fatty layers of the skin. Take the following steps: 1) Try diluting the oils first (1-3 drops of oil to ½ tsp. V-6 Mixing Oil), 2) reduce the number of oils used with each application (use oils one at a time), 3) reduce the amount of oils (number of drops) used, 4) reduce the frequency of application (more time between applications). Drinking pure (steam distilled) water helps promote the elimination of accumulated toxins from the body. Initiating programs to cleanse the bowels and blood will also help remove accumulated toxins and reduce the possible recurrences of the rash. If the rashes persist, discontinue use of the oils and consult your health care professional.

three years on the side of the face and arms and the eyes were weeping. They had gone to five physicians for treatments and had no success. Dr. Friedmann did the following: 1) Did a culture of the eye and face and determined that the patient had staphylococcus. 2) Had the patient apply Melrose and lavender alternately morning and night. 3) Had the patient take Mineral Essence and Colloidal Essence (a colloidal silver product). After a short period of time, the patient's face and eyes totally cleared up and their arms were healing.

Raynaud's Disease (feel cold; hands and feet turn blue): Aroma Life, clove, cypress, fennel, geranium, helichrysum, lavender, nutmeg, rosemary.

Regenerating: Helichrysum, lavender, Melrose, or equal parts of Thieves and V-6 Mixing Oil. *SUPPLEMENTS*—Bodygize, ImmuneTune, Power Meal.

Rejection: Acceptance, Joy.

Relationships:
> *BATH & SHOWER GELS*—Sensation Bath & Shower Gel contains oils used by Cleopatra to enhance love and increase the desire to be close to that someone special.
> *MASSAGE OILS*—Sensation creates an exotic arousal; increases sexual desire. The fragrance creates a peaceful and harmonious feeling that is helpful in easing relationship stress.
> *PERSONAL CARE*—Sensation Hand & Body Lotion.
> *ENHANCING*—Lady Love or Lady Sclareol (especially for the woman - best if applied by male partner), Ylang ylang.
> *ENDING RELATIONSHIPS*—Basil.

Relaxation: Citrus Fresh, Clary sage, frankincense, Gentle Baby, geranium, jasmine, lavender, Peace & Calming, Roman chamomile, sandalwood, Trauma Life (calming), ylang ylang.
> *BATH & SHOWER GELS*—Evening Peace Bath & Shower Gel.
> *DIFFUSION*—*See Negative Ions* for oils that produce negative ions when diffused to help promote relaxation. Lavender, Peace & Calming.
> *MASSAGE OILS*—Relaxation Massage Oil.
> *TINCTURES*—Ner-Vus (available through Creer Labs 801-418-8870).
> *SENSE OF*—Ylang ylang.
> *BLEND*—1 bergamot, 2 lavender, 2 marjoram, and 4 rosewood.

Release Negative Trauma: Inspiration, Release, Transformation.

Resentment: Forgiveness, Harmony, Humility, Idaho tansy, jasmine, Release, rose, White Angelica.

Respiratory System: <u>Abundance</u>, anise, basil (restorative), bergamot (infections), cajeput (infections), Clary sage (strengthens), clove, <u>Di-Gize</u>, <u>EndoFlex</u>, ^Feucalyptus (general stimulant and strengthens), *Eucalyptus radiata*, fennel (stimulant),

> *Vita Flex points for the bronchial tubes are located between the bones on the tops of the feet. The sinuses are located at the base of the middle three toes on the bottom of the feet. One of the most effective ways of handling a respiratory problem is by doing rectal implants. There is a nerve that goes from the rectum to the lungs. The oils will travel in this manner in 3 seconds. The next best method is through inhalation.*

^Ffir (opens respiratory tract, increases oxygenation, decongests and balances), frankincense, goldenrod (discharges mucus), <u>GLF</u>, helichrysum (relieves), hyssop (opens respiratory system and discharges toxins and mucus), <u>JuvaFlex</u>, ledum (supports), lemon, marjoram (calming), melaleuca, *Melaleuca ericifolia*, <u>Melrose</u>, ^Fmyrtle, oregano (antiseptic), ^Fpeppermint (aid), pine (dilates and opens bronchial tract), <u>RC</u>, <u>Raven</u> (all respiratory problems), ravensara, rosemary verbenon, <u>Sacred Mountain</u> (soothing), ^Fspearmint, spruce (combine with any Eucalyptus oils; especially *Eucalyptus polybractea*), <u>Thieves</u> (diffuse with *Eucalyptus radiata*; add spruce to help push the oils deeper into the lungs), tsuga (dilates and opens tract).

> *My 18 year old daughter has had **respiratory problems** for years and finally the doctors put her on inhalers. These helped, but she did not like the way they made her feel. Soon after I started using therapeutic grade essential oils we began using them on her. After a few weeks she was off her inhalers and has never needed them since. She has, however, had the occasional upper respiratory infection, which in the past has always led to a bout with bronchitis and several months of coughing. Now, we apply oils and the infection goes away without bronchitis ever showing up. This has saved vacations and more! We apply the oils to her chest, back and feet twice a day. The oils we use are hyssop, myrrh, and two Young Living blends - <u>RC</u> and <u>Raven</u>.*
>
> **-Submitted by Lauren Martin (July 2004)**

SUPPLEMENTS—Super C / Super C Chewable.

RECIPE #1—Dr. Young alternates the oils of <u>Raven</u> and <u>RC</u> in rectal implants. He uses 20 drops of the oil in 1 Tbs. of V-6 Mixing Oil and implants it rectally using a pipet (glass dropper) or syringe with rectal insertion tip (*available at Abundant Health*).

BLEND #1—3 drops birch/wintergreen, 8 eucalyptus, 6 fir, 6 frankincense, 1 peppermint, 10 ravensara and 1 oz. V-6 Mixing Oil.

BLEND #2—3 drops German chamomile, 10 fir, and 5 lemon.

ACUTE—<u>RC</u> and <u>Raven</u>, <u>Thieves</u>.

BLEND #3—5 drops eucalyptus, 8 frankincense, and 6 lemon. Add to 1 oz. V-6 Mixing Oil for a hot compress on chest and rub neat (without V-6) on bottom of feet under toes.

BLEND #4—3 tsp. *Eucalyptus radiata* (or any oil from the Myrtaceae botanical family), 1 tsp. Balsam fir (or any conifer oil). Apply to Vita Flex points on the feet, add to V-6 Mixing Oil and apply to chest area, or diffuse.

BLEND #5—10 drops each of *Eucalyptus radiata* and myrrh. Add to 1 Tbs. of V-6 Mixing Oil and insert rectally with syringe for overnight retention enema. Works well for all lung conditions including emphysema, pneumonia, and tuberculosis.

Restlessness: <u>Acceptance</u>, angelica, basil, bergamot, cedarwood, frankincense, <u>Gathering</u>, geranium, <u>Harmony</u>, <u>Inspiration</u>, <u>Joy</u>, lavender, orange, <u>Peace & Calming</u>, rose, rosewood, <u>Sacred Mountain</u>, spruce, <u>Trauma Life</u>, valerian, <u>Valor</u>, ylang ylang.
TINCTURES—Ner-Vus (available through Creer Labs 801-418-8870).

Rheumatic Fever: Ginger, ᶠtarragon. Both help with pain.

Rheumatism: *See Arthritis.*

Rhinitis: Basil, sage lavender.

> *Rhinitis is an inflammation of the nasal mucus membrane.*

Rhinopharyngitis: ᶠRavensara.

Ringworm: *See Anti-fungal.* Geranium, lavender, melaleuca (Tea Tree), <u>Melrose</u>, myrrh, peppermint, <u>Purification</u>, <u>RC</u>, <u>Raven</u>, rosemary verbenon, thyme.
    BLEND #1—2 lavender, 2 melaleuca, and 2 thyme, or
    BLEND #2—3 melaleuca, 2 peppermint, and 3 spearmint. Apply 1-2 drops of blend (#s 1 or 2 above) or <u>Melrose</u> on ringworm three times a day for ten days. Then mix 30 drops of melaleuca (Tea Tree) or <u>Melrose</u> with 2 Tbs. V-6 Mixing Oil and use daily until ringworm is gone.
    MASSAGE OILS—Ortho Ease or Ortho Sport.
    PERSONAL CARE—Rose Ointment.

> *My friend's eight month old little boy had a **ringworm** the size of a quarter on his head. After putting lavender neat on it several times it started to go away and after a few more times it was gone altogether. Shortly after that he got a **tick** in his head and by putting peppermint right on the back of the tick that nasty thing backed right out. I guess he could not breath–whatever it was, it got the tick out without us trying to pull it out and perhaps getting only part of the critter out.*
>
> **-Submitted by V. Frierdich**
> **Overland Park, Kansas (July 2004)**

Romantic Touches: Jasmine, <u>Lady Sclareol</u>, patchouli, <u>Sensation</u>, ylang ylang; use these in small amounts.
    BATH & SHOWER GELS— Sensation Bath & Shower Gel.
    MASSAGE OILS—Sensation Massage Oil.
    PERSONAL CARE—Sensation Hand & Body Lotion.

Rosacea (Acne Rosacea): Lavender. Dilute with V-6 Mixing Oil and apply daily after washing face with Orange Blossom Facial Wash

> *Rosacea is a chronic, acne-like condition of the facial skin which typically first appears as a flushing or subtle redness on the cheeks, nose, chin or forehead that comes and goes. Left untreated, the condition progresses and the redness becomes more persistent, bumps and pimples appear, and small dilated blood vessels may become visible. In some cases the eyes may be affected, causing them to be irritated and bloodshot and, according to some doctors, can even cause blindness. In the more advanced cases, the nose becomes red and swollen from excess tissue. Currently, this condition can only be controlled.*

and before applying Sandalwood Moisture Creme. Can also add extra lavender oil to Sandalwood Moisture Creme.

PERSONAL CARE—Essential Beauty Serum - Acne-Prone Skin Blend, Orange Blossom Facial Wash, Sandalwood Moisture Creme.

Sacredness: Sacred Mountain (sacred place of protection within self).

Sadness: Acceptance, helichrysum, Inspiration, Joy (over heart), onycha (combine with rose in V-6 Mixing Oil for calming/uplifting massage), orange (overcome), 3 Wise Men, Transformation, Valor. Wear as cologne or diffuse.

Saint Vitus Dance (Chorea):
BLEND—5 drops Aroma Siez, 3 basil, 6 juniper, and 8 peppermint.

Sanitation: Citronella, lemongrass, Purification.

Scabies: Bergamot, laurel, lavender and peppermint, pine, Thieves (needs to be diluted).

Scarring: Frankincense (prevents), Gentle Baby, geranium, helichrysum (reduces), hyssop (prevents), Flavender (burns), Melrose, rose (prevents), rosehip (reduces).

PERSONAL CARE—A·R·T Skin Care System, Satin Hand & Body Lotion (moisturizes skin and promotes healing).

BLEND #1—Equal parts helichrysum and lavender mixed with liquid lecithin.

BLEND #2—3 drops rosemary, 15 rosewood, and 1¾ oz. Hazel Nut Oil.

BLEND #3—6 drops lavender, 3 patchouli, 4 rosewood, and Vitamin E Oil.

PREVENT FORMATION—Frankincense, helichrysum, hyssop, myrrh, rose, rosehip seed.

BLEND #4—5 drops helichrysum, 2 patchouli, 4 lemongrass, 3 lavender in ¼ to ½ oz. V-6 Mixing Oil.

BLEND #5—Equal parts lavender, lemongrass, and geranium.

Schmidt's Syndrome: *See Addison's Disease.*
En-R-Gee, EndoFlex, Joy, nutmeg (increases energy; supports adrenal glands), sage (combine with nutmeg).

> *Schmidt's Syndrome is the same as Addison's Disease with the additional problem of low thyroid hormone production.*

SUPPLEMENTS—ImmuPro, Master Formula His/Hers (3 times a day), Mineral Essence (help supplement mineral loss), **Sulfurzyme** (shown to slow or reverse autoimmune diseases), Super B (after each meal), Thyromin (first thing in morning), VitaGreen.

Sciatica: Aroma Life, cardamom, **cistus (followed by peppermint)**, fir, Fhelichrysum, Gentle Baby, hyssop, M-Grain, PanAway, peppermint, Relieve It, sandalwood, spruce (alleviates pain), Ftarragon (with Idaho tansy - can promote sciatic regeneration), Fthyme, Valor.

Apply a cold compress and lightly massage with Roman chamomile or lavender, and birch/wintergreen. Relief can also be obtained by applying <u>Joy</u> and lavender to the bottoms of the feet.

BLEND—Tarragon, Balsam fir, and spearmint (small amount) or tarragon, basil, and peppermint.

MASSAGE OIL—Ortho Ease.

RECIPE #1—Apply frankincense to the top of the spine (at the base of the skull) and work it in. Then apply 3-5 drops of each of the following oils, one at a time, up the back of the neck, and work each one in individually: valerian, vetiver, Balsam fir, and tarragon. When working each one into the spine, a glass probe or glass dropper can be used to stimulate the tops of each of the vertebrae.

Scoliosis: May be caused by a virus. **Do the raindrop technique!**

    ****COMMENT—The videos, listed in the Bibliography, are highly recommended for a professional visual presentation of the Raindrop Technique!*

    BLEND—8 drops basil, 12 birch/wintergreen, 5 cypress, 10 marjoram, and 2 peppermint.

CORRECT—Do the following (a variation of the Raindrop Technique) every seven to ten days for a minimum of eight times to help get rid of **scoliosis**:

1. Rub <u>Valor</u> on feet.
2. Apply oregano and thyme using the Raindrop Technique up the spine.
3. Apply **blend** along the spine. Push or pull in the direction that the spine needs to be strengthened. Knead fingers clockwise three times. Then work two fingers up the spine with the other hand on top of the hand that is doing the kneading (do this three times).
4. Apply <u>Aroma Siez</u> and marjoram on the muscles on each side of the spine. Apply warm wet towel to back and have individual lay on their back.
5. Work the Vita Flex areas down the leg to the feet with basil, birch/wintergreen, cypress, and peppermint in V-6 Mixing Oil.
6. Work the spine Vita Flex areas on the feet then give feet a mild pull.
7. Put one hand under their chin and the other hand at the back of their neck. Have them breathe in and out as you gently rock and pull the neck in time with their breathing.
8. Take towel off. If the back gets too hot during massage apply V-6 Mixing Oil.
9. Measure the spine to see how much it has changed.

Scrapes: Lavender, ravensara.

Scurvy: [F]Ginger. Apply over kidneys, liver, and on corresponding Vita Flex points on the feet.

    SUPPLEMENTS—Super C / Super C Chewable.

Security: <u>Christmas Spirit</u>, <u>Sacred Mountain</u>.

    CREATING—<u>Acceptance</u>, Roman chamomile.

FEELING OF—Cypress (aromatic).
IN THE HOME—Bergamot.
SELF SECURE—Oregano.

Sedative: Among the most effective sedatives are: Bergamot, <u>Citrus Fresh</u>, lavender, neroli, and <u>Peace & Calming</u>. Other oils that may also help are: Angelica, cedarwood, Clary sage, coriander, cypress, elemi, frankincense, geranium, hyssop, jasmine, juniper, lavender, lemongrass, melissa, marjoram, onycha (benzoin), orange, patchouli, Roman chamomile, rose, sandalwood, tangerine, <u>Trauma Life</u>, valerian, vetiver (nervous system), ylang ylang. Use intuition as to which one may be best for the given situation. In addition, check the safety data for each of the oils in the Appendix of this book.

   ***COMMENTS—*Refer to* BLEND #3 *under* Insomnia *for a blend of oils that can either be taken internally in water or applied to the back of the neck to help relax the body.*

Seizure: *See Epilepsy.*

   GRAND MAL—Need to support the body. <u>Aroma Siez</u> (apply using the Raindrop Technique up the spine), <u>Brain Power</u> and <u>Peace & Calming</u> (diffuse and put around naval), <u>Joy</u> (over the heart), <u>Sacred Mountain</u> (back of neck and crown), and <u>Valor</u> (on feet).

   SUPPLEMENTS—Cleansing Trio (ComforTone, Essentialzyme, and ICP), JuvaPower, Omega Blue.

   ***COMMENTS—*Grand Mal seizures can sometimes be caused by zinc and copper imbalance. Mineral Essence provides zinc and copper in both ionic and colloidal form for optimal assimilation.*

Self Adjustment: <u>Awaken</u>.

Self Esteem: <u>Acceptance</u>, <u>Forgiveness</u>, <u>Joy</u>, <u>Valor</u>.

   BUILD—<u>Joy</u>, <u>Transformation</u>, <u>Valor</u>.

   SELF LOVE—<u>Joy</u>, <u>Valor</u>.

Self Hypnosis: Clary sage, geranium, patchouli.

Self Pity: Acceptance, Motivation, Transformation, Valor.

Sensory System (Senses): *See Awareness.* Birch/wintergreen.

Sexual Abuse: <u>SARA</u> has a fragrance that when inhaled may enable one to relax into a mental state whereby one may be able to release and let go of the memory trauma of sexual and or ritual abuse.

Sex Stimulant: Chivalry, ^Fcinnamon bark (general), ginger, goldenrod, Lazarus, rose, SclarEssence, Sensation, ^Fylang ylang (sex drive problems).

> *BATH & SHOWER GELS*—Sensation Bath & Shower Gel contains oils used by Cleopatra to enhance love and increase the desire to be close to that someone special.

> *MASSAGE OILS*—Sensation creates an exotic arousal and increases sexual desire. The fragrance creates a peaceful and harmonious feeling that helps to ease relationship stress.

> *PERSONAL CARE*—PD 80/20, Prenolone/Prenolone+ (for both males and females), Progessence (for females only), Sensation Hand & Body Lotion.

> *SUPPLEMENTS*—Master Formula His/Hers, Mineral Essence, VitaGreen.

> *TINCTURES*—SE-6 Tincture (available through Creer Labs 801-418-8870). Use 10-50 drops of SE-6 Tincture three times a day plus 2 droppers at bedtime for three to five days.

> Arousing Desire—Clary sage, Lady Love, Lady Sclareol.

> Frigidity—*See Frigidity.* Lady Sclareol, nutmeg (overcome).

> Impotence—Goldenrod, SclarEssence (use capsules to take internally).

> Influences—Lady Love, Lady Sclareol, patchouli (aromatic).

Shingles: Australian Blue, Bergamot, Blue cypress, eucalyptus, geranium, lavender, lemon, melaleuca (Tea Tree), tamanu, ^Fravensara, Roman chamomile.

> *BLEND*—10 drops lavender, 10 melaleuca (Tea Tree), and 10 thyme mixed in Genesis Hand & Body Lotion. Rub on feet.

> *MASSAGE OILS*—Ortho Sport.

> *PERSONAL CARE*— PD 80/20, Prenolone/ Prenolone+, Progessence.

> *SUPPLEMENTS*—Cleansing Trio (ComforTone, Essentialzyme, and ICP).

> Herpes Zoster—Australian Blue, Bergamot, Blue cypress, *Eucalyptus radiata*, geranium, lavender, melaleuca (Alternative Medicine—The Definitive Guide, p. 972), Roman chamomile.

> *Shingles is an acute viral infection with inflammation of certain spinal or cranial nerves and the eruption of vesicles along the affected nerve path. It usually strikes only one side of the body is often accompanied by severe neuralgia. Also called herpes zoster. Some say it is necessary to cleanse the liver.*
>
> *Dr. Schnaubelt says that his greatest success in helping individuals with shingles came from applying a blend of 50 percent Ravensara aromatica and 50 percent Calophyllum inophyllum (Tamanu). "Drastic improvements and complete remission occur within seven days." (Alternative Medicine—The Definitive Guide, p. 56).*

Shock: *See Fainting.* Aroma Life, Australian Blue, basil, Clarity (to keep from going into shock), Gathering, Grounding, helichrysum, Highest Potential, Inspiration, Joy, melaleuca, melissa, myrrh, neroli, ^Fpeppermint, ^FRoman chamomile, rosemary, Valor, ylang ylang.

S

Shoulder (Frozen): Basil, birch/wintergreen, lemongrass, oregano, peppermint, White fir. Begin by applying White fir to shoulder Vita Flex point on foot (same side of body as frozen shoulder) to deal with any inflammation. Work it in with Vita Flex technique. Then check for improvement in pain reduction and/or range of motion (check after each oil to help determine what problem really was). In a similar manner apply lemongrass (for torn or pulled ligaments), basil (for muscle spasms), and birch/wintergreen (for bone problems) on the same Vita Flex point on the foot. After applying the oils to the foot and determining which oil(s) get the best results, apply same oil(s) on the shoulder and work it into the area with Vita Flex. Then apply peppermint (for nerves) and oregano (create thermal reaction to enhance elasticity of muscle and help it to stretch) on the shoulder and work each one into the area with Vita Flex. Finally, apply White fir to the other shoulder to create balance as the opposite shoulder will compensate for the sore one. Drink lots of water.

   PERSONAL CARE—Regenolone.

   SUPPLEMENTS—Sulfurzyme.

Sinus: Cedarwood, eucalyptus, ^Fhelichrysum, ^Fmyrtle, <u>PanAway</u>, peppermint, <u>RC</u>, or <u>Thieves</u> on feet.

   ***COMMENTS**—Eucalyptus and other sinus oils work really well when rubbed on each side of the nose. It seems to clear the sinuses almost immediately.*

Sinusitis: *See Respiratory System.* Cajeput, elemi, ^Feucalyptus, *Eucalyptus radiata*, fir, ginger, *Melaleuca ericifolia*, myrtle, ^Fpine, peppermint, ravensara, <u>RC</u>, ^Frosemary, sage lavender.

   SUPPLEMENTS— ImmuneTune.

Skeletal System: *See Scoliosis.* <u>Valor</u> ("chiropractor in a bottle"). Also try the **raindrop technique**.

Skin: *See Acne, Allergies, Bruises, Cuts, Dermatitis, Eczema, Facial Oils, Psoriasis, Wrinkles.* <u>Acceptance</u>, <u>Aroma Life</u>, cajeput, cedarwood, Roman and German chamomile (inflamed skin), <u>Clarity</u>, cypress, <u>Dragon Time</u>, frankincense, <u>Gentle Baby</u> (youthful skin), geranium, helichrysum, <u>Inner Child</u>, jasmine (irritated skin), juniper, lavender, ledum (all types of problems), lemon, marjoram, ^Fmelaleuca (healing), <u>Melrose</u>, <u>Mister</u>, <u>M-Grain</u>, myrrh (chapped and cracked), ^Fmyrtle (antiseptic), orange, palmarosa (rashes, scaly, and flaky

> ***Contact-sensitization** is a type of allergic reaction which can occur when a substance comes into contact with the body. A few essential oils applied to the skin may cause sensitization, perhaps only after repeated application (the amount used is not significant). The skin reaction appears as redness, irritation, or vesiculation. A rule of thumb when applying oils to someone is that people with darker hair usually have less sensitive skin while those with blond or red hair are generally more sensitive.*
>
> ***Single oils:** Bergamot, cassia, cinnamon bark, citronella, clove, fennel, Laurus nobilis, ylang ylang.*
>
> *(For a list of possible skin irritants, please see the Appendix of this book.)*

skin), patchouli (chapped; tightens loose skin and prevents wrinkles), [F]peppermint (itching skin), <u>Relieve It</u>, rosehip, rosemary, rosewood (elasticity and candida), sage, sandalwood (regenerates), <u>Sensation</u>, <u>Valor</u>, vetiver, Western Red cedar (nourishing), and ylang ylang.

PERSONAL CARE—Essential Beauty Serums (Dry, Oily & Acne-Prone Skin Blends)

AFTERSHAVE—<u>Awaken</u> can be used instead of aftershave lotion. Try adding <u>Awaken</u> to Sandalwood Moisture Creme, Satin Hand & Body Lotion, Sensation Hand & Body Lotion, or Genesis Hand & Body Lotion as an aftershave. KidScents Lotion makes a great aftershave as it soothes and rehydrates the skin (and smells good too).

BAR SOAPS—Lavender Rosewood Moisturizing Soap, Lemon Sandalwood Cleansing Soap, Peppermint Cedarwood Moisturizing Soap, Sacred Mountain Moisturizing Soap for Oily Skin, Thieves Cleansing Soap.

BATH & SHOWER GELS—Dragon Time (for women who have lower back pain, stress and sleeping problems due to menstruation), Evening Peace (relaxes tired, fatigued muscles and helps to alleviate tension), Morning Start (dissolves oil and grease), and Sensation (aphrodisiac).

PERSONAL CARE—**A·R·T Skin Care System**, Boswellia Wrinkle Creme, Genesis Hand & Body Lotion (hydrates, heals, and nurtures the skin), Satin Facial Scrub Mint (eliminates layers of dead skin cells and slows down premature aging of the skin), NeuroGen (provide nutrients and moisturizers to deeper layers of the skin), Orange Blossom Facial Wash combined with Sandalwood Moisture Creme (cleans and moisturizes dry or prematurely aging skin), Prenolone , Progessence, Regenolone (helps moisturize and regenerate tissues), Rose Ointment (for skin conditions and chapped skin), Satin Hand & Body Lotion (moisturizes skin leaving it feeling soft, silky, and smooth), Sensation Hand & Body Lotion (moisturizes, softens, and protects the skin from weather, chemicals, and household cleaners).

SUPPLEMENTS FOR SKIN—JuvaTone, Sulfurzyme, Ultra Young (helps firm and tighten skin by activating the production of skin proteins, collagen, and elastin).

TINCTURES—AD&E

AGING/WRINKLES—Carrot, frankincense, patchouli (prevents wrinkles), rose, rosehip (retards), rosewood (slows).

BATH & SHOWER GELS—Bath Gel Base (cleanses the pores of the skin) plus use your own choice of oils or blends to create the fragrance or therapeutic action you desire.

PERSONAL CARE—Boswellia Wrinkle Creme, Genesis Hand & Body Lotion, Satin Facial Scrub - Mint, PD 80/20, Prenolone/Prenolone+, Progessence, Rose Ointment, Sandalwood Moisture Creme.

SUPPLEMENTS—Ultra Young (helps firm and tighten skin by activating the production of skin proteins, collagen, and elastin).

CHAPPED/CRACKED—Davana, elemi, myrrh, onycha (benzoin), patchouli.

BLEND #1—1 geranium, 1 patchouli, and 1 rosemary in Genesis Hand & Body Lotion or Satin Hand & Body Lotion.

BLEND #2—1-3 drops of both onycha (benzoin) and rose in Genesis Hand & Body Lotion, Satin Hand & Body Lotion (makes a wonderful hand cream), or Rose Ointment. May also add lemon and/or lavender for their additional healing properties.

PERSONAL CARE—Cinnamint Lip Balm.

DISEASE—Rose, Melrose.

DRY—Davana, Gentle Baby, geranium, jasmine, lavender, lemon, neroli, patchouli, Roman chamomile, Frosewood, sandalwood.

MASSAGE OILS—Sensation Massage Oil (silky and youthful skin).

PERSONAL CARE—Genesis Hand & Body Lotion (hydrates, heals, and nurtures), NeuroGen, Orange Blossom Facial Wash (gently cleanses the skin), PD 80/20, Prenolone/Prenolone+, Progessence, Sandalwood Moisture Creme (hydrates), Satin Hand & Body Lotion (nourishes and moisturizes)

> *For years, I had been troubled with an **actinic keratosis** on the back of my hand. It had been caused by excessive sun exposure when I was younger. Farmers often get them on their foreheads. My dermatologist said there was no way to get rid of it - unless I wanted to freeze it off with liquid nitrogen. He didn't want to do that because it was over 1/2 inch in diameter and would have made a hole in my hand. The growth continued to bother me. It was red, scaly, and itchy. One day, in desperation, I put some "Thieves" blend on it. The Thieves seemed to make it feel better so I continued to apply it once a day. It is now several months later and the growth has almost disappeared. I intend to continue using Thieves on it until it is gone. It doesn't bother me anymore and the redness and itching have disappeared.*
>
> *-Submitted by Judy Brown Geneva, New York (July 2004)*

FACIAL MASK—Myrrh, patchouli, sandalwood, vetiver. Can use individually or together. Frankincense is too drying to the skin alone, but can be combined with any or all of these others.

PERSONAL CARE—Orange Blossom Facial Wash, Satin Facial Scrub - Mint.

FEEDS SKIN AND SUPPLIES NUTRIENTS—All applicable essential oils, Boswellia Wrinkle Creme, NeuroGen (deeper layers of the skin), Rose Ointment.

ITCHING—Peppermint.

PERSONAL CARE— ClaraDerm (essential oil spray), Satin Hand & Body Lotion.

OILY (GREASY) COMPLEXION—Bergamot, cajeput, Clary sage, cypress, jasmine, lavender, lemon, nutmeg, orange, ylang ylang.

SAGGY SKIN—Combine 8 drops each of sage, pine, lemongrass, and 1 oz. V-6 Mixing Oil. Rub on areas.

SENSITIVE—Geranium, German chamomile, jasmine, lavender, neroli.

PERSONAL CARE—Satin Hand & Body Lotion.

SUNBURN—Add a little lavender or tamanu oil to some Satin Hand & Body Lotion. Australian Blue.

PERSONAL CARE—LavaDerm Cooling Mist (use as often as necessary to keep skin cool and moist). May also use Satin Hand & Body Lotion later to help maintain moisture.

TONES—Patchouli.

MASSAGE OILS—Cel-Lite Magic.

PERSONAL CARE—Satin Facial Scrub - Mint, Sandalwood Moisture Creme.

SUPPLEMENTS—Ultra Young (helps firm and tighten skin by activating the production of skin proteins, collagen, and elastin).

WRINKLES—(*see Wrinkles for recipes/blends*) Carrot, cistus, Clary sage, cypress, elemi, fennel, frankincense, galbanum, geranium, helichrysum, lavender, lemon, lime, myrrh, neroli, orange, oregano, patchouli, rose, rosemary, rosewood, sandalwood, spikenard, thyme, ylang ylang.

PERSONAL CARE—**A·R·T Skin Care System** (repairs DNA damage, builds collagen), Boswellia Wrinkle Creme (collagen builder), NeuroGen (helps moisturize deep tissues), Rose Ointment, Sandalwood Moisture Creme, Satin Hand & Body Lotion, Satin Facial Scrub - Mint, Wolfberry Eye Creme. The following three items can be used together to help tone the skin and prevent wrinkles: Orange Blossom Facial Wash, Sandalwood Moisture Creme.

SUPPLEMENTS—Essentialzyme, PD 80/20, Prenolone/Prenolone+, Progessence, Thyromin (thyroid function affects the skin), Ultra Young.

Sleep: Lavender (on spine), marjoram (aromatic), Peace & Calming, Roman chamomile (aromatic), valerian (disturbances).

DIFFUSION—*See Negative Ions* for oils that produce negative ions when diffused to help promote sleep. Lavender, Peace & Calming.

SUPPLEMENTS—Ultra Young (restores deep sleep).

ANIMALS—Oils can be used on the paws of animals to help them relax and sleep when in pain. Peace & Calming, Trauma Life.

GOOD NIGHT'S SLEEP—(*See Insomnia for recipe*) ¼ cup bath salts, 10 drops geranium or lavender in bath and soak. Bath with Evening Peace Bath Gel.

RESTLESS—(*See Legs, Restless for recipe*) Lavender and Gathering.

SLEEPING SICKNESS—Geranium, juniper, Peace & Calming (on big toes, back of neck and navel), peppermint, or Valor (on feet).

Slimming and Toning Oils: Basil, grapefruit, lavender, lemongrass, orange, rosemary, sage, thyme.

Slivers (Splinters): Mix 10 drops Thieves with 4 Tbs. V-6 Mixing Oil and massage bottom of feet, arm pits, throat, and lower stomach. Put 30 drops of Thieves in Bath Gel Base and use in shower each day (this helps pull the slivers to gently massage them out).

Smell-loss of: Basil (helps when loss of smell is due to chronic nasal catarrh), peppermint.

STIMULATE SENSORY CORTEX—Brain Power. Place under the tongue, behind the ears, and on the forehead. Can also place a couple drops of

*Just smelling the oils helps stimulate the sense of smell. **To smell the oils**, first close the eyes, hold the left nostril closed, breathe in the smell of the oil through the right nostril, then breathe out through the mouth. Breathing in the fragrance of the oils in this manner stimulates every endocrine gland in the brain. Next hold the right nostril closed and repeat the process.*

oil in the hands, rub them together in a clockwise motion, cup over nose and mouth, and breathe deeply.

   ***COMMENTS—*According to the* <u>Essential Oils Desk Reference</u>, *"Massage 1 or 2 drops [of Brain Power] with a finger on the insides of cheeks in the mouth. Doing this 1 or 2 times a day will immediately improve the smell sensory cortex." (EDR-June 2002; Ch. 8; Brain Power; Application)*

Smoking: <u>Purification</u>.
   CIGARETTE—<u>Purification</u>.
   STOP SMOKING—*See Addictions.* Clove (removes desire), <u>Present Time</u> (helps with insecurity), Thieves (on tongue before lighting up helps remove desire).
   SUPPLEMENTS—JuvaTone, Super C / Super C Chewable.
   ***COMMENTS—*One individual used JuvaTone to break a habit of smoking 2½ packs of cigarettes a day for 20 years. Another individual who used JuvaTone went from smoking a pack a day to 1 cigarette in 1½ weeks.*

Snoring: <u>RC</u>. Rub on throat before sleeping to help keep the airway open.

Soothing: <u>Gentle Baby</u>, myrrh, onycha (benzoin), <u>Release</u>, Roman chamomile.

Sores: Melaleuca, pine, <u>Thieves</u>.

Sore Throat: *See Throat.*

Spacing Out: <u>Grounding</u>, <u>Acceptance</u>, <u>Present Time</u>, <u>Sacred Mountain</u>.

Spasms: *See Muscles, Antispasmodic.* <u>Aroma Siez</u>, **basil**, calamus, ᶠcypress, jasmine (muscle), lavender (antispasmodic), marjoram (relieves), oregano, <u>Peace & Calming</u>, peppermint, Roman chamomile, spikenard, tarragon, and thyme.
   SPASTICITY—Cypress, ginger, juniper, lavender, lemon, rosemary, sandalwood.

Spina Bifida: Work on the nervous system with eucalyptus, lavender, lemon, nutmeg, orange, Roman chamomile, rosemary, <u>3 Wise Men</u>. Apply oil(s) to bottom of feet, along spine, forehead, back of neck, and diffuse. Do the Raindrop Technique.

> *Spina Bifida is a congenital defect of the back bone, usually the lower vertebrae varies from a small area of numbness to paralysis from the waist down. A mental handicap can occur.*

Spine: *See Back.* Oils can be applied along the Vita Flex spine points on the feet as an alternative to working directly on the spine.
   SUPPLEMENTS—BLM
   CALCIFIED—Geranium, <u>PanAway</u> (on spine), rosemary.

MASSAGE OILS—Ortho Ease for body massage.

SUPPLEMENTS—Super C / Super C Chewable.

DETERIORATING—PanAway.

MASSAGE OILS—Ortho Ease.

SUPPLEMENTS—BLM, Super C / Super C Chewable.

PAIN—Valor and PanAway may relieve pain along the spine when applied to spine and Vita Flex points on feet.

MASSAGE OILS—Ortho Sport.

STIFFNESS—Marjoram, Valor. Do the Raindrop Technique.

MASSAGE OILS—Ortho Sport.

VIRUS—*Eucalyptus radiata*, ImmuPower, oregano, and Ortho Ease on Spine. Viruses tend to hibernate along the spine.

Spiritual: Awaken, Believe, Dream Catcher, Gathering, Gratitude, Humility, Inspiration.

AWARENESS—Acceptance, Western Red cedar, cedarwood, juniper, myrrh, 5, spruce, Transformation, White Angelica (Aromatic), White lotus.

BALANCING—Joy, Into the Future, spruce.

INCREASE—Believe, cedarwood (enhances), frankincense (opening and enhancing spiritual receptivity; aromatic), Gratitude, Transformation.

INNER AWARENESS—Believe, Gratitude, Inner Child, Inspiration.

MEDITATION—Believe, Western Red cedar, frankincense, Inspiration, tsuga, White Angelica.

PRAYER—Gratitude, Inspiration, White Angelica.

PROTECTION—3 Wise Men (on crown and shoulders).

PURITY OF SPIRIT—Myrrh.

SPIRITUALLY UPLIFTING—Believe, Gratitude, Sacred Mountain, Transformation.

Spleen: is a major receptor for infections. Laurel, marjoram.

Sports: *See Aches/Pains, Bones, Injuries, Muscles, Tissue.*

EXCEL IN—Clarity (on forehead), Peace & Calming (back of neck), PanAway (injuries), Valor (on feet for courage and confidence).

INJURIES—Helichrysum, lemongrass, Melrose, PanAway, Peace & Calming.

SUPPLEMENTS—BLM

TRACK COMPETITION—

BLEND—5 basil, 5 bergamot, and 2 tsp. V-6 Mixing Oil.

MASSAGE OILS—Ortho Ease, Ortho Sport. Massage into the muscles to increase the oxygen and elasticity in the tissues to prevent the muscles and ligaments from tearing during strenuous exercise. It may also be used after to prevent the muscle from cramping.

SUPPLEMENTS—VitaGreen.

S

Sprains: <u>Aroma Siez</u>, ginger, jasmine, lavender, ^Fmarjoram, <u>PanAway</u>, <u>Peace & Calming</u>, rose, sage. Make a cold compress with eucalyptus, lavender, Roman chamomile, or rosemary.

Spurs, Bone: *See Bones.* Lavender, <u>RC</u> (dissolves). Apply directly on location.

Stains: Lemon (removes).

Staph Infection: *See MRSA.* Black pepper or peppermint will make it more painful. Use oregano and hyssop; alternate with oregano and thyme to relieve the pain. Helichrysum, lavender, <u>Purification</u>.

Sterility: Clary sage, ^Fgeranium, rose (wonderful for both men and women). Can also try jasmine, neroli, sage lavender, sandalwood, <u>SclarEssence</u> (taken internally, helps increase estradiol and testosterone levels), rosewood, and vetiver. Apply several together (or alternate individually) by massage or aromatic baths.
   PERSONAL CARE—Prenolone/Prenolone+, Progessence.
   SUPPLEMENTS—Bodygize, Power Meal.

Stimulating: Basil, Black pepper, <u>En-R-Gee</u>, eucalyptus, fir, ginger, grapefruit, orange, patchouli, ^Fpeppermint, rose, rosemary, ^Fsage, <u>Transformation</u>. Dilute with Massage Oil for stimulating massage. Adding a little Black pepper to an oil like rosemary can give it a little more power. Can also add a few drops of an oil or a couple oils to Bath Gel Base then add to bath water as the tub is filling.

Stings: *See Bites.*

Stomach: ^FBasil, calamus (supports), ginger, peppermint. Apply to stomach Vita Flex points on feet or use with a hot compress over the stomach area.
   ACHE—<u>Di-Gize</u> (behind ears and down jaw bone), eucalyptus, geranium, lavender, peppermint, or rosemary.
   ACID—Peppermint (put drop on finger and place on tongue). Put several drops of fresh lemon juice in warm water and sip slowly.
      SUPPLEMENTS—AlkaLime (acid-neutralizing mineral formula).
   BACTERIA OR GERMS—Peppermint.
   BLOATING—Fennel (1-2 drops in liquid as dietary supplement).
   CRAMPS—Blue cypress, ginger, ^Fhelichrysum, lavender, onycha (benzoin), rosemary cineol, ^Fthyme (general tonic for). Flavor water with 5 drops of <u>Di-Gize</u> and drink for stomach pains **or** add 3 drops basil in capsule with <u>Di-Gize</u>.
   TONIC—Tangerine.
   UPSET—<u>Di-Gize</u>. Apply over stomach and colon, behind the ears, on Vita Flex points on the feet, and/or add 1 drop to 8 oz. rice or almond milk and drink. Can also place a couple of drops on the palms of the hands, rub together clockwise, then cup over nose and mouth and breathe deeply.

Strength: Cypress (aromatic), <u>Hope</u>, oregano, patchouli, ^Fpeppermint, <u>Raven</u>, Roman chamomile (strengthens positive imprinting in DNA), <u>Sacred Mountain</u>, <u>White Angelica</u>.

    SUPPLEMENTS—Be-Fit (enhances strength by promoting muscle formation), NingXia Red, Power Meal, Pure Protein Complete, WheyFit (provides three high-quality sources of protein for enhanced strength), Wolfberry Crisp Bars.

Strep Throat: *See Throat: STREP.*

Stress: <u>Aroma Life</u>, basil, <u>Believe</u>, ^Fbergamot, <u>Clarity</u>, Clary sage, cypress, elemi, <u>Evergreen Essence</u>, frankincense, geranium, grapefruit, <u>Harmony</u>, <u>Inspiration</u>, <u>Joy</u>, lavender (aromatic), <u>Lazarus</u> (available through Creer Labs 801-418-8870), marjoram, neroli, onycha (benzoin), <u>Peace & Calming</u>, pine, Roman chamomile (relieves stress), rosewood, <u>Sacred Mountain</u>, spruce, <u>Surrender</u>, tangerine, <u>3 Wise Men</u>, <u>Valor</u>, <u>White Angelica</u> and ylang ylang.

    BATH & SHOWER GELS—Evening Peace or Sensation Shower Gel.

    MASSAGE OILS—Relaxation or Sensation Massage Oil.

    PERSONAL CARE—Sensation Hand & Body Lotion.

    SUPPLEMENTS—ImmuPro, Master Formula His/Hers, Thyromin, Super B, and Super Cal.

    ***COMMENTS**—You can't change the stressful situations that come, but you can change your response to those situations. Focus on resolution not recrimination! (See Forgive)*

    CHEMICAL—Clary sage, geranium, grapefruit, lavender, lemon, patchouli, rosemary.

    EMOTIONAL STRESS—Bergamot, Clary sage, <u>Evergreen Essence</u>, <u>Forgiveness</u>, <u>Gathering</u>, geranium, <u>Joy</u>, ravensara, sandalwood (layer on navel and chest), <u>Surrender</u>, <u>Transformation</u>, <u>Trauma Life</u>.

    ENVIRONMENTAL STRESS—Basil, bergamot, cedarwood, cypress, geranium, Roman chamomile.

    MENTAL STRESS—Basil, bergamot, <u>Evergreen Essence</u>, geranium, grapefruit, lavender, patchouli, pine, sandalwood, <u>Surrender</u>.

    PERFORMANCE STRESS—Bergamot, ginger, grapefruit, rosemary.

    PHYSICAL STRESS—<u>Believe</u>, bergamot, fennel, <u>Gentle Baby</u>, geranium, <u>Harmony</u>, lavender, marjoram, <u>Peace & Calming</u>, Roman chamomile, rosemary, thyme, <u>Trauma Life</u> (calming).

    SUPPLEMENTS—ImmuPro.

    RELATIONSHIP STRESS—*See Sex Stimulant.*

    BATH & SHOWER GELS—Sensation Bath & Shower Gel.

    MASSAGE OILS—Sensation Massage Oil creates an exotic arousal, increasing sexual desire. The fragrance creates a peaceful and harmonious feeling that helps ease relationship stress. Relaxation Massage Oil also creates a peaceful and harmonious feeling. You may want to add jasmine and ylang ylang.

    PERSONAL CARE—Sensation Hand & Body Lotion.

    STRESS THAT STARTS WITH TIREDNESS, IRRITABILITY, OR INSOMNIA—

    BLEND—15 Clary sage, 10 lemon, 5 lavender, and 1 oz. V-6 Mixing Oil.

    SUPPLEMENTS—ImmuPro, Super B.

S

Stretch Marks: *See Pregnancy.* <u>Gentle Baby</u>, ᶠlavender, mandarin, ᶠmyrrh, neroli.
      Bʟᴇɴᴅ #1—3 drops rosemary, 15 rosewood, and 1¾ oz. Hazel Nut Oil.
      Bʟᴇɴᴅ #2—6 drops lavender, 4 rosewood, 3 patchouli, and Vitamin E Oil.
     ***Cᴏᴍᴍᴇɴᴛs—*Patricia Davis recommends adding mandarin and neroli to either rosehip seed oil or Almond oil to massage over tummy and hips.*

Stroke: *See Blood:* Cʟᴏᴛs *and Blood:* Bʀᴏᴋᴇɴ Bʟᴏᴏᴅ Vᴇssᴇʟs. <u>Aroma Life</u>, calamus, cypress, helichrysum. Breathe deeply and apply to neck and forehead. *See* Cᴏᴍᴍᴇɴᴛs *under Asthma for a discussion on using* **plastic nasal inhalers**.
    Sᴜᴘᴘʟᴇᴍᴇɴᴛs—Master Formula His/Hers, NingXia Red, Power Meal, Sulfurzyme, Ultra Young, Wolfberry Crisp Bars.
    Hᴇᴀᴛ—Lavender or peppermint (rub on neck and forehead).
    Mᴜscᴜʟᴀʀ Pᴀʀᴀʟʏsɪs—Lavender.
    *Bʟᴇɴᴅ—*Mix together equal parts of basil, lavender, and rosemary. Rub spinal column and paralyzed area (<u>Alternative Medicine—The Definitive Guide</u>, p. 978).

Structural Alignment: <u>Aroma Siez</u>, basil, birch, cypress, peppermint, <u>Valor</u>, wintergreen (apply on feet to reduce time and effort necessary for alignments and to increase amount of time the alignment remains effective). **Do the Raindrop Technique**.
    *Mᴀssᴀɢᴇ Oɪʟs—*Ortho Ease.

> *Valor is considered a "chiropractor in a bottle." It may help to realign the spine and keep the body in balance.*

Subconscious: <u>Believe</u>, Balsam fir, <u>Gratitude</u>, helichrysum (uplifts when diffused), <u>Transformation</u>, Western Red cedar.

Sudorific: Hyssop, juniper, lavender, Roman chamomile, rosemary, thyme.

> *A sudorific is an agent that causes sweating. It may be helpful in times of fever or when toxins need to be released through the skin.*

Sugar: White sugar creates acid in the body.
    Sᴜᴘᴘʟᴇᴍᴇɴᴛs—Allerzyme (aids the digestion of sugars, starches, fats, and proteins). NingXia Red (contains 4 of the 8 essential sugars that heal the body and are necessary for cell-to-cell communication).
    Rᴇᴍᴏᴠᴇ Aᴅᴅɪᴄᴛɪᴏɴs ᴛᴏ Sᴜɢᴀʀ—Dill (on wrists).
    Sᴛᴏᴘ Eᴀᴛɪɴɢ—<u>Peace & Calming</u>, <u>Purification</u>.
      Sᴜᴘᴘʟᴇᴍᴇɴᴛs—JuvaTone.
    Sᴜʙsᴛɪᴛᴜᴛᴇ—Stevia (liquid).

> *Honey goes into the blood stream faster than sugar and can be harder on the system than sugar. Maple syrup is one of the most perfect sugars because it has equal proportions of positive and negative ions. It also has the same pH as the blood and it doesn't go into the blood as fast as honey or sugar. Diabetics and pre-diabetics should use black strap molasses instead of maple syrup.*

Suicide: *See Depression and Emotions.*

Sunburn: *See Burns.* <u>Australian Blue</u>,
[F]melaleuca, peppermint. Spray
or rub with Roman chamomile
and lavender. 5-6 drops of
Roman chamomile added to
lukewarm bath water helps
reduce the burning sensation.
SUPPLEMENTS—Mineral Essence (can
apply directly on affected area).
PERSONAL CARE—LavaDerm Cooling

> *My niece came to me in a panic. She had been at the beach all day and acquired a nasty sunburn on her face, chest, and arms. She was planning to go to a fancy party the next day and decided that she absolutely could not go to the party unless the sunburn was gone. I immediately applied a layer of lavender oil, followed a few minutes later by a layer of peppermint oil. The next day to her amazement the sunburn had vanished and she was able to enjoy her party.*
>
> *-Submitted by J. S., Florida (July 2004)*

Mist (use as often as needed to keep skin cool and moist), Satin Hand & Body
Lotion.
PREVENT BLISTERING—Apply 2-3 drops of lavender with Satin Hand & Body Lotion.

Sun Screen: [F]Helichrysum, Tamanu (used by Polynesians as a natural sunscreen for centuries).
PERSONAL CARE—A·R·T Skin Care System.

Supportive: Myrrh.

Swelling: *See Edema (for swelling from water retention).* Helichrysum, lemongrass, **tangerine**.
BLEND—Layer myrrh, frankincense, Balsam fir, and helichrysum directly on location.

Sympathetic Nervous System: Black pepper,
<u>Brain Power</u>, <u>Clarity</u>, *Eucalyptus radiata*, ginger, peppermint.
Stimulation of certain areas
of the Sympathetic Nervous

> *The **Sympathetic Nervous System** is responsible for preparing our bodies for action by stimulating the heart, dilating the bronchi, contracting the arteries, and inhibiting the digestive system.*

System can be achieved by application of any of the above oils at the appropriate
places along the spinal column (*refer to the Autonomic Nervous System chart in the
Science and Application section of the <u>Reference Guide for Essential Oils</u>*).
SUPPLEMENTS—Mineral Essence, Power Meal, Sulfurzyme, Super Cal, Ultra Young.
***COMMENTS—*Stress can create a condition that has been termed as "Sympathetic
System Override" where the production of cortisol, adrenalin, and 5HT
(serotonin) skyrockets, and heavily overloads the lymphatic and cardiovascular
systems. Essential oils can help suppress "Sympathetic System Override" and the
following recipe has been used to do just that, and to bring the body back into a
parasympathetic state.*
RECIPE #2—Apply frankincense to the top of the spine (at the base of the skull) and work
it in. This is the "gatekeeper" and helps prepare the body to more effectively transmit

and utilize the oils that follow. Then apply 3-5 drops of each of the following oils, one at a time, up the back of the neck, and work each one in individually: valerian, vetiver, and Balsam fir. Other oils can be added, such as Roman chamomile, helichrysum, clove, and peppermint.

Sympathy: Acceptance, Awaken, Present Time.

Tachycardia (Rapid Heartbeat): *See Anxiety, Heart, Shock, or Stress.* Aroma Life (combine with ylang ylang), Australian Blue, goldenrod, Idaho tansy, lavender, neroli, orange, PanAway, Relieve It, Roman chamomile, rose, ^Frosemary, ^Fylang ylang (smell on tissue or straight from bottle in emergency). Apply over heart and to heart Vita Flex points on the left hand and elbow (*see illustration under Heart*) and on the left foot. Add oils to V-6 Mixing Oil or Massage Oil for massage, or add them to Bath Gel Base for an aromatic bath. Continue to use regularly to help prevent recurrence.
    TINCTURES—HRT.
    SUPPLEMENTS—CardiaCare, Sulfurzyme.

Talkative: Cypress (for over-talkative).

Taste: Helichrysum (1 drop on tongue), peppermint (for impaired taste).
    SUPPLEMENTS—Mineral Essence, Super B, Super C / Super C Chewable (enhances flavor).

Teeth: *See Dental Infection.*
    CAVITIES—Brush teeth with Thieves. *Put a drop on your toothpaste if you can't handle it straight.*
        PERSONAL CARE—Dentarome/Dentarome Plus Toothpaste (contains Thieves), Fresh Essence Plus Mouthwash (contains Thieves), KidScents Toothpaste (for children).
        ***COMMENTS*—*People have had regeneration of their teeth in as little as four months by brushing their teeth with Thieves.*
    FILLINGS—(to help eliminate toxins from mercury in the system) Balsam fir (22 drops in a capsule, once in morning, once at night). Can also combine Balsam fir with helichrysum and/or frankincense.
        SUPPLEMENTS—Super C / Super C Chewable, Cleansing Trio (ComforTone, Essentialzyme, and ICP), Detoxzyme (5 in morning and 5 at night until body says stop! Then back off to 1 or 2 per day).
    GUM SURGERY—Helichrysum every 15 minutes for the pain.
    TEETHING PAIN—German chamomile, Thieves.
    TOOTHACHE—Cajeput, ^F**clove**, melaleuca, Purification (anti-bacterial), Roman chamomile. Apply on location (on gums) and along jawbone.
        PERSONAL CARE—Dentarome / Dentarome Plus Toothpaste (contains Thieves), Fresh Essence Plus Mouthwash (contains Thieves).
    TOOTHPASTE—Thieves.

***COMMENTS**—You may want to put
10-12 drops of <u>Thieves</u> in a 2 oz.
spray bottle filled with distilled
water. Shake well, then mist in
mouth or on toothbrush and
brush.*

PERSONAL CARE— Dentarome /
Dentarome Plus/Dentarome
Ultra Toothpaste (contains
<u>Thieves</u>), Fresh Essence Plus
Mouthwash (contains <u>Thieves</u>),
KidScents Toothpaste (for
children).

RECIPE—Combine 4 tsp. green or
White clay, 1 tsp. salt, 1 to 2
drops peppermint, 1 to 2 drops
lemon, mix clockwise.

NERVE PAIN—Melaleuca (put 1 drop in
small amount of water and hold
in mouth for one to two minutes
to help calm nerves).

> *My husband has very cavity prone teeth that have needed much dental work in the past 5 years. He has been going in for cleanings every 3 months. His dentist had once pre-scribed a special mouth wash that was supposed to help his decaying teeth. He didn't use the mouthwash regularly enough to see any improvement. About a year ago, he started using Dentarome Plus toothpaste instead of the brand he had been using from the local grocer. That was the only change he made to his dental hygiene routine. At his cleaning in March, his dentist wanted to know what he was doing differently, because his x-rays showed no dental work needed to be done and they didn't have to work as hard to polish his teeth. He told them that all he changed was the toothpaste he was using. They wanted to know if it had fluoride in it, because to be any good (in their eyes) it must have fluoride in it; he brushed them off not wanting to get into the dangers of fluoride with them that day. Then at his cleaning just last week, the dentist had to look at his x-rays twice as well as call on two other colleagues to look at his x-rays to be sure that nothing was being missed because they could not find anything that needed to be fixed. They also told him to come back in six months (instead of 3) for his next cleaning. Now, if I could only get him to use the Fresh Essence Plus mouthwash...*
> *-Submitted by A. Corn*
> *Machesney Park, Illinois (July 2004)*

Temperature: *See Fever or Thyroid.*

SUPPLEMENTS—Thyromin (balances the temperature in the body).

LOWER—Bergamot, eucalyptus, lavender, melissa, peppermint. Cypress and rosemary induce
sweating to lower temperature indirectly. Use oils in baths or mix with cool water
and sponge over body or area.

RAISE—Marjoram, onycha (benzoin), thyme. Add to V-6 Mixing Oil for brisk massage.
Locally warming (rubefacient) oils like Black pepper, juniper, and rosemary help
raise temperature in cold extremities.

Tendonitis: Basil, Fbirch, cypress, Balsam fir,
ginger, lavender, <u>PanAway</u>,
peppermint, <u>Relieve It</u>,
rosemary, wintergreen. Apply
oils in Raindrop fashion on
location and ice pack.

SUPPLEMENTS—BLM

PAIN RELIEF—Birch/wintergreen,
Balsam fir, frankincense,
and peppermint. If pain and
inflammation is a result of torn

> ***Tendonitis Blend***
> *This has worked for my tendonitis and for several other people I have given it to. In a 15 ml amber glass bottle I mix the following essential oils: 3 drops each of helichry-sum, pepper, bergamot, and geranium, 5 drops each of Idaho Balsam fir and lemongrass, then 3 drops each of hyssop, Blue tansy, pine, and myrtle. Then I fill the bottle with V-6 Mixing Oil. This is applied to the area where the pain is and followed with a layer of peppermint oil. This can be done several times per day. If a sensitivity devel-ops, stop using it for a few weeks.*
> *-Submitted by J. S.*
> *West Saint Paul, Minnesota (July 2004)*

or infected ligaments or tendons, then lemongrass and helichrysum can be helpful when added to any of these oils.

T

Tennis Elbow: Birch, eucalyptus, helichrysum, PanAway, peppermint, rosemary, wintergreen.

> *Tennis Elbow is the painful inflammation of the tendon on the outer side of the elbow that usually results from excessive strain on and twisting of the forearm.*

BLEND #1—10 drops eucalyptus, 10 peppermint, 10 rosemary, and 1 Tbs. V-6 Mixing Oil. Mix and apply, then ice pack. Can also try alternating cold and hot packs.

BLEND #2—Equal parts lemongrass, helichrysum, marjoram, and peppermint. Mix and apply, then ice pack.

Tension: Basil (nervous), bergamot (nervous), ^Fcedarwood, frankincense, Harmony, lavender, *Melaleuca ericifolia* (nervous), Peace & Calming, Trauma Life (balances and calms), valerian, ylang ylang. Apply on hands, cup over nose and mouth and breathe deeply or diffuse. Mix a few drops of oil, or oils of choice, in ½ cup Epsom salts and add to bath water. *See COMMENTS under Asthma for a discussion on using* **plastic nasal inhalers**.

AQUA ESSENCE BATH PACKS—Finally, some of the most popular essential oil blends have been combines with the latest hydro-diffusion technology to create the perfect solution for adding oils to your bath water. Just place a packet in the tub while hot water is being added and the oils are perfectly dispersed into the water. The packets contain 10 ml of oil and are reusable. Try either Valor or Peace & Calming.

RELIEVE—Grapefruit, Roman chamomile, Transformation.

MASSAGE OILS—Ortho Ease, Relaxation.

PERSONAL CARE—Prenolone/Prenolone+, Progessence.

Testicles: ^FRosemary.

REGULATION—Aroma Siez (combine with Mister), Clary sage, geranium, sandalwood, yarrow.

PERSONAL CARE—Prenolone+.

SUPPLEMENTS—Mineral Essence, ProGen, Ultra Young+.

Thoughts: Inspiration (relieves negative), ravensara (lifts emotions).

Throat: Calamus (helps remove phlegm), ^Fcypress, oregano. Myrrh and peppermint are also very effective for removing phlegm and mucus from the throat area.

DRY—Grapefruit, lemon.

INFECTION IN—Clary sage, ^Flemon, oregano, ^Fpeppermint.

LARYNGITIS—*See Laryngitis*.

SORE—Rub one of the following on the throat: Bergamot, cajeput, geranium, ginger, ImmuPower, ^Fmelaleuca, myrrh, oregano, RC, sandalwood, Thieves, or put 1 drop of

Thieves in 32 oz. water and drink. Inhalations with Clary sage, eucalyptus, lavender, sandalwood, thyme.

PERSONAL CARE—Gargle with Fresh Essence Plus Mouthwash.

SUPPLEMENTS—Thieves Lozenges.

STREP—Geranium, ginger, or Thieves (rub on throat every time it feels sore; dilute well!). Also hyssop, laurel, melaleuca (combine with Thieves and dilute), oregano, ravensara (combine with Melrose).

PERSONAL CARE—Gargle with Fresh Essence Plus Mouthwash (every hour).

SUPPLEMENTS—ImmuneTune, ImmuPro, Super C / Super C Chewable, Thieves Lozenges.

Thrush: Bergamot, eucalyptus, Flavender, marjoram, rose, thyme.

VAGINAL—Geranium, Fmelaleuca, Fmyrrh, patchouli, rosemary.

Thymus: Elemi, ImmuPower (apply on throat and chest), ravensara, Thieves (dilute with V-6 Mixing Oil and apply over thymus or apply neat on bottom of feet).

STIMULATES—ImmuPower, Fspruce.

SUPPLEMENTS—Ultra Young (reverses aging of the thymus gland).

Thyroid:

DYSFUNCTION—Clove.

NORMALIZES HORMONAL IMBALANCE OF—Myrtle.

HYPERTHYROIDISM—EndoFlex, Fmyrrh, myrtle, Fspruce.

SUPPLEMENTS— Sulfurzyme.

BLEND #1—Equal parts lemongrass and myrrh. Can apply undiluted on thyroid and parathyroid Vita Flex points under big toes or dilute with small amount of V-6 Mixing Oil and apply on throat just under the Adam's apple.

BLEND #2—Equal parts myrrh and spruce. Apply as directed in BLEND #1 above.

HYPOTHYROIDISM—Clove, EndoFlex (apply on top of big toes), Fmyrtle, peppermint, spearmint. Combine lemongrass with any or all of these oils and apply as directed in BLEND #1 above.

> The **thyroid gland** *is situated in the neck and regulates the body's metabolic rate.*
>
> *To determine whether or not the thyroid needs help, you must monitor your basal cell temperature. Place a thermometer under your arm pit before getting out of bed in the morning and rest quietly for 10 minutes. A temperature below 97.6° F (36.5° C) may indicate hypothyroidism (low thyroid function) and a temperature above 98° F (36.7° C) may indicate hyperthyroidism.*

SUPPLEMENTS—Thyromin (regulates metabolism, balances body temperature, prevents fatigue; *follow directions for use as specified in the Supplements section of the* Reference Guide for Essential Oils *under Thyromin*).

***COMMENTS—*One of the signs of thyroid deficiency is rough, dry skin on the bottoms of the feet.*

REGULATION—Ledum.

SUPPORTS—EndoFlex, myrrh (rub on hands and feet), myrtle.

T

> SUPPLEMENTS—Cleansing Trio (ComforTone, Essentialzyme, and ICP), Power Meal, VitaGreen (enhances effect of Thyromin), Thyromin (regulates metabolism, balances body temperature, prevents fatigue; *follow directions for use as specified in the Supplements section of the <u>Reference Guide for Essential Oils</u> under Thyromin*).

Tinnitus: (Ringing in the ears) *See Ears.* Juniper & helichrysum (along mastoid bone behind ear).

Tired: *See Energy, Exhaustion, and Fatigue.*

Tissue: Basil, elemi (rejuvenates), helichrysum, lavender, lemongrass, lime (tightens connective tissue), marjoram, <u>Melrose</u>, Roman chamomile, sandalwood.
> PERSONAL CARE—Essential Beauty Serums (Dry, Oily & Acne-Prone Skin Blends)
> SUPPLEMENTS—Be-Fit (builds muscle tissue), Bodygize (for elasticity in tissues), Power Meal (pre-digested protein), Pure Protein Complete, WheyFit. Biotin (found in Bodygize) is important for damaged tissue.

ANTI-INFLAMMATORY—Myrrh.

BONE AND JOINT REGENERATION—
> BLEND—5 drops birch/wintergreen, 2 German chamomile, 1 Blue tansy, 7 fir, 5 hyssop, 5 helichrysum, 4 lemongrass, 8 sandalwood, 8 spruce, and 1 oz. V-6 Mixing Oil.

CLEANSES TOXINS FROM—Fennel.

CONNECTIVE TISSUE, WEAK—Aroma Siez, helichrysum, lavender, lemongrass, patchouli.
> MASSAGE OILS—Ortho Ease.

DEEP TISSUE PAIN—Helichrysum, palo santo, <u>PanAway</u>, <u>Relieve It</u>.
> MASSAGE OILS—Ortho Ease and Ortho Sport.

REPAIR—Elemi (builds), helichrysum (scar tissue and reduces tissue pain), hyssop (scars), lemongrass (repairs connective tissue), orange, rosewood, sage (firms tissue), <u>Relieve It</u> (deep tissue damage).
> PERSONAL CARE—A·R·T Skin Care System (unique enzymes that work to repair DNA damage), Rose Ointment (to help maintain, protect, and keep the scab soft), Satin Hand & Body Lotion (to moisturize and promote healing).

REGENERATE—Geranium, helichrysum, lemongrass, <u>Melrose</u>, [F]patchouli, rosehip.
> ***COMMENTS—*Use helichrysum and <u>Melrose</u> together for traumatized tissue (cuts, wounds, and abrasions).*

TMJ (Temporomandibular Joint Disorder or TMD): <u>3 Wise Men</u>. Apply on temple and side of face, in front of ear and down to the jaw. Cover with ice packs for 10 minutes at a time, 3-4 times a day. May be best to seek advise from a health care professional, especially a dentist.

Tonic:
> DIGESTIVE— [F]German chamomile, *Melaleuca quinquenervia.*
> SUPPLEMENTS—Digest + Cleanse (very soothing to the digestive system)

GENERAL—Angelica, basil, cajeput, cardamom, cinnamon bark, cistus, Clary sage, cumin, galbanum, geranium, ginger, grapefruit, juniper, lemon, lemongrass, lime, mandarin, marjoram, melissa, Roman chamomile, Mountain savory, myrrh, neroli, nutmeg, orange, palmarosa, patchouli, sandalwood, spruce, ylang ylang. Best way to restore tone in a body that is run-down is to apply oils by massage when possible. Baths are next in effectiveness to massage if not possible or between massages.

HEART—Lavender, thyme.

NERVE—Carrot, Clary sage, melaleuca, [F]ravensara, thyme.

SKIN—Lemon, lime, spearmint, spikenard.

  PERSONAL CARE—Essential Beauty Serums (Dry, Oily & Acne-Prone Skin Blends)

STOMACH—Tangerine.

UTERINE—Jasmine, thyme.

Tonsillitis: (Inflamed tonsils, most often due to streptococcal infection.) *See Throat:* STREP. Bergamot, clove, goldenrod, [F]ginger, lavender, lemon (gargle), [F]melaleuca, Roman chamomile, Thieves. Apply on throat, lungs, and Vita Flex points.

  DIFFUSE—Bergamot, clove, geranium, lavender, lemon, melaleuca (Tea Tree), onycha (benzoin), Thieves, thyme. Breathe deeply through mouth.

  PERSONAL CARE—Fresh Essence Plus Mouthwash.

  SUPPLEMENTS—Thieves Lozenges.

  ***COMMENTS—*Use caution when considering surgery (tonsillectomy) for recurring tonsillitis as doctors have discovered that the only area of the body that can synthesize the antibody to poliomyelitis (polio) is the tonsils.*

Toothache: *See Teeth.*

Toxemia: Aroma Life, cypress.

  SUPPLEMENTS—Essential Manna, Exodus.

  TINCTURES—Rehemogen.

> *Toxemia—poisoned condition of the blood caused by the presence of toxic materials, usually bacterial but occasionally chemical or hormonal in nature. When bacteria themselves find entrance into the bloodstream, the condition is known as bacteremia. The term toxemia is also sometimes applied to pre-eclampsia, a condition that occasionally occurs in late pregnancy and is characterized by high blood pressure and kidney malfunction.*
> *(Microsoft® Encarta® Online Encyclopedia 2000)*

Toxins: Fennel, fir, hyssop (opens respiratory system and discharges toxins and mucus), lemongrass (helps increase lymphatic circulation for enhanced toxin removal), patchouli (digests toxic wastes).

  SUPPLEMENTS—Balance Complete, Cleansing Trio (ComforTone, Essentialzyme, and ICP), Digest + Cleanse. These cleansing products may help remove toxic by-products from the body. Also, take Detoxzyme between meals to break down toxins.

  ***COMMENTS—*Another way to help remove toxins through the skin is to add 2 cups of Apple Cider Vinegar to warm bath water and soak for 25 minutes.*

T

Transition in Life: <u>Acceptance</u>, <u>Awaken</u> (into achieving success), basil, cypress, **Transformation**. May also want to concentrate on the emotional blends of <u>Valor</u>, <u>Motivation</u>, <u>Grounding</u>, <u>Release</u>, <u>Hope</u>, and <u>Joy</u> (*refer to the pages on "Auricular Emotional Therapy" and "Emotional Release" in the Science and Application section of the <u>Reference Guide for Essential Oils</u>*).

Trauma: *See Shock.* <u>Release</u> (feet and liver), <u>Joy</u> (heart), <u>3 Wise Men</u> (crown); use all three blends in succession. May also diffuse. <u>Australian Blue</u>, <u>Envision</u>, <u>Forgiveness</u>, <u>Hope</u>, and <u>Release</u> can also aid in releasing emotional trauma (*Refer to each blend separately in the Blends section of the <u>Reference Guide for Essential Oils</u> for possible applications*). <u>Trauma Life</u> is an excellent blend for helping to cope with shock or emotional trauma. Apply on forehead and on palms then rub palms together, cup over nose and mouth, and inhale deeply. Others that may help are <u>Valor</u> (on the feet), <u>SARA</u> (on temples), <u>Peace & Calming</u> (on palms; place hands together over heart in prayer position).
  COMMENTS— *Concentrate on relaxing to help release the trauma. Also, if after an emotional or physical trauma you find you don't like the smell of a particular oil, it may be the one you need most to help unlock the trauma. Try exposing yourself to it a little at a time until the healing is finished.*
  SUPPLEMENTS—ImmuPro, Mineral Essence, Super C / Super C Chewable.

Travel Sickness: *See Motion Sickness.*

Tuberculosis (T. B.): *See Respiratory System (BLEND #5).* Cajeput, ᶠcedarwood, ᶠcypress, ᶠ*Eucalyptus radiata*, lemon, **melissa**, ᶠmyrtle, peppermint, rosemary verbenon, sandalwood, or ᶠthyme linalol. <u>Exodus II</u> (on spine and Raven on back with a hot compress), <u>ImmuPower</u> (on spine daily), <u>Raven</u> (1-2 drops in V-6 Mixing Oil as a rectal implant), <u>RC</u> (on chest and back– reverse each night with Raven), rose, rosemary, <u>Thieves</u> (on feet). A hot compress can be used when applying oils to the chest or back. **Do the raindrop technique**.
  SUPPLEMENTS—Exodus, ImmuneTune, ImmuPro, Super C / Super C Chewable, VitaGreen. Do a colon and liver cleanse with Balance Complete or the Cleansing Trio (ComforTone, Essentialzyme, and ICP), and JuvaTone.
  TINCTURES—Rehemogen.
  BLEND—1-2 drops each of *Eucalyptus radiata*, myrtle, Mountain savory, and ravensara in 1 Tbs. V-6 Mixing Oil. Apply as a rectal implant.
  COMMENTS— *Refer to the chapter entitled "How to Use - The Personal Usage Reference" in the <u>Essential Oils Desk Reference</u> under "Tuberculosis" for a specific regimen using the blends and supplements.*
  AIRBORNE BACTERIA—<u>Purification</u>, <u>Raven</u>, <u>RC</u>, <u>Sacred Mountain</u>, <u>Thieves</u>. Alternate diffusing different oils to help control spread of bacteria like *Mycobacterium tuberculosis*.
  BLEND—Equal amounts of cypress and <u>Sacred Mountain</u>. Diffuse.

PULMONARY—Cypress, eucalyptus, Inspiration, [F]oregano, ravensara.
> BLEND—Equal amounts of frankincense and ImmuPower. Diffuse or dilute with V-6 Mixing Oil and massage on chest or back. Can also apply to Vita Flex lung points on hands and feet.

Tumors: *See Cancer.*
> ANTI-TUMORAL—Clove (inhibits tumor growth), [F]frankincense (can combine with Balsam fir), ledum (may be more powerful than frankincense). Apply directly on tumor.
>> SUPPLEMENTS—Longevity Capsules (contains clove, orange-high limonene, and frankincense essential oils)
> LIPOMA–Frankincense and clove, grapefruit, ginger, ledum.
>> PERSONAL CARE—Prenolone/Prenolone+, Progessence.

Typhoid: (Fever from contamination of the Salmonella typhosa bacteria) *See Anti-bacterial.*
> [F]Cinnamon bark, lemon, Melrose, Mountain savory, peppermint, Purification, Raven, ravensara, RC. Diffuse or dilute with V-6 Mixing Oil and apply over intestines and on Vita Flex points on the feet.

Ulcers: Bergamot, cinnamon bark, clove, elemi, [F]frankincense, geranium, [F]German chamomile, lemon, [F]myrrh, oregano, rose, thyme, vetiver. Add one drop of oil to rice or almond milk and take as dietary supplement. May also be applied over stomach by hot compress.

> *While some sources claim that sixty percent of all **ulcers** are caused by bacteria, F. Batmanghelidj, M.D. maintains that the majority of ulcers are only dehydration of the stomach lining. In his book, Your Body's Many Cries for Water, Dr. Batmanghelidj shows that rehydration is the simplest cure for this and many other adverse health conditions.*

> SUPPLEMENTS—Use ComforTone to help destroy the bacteria, then use Essentialzyme, Master Formula His/Hers.
> DUODENAL—(Damaged mucous membrane in a portion of the small intestine). Same oils as listed above.
>> SUPPLEMENTS—AlkaLime.
> GASTRIC—*See Gastritis.* [F]Geranium.
> LEG—(From lack of circulation in lower extremities and possible bacterial, fungal, or viral infection). Gentle Baby, geranium, German chamomile, lavender, Melrose, patchouli, Purification, Roman chamomile, rosewood, Sensation.
>> ***COMMENTS—*Dilute oils with V-6 Mixing Oil and massage lower extremities to stimulate circulation. Thyromin may be needed to help with overall circulation.*
>> MASSAGE OILS—Sensation.
>> PERSONAL CARE—Rose Ointment.
>> BLEND—Equal drops of lavender and either Melrose or Purification applied to location. Can cover with Rose Ointment.

MOUTH—*See Cankers*. Basil (mouthwash), myrrh, orange.

> **BLEND #1**—1 drop each of sage and clove and 1-3 drops lavender. Apply directly on location.

PEPTIC—Flavor a quart of water with 1 drop of cinnamon bark oil and sip all day.

> *SUPPLEMENTS*—AlkaLime.

STOMACH—Bergamot, frankincense, geranium, manuka, orange, peppermint. Use as food flavoring, apply to stomach, and Vita Flex points.

> *SUPPLEMENTS*—AlkaLime, Cleansing Trio (ComforTone, Essentialzyme, and ICP), Master Formula His/Hers.
>
> ***COMMENTS—*Manuka Honey is said to naturally kill Helicobacter pylori.*

ULCERATIONS—Cleanse liver and colon (*See Cleansing*). Lavender, Melrose, rose.

> *PERSONAL CARE*—Rose Ointment.

VARICOSE ULCERS—*See Varicose Ulcers*.

Unwind: *See Massage*. Lavender, Peace & Calming. Diffuse, rub between hands and inhale deeply, or combine with V-6 Mixing Oil or Massage Oil for massage. *See COMMENTS under Asthma for a discussion on using* **plastic nasal inhalers**.

> *MASSAGE OILS*—Relaxation.
>
> *BATH & SHOWER GELS*—Evening Peace.

Uplifting: Believe, bergamot, birch, Brain Power, fir (emotionally uplifting), Balsam fir, grapefruit, helichrysum, Idaho tansy, jasmine, lavender, myrrh, orange, Live with Passion, ravensara, Sacred Mountain, Sensation, spruce, 3 Wise Men, Transformation, tsuga, wintergreen. Diffuse or wear as perfume or cologne. *See COMMENTS under Asthma for a discussion on using* **plastic nasal inhalers**.

> *BLEND*—3 birch/wintergreen, 3 lavender, 3 orange, 3 spruce and 1 oz. V-6 Mixing Oil. Wear a few drops of this blend as a perfume or cologne or apply over the heart, on the chest, neck, and/or shoulders, and behind the ears. Can also apply a few drops on both hands, rub together, cup over nose and mouth and breathe deeply.
>
> *BATH & SHOWER GELS*—Morning Start, Sensation.

Ureter:

> INFECTION IN—*See Bladder: INFECTION or Kidneys: INFECTION.* ^FLemon, ^Fmyrtle. Apply as specified below in Urinary Tract Infection.

> *The **ureter** is the duct that carries the urine away from the kidneys to the bladder.*

Urinary Tract: Bergamot, ImmuPower, lavender, ledum, melaleuca (Tea Tree), pine (antiseptic), ^Fsage, ^Fsandalwood, rosemary, tarragon, ^Fthyme (infection).

> GENERAL—Bergamot, ^Feucalyptus (general stimulant).
>
> INFECTION—*See Bladder: INFECTION*. Bergamot, cajeput, ^Fcedarwood, Di-Gize, EndoFlex, geranium, hyssop, ImmuPower, Inspiration (effective by itself), juniper, lemongrass, Melrose, onycha, Purification (effective by itself), tarragon. Apply 2-3 drops of oil directly over bladder. May also apply a hot compress.

BLEND #1—Equal parts sage and <u>Purification</u>.

BLEND #2—Equal parts thyme and <u>Melrose</u>.

BLEND #3—Equal parts oregano and <u>Thieves</u>.

BLEND #4—Equal parts juniper and <u>EndoFlex</u>.

> *With any of these blends, dilute with V-6 Mixing Oil and massage over lower back and pubic area or apply with hot compress.*

SUPPLEMENTS—AlkaLime.

TINCTURES—K&B.

RECIPE #1—Add 1 drop of Mountain savory to 3 droppers of K&B tincture in distilled water and drink every few hours.

***COMMENTS—*Refer to the chapter entitled "How to Use - The Personal Usage Reference" in the* <u>Essential Oils Desk Reference</u> *under "Urinary Tract/Bladder Infection" for a unique blend of 14 different oils to specifically help with infection.*

STONES IN—^FFennel, ^Fgeranium. Apply oils over pubic area and lower back with hot compress. *See MASTER CLEANSER under Cleansing.*

SUPPORT—Cypress, geranium, goldenrod, juniper, laurel, melaleuca.

TINCTURES—K&B.

Uterus: Cedarwood, frankincense, geranium, jasmine, lemon, myrrh.

INFLAMMATION—Elemi.

REGENERATION OF TISSUE—Frankincense, sage, tarragon. Add 1-3 drops of each to 1 tsp. V-6 Mixing Oil, insert into vagina, and retain overnight.

PERSONAL CARE—PD 80/20, Prenolone/Prenolone +, Progessence.

SUPPLEMENTS—Bodygize, FemiGen.

UTEROTONIC—Thyme.

UTERINE CANCER—*See Cancer.* Cedarwood, frankincense, geranium, <u>Gratitude</u>, <u>ImmuPower</u>, lemon, myrrh. Oils can be applied to the reproductive Vita Flex points on the feet, mostly around the front of the ankle, on either side of the ankle under the ankle bone, and up the Achilles tendon. The most effective application of oils is by vaginal retention implant. Add 2-5 drops of any of these single oils or a combination of any of them to 1 tsp. V-6 Mixing Oil, insert into vagina and retain overnight. A tampon may be used if necessary to help retain the oil.

UTERINE CYSTS—*See Ovaries: OVARIAN CYSTS.*

Vaginal:

APPLICATION METHODS—Mix desired oil(s) with water and either use in a douche or sitz bath. Desired oil(s) may also be mixed with V-6 Mixing Oil and either applied directly, inserted with a vaginal syringe (available from Abundant Health) and retained with a tampon, or by soaking a tampon in mixture, inserting, and leaving in all day or night.

CANDIDA (thrush)— ^FBergamot, lavender, laurel, ^Fmelaleuca, ^Fmyrrh, rosemary, spikenard, ^Fthyme. *See APPLICATION METHODS above.*

SUPPLEMENTS—AlkaLime, Royaldophilus. Yogurt, mixed with a little bit of water, may be applied directly to relieve the pain associated with candida.

***COMMENTS—*Focus on the underlying problem of system-wide yeast infection. See Candida. Also, refer to the chapter entitled "How to Use - The Personal Usage Reference" in the Essential Oils Desk Reference under "Fungal Infections" for some excellent blend recipes for dealing with vaginal yeast infections.*

INFECTION— ᶠCinnamon bark (be extremely careful; dilute well), Clary sage, cypress, eucalyptus, hyssop, Inspiration, juniper, lavender, laurel, melaleuca, Melrose, myrrh, Mountain savory, oregano, ᶠrosemary, ᶠrosewood, sage, 3 Wise Men, thyme. Apply oregano and thyme along the spine using the Raindrop Technique. *See also APPLICATION METHODS above.*

BLEND #1—Equal parts oregano, thyme, and Melrose. Dilute with V-6 Mixing Oil and apply as described in *APPLICATION METHODS* above.

BLEND #2—3 drops rosemary, 2 *Melaleuca quinquenervia*, 2 oregano, and 1 thyme. Dilute with V-6 Mixing Oil and apply as described in *APPLICATION METHODS* above. Can also apply as hot compress over lower abdominal area.

BLEND #3—5 drops Melrose, 2 oregano, and 1 thyme in 1 Tbs. V-6 Mixing Oil. Use as douche or vaginal retention implant as described in *APPLICATION METHODS* above.

INFLAMMATION OF VAGINA—Eucalyptus, lavender, melaleuca, yarrow.

RETENTION IMPLANT—Used to cleanse and nourish the female reproductive system or as a support when taking products like the FemiGen supplement. Best when done after a colon and liver cleanse using the Cleansing Trio (ComforTone, Essentialzyme, ICP). The following blends can be inserted directly into the vagina with a vaginal syringe (available from Abundant Health). A tampon may be necessary to help retain.

BLEND #4—Dilute 2 drops *Melaleuca quinquenervia*, 1 lavender, and 1 bergamot in 1 Tbs. V-6 Mixing Oil. Insert and retain overnight.

BLEND #5—Dilute 2 drops frankincense and 7 Purification in 1 Tbs. V-6 Mixing Oil. Insert and retain overnight.

VAGINITIS— ᶠCinnamon bark (be extremely careful; dilute well), *Eucalyptus radiata*, ᶠrosemary, ᶠrosewood. Valerie Worwood suggests the following douche recipe that should be used daily for three days a week only.

RECIPE #1—1 lavender, 1 melaleuca (Tea Tree), 1 tsp. of vinegar, ½ tsp. lemon juice, and 2½ cups of warm water. Mix thoroughly.

Varicose Ulcers: Eucalyptus, geranium, lavender, melaleuca (Tea Tree), thyme, yarrow.

Varicose Veins: Aroma Life, Aroma Siez, basil, bergamot, Citrus Fresh, ᶠcypress (as bath oil), geranium, helichrysum (especially during pregnancy), Idaho tansy (helps weak veins), juniper, lavender, ᶠlemon (tonic for circulatory system), ᶠlemongrass, orange, ᶠpeppermint, rosemary, spikenard, tangerine, yarrow.

MASSAGE OILS—Cel-Lite Magic (strengthens vascular walls).

SUPPLEMENTS—Super B, Thyromin, VitaGreen.

TINCTURES—Rehemogen.

BLEND #1—1-3 drops each of lemongrass and Aroma Life with Cel-Lite Magic.

BLEND #2—1-3 drops each of basil and Aroma Siez. Massage above the affected vein toward the heart.

***COMMENTS—*Refer to the chapter entitled "How to Use - The Personal Usage Reference" in the Essential Oils Desk Reference under "Varicose Veins" for more specific blend recipes and instructions regarding treatment.*

> *Varicose veins are abnormal swelling of the veins in the legs. It is most often a symptom of poor circulation and a loss of elasticity of the vascular walls and particularly their valves. If the valves do not work properly, blood accumulates in the veins instead of flowing back to the heart. This accumulation of blood causes the vein to become swollen and twisted. Hemorrhoids are varicose veins of the anus or rectum usually resulting from constipation. Cleanse the colon.*
>
> *Helichrysum dissolves the coagulated blood inside and outside of the veins. Cypress strengthens the veins. Massage **above** the affected vein toward the heart with helichrysum and cypress every morning and night; wear support hose until healed; it may take from three months to a year to heal completely. It is important to vary the essential oils being used. Try using lavender, juniper or rosemary instead of cypress and helichrysum. See Diet, Circulatory System.*
>
> *Caution: Do not rub below the affected area as it may increase the pressure on the vein*

Vascular System: Aroma Life, cypress, frankincense, helichrysum, ᶠlemongrass (strengthens vascular walls). Apply as a full body massage, over heart, and on bottom of the feet.

> *The **vascular system** refers to the vessels or veins that carry and circulate fluids (blood and lymph) throughout the body.*

MASSAGE OILS—Cel-Lite Magic (strengthens vascular walls).

CLEANSING—*See Chelation and Metals.* Juva Cleanse.

SUPPLEMENTS—JuvaTone, and VitaGreen work very well together. Others include AD&E, Essentialzyme, ImmuneTune, and Super C.

TINCTURES—HRT, K&B, Rehemogen.

BLEND—1-3 drops each of helichrysum and Aroma Life with Cel-Lite Magic Massage Oil. Massage on the body to help dilate the blood vessels and enhance the chelation of metallics.

Vasodilator: *See Blood: VESSELS.* Lemongrass, marjoram.

Veins: *See Vascular System above.*

CIRCULATION IN VASCULAR WALLS OF VEINS—Aroma Life, cypress, lemon.

BLOOD CLOT IN VEIN—Cypress and helichrysum (rub neat on location to dissolve).

Vertigo: *See Ears, Equilibrium and Dizziness.* Ginger.

Viral Disease: Cinnamon bark.

SUPPLEMENTS—ParaFree, Super C/Super C Chewable, ImmuneTune, ImmuPro.

ANTI-VIRAL—Oregano.

INFECTION—Cajeput, melaleuca, oregano, ravensara, thyme. Apply along spine, bottom of feet, and diffuse.

BLEND—Mix one drop each of lavender, orange, and spruce and apply to chest. Then put 10 drops of frankincense in a cap full of Evening Peace Bath Gel and add to bath as a bubble bath and soak.

Viruses: (often hibernate along the spine) Massage ImmuPower and oregano along the spine. Also use bergamot, Blue cypress (especially for HPV), cypress, Egyptian Gold, *Eucalyptus radiata*, lavender, *Melaleuca quinquenervia* (viral and fungal infection), myrrh (both internally and externally - reported 75% effective), ravensara (viral infection), ^Frosemary, Thieves (diffuse with extra cinnamon bark to help fight viral conditions). **Do the raindrop technique!**

> *When my friend contracted the* **West Nile virus** *from a mosquito bite last summer, her neck became stiff, and she had swelling in her ears and behind her ears at the base of her brain. She was in great pain and her ears felt "full" all of the time. We applied an oil blend from Young Living Oils called* Thieves. *She placed the oil at the base of her head and down both sides of her neck and jaw area. This gave her relief from the intense pain in her neck and reduced the swelling in her ears and head. She also drank a couple of drops of the* Thieves *oil blend in fluids several times a day. She continued doing this for at least a month while she fought this disease. We both agree this probably kept her from more serious complications due to the severity of the illness. We also believe it kept her out of the hospital.*
>
> *-Submitted by C. Ness*
> **Rapid City, South Dakota (July 2004)**

SUPPLEMENTS—ImmuPro, Royaldophilus (up to 2 a day), Thieves Lozenges.

AIRBORNE VIRUSES—ImmuPower on throat and chest, Thieves on feet. Diffuse.

ASTHMA—*See Asthma.*

EBOLA VIRUS—This virus cannot live in the presence of cinnamon bark or oregano.

EPSTEIN BARR VIRUS—*See Epstein Barr.* Strengthen immune system, ensure proper thyroid function, and work on hypoglycemia. ImmuPower, Thieves.

SUPPLEMENTS—Exodus, ImmuneTune, ImmuPro, NingXia Red, Wolfberry Crisp Bars.

RESPIRATORY—*Eucalyptus radiata* (diffuse with Thieves; add spruce to push lower in lungs).

SPINE—5 drops oregano and 5 thyme. Put on bottom of the feet and up the spine using the Raindrop Technique.

Visualization: Awaken, Dream Catcher, helichrysum, palo santo, PanAway. Diffuse or wear as perfume or cologne.

Vital Centers: Oregano and sage may strengthen the vital centers of the body.

Vitamins: *See the Supplements section of the* <u>Reference Guide for Essential Oils</u>.
  SUPPLEMENTS—Bodygize, Power Meal, Sulfurzyme (sulfur necessary for proper assimilation of Vitamin C), Super B, Super C / Super C Chewable, Super Cal.
  TINCTURES—AD&E.
  CHILDREN'S SUPPLEMENTS—KidScents Mighty Mist (vitamin spray), KidScents Mighty Vites (chewable vitamin tablets), KidScents MightyZyme (chewable enzymes).

Vitiligo: Frankincense, <u>Melrose</u>, myrrh, <u>Purification</u>, sage, sandalwood, vetiver. Apply behind ears and to back of neck. Then rub hands together, cup over nose and mouth, and breathe deeply. Can also be applied to Vita Flex points relating to the pineal and pituitary glands on the feet and hands.

> *Vitiligo is a disease in which the skin pigmentation is absent in certain areas of the body. It looks as if patches of skin have been bleached white. This may be due to a malfunction of the pineal gland and possibly the pituitary gland as well. See* Pineal *and* Pituitary *for oils and products that can help oxygenate these glands. Another possible remedy includes daily exposure of the eyes to full-spectrum light without contacts or eyeglasses.*

Voice (Hoarse): Bergamot, jasmine.
  BLEND—Add one drop each of <u>Melrose</u> and lemon to 1 tsp. honey. Swish around in mouth for a couple of minutes to liquefy then swallow.

Void: <u>3 Wise Men</u> (replaces the void; place on crown).

Vomiting: *See Nausea.* ᶠFennel, nutmeg, ᶠpeppermint (aromatic).
  MASSAGE OR COMPRESS (over stomach)—Black pepper, fennel, lavender, peppermint, Roman chamomile, rose.

Warming: Cinnamon bark, onycha (benzoin), oregano, thyme.

Warts: Cinnamon bark, colloidal silver, clove, cypress, frankincense (excellent for more stubborn warts), jasmine, lavender, lemon (may dilute in 2 tsp. apple cider vinegar), <u>Melrose</u>, oregano, <u>Thieves</u>. Dilute 1 to 2 drops of oil in a few drops of V-6 Mixing Oil and apply on location.

> *My son had a really big* **wart** *on his hand and I started using Lavender and* <u>Melrose</u> *and it seemed to help. Then I decided to try something new. I used* <u>Melrose</u>, <u>Purification</u>, <u>Thieves</u>, *and Clove–one drop each–and rubbed them in one by one and within a few days the wart was gone. I was so impressed and happy!*
>
> *-Submitted by Caroline Rood*
> *Toledo, Ohio (July 2004)*

  BLEND—5 drops cypress, 10 lemon, 2 Tbs. apple cider vinegar, and AD&E tincture. Apply twice daily and bandage. Keep a bandage on it until wart is gone.
  TINCTURES—AD&E.

GENITAL—Frankincense (excellent
for more stubborn warts),
hyssop, melaleuca, oregano,
Thieves, thyme. Dilute 1-2
drops of oil in a few drops of
V-6 Mixing Oil and apply on
location.
PLANTAR—Oregano.

Waste: *Refer to the chapter entitled, "Cleansing
and Diets" in the Essential
Oils Desk Reference for lots of
information on cleansing.*
ELIMINATING—[F]Lavender (through
lymphatic system).
SUPPLEMENTS—Balance Complete,
Cleansing Trio (ComforTone, Essentialzyme, and ICP), Digest + Cleanse. These
cleansing products help eliminate toxic waste from the body.

*In late October of last year, Cathy brought her 15 year
old daughter to see me for massage therapy. Amanda
was dealing with a huge **plantar's wart** grown deep into
the ball of her foot. She was dealing with a great deal of
pain with every step, and Cathy was planning to make an
appointment for her to see a medical doctor. Cathy also
suffered from these warts and had undergone months of
treatment at her doctor's office having them repeatedly
cut and burned with liquid nitrogen. She was also told you
could never get rid of them. I suggested that Amanda rub
essential oil of oregano on the infected area which
Amanda did diligently each day, covering it with a bandage. They were amazed that the wart had completely
disappeared in 6 weeks and has had no recurrence of the
virus. Amanda's only complaint was she got tired of going
to school every day smelling like a pizza.*
-Submitted by Ellie Ayers (July 2004)

Water Distillation: Add 3-5 drops of your favorite oil to the post-filter on your distiller. The oils will
help increase the oxygen and frequency of the water. Try lemon or peppermint.

Water Purification: [F]Lemon, orange. H2Oils packets are wonderful for purifying and flavoring
drinking water at the same time. Packets can be left in a container of water overnight
to allow the oils to be effectively dispersed throughout the water. Try lemon, lemon/
grapefruit, or lemon/orange.
REMOVE NITRATES—Peppermint.

Water Retention: *See Edema, Diuretic, and Hormonal Imbalance.*

Weakness:
AFTER ILLNESS—Thyme (physical).

Wealth: Abundance, bergamot.
ATTRACTS—Cinnamon bark (aromatic).
MONEY—Ginger, patchouli.

Weight: *See Hormonal Imbalance and pH
Balance.* **Proper exercise** is
absolutely important! *Refer to
the Supplements section of the Reference Guide for Essential Oils for instructions on
how to use Bodygize and ThermaBurn for different weight problems.*

***Weight gain** is often attributed to slow metabolism, lack
of exercise, low fiber, poor diet, stress, enzyme deficiency,
hormonal imbalance, low thyroid function, and poor digestion and assimilation. It can also result from too much
insulin being produced by the body.*

SUPPLEMENTS—Enzyme products: Allerzyme (aids the digestion of sugars, starches, fats, and proteins), Carbozyme (aids the digestion of carbohydrates), Detoxzyme (helps maintain and support a healthy intestinal environment), Digest + Cleanse, Polyzyme (aids the digestion of protein and helps reduce swelling and discomfort), and Lipozyme (aids the digestion of fats). Balance Complete (an excellent meal replacer, nutritive cleanser providing 11 grams of fiber per serving), Body Balancing Trio (Bodygize, Master Formula His/Hers, VitaGreen), Cleansing Trio (ComforTone, Essentialzyme, and ICP), JuvaPower/JuvaSpice, NingXia Red, Pure Protein Complete.

CONTROL—EndoFlex (while taking Thyromin, a drop of EndoFlex under the tongue two or three times a day can help).

SUPPLEMENTS—Balance Complete, Digest + Cleanse, Pure Protein Complete, Thyromin, Wolfberry Crisp Bars.

EMOTIONS—Excessive weight may be due to unresolved childhood emotions. Any or all of the following may help: Acceptance, Forgiveness, Inner Child, SARA (*Refer to the "Emotional Release" part of the Science and Application section or to the Blend section of the Reference Guide for Essential Oils for more information on each of these blends*).

WEIGHT LOSS—EndoFlex (on throat, under big toes), Joy, and Motivation.

BLEND #1—Put 5 lemon and 5 grapefruit in 1 gallon of water and drink during the day. Add more grapefruit to dissolve fat faster. This same thing can now be done easier and more effectively by using the H2Oils packet with lemon/grapefruit. Just leave the packet in a gallon of purified drinking water overnight and the oils will disperse throughout the water.

BLEND #2—4 lavender, 4 basil, 3 juniper, 8 grapefruit, 5 cypress. Mix and apply to feet, on location, as a body massage, or use in bath. Blend is used to emulsify fat.

MASSAGE OILS—Massage whole body with Cel-Lite Magic after showering.

PERSONAL CARE—If the weight problem is related to a hormonal imbalance, Prenolone/ Prenolone+ / Progessence combined with Thyromin and EndoFlex may help.

SUPPLEMENTS—Use Balance Complete (to replace 2 meals and promote proper elimination) or Bodygize (helps to be at ideal weight) to replace breakfast and dinner, ComforTone, Digest + Cleanse, ICP, and Essentialzyme to promote proper elimination of waste material from the bowels, ThermaBurn to naturally suppress the appetite and regulate the metabolism, and Thyromin to ensure proper thyroid function. Eat a normal meal at lunch, but watch fat intake. Other products that may help are AlkaLime (improves digestion), JuvaPower/ JuvaSpice, Power Meal, Sulfurzyme, Ultra Young (may help improve fat-to-lean ratios), and WheyFit (high quality, lactose-free proteins from three different sources), Wolfberry Crisp Bars. Master Formula His/Hers is also important to use.

UNDERWEIGHT—Pure Protein Complete. Drink Bodygize with meals. Feed cells with Mineral Essence.

Well Being: Citrus Fresh, Idaho tansy, Release (emotional), rose, Transformation.
> FEELING OF—Harmony, spearmint.
> PROMOTES—Eucalyptus, geranium, lavender, lemon, lime.
> > SUPPLEMENTS—Cleansing Trio (ComforTone, Essentialzyme, and ICP).

Whiplash: *See Trauma or Shock.* Aroma Siez, basil, birch, helichrysum (bruising), hyssop (inflammation), juniper, lemongrass (strained ligaments), marjoram (muscles), PanAway, Relieve It, Roman chamomile, spruce, wintergreen (bones). Can also apply valerian, vetiver, helichrysum, clove, and peppermint to the back of the neck (up to the base of the skull) to help calm the sympathetic nervous system and reduce pain and swelling.
> SUPPLEMENTS—Sulfurzyme, Super C / Super C Chewable.

***COMMENTS—*Remember to think through every physical aspect of the injury (i.e. muscle damage, nerve damage, inflammation, ligament strain, bone injury, fever, and emotions). Select oils for each area of concern.*

Wholeness: Ones own spirituality and oneness with the Creator. Apply each of the following blends, one right after the other: Awaken over the heart and on the forehead, Sacred Mountain on the crown of the head and over the thymus, and White Angelica on the shoulders. Then rub hands together, cup over nose and mouth, and breathe deeply to inhale the aroma of all three blends together.

Whooping Cough: *See Childhood Diseases.* Cinnamon bark, Clary cage, cypress, grapefruit, hyssop, lavender, ᶠoregano. Apply on chest, throat, and Vita Flex points. Use a hot compress for deeper penetration.
> DIFFUSE—Basil, eucalyptus, lavender, melaleuca, peppermint, Roman chamomile, rose, thyme.

Withdrawal: *See Addictions.*

Workaholic: Basil, geranium, lavender, marjoram. Rub a couple drops between hands, cup over nose and mouth and breathe deeply. Can also be diffused.

Worms: *See Ringworm or Parasites.* Bergamot, Di-Gize (helps expel intestinal worms), lavender, melaleuca, peppermint, Roman chamomile, rosemary verbenon, thyme. For intestinal worms, apply a few drops over abdomen with a hot compress or add to V-6 Mixing Oil (½ to 1 oz.) and use as a retention enema for 15 minutes or more. Can also apply on intestine and colon Vita Flex points on the feet.
> BLEND—Mix 6 drops Roman chamomile, 6 eucalyptus, 6 lavender, and 6 lemon with 2 Tbs. V-6 Mixing Oil. Apply 10-15 drops of blend over abdomen with a hot compress and on intestine and colon Vita Flex points on the feet.
> SUPPLEMENTS—Cleansing Trio (ComforTone, Essentialzyme, and ICP), Digest + Cleanse, ParaFree.

Worry: Bergamot. Diffuse.

Wounds: Bergamot, cajeput, cistus (to help reduce scarring), [F]clove (infected wounds), cypress, elemi (infected), eucalyptus, frankincense, galbanum, geranium, juniper, lavender (combine with any of these other oils), melaleuca (Tea Tree), myrrh (infected), onycha (benzoin), peppermint (when wound has closed, will soothe, cool, and reduce inflammation), Roman chamomile (add to Rose Ointment for an excellent first aid salve), rose, rosemary, rosewood, sandalwood (for DNA repair), thyme, tsuga.

> BLEND #1—Lavender with Purification or Melrose.

> RECIPE #1—First, 1-3 drops of helichrysum on the fresh wound will help stop the bleeding and a drop of clove will help with pain. Once bleeding is stopped, a drop of lavender (to help start the healing), a drop of Melrose (to help fight infection), and a drop of lemongrass (for possible ligament damage) can be applied. Other oils such as birch/wintergreen, thyme, or sage may also be applied depending on the extent of the injury. Rose Ointment can then be applied to help seal the wound and extend the effectiveness of the applied oils, and then cover it all with a bandage. When changing the bandage, cistus, myrrh, onycha, sandalwood (for DNA repair), or patchouli can be applied to help promote further healing. Thieves, myrrh, or Purification may be necessary to help fight any occurrence of infection.

One Sunday morning I tripped and rammed my foot into a dirty pair of grass clippers, cutting my 4th toe at the base where it joins my foot. I washed it out as best I could with hydrogen peroxide, and then applied lavender oil and a bandage, and went on to church. When I came home, I kept my foot elevated and applied more lavender oil throughout the day. My friend looked at my wound and commented that it wasn't just a gash, it was punctured. That evening I also applied clove oil, along with the lavender oil. I slept with it unbandaged, and then bandaged it during the day while I was at work. I applied the oils morning and night. I had no infection, and by the following Sunday evening, it was almost totally healed. My friend who looked at it again was amazed, and she's an EMT!

-Submitted by C. Ness
Rapid City, South Dakota (July 2004)

> PERSONAL CARE—Rose Ointment (seals and protects).

> SUPPLEMENTS—Stevia extract (apply on closed wound to help reduce scarring).

> CHILDREN (AND INFANTS)—Lavender and/or Roman chamomile. Helichrysum and peppermint are best diluted with lavender or Rose Ointment first to help minimize stinging effect on open wounds.

> BLEND #2—(for Bruises or Wounds) 1-3 drops each of helichrysum and lavender diluted in 1/8 oz. V-6 Mixing Oil.

> BLEEDING—Rose, helichrysum, lemon, lavender.

> BLEND #3—Equal amounts of Roman chamomile, geranium, and lemon. Can alternate with cypress, hyssop, palmarosa, and rose. Apply directly with a compress 2-3 times a day for 3-4 days then reduce to once a day until healed.

DISINFECT—Hyssop, Idaho tansy, lavender, melaleuca, Mountain savory, thyme (thymol and linalol). Apply 1-2 drops directly on wound.

HEALING—*See Scarring*. Helichrysum, Idaho tansy, lavender, melaleuca (pus-filled wounds), myrrh, neroli, onycha (benzoin), patchouli, ravensara, sandalwood, tsuga, yarrow. Apply directly on wound followed by Rose Ointment.

> Dr. Marcy Foley maintains that "Each person will have a unique picture which created their healing challenges, and will require that each of these areas be addressed for a complete healing to take place." This is especially true for surface **wounds** where each aspect of the trauma must be considered. For example, there may also be damage to muscles, nerves, ligaments, or bones; there may be infection or inflammation; and there may be an emotion or even fever to deal with. Oils should be considered for each of these different areas as well.

INFLAMMATION—German chamomile (helps reduce).

SURGICAL—Melrose, peppermint (cooling and soothing), Purification, Thieves.

BLEND #4—3 drops helichrysum, 3 frankincense, 4 lavender in 2 tsp. V-6 Mixing Oil. Reapply a few drops of blend when changing bandages.

> My husband, Tom, was taking apart a rabbit cage and the roof with the nails poking through fell on his hand and punctured it. Blood was dripping everywhere and he was becoming sick with pain and weakness. He applied pressure to the wounds but it still bled until I applied lavender and *PanAway*. Before our very eyes it immediately stopped bleeding. It did swell up, but he kept applying lavender and *PanAway* and it would take away the pain and bring the swelling down. It was healed in a matter of three days without a trip to the doctor. We feel so blessed to have oils on hand to treat emergencies like this one.
> **-Submitted by Diana Wolford**
> **Olive Branch, Mississippi (July 2004)**

WEEPING—Juniper, myrrh, patchouli, tarragon.

BLEND #5—5 drops Roman chamomile, 10 lavender, 3 tarragon, and 2 oz. V-6 Mixing Oil. Apply as a hot compress.

Wrinkles: Carrot, cistus, Clary sage, cypress, elemi, fennel, frankincense, galbanum, geranium, helichrysum, lavender, lemon, myrrh, neroli, orange, oregano, patchouli, rose, rosemary, rosewood, sandalwood, spikenard, thyme, ylang ylang.

> **Wrinkles** occur as we mature and as we lose oxygen to the tissues. Essential oils oxygenate the tissues and thereby slow down the premature aging of the skin.

AFTERSHAVE—Awaken can be used instead of aftershave lotion. KidScents Lotion works well to rehydrate the skin after shaving.

BLEND #1—3 drops lavender, 4 geranium, 2 patchouli, 6 rosewood, and 1 oz. V-6 Mixing Oil. Rub on wrinkles in an upward, lifting motion.

BLEND #2—1 drops frankincense, 1 lavender, and 1 lemon. It's like magic for wrinkles. Rub on morning and night around the eyes.

BLEND #3—5-10 drops frankincense added to Sandalwood Moisture Creme.

BLEND #4—Equal amounts of sandalwood, helichrysum, geranium, lavender, and frankincense. Combine with either Genesis Hand & Body Lotion or Satin Hand & Body Lotion and apply.

PERSONAL CARE—**A·R·T Skin Care System** (smooths wrinkles by repairing DNA, building collagen and fibroconectin, and moisturizing deeper layers), Essential Beauty Serums (Dry, Oily & Acne-Prone Skin Blends), Rose Ointment, Sandalwood Moisture Creme, Satin Hand & Body Lotion.

SUPPLEMENTS—Essentialzyme, PD 80/20, Prenolone/Prenolone+, Progessence, Thyromin (thyroid function affects the skin), Ultra Young.

PREVENT—Gentle Baby and patchouli (prevents and retards).

PERSONAL CARE—**A·R·T Skin Care System**, Boswellia Wrinkle Creme (collagen builder), Essential Beauty Serums (Dry, Oily & Acne-Prone Skin Blends), Satin Facial Scrub - Mint, NeuroGen (helps moisturize deep tissues), Wolfberry Eye Creme. The following three items can be used together to help tone the skin and prevent wrinkles: Orange Blossom Facial Wash, Sandalwood Moisture Creme.

SMOOTH—Add 2 drops frankincense to a little Genesis Hand & Body Lotion or Satin Hand & Body Lotion and apply.

PERSONAL CARE—**A·R·T Skin Care System**, Boswellia Wrinkle Creme (collagen builder), Essential Beauty Serums (Dry, Oily & Acne-Prone Skin Blends).

Yeast: *See Candida.*

Yin and Yang: Ylang ylang (balances)

Yoga: Cedarwood, sandalwood, spruce, tsuga.

Zest (for life): En-R-Gee, Motivation, nutmeg, Legacy, Live with Passion. Diffuse.

Peace & Calming Saves the Day

My husband works at an elementary school as a LAN technician. Last spring the secretaries union went on strike for 2 weeks. All the other unions in the school district, in a show of support for the secretaries, forbade any of their members helping out with the secretarial duties. That left 3 people in my husband's school (my husband included) who were not union and able to attempt to keep the school running normally. After his first day of secretarial duties he took in a travel diffuser soaked in Peace & Calming, to help calm the kids who were sent to the office because they were trouble makers in their classes as well as to keep himself calm. He still is not sure who the Peace & Calming helped more (him or the kids), but the rest of the 2 weeks were less stressful thanks to the Peace & Calming.

-Submitted by A. Cornn, Machesney Park, Illinois (July 2004)

Appendix

BODY SYSTEMS CHART

The following chart lists all of the products discussed within this book and indicates which body systems they primarily affect. While this chart does not include every system that could possibly be affected by each product, it attempts to list the primary systems that are most often affected. It is provided to give the beginning aromatherapy student a starting point for personal use and analysis.

Essential Oil	Cardiovascular System	Digestive System	Emotional Balance	Hormonal System	Immune System	Muscles and Bones	Nervous System	Respiratory System	Skin and Hair
3 Wise Men			X						
Abundance			X		X			X	
Acceptance			X				X		
AD&E					X		X		X
AlkaLime	X	X				X			
Allerzyme		X						X	
Angelica			X				X		
Animal Scents Products									X
Anise	X	X		X				X	
Anti-Cana					X				
Aroma Life	X								
Aroma Siez						X		X	
AromaGuard Deodorants									X
Australian Blue			X						
Awaken			X						
Balance Complete		X							
Basil	X					X			
Be-Fit						X			
Believe			X						
Bergamot		X	X						X
Berry Young Juice					X				
Birch						X			

Essential Oil	Cardiovascular System	Digestive System	Emotional Balance	Hormonal System	Immune System	Muscles and Bones	Nervous System	Respiratory System	Skin and Hair
BLM						X			
Blue Agave				X		X			
Bodygize		X			X	X			
Boswellia Wrinkle Creme									X
Brain Power			X				X		
Cajeput	X							X	
Carbozyme		X							
Cardamom		X							
CardiaCare	X								
Carrot	X						X		X
Cedar, Western Red									X
Cedarwood							X	X	
Cel-Lite Magic									X
Celery Seed		X				X	X		
Chamomile, German			X				X		X
Chamomile, Roman			X				X		X
Chelex					X				
Chivalry			X						
Christmas Spirit	X		X				X		
Cinnamint Lip Balm									X
Cinnamon Bark					X				
Cistus					X				X
Citronella						X			X
Citrus Fresh			X		X				
ClaraDerm									X
Clarity			X				X		
Clary Sage				X					
Clove	X	X			X			X	
ComforTone		X			X				
Coriander		X		X					
CortiStop				X					
Cumin		X			X				
Cypress	X						X		
Cypress, Blue		X			X				
Davana				X					

Essential Oil	Cardiovascular System	Digestive System	Emotional Balance	Hormonal System	Immune System	Muscles and Bones	Nervous System	Respiratory System	Skin and Hair
Detoxzyme		X			X				
Di-Gize		X							
Digest + Cleanse		X							
Dill		X							
Dragon Time			X	X					
Dream Catcher			X						
Elemi									X
Egyptian Gold			X		X				
En-R-Gee			X				X		
EndoFlex				X					
Envision			X						
Essential Manna		X			X	X			
Essentialzyme		X							
Estro				X					
Eucalyptus						X		X	
Eucalyptus citriodora								X	
Eucalyptus radiata								X	X
Eucalyptus staigeriana						X		X	X
Evening Peace									X
Evergreen Essence			X						
Exodus					X				
Exodus II					X				
FemiGen				X					
Fennel		X		X					
FHS				X					
Fir								X	
Fir, Balsam						X	X		
Fir, Douglas						X		X	
Fir, White			X			X		X	
Fleabane (Conyza)	X			X					
Forgiveness			X						
Frankincense			X		X		X		X
Galbanum					X				
Gathering			X						
Genesis Lotion			X						X

Essential Oil	Cardiovascular System	Digestive System	Emotional Balance	Hormonal System	Immune System	Muscles and Bones	Nervous System	Respiratory System	Skin and Hair
Gentle Baby			X						X
Geranium			X						X
Ginger		X					X		
GLF		X							
Goldenrod	X			X					
Grapefruit	X								
Gratitude			X						
Grounding			X						
Harmony			X						
Helichrysum	X						X		
Highest Potential			X						
Hope			X						
HRT	X								
Humility			X						
Hyssop	X						X	X	
ICP	X	X							
ImmuneTune					X				
ImmuPower					X				
ImmuPro					X				
Inner Child			X						
Inspiration			X						
Into the Future			X						
Jasmine			X	X					
Joy			X						
Juniper		X	X				X		X
Juva Cleanse		X							
JuvaFlex		X							
JuvaPower		X							
JuvaSpice		X							
JuvaTone		X			X				
K&B		X							
KidScents Mighty Mist	X		X		X		X		
KidScents Mighty Vites	X		X		X		X		
KidScents MightyZyme		X							
KidScents Royaldophilus		X			X				
Lady Flash			X	X					

Essential Oil	Cardiovascular System	Digestive System	Emotional Balance	Hormonal System	Immune System	Muscles and Bones	Nervous System	Respiratory System	Skin and Hair
Lady Love			X	X					
Lady Sclareol			X						X
Laurel		X			X			X	
LavaDerm Cooling Mist			X						X
Lavandin	X					X		X	
Lavender	X		X				X		X
Laxarus			X						
Ledum		X			X				X
Legacy			X						
Lemon		X			X			X	
Lemongrass					X	X			
Lime		X			X			X	
Lipozyme		X							
Live with Passion			X				X		
Longevity	X		X						
Longevity Capsules	X				X		X		X
M-Grain						X	X		
Magnify Your Purpose			X				X		
Male-Pro				X					
Mandarin		X							X
Manuka						X		X	X
Marjoram	X					X			
Master Formula	X		X		X		X		
MegaCal	X					X	X		
Melaleuca					X	X			X
Melaleuca Ericifolia								X	X
Melaleuca Quinquenrvia							X	X	
Melissa			X						X
Melrose								X	X
Mineral Essence	X		X	X	X	X	X		
Mister				X					
Morning Start			X						X
Motivation			X				X		
Mountain Savory					X				

Essential Oil	Cardiovascular System	Digestive System	Emotional Balance	Hormonal System	Immune System	Muscles and Bones	Nervous System	Respiratory System	Skin and Hair
Myrrh				X	X		X		X
Myrtle		X		X		X		X	
Ner-Vus							X		
Neroli		X							X
Nerv-Cal							X		
NeuroGen				X		X	X		
NingXia Red					X				
Nutmeg				X	X		X		
Omega Blue	X						X		
Onycha	X		X						X
Orange		X	X		X				X
Orange Blossom Facial Wash									X
Oregano					X	X		X	
Ortho Ease						X			
Ortho Sport						X			
Palmarosa	X		X						X
Palo Santo			X		X		X		
PanAway						X	X		
ParaFree		X			X				
Patchouli									X
PD 80/20			X	X		X			
Peace & Calming			X				X		
Pepper, Black		X					X		
Pepper, Pink					X			X	X
Peppermint		X				X	X	X	X
Petitgrain			X						
Pine			X					X	
Polyzyme		X				X			
Power Meal	X	X			X	X			
Prenolone			X	X		X	X		X
Present Time			X						
ProGen				X					
Progessence			X	X		X	X		X
Protec				X					
Pure Protein Complete						X			
Purification		X	X						X
Raven								X	X

Essential Oil	Cardiovascular System	Digestive System	Emotional Balance	Hormonal System	Immune System	Muscles and Bones	Nervous System	Respiratory System	Skin and Hair
Ravensara					X			X	
RC								X	
Regenolone				X		X	X		X
Rehemogen	X	X							
Relaxation			X			X			X
Release			X						
Relieve It						X			
Rose			X						X
Rose Ointment									X
Rosemary camphor	X	X				X			
Rosemary cineol					X		X	X	
Rosemary verbanon		X		X					X
Rosewood									X
Royaldophilus		X			X				
Sacred Mountain			X						
Sage				X	X				
Sage Lavender			X	X		X	X	X	X
Sandalwood			X			X	X		X
Sandalwood Moisture Creme									X
SARA			X						
Satin Hand & Body Lotion									X
Satin Facial Scrubs									X
SclarEssence		X		X					
SE-6				X					
Sensation Lotion									X
Sensation Oil Blend			X	X					
Spearmint		X	X						
Spikenard			X						X
Spruce			X				X	X	
Stevia	X	X			X				
Sugar-Up		X							
Sulfurzyme					X	X	X		X
Super B	X					X	X		

Essential Oil	Cardiovascular System	Digestive System	Emotional Balance	Hormonal System	Immune System	Muscles and Bones	Nervous System	Respiratory System	Skin and Hair
Super C					X			X	
Super C Chewable					X	X			
Super Cal	X		X			X	X		
Surrender			X				X		
Tangerine			X		X				X
Tansy, Blue							X		
Tansy, Idaho					X				
Tarragon		X					X		
ThermaBurn						X			
Thieves					X				
Thieves Cleaning Prod					X				
Thieves Lozenges					X				
Thyme					X	X			
Thyme linalol								X	X
Thyromin				X					
Transformation			X						
Trauma Life			X						
Tsuga	X							X	
Ultra Young				X	X				
Valerian							X		
Valor			X			X	X		X
Vetiver			X	X			X		X
VitaGreen	X	X			X	X	X		
WheyFit						X			
White Angelica			X						
White Lotus					X				
Wintergreen						X			
Wolfberry Crisp Bars		X			X	X			
Wolfberry Eye Creme									X
Yarrow				X	X				X
Ylang Ylang	X		X	X					

SINGLE OIL PROPERTY CHART

The following chart presents some of the properties of each of the single oils. An attempt has been made to indicate the effectiveness of the oils for each property, where supporting information existed. However, this information should not be considered conclusive. It is provided to give the beginning aromatherapy student a starting point for personal use and analysis. Also, keep in mind the applicable safety data when applying an oil for its property. For example, cinnamon bark is one of the best known antiseptics, but it is also extremely irritating to the skin. It may work well to sanitize the bathroom with, but should be used with extreme caution on the skin.

Essential Oil	A-Bac	A-Cat	A-Dep	A-Fun	A-Inf	A-Infl	A-Mic	A-Par	A-Rhe	A-Sep	A-Spa	A-Vir	Analg	Imm
Angelica		+										+		
Basil	++	+	+		+	+++				+	+	+		
Bergamot					+	+++	+			+	+		+	
Birch						++			++	+	+++		++	
Cajeput	+	+			+					+	+		+	
Cardamom										+	+			
Cedarwood				+	+					+				
Chamomile, German	+		+		+	+++				+	+		++	
Chamomile, Roman	+					++		+++			+++		+	
Cinnamon Bark	+		+	+	+	+	++	+		++++	+	+		
Cistus							+			+				+
Citronella	+			+	+					+++	+			
Clary Sage	+		+		+					+	+			
Clove	+++	+		++	+			++	+	+			+++	
Coriander	++		++		++			+			+		+	
Cumin	+							+		+	++	+		+
Cypress	+				+			+	+	+	+			
Davana					++									
Dill	+	+									+			
Elemi		++	++		+					+				
Eucalyptus	++	++++			+	+		+	++	+	++	+++	++	
Eucalyptus, citriodora	++	++		+	++					+		++		
Eucalyptus, radiata	++	++			+	+						+++	++	+
Fennel	+	++				+	+	+		+	+			
Fir		+								++			+	
Frankincense		++	++				+			+				+++

Essential Oil	A-Bac	A-Cat	A-Dep	A-Fun	A-Inf	A-Infl	A-Mic	A-Par	A-Rhe	A-Sep	A-Spa	A-Vir	Analg	Imm
Galbanum		+			+	+	+			+	+	++	++	
Geranium	+++		++	++	+	+				+				
Ginger		++								++			++	
Grapefruit	++									++				
Helichrysum	++	+++		+		++	++			+	+++			
Hyssop	++	++++			+	++		+	+	+	+	+++		
Jasmine		+	++				++				+	+	+	
Juniper					+			+	++	+	+			
Laurel				+						+				
Lavender			++		+	++	+	+	+	+	++		++	
Lavandin	+			+		++				+++	++		++	
Lemon	++				+		++		+	+++	+			++
Lemongrass	+		+	+		++	+			+			++	
Lime	++									++		+		
Mandarin				+						++	+			
Marjoram	+	+		+	+					++	++	+	++	
Melaleuca	+++			++++	+	+		+		+		+++		++
Melaleuca Ericifolia	+			+	+		+++							
Melaleuca Quinquenrvia	+++			++++		+				+		+++		
Melissa	+		++				+				++	++		
Mountain Savory	+++	+		+	++		+++	++		+	+	++	++	++
Myrrh		+		+	+	+++	++	+		+		+++		
Myrtle	+	+++			+					+				
Neroli	+		++		+			+		++	++	+		
Nutmeg						+		+		+				
Orange	++		++	+		+				++				
Oregano	+++	+		+++	+++			+++	++	+	+	++	++	++
Palmarosa	+			+			+			+		+		
Patchouli	+		+	+	+	+	+			+		+		
Pepper, Black	+						+			+	+		++	
Peppermint	+	+		+	+	++	+			+	+	+	++	
Petitgrain	+				++	++				+	++			
Pine	+	+		+	++		+			+		+	+	
Ravensara	+	+++		+	+					++		++++		
Rose			++		++	+								
Rosemary	+	+++		+	+		++	+	++	+	+	+	++	
Rosewood	+++		+	++	+		+	+		+		++	+	+
Sage	+	+	+	++	+	+	++			+	+	+++		

Essential Oil	A-Bac	A-Cat	A-Dep	A-Fun	A-Inf	A-Infl	A-Mic	A-Par	A-Rhe	A-Sep	A-Spa	A-Vir	Analg	Imm
Sandalwood	+	+++	++	+						++	+			
Spearmint	+			++		++				+	+			
Spikenard	+			+	++	++		++		++				+
Spruce		+		+		+++	+		+	+				+
Tangerine														
Tarragon	++				++	++		+		+	++	++		
Thyme	+	+		+++			++	+	++	+	+			++
Valerian	+										++			
Vetiver					+					+	+			+
Idaho Tansy	++				++	++				+		++		+
Yarrow						++				++				
Ylang Ylang			+		+					+	+			

Glossary

A-Bac (Anti-bacterial): an agent which prevents the growth of, or destroys, bacteria.

A-Cat (Anti-catarrhal): an agent which helps remove excess catarrh from the body. Expectorants help promote the removal of mucus from the respiratory system.

A-Dep (Anti-depressant): an agent which helps alleviate depression.

A-Fun (Anti-fungal): an agent which prevents and combats fungal infection.

A-Inf (Anti-infectious): an agent which prevents and combats the spread of germs.

A-Infl (Anti-inflammatory): an agent which alleviates inflammation.

A-Mic (Antimicrobial): an agent which resists or destroys pathogenic micro-organisms.

A-Par (Anti-parasitic): an agent which prevents and destroys parasites.

A-Rhe (Anti-rheumatic): helps prevent and relieve rheumatism.

A-Sep (Antiseptic): destroys and prevents the development of microbes.

A-Spa (Antispasmodic): prevents and eases spasms or convulsions.

A-Vir (Anti-viral): a substance which inhibits the growth of a virus.

Analg (Analgesic): a substance which relieves pain.

Imm (Immune-stimulant): an agent which stimulates the natural defense mechanism of the body.

SINGLE OIL SUMMARY INFORMATION

The following chart displays summary information about each of the single oils, including: botanical name, safety data, and the products (blends, personal care products, bath and shower gels, tinctures, massage oils, and supplements) that contain the single oil. The safety data includes possible skin reactions and conditions during which use of that particular oil should be limited or completely avoided (refer to the legend following the Blend Summary Information). **Note:** This safety data is provided for **external use only!**

Single Oil Name	Botanical Name	Safety Data	Products containing Single Oil
Angelica	*Angelica archangelica* (Umbelliferae)	(GRAS), D, P, PH Dilute 1:1	Awaken, Forgiveness, Grounding, Harmony, Legacy, Live with Passion, Surrender
Anise	*Pimpinella anisum* (Umbelliferae)	(GRAS), CS Dilute 1:1	Awaken, Di-Gize, Dream Catcher, Allerzyme, Carbozyme, ComforTone, Detoxzyme, Digest + Cleanse, Essentialzyme, ICP, JuvaPower, JuvaSpice, Lipozyme, ParaFree, Polyzyme, Power Meal
Basil	*Ocimum basilicum* (Labiatae)	(GRAS), E*, P*, SI, Dilute 1:1	Aroma Siez, Clarity, Lazarus, Legacy, M-Grain, Sugar-Up Tincture
Bergamot	*Citrus bergamia* (Rutaceae)	(GRAS), CS*, PH* Dilute 1:1	Awaken, Clarity, Dream Catcher, Forgiveness, Gentle Baby, Harmony, Joy, Lady Flash, Lady Love, Legacy, White Angelica, Genesis Hand & Body Lotion, Prenolone, Prenolone+, Progessence, Rosewood Moisturizing Shampoo, Rosewood Moisturizing Conditioner, Sandalwood Moisture Creme, Joy Aqua Essence, Dragon Time Bath Gel, Evening Peace Bath Gel
Birch	*Betula alleghaniensis* (Betulaceae)	E*, P* Dilute 1:1	
Black Cumin	*Nigella sativa*		ParaFree
Buplevere	*Bupleurum fruticosum*		Legacy
Cajeput	*Melaleuca leucadendra* (Myrtaceae)	(FA/FL), SI Dilute 1:1	Legacy
Calamus	*Acorus calamus (Araceae)*	Dilute 1:4	Exodus II
Caraway	*Carum carvi* (Umbelliferae)	(GRAS), CS, SI, P* Dilute 1:1	Digest + Cleanse

Single Oil Name	Botanical Name	Safety Data	Products containing Single Oil
Cardamom	*Elettaria cardamomum* (Zingiberaceae)	(GRAS) Dilute 1:1	Clarity, Lazarus, Legacy, Transformation, Male-Pro Tincture, SE-6 Tincture
Carrot	*Daucus carota* (Umbelliferae)	(GRAS) Dilute 1:1	Legacy, Animal Scents Pet Ointment, Rose Ointment
Cassia	*Cinnamomum cassia* (Lauraceae)	(GRAS), CS*, SI*, Dilute 1:4	Exodus II
Cedar	*Cedrus canadensis* (Cupressaceae)		Evergreen Essence
Cedar, Western Red	*Thuja plicata* (Cupressaceae)	Dilute 1:1	Legacy, KidScents Lotion
Cedar Leaf	*Thuja occidentalis* (Cupressaceae)	Dilute 1:1	Legacy
Cedarwood	*Cedrus atlantica* (Pinaceae)	P	Australian Blue, Brain Power, Egyptian Gold, Grounding, Inspiration, Into the Future, Legacy, Live with Passion, Sacred Mountain, SARA, AromaGuard Deodorants, Essential Beauty Serums - Dry Skin Blend & Acne-Prone Skin Blend, KidScents Bath Gel, KidScents Lotion, Sacred Mountain Aqua Essence, Sacred Mountain Bar Soap, Peppermint Cedarwood Bar Soap, Cel-Lite Magic Massage Oil
Celery Seed	*Apium graveolens* (Umbeliferae)	(GRAS), CS, SI, P, Dilute 1:1	GLF, Juva Cleanse
Chamomile (German/ Blue)	*Matricaria chamomilla/ recutita* (Compositae)	(GRAS), P, SI	EndoFlex, Legacy, Surrender, K&B Tincture, ComforTone, JuvaTone, Omega Blue
Chamomile (Roman)	*Chamaemelum nobile* (Compositae)	(GRAS), SI	Clarity, Forgiveness, Gentle Baby, Harmony, Joy, JuvaFlex, Lady Flash, Lady Love, Legacy, M-Grain, Motivation, Surrender, ClaraDerm, Genesis Hand & Body Lotion, KidScents Tender Tush, Lemon Sage Clarifying Shampoo, Lemon Sage Clarifying Conditioner, Satin Hand & Body Lotion, Wolfberry Eye Creme, Joy Aqua Essence, Dragon Time Bath Gel, Evening Peace Bath Gel, Chelex Tincture, K&B Tincture, Rehemogen Tincture

Single Oil Name	Botanical Name	Safety Data	Products containing Single Oil
Cinnamon Bark	*Cinnamomum verum* (Lauraceae)	CS*, P*, SI* Dilute 1:4	Christmas Spirit, Egyptian Gold, Exodus II, Gathering, Lazarus, Legacy, Magnify Your Purpose, Thieves, Cinnamint Lip Balm, Fresh Essence Plus Mouthwash, Thieves Bar Soap, Anti-Cana Tincture, Mineral Essence
Cistus	*Cistus ladanifer* (Cistaceae)	(FA/FL), P	ImmuPower, Legacy, ImmuneTune, KidScents Tender Tush
Citronella	*Cymbopogon nardus* (Gramineae)	(GRAS), CS*, P, SI, Dilute 1:1	Legacy, Purification, Animal Scents Pet Shampoo
Clary Sage	*Salvia sclarea* (Labiatae)	(GRAS), A, P Dilute 1:1	Dragon Time, Into the Future, Lady Flash, Lady Love, Lady Sclareol, Legacy, Live with Passion, SclarEssence, Transformation, Lavender Volume Shampoo, Lavender Volume Conditioner, Prenolone, Prenolone+, Progessence Cream, Rosewood Moisturizing Shampoo, Rosewood Moisturizing Conditioner, Dragon Time Bath Gel, Evening Peace Bath Gel, Estro Tincture, FHS Tincture, Cel-Lite Magic Massage Oil, Dragon Time Massage Oil, CortiStop (Women's), FemiGen
Clove	*Syzygium aromaticum* (Myrtaceae)	(GRAS), CS*, P, SI Dilute 1:4	Abundance, En-R-Gee, ImmuPower, Legacy, Longevity, Melrose, PanAway, Thieves, AromaGuard Deodorants, Dentarome Plus Toothpaste, Essential Beauty Serum - Dry Skin Blend, Fresh Essence Plus Mouthwash, KidScents Toothpaste, Thieves Bar Soap, K&B Tincture, BLM, Essentialzyme, Longevity Capsules, Omega Blue, ParaFree
Coriander	*Coriandrum sativum* L. (Umbelliferae)	(GRAS), ST Dilute 1:1	Legacy
Cumin	*Cuminus cyminum* (Umbelliferae)	(GRAS), P, PH* Dilute 1:1	ImmuPower, Legacy, Detoxzyme, Protec
Cypress	*Cupressus sempervirens* (Cupressaceae)	P Dilute 1:1	Aroma Life, Aroma Siez, Lady Flash, Legacy, RC, HRT Tincture, Cel-Lite Magic Massage Oil, Bodygize, Power Meal, Super Cal
Cypress, Blue	*Callitris intratropica* (Cupressaceae)		Australian Blue, Brain Power, AromaGuard Deodorants, Essential Beauty Serum - Dry Skin Blend

Single Oil Name	Botanical Name	Safety Data	Products containing Single Oil
Davana	*Artemisia pallens* (Compositae)	(FA/FL), P Dilute 1:1	Trauma Life , Essential Beauty Serum - Oily Skin Blend
Dill	*Anethum graveolens* (Umbelliferae)	(GRAS), E Dilute 1:1	Legacy
Elemi	*Canarium luzonicum* (Burseraceae)	(FA/FL)	Legacy, Ortho Sport Massage Oil
Eucalyptus	*Eucalyptus globulus* (Myrtaceae)	(FA/FL) Dilute 1:1	Legacy, RC, Chelex Tincture, Ortho Sport Massage Oil
Eucalyptus Citriodora	*Eucalyptus citriodora* (Myrtaceae)	CS Dilute 1:1	Legacy, RC
Eucalyptus Dives	*Eucalyptus dives* (Myrtaceae)	Dilute 1:1	Legacy
Eucalyptus Polybractea	*Eucalyptus polybractea* (Myrtaceae)	Dilute 1:1	Legacy
Eucalyptus Radiata	*Eucalyptus radiata* (Myrtaceae)	Dilute 1:1	Legacy, Raven, RC, Thieves, Fresh Essence Plus Mouthwash, Thieves Bar Soap
Eucalyptus Staigeriana	*Eucalyptus staigeriana* (Myrtaceae)	Dilute 1:1	Essential Beauty Serum - Acne-Prone Skin Blend
Fennel	*Foeniculum vulgare* (Umbelliferae)	(GRAS), CS, E, P Dilute 1:1	Di-Gize, Dragon Time, JuvaFlex, Lady Flash, Legacy, Mister, SclarEssence, Allerzyme, Carbozyme, Detoxzyme, Essentialzyme, JuvaPower, JuvaSpice, Lipozyme, Prenolone, Prenolone+, Progessence Cream, Dragon Time Bath Gel, Estro Tincture, FHS Tincture, K&B Tincture, SE-6 Tincture, Sugar-Up Tincture, Dragon Time Massage Oil, CortiStop (Women's), Digest + Cleanse, FemiGen, ICP, ParaFree, Power Meal, ProGen
Fir	*Abies alba* (Pinaceae)	(FA/FL), SI Dilute 1:1	En-R-Gee, Grounding, Into the Future, ImmuneTune
Fir, Balsam (Idaho Balsam Fir)	*Abies balsamea* (Pinaceae)	(FA/FL), SI Dilute 1:1	Egyptian Gold, Legacy, Sacred Mountain, Transformation, Sacred Mountain Aqua Essence, Animal Scents Pet Ointment, Sacred Mountain Bar Soap, BLM
Fir, Douglas	*Pseudotsuga menziesii* (Pinaceae)	SI Dilute 1:1	Legacy, Regenolone
Fir, Red	*Abies magnifica* (Pinaceae)	SI Dilute 1:1	Evergreen Essence, Legacy

Single Oil Name	Botanical Name	Safety Data	Products containing Single Oil
Fir, White	*Abies grandis* (Pinaceae)	SI Dilute 1:1	Australian Blue, Believe, Evergreen Essence, Gratitude, Legacy
Fleabane	*Conyza canadensis* (Compositae)	Dilute 1:1	Legacy, CortiStop (Women's), Progessence Cream, ThermaBurn, Ultra Young, Ultra Young Plus
Frankincense	*Boswellia carteri* (Burseraceae)	(FA/FL)	Abundance, Acceptance, Believe, Brain Power, Egyptian Gold, Exodus II, Forgiveness, Gathering, Gratitude, Harmony, Humility, ImmuPower, Inspiration, Into the Future, Lazarus, Legacy, Longevity, 3 Wise Men, Transformation, Trauma Life, Valor, A·R·T Purifying Toner, Boswellia Wrinkle Creme, ClaraDerm, KidScents Tender Tush, Protec, Wolfberry Eye Creme, Valor Bar Soap, Valor Aqua Essence, CortiStop (Women's), Exodus, Longevity Capsules, ThermaBurn
Galbanum	*Ferula gummosa* (Umbelliferae)	(FA/FL)	Exodus II, Gathering, Gratitude, Legacy
Geranium	*Pelargonium graveolens* (Geraniaceae)	(GRAS), CS	Acceptance, Clarity, EndoFlex, Envision, Forgiveness, Gathering, Harmony, Humility, Joy, Joy Aqua Essence, JuvaFlex, Lady Flash, Lady Love, Lady Sclareol, Legacy, Release, SARA, Trauma Life, White Angelica, Animal Scents Pet Ointment, AromaGuard Deodorants, Boswellia Wrinkle Creme, Genesis Hand & Body Lotion, Lemon Sage Clarifying Shampoo, Lemon Sage Clarifying Conditioner, Prenolone, Prenolone+, Progessence Cream, Rosewood Moisturizing Shampoo, Rosewood Moisturizing Conditioner, Satin Hand & Body Lotion, Wolfberry Eye Creme, Animal Scents Pet Shampoo, Dragon Time Bath Gel, Evening Peace Bath Gel, KidScents Bath Gel, KidScents Lotion, Melaleuca Geranium Bar Soap, K&B Tincture, JuvaTone
Geranium, Rose	*Pelargonium x asperum* (Geraniaceae)		Gentle Baby

Single Oil Name	Botanical Name	Safety Data	Products containing Single Oil
Ginger	*Zingiber officinale* (Zingiberaceae	(GRAS), CS, PH Dilute 1:1	Abundance, Di-Gize, Lazarus, Legacy, Live with Passion, Magnify Your Purpose, Nerv-Cal Tincture, Allerzyme, Carbozyme, ComforTone, Digest + Cleanse, ICP, Lipozyme
Goldenrod	*Solidago canadensis* (Asteraceae)	Dilute 1:1	Legacy
Grapefruit	*Citrus x paradisi* (Rutaceae)	(GRAS) Dilute 1:1	Citrus Fresh, GLF, Legacy, Cel-Lite Magic Massage Oil, Bodygize, Power Meal, Super C
Helichrysum	*Helichrysum italicum* (Compositae)	(GRAS)	Aroma Life, Brain Power, Forgiveness, GLF, Juva Cleanse, JuvaFlex, Legacy, Live with Passion, M-Grain, PanAway, Trauma Life, ClaraDerm, Chelex Tincture, CardiaCare
Hyssop	*Hyssopus officinalis* (Labiatae)	(GRAS), E*, HBP*, P*, D-1:1	Egyptian Gold, Exodus II, GLF, Harmony, ImmuPower, Legacy, Relieve It, White Angelica, Exodus
Jasmine	*Jasminum officinale* (Oleaceae)	(GRAS)	Clarity, Dragon Time, Forgiveness, Gentle Baby, Harmony, Highest Potential, Inner Child, Into the Future, Joy, Lady Flash, Lady Love, Lady Sclareol, Legacy, Live with Passion, Sensation, Genesis Hand & Body Lotion, Lavender Volume Shampoo, Lavender Volume Conditioner, Satin Hand & Body Lotion, Sensation Hand & Body Lotion, Joy Aqua Essence, Dragon Time Bath Gel, Evening Peace Bath Gel, Sensation Bath Gel, Dragon Time Massage Oil, Sensation Massage Oil
Juniper	*Juniperus osteosperma* and/or *J. scopulorum* (Cupressaceae)	Dilute 1:1	Di-Gize, Dream Catcher, En-R-Gee, Grounding, Hope, Into the Future, Lazarus, Legacy, 3 Wise Men, Allerzyme, Carbozyme, Lipozyme, NeuroGen, Morning Start Bath Gel, Morning Start Bar Soap, K&B Tincture, Cel-Lite Magic Massage Oil, Ortho Ease Massage Oil
Laurel	*Laurus nobilis* (Lauraceae)	(GRAS), CS, P* Dilute 1:1	Legacy, Exodus, ParaFree
Lavandin	*Lavandula x hybrida* (Labiatae)	(GRAS), E, P*	Purification, Release, Animal Scents Pet Shampoo

Single Oil Name	Botanical Name	Safety Data	Products containing Single Oil
Lavender	*Lavandula angustifolia* CT linalol (Labiatae)		Aroma Siez, Brain Power, Dragon Time, Egyptian Gold, Envision, Forgiveness, Gathering, Gentle Baby, Harmony, Legacy, M-Grain, Mister, Motivation, RC, SARA, Surrender, Trauma Life, AromaGuard Deodorants, ClaraDerm, Essential Beauty Serum - Dry Skin Blend, LavaDerm Cooling Mist, Lavender Volume Shampoo, Lavender Volume Conditioner, KidScents Tender Tush, Orange Blossom Facial Wash, Sandalwood Moisture Creme, Wolfberry Eye Creme, Dragon Time Bath Gel, Lavender Rosewood Bar Soap, Estro Tincture, Dragon Time Massage Oil, Relaxation Massage Oil, ProGen
Ledum	*Ledum groenlandicum* (Ericaceae)		GLF, Juva Cleanse, Legacy
Lemon	*Citrus limon* (Rutaceae)	(GRAS), PH*, SI* Dilute 1:1	Citrus Fresh, Clarity, Forgiveness, Gentle Baby, Harmony, Joy, Lady Flash, Lady Love, Legacy, Raven, Surrender, Thieves, Transformation, A·R·T Purifying Toner, AromaGuard Deodorants, Genesis Hand & Body Lotion, Animal Scents Pet Shampoo, Fresh Essence Plus Mouthwash, KidScents Shampoo, Lavender Volume Shampoo, Lavender Volume Conditioner, Lemon Sage Clarifying Shampoo, Lemon Sage Clarifying Conditioner, Orange Blossom Facial Wash, Joy Aqua Essence, Dragon Time Bath Gel, Evening Peace Bath Gel, Thieves Bar Soap, Lemon Sandalwood Bar Soap, HRT Tincture, Ner-Vus Tincture, AlkaLime, Berry Young Juice, Bodygize, CardiaCare, Digest + Cleanse, ImmuneTune, JuvaTone, MegaCal, Mineral Essence, NingXia Red, Power Meal, Super C, Super C Chewable, VitaGreen, WheyFit
Lemongrass	*Cymbopogon flexuosus* (Gramineae)	(GRAS), SI* Dilute 1:4	Di-Gize, En-R-Gee, Inner Child, Lazarus, Legacy, Purification, Allerzyme, Carbozyme, Lipozyme, NeuroGen, Morning Start Bath Gel, Morning Start Bar Soap, Ortho Ease Massage Oil, Ortho Sport Massage Oil, Be-Fit, Bodygize, ICP, Omega Blue, VitaGreen

Single Oil Name	Botanical Name	Safety Data	Products containing Single Oil
Lime	*Citrus aurantifolia* (Rutaceae)	(GRAS), PH* Dilute 1:1	Legacy, Lemon Sage Clarifying Shampoo, Lemon Sage Clarifying Conditioner, AlkaLime, KidScents Mighty Vites, Super C
Limette (Combava)	Citrus hystrix (Rutaceae)	PH* Dilute1:1	Trauma Life
Mandarin	*Citrus reticulata* (Rutaceae)	(GRAS), PH Dilute 1:1	Citrus Fresh, Joy, Lady Love, Legacy, Joy Aqua Essence, Dragon Time Bath Gel, KidScents Mighty Vites, Super C
Manuka	*Leptospermum scoparium* (Myrtaceae)	Dilute 1:1	Essential Beauty Serum - Acne-Prone Skin Blend
Marjoram	*Origanum majorana* (Labiatae)	(GRAS), P Dilute 1:1	Aroma Life, Aroma Siez, Legacy, M-Grain, RC, Male-Pro Tincture, Ortho Ease Massage Oil, Ortho Sport Massage Oil, CardiaCare, Super Cal
Melaleuca (Tea Tree)	*Melaleuca alternifolia* (Myrtaceae)	(FA/FL), CS Dilute 1:1	Legacy, Melrose, Purification, Animal Scents Pet Ointment, AromaGuard Deodorants, ClaraDerm, Essential Beauty Serum - Acne-Prone Skin Blend, Rose Ointment, Melaleuca Geranium Bar Soap, Anti-Cana Tincture, Rehemogen Tincture, ParaFree
Melaleuca ericifolia (Rosalina)	*Melaleuca ericifolia* (Myrtaceae)	(FA/FL) Dilute 1:1	Legacy, Melaleuca Geranium Bar Soap
Melaleuca quinquenervia (Niaouli)	*Melaleuca quinquenervia* (Myrtaceae)	(FA/FL), CS Dilute 1:1	Melrose, AromaGuard Deodorants
Melissa	*Melissa officinalis* (Labiatae)	(GRAS)	Brain Power, Forgiveness, Hope, Humility, Legacy, Live with Passion, White Angelica, VitaGreen
Mountain Savory	*Satureja montana* (Labiatae)	(GRAS), P*, SI* Dilute 1:4	ImmuPower, Legacy, Surrender
Mugwort	*Artemisia vulgaris* (Asteraceae)	P* Dilute 1:1	FHS Tincture
Myrrh	*Commiphora myrrha* (Burseraceae)	(FA/FL), P	Abundance, Egyptian Gold, Exodus II, Gratitude, Hope, Humility, Legacy, 3 Wise Men, White Angelica, Animal Scents Pet Ointment, Boswellia Wrinkle Creme, ClaraDerm, Essential Beauty Serum - Dry Skin Blend, Protec, Rose Ointment, Sandalwood Moisture Creme, Omega Blue, Thyromin

Single Oil Name	Botanical Name	Safety Data	Products containing Single Oil
Myrtle	*Myrtus communis* (Myrtaceae)	Dilute 1:1	EndoFlex, Inspiration, Legacy, Mister, Purification, RC, JuvaTone, ProGen, ThermaBurn, Thyromin
Myrtle, Lemon	*Backhousia citriodora* (Myrtaceae)	CS, SI Dilute 1:4	
Neroli	*Citrus aurantium bigaradia* (Rutaceae)	(GRAS) Dilute 1:1	Acceptance, Humility, Inner Child, Legacy, Live with Passion, Present Time
Nutmeg	*Myristica fragrans* (Myristicaceae)	(GRAS), E*, P Dilute 1:2	EndoFlex, En-R-Gee, Legacy, Magnify Your Purpose, Essential Beauty Serum - Oily Skin Blend, Be-Fit, ParaFree, Power Meal, ThermaBurn
Onycha	*Styrax benzoin* (Styracaceae)	(FA/FL)	
Orange	*Citrus sinensis* (Rutaceae)	(GRAS), PH* Dilute 1:1	Abundance, Christmas Spirit, Citrus Fresh, Envision, Harmony, Inner Child, Lady Sclareol, Legacy, Longevity, Peace & Calming, SARA, Essential Beauty Serum - Oily Skin Blend, Peace & Calming Aqua Essence, Balance Complete, Berry Young Juice, Bodygize, ImmuneTune, ImmuPro, Longevity Capsules, Pure Protein Complete, KidScents Mighty Vites, NingXia Red, Power Meal, Super C
Oregano	*Origanum compactum* (Labiatae)	(GRAS), SI* Dilute 1:4	ImmuPower, Legacy, Regenolone, Ortho Sport Massage Oil
Palmarosa	*Cymbopogon martinii* (Gramineae)	(GRAS) Dilute 1:1	Clarity, Forgiveness, Gentle Baby, Harmony, Joy, Lady Flash, Lady Love, Legacy, Animal Scents Pet Ointment, Genesis Hand & Body Lotion, Rose Ointment, Joy Aqua Essence, Dragon Time Bath Gel, Evening Peace Bath Gel
Palo Santo	*Bursera graveolens* (Burseraceae)		
Patchouli	*Pogostemon cablin* (Labiatae)	(FA/FL)	Abundance, Di-Gize, Legacy, Live with Passion, Peace & Calming, Allerzyme, Carbozyme, Lipozyme, Peace & Calming Aqua Essence, Animal Scents Pet Ointment, Orange Blossom Facial Wash, Rose Ointment
Pepper, Black	*Piper nigrum* (Piperaceae)	(GRAS), SI* Dilute 1:1	Dream Catcher, En-R-Gee, Legacy, Relieve It, Cel-Lite Magic Massage Oil

Single Oil Name	Botanical Name	Safety Data	Products containing Single Oil
Pepper, Pink	*Schinus molle* (Anacardiaceae)	(GRAS), P* Dilute 1:1	Essential Beauty Serum - Oily Skin Blend
Peppermint	*Mentha piperita* (Labiatae)	(GRAS), CS, HBP, P Dilute 1:2	Aroma Siez, Clarity, Di-Gize, Lady Flash, Lazarus, Legacy, M-Grain, Mister, PanAway, Raven, RC, Relieve It, SclarEssence, Transformation, A·R·T Purifying Toner, Cinnamint Lip Balm, Dentarome/Dentarome Plus Toothpaste, Fresh Essence Plus Mouthwash, Mint Satin Facial Scrub, NeuroGen, Regenolone, Satin Hand & Body Lotion, Morning Start Bath Gel, Peppermint Cedarwood Bar Soap, Morning Start Bar Soap, Nerv-Cal Tincture, SE-6 Tincture, Ortho Ease Massage Oil, Ortho Sport Massage Oil, Relaxation Massage Oil, Allerzyme, Carbozyme, ComforTone, CortiStop (Women's), Digest + Cleanse, Essential Manna (Carob Mint Flavor), Essentialzyme, Lipozyme, Mineral Essence, Polyzyme, ProGen, Thyromin
Petitgrain	*Citrus aurantium* (Rutaceae)	(GRAS) Dilute 1:1	Legacy
Pine	*Pinus sylvestris* (Pinaceae)	(FA/FL), SI Dilute 1:1	Evergreen Essence, Grounding, Legacy, RC, Lemon Sage Clarifying Shampoo, Lemon Sage Clarifying Conditioner, Ner-Vus Tincture, ImmuneTune
Pine, Black	*Pinus nigra* (Pinaceae)	SI	Evergreen Essence
Pine, Lodge Pole	*Pinus contorta* (Pinaceae)	SI	Evergreen Essence
Pine, Piñon	*Pinus edulis* (Pinaceae)	SI	Evergreen Essence
Pine, Ponderosa (Yellow Pine)	*Pinus ponderosa* (Pinaceae)	SI	Evergreen Essence, Legacy
Ravensara	*Ravensara aromatica* (Lauraceae)		ImmuPower, Legacy, Raven, ImmuneTune
Rose (Bulgarian)	*Rosa damascena* (Rosaceae)	(GRAS), P	Egyptian Gold, Envision, Forgiveness, Gathering, Gentle Baby, Harmony, Humility, Joy, Joy Aqua Essence, Legacy, SARA, Trauma Life, White Angelica, Rose Ointment

Single Oil Name	Botanical Name	Safety Data	Products containing Single Oil
Rosehip	*Rosa canina* (Rosaceae)	(GRAS)	Legacy, Animal Scents Pet Ointment, Rose Ointment, Sandalwood Moisture Creme, Wolfberry Eye Creme
Rosemary Cineol	*Rosmarinus officinalis* CT 1,8 cineol (Labiatae)	(GRAS), E*, HBP*, P* Dilute 1:1	En-R-Gee, JuvaFlex, Legacy, Melrose, Purification, Thieves, Transformation, AromaGuard Deodorants, Fresh Essence Plus Mouthwash, Morning Start Bath Gel, Thieves Bar Soap, Morning Start Bar Soap, Anti-Cana Tincture, Chelex Tincture, Rehemogen Tincture, Sugar-Up Tincture, Be-Fit, ComforTone, ICP, JuvaTone, Polyzyme, VitaGreen
Rosemary Verbenon	*Rosmarinus officinalis* CT verbenon (Labiatae)	(GRAS), E*, HBP, P Dilute 1:1	Clarity, Orange Blossom Facial Wash, Sandalwood Moisture Creme
Rosewood	*Aniba rosaeodora* (Lauraceae)	(GRAS)	Acceptance, Believe, Clarity, Forgiveness, Gentle Baby, Gratitude, Harmony, Humility, Inspiration, Joy, Lady Flash, Lady Love, Lady Sclareol, Legacy, Magnify Your Purpose, Sensation, Valor, White Angelica, Animal Scents Pet Ointment, AromaGuard Deodorants, Genesis Hand & Body Lotion, KidScents Lotion, KidScents Tender Tush, Rose Ointment, Rosewood Moisturizing Shampoo, Rosewood Moisturizing Conditioner, Sandalwood Moisture Creme, Satin Hand & Body Lotion, Sensation Hand & Body Lotion, Wolfberry Eye Creme, Joy Aqua Essence, Valor Aqua Essence, Dragon Time Bath Gel, Evening Peace Bath Gel, Sensation Bath Gel, Lavender Rosewood Bar Soap, Valor Bar Soap, HRT Tincture, Relaxation Massage Oil, Sensation Massage Oil
Sage	*Salvia officinalis* (Labiatae)	(GRAS), E*, HBP*, P* Dilute 1:1	EndoFlex, Envision, Lady Flash, Lady Love, Legacy, Magnify Your Purpose, Mister, Progessence Cream, Protec, Lemon Sage Clarifying Shampoo, Lemon Sage Clarifying Conditioner, Dragon Time Bath Gel, K&B Tincture, Dragon Time Massage Oil, FemiGen, ProGen
Sage, Spanish (Sage Lavender)	*Salvia lavandulifolia* (Labiatae)	(GRAS) Dilute 1:1	Harmony, Lady Sclareol, SclarEssence

Single Oil Name	Botanical Name	Safety Data	Products containing Single Oil
Sandalwood	*Santalum album* (Santalaceae)	(FA/FL)	Acceptance, Brain Power, Dream Catcher, Forgiveness, Gathering, Harmony, Inner Child, Inspiration, Lady Sclareol, Legacy, Live with Passion, Magnify Your Purpose, Release, 3 Wise Men, Transformation, Trauma Life, White Angelica, A·R·T Purifying Toner, Boswellia Wrinkle Creme, Essential Beauty Serum - Dry Skin Blend, KidScents Tender Tush, Rosewood Moisturizing Shampoo, Rosewood Moisturizing Conditioner, Sandalwood Moisture Creme, Satin Hand & Body Lotion, Evening Peace Bath Gel, Lemon Sandalwood Bar Soap, SE-6 Tincture, Ultra Young, Ultra Young Plus
Spearmint	*Mentha spicata* (Labiatae)	(GRAS), P Dilute 1:2	Citrus Fresh, EndoFlex, GLF, Legacy, Cinnamint Lip Balm , Essential Beauty Serum - Oily Skin Blend, Fresh Essence Plus Mouthwash, Nerv-Cal Tincture, Ner-Vus Tincture, Relaxation Massage Oil, ThermaBurn, Thyromin
Spikenard	*Nardostachys jatamansi* (Valerianaceae)		Egyptian Gold, Exodus II, Humility, Legacy, Exodus, Animal Scents Pet Shampoo
Spruce	*Picea mariana* (Pinaceae)	(FA/FL) Dilute 1:1	Abundance, Christmas Spirit, Envision, Gathering, Grounding, Harmony, Hope, Inner Child, Inspiration, Legacy, Motivation, Present Time, RC, Relieve It, Sacred Mountain, Sacred Mountain Aqua Essence, Surrender, 3 Wise Men, Trauma Life, Valor, Valor Aqua Essence, White Angelica, Sacred Mountain Bar Soap, Valor Bar Soap
Spruce, Colorado Blue	*Picea pungens* (Pinaceae)		Evergreen Essence
Tangerine	*Citrus nobilis* (Rutaceae)	(GRAS) Dilute 1:1	Citrus Fresh, Dream Catcher, Inner Child, Legacy, Peace & Calming, KidScents Shampoo, Peace & Calming Aqua Essence, Relaxation Massage Oil, ComforTone
Tansy, Blue	*Tanacetum annum* (Compositae)	Dilute 1:1	Acceptance, Australian Blue, Dream Catcher, JuvaFlex, Legacy, Peace & Calming, Release, SARA, Valor, KidScents Shampoo, KidScents Tender Tush, Peace & Calming Aqua Essence, Valor Aqua Essence, Dragon Time Bath Gel, Evening Peace Bath Gel, Valor Bar Soap, JuvaTone

Single Oil Name	Botanical Name	Safety Data	Products containing Single Oil
Tansy, Idaho	*Tanacetum vulgare* (Compositae)	Dilute 1:1	ImmuPower, Into the Future, Lady Sclareol, Legacy, ParaFree
Tarragon	*Artemisia dracunculus* (Compositae)	(GRAS), E*, P* Dilute 1:1	Di-Gize, Legacy, Allerzyme, Carbozyme, ComforTone, ICP, Lipozyme, Essentialzyme
Thyme	*Thymus vulgaris* (Labiatae)	(GRAS), HBP Dilute 1:4	Longevity, Dentarome Plus Toothpaste, Essential Beauty Serum - Acne-Prone Skin Blend, KidScents Toothpaste, Rehemogen, Longevity Capsules, ParaFree
Thyme linalol	*Thymus vulgaris* CT Linalol (Labiatae)	(GRAS) Dilute 1:2	Legacy
Thyme, Red	*Thymus serpyllum* (Labiatae)	(GRAS)	Ortho Ease
Tsuga	*Tsuga canadensis* (Pinaceae)	(FA/FL), SI* Dilute 1:1	Legacy
Valerian	*Valeriana officinalis* (Valerianaceae)	(FA/FL), CS	Legacy, Trauma Life
Vetiver	*Vetiveria zizanoides* (Gramineae)	P	Lady Sclareol, Legacy, Fresh Essence Plus Mouthwash, Melaleuca Geranium Bar Soap, Ortho Ease Massage Oil, Ortho Sport Massage Oil, ParaFree
White Lotus	*Nymphaea lotus* (Nymphaeaceae)		SARA
Wintergreen	*Gaultheria procumbens* (Ericaceae)	E*, P* Dilute 1:2	Legacy, PanAway, Raven, Dentarome/ Dentarome Plus Toothpaste, Regenolone, Rosewood Moisturizing Shampoo, Rosewood Moisturizing Conditioner, Ortho Ease Massage Oil, Ortho Sport Massage Oil, Be-Fit, BLM, Super Cal
Yarrow	*Achillea millefolium* (Compositae)	CS, P Dilute 1:1	Dragon Time, Legacy, Mister, Prenolone/ Prenolone+, Progessence Cream, Dragon Time Massage Oil, ProGen

Single Oil Name	Botanical Name	Safety Data	Products containing Single Oil
Ylang Ylang	*Cananga odorata* (Annonaceae)	(GRAS), CS Dilute 1:1	Aroma Life, Australian Blue, Clarity, Dream Catcher, Forgiveness, Gathering, Gentle Baby, Gratitude, Grounding, Harmony, Highest Potential, Humility, Inner Child, Into the Future, Joy, Lady Flash, Lady Love, Lady Sclareol, Legacy, Motivation, Peace & Calming, Present Time, Release, Sacred Mountain, SARA, Sensation, White Angelica, Boswellia Wrinkle Creme, Genesis Hand & Body Lotion, Lemon Sage Clarifying Shampoo, Lemon Sage Clarifying Conditioner, Prenolone/Prenolone+, Progessence Cream, Satin Hand & Body Lotion, Sensation Hand & Body Lotion, Joy Aqua Essence, Peace & Calming Aqua Essence, Sacred Mountain Aqua Essence, Dragon Time Bath Gel, Evening Peace Bath Gel, Sensation Bath Gel, Sacred Mountain Bar Soap, HRT Tincture, Ner-Vus Tincture, SE-6 Tincture, Dragon Time Massage Oil, Relaxation Massage Oil, Sensation Massage Oil, CardiaCare, FemiGen

Safety Data Legend:

A	**Avoid** during and after consumption of **alcohol**
CS	Could possibly result in **contact sensitization** (redness or irritation of the skin due to repeated application of a substance) (rotate or use different oils)
CS*	Repeated use can result in **extreme contact sensitization** (rotate between different oils)
D	**Avoid** if **diabetic**
E	Use with **caution** if susceptible to **epilepsy** (small amounts or in dilution)
E*	**Avoid** if susceptible to **epilepsy** (can trigger a seizure)
HBP	Use with **caution** if dealing with **high blood pressure** (small amounts)
HBP*	**Avoid** if dealing with **high blood pressure**
P	Use with **caution** during **pregnancy** (small amounts or in dilution)
P*	**Avoid** during **pregnancy**
PH	**Photosensitivity**–direct exposure to sunlight after use could cause dermatitis (test first)
PH*	**Extreme Photosensitivity**–direct exposure to sunlight after use can cause severe dermatitis (avoid exposing affected area of skin to direct sunlight for 12 hours)
SI	Could possibly result in **skin irritation** (dilution may be necessary)
SI*	Can cause **extreme skin irritation** (dilution highly recommended)
ST	Can cause **stupification** in high doses (use only small amounts or in dilution)

Dilute - Dilution ratios shown equal Essential Oil:Vegetable Oil

BLEND SUMMARY INFORMATION

The following chart displays summary information about each of the oil blends, including: single oils contained in the blend, possible uses or areas of application, and safety data. The safety data includes possible skin reactions and conditions during which use of that particular blend should be limited or completely avoided (refer to the legend following the chart). **Note:** This safety data is provided for **external use only!**

Blend Name	Single Oil Contents	Uses/Application Areas	Safety Data
Abundance	Myrrh, frankincense, patchouli, orange, clove, ginger, spruce	Diffuse; Wrists, ears, neck, face; Wallet/Purse; Painting; Perfume	CS*, SI Dilute 1:1
Acceptance	Geranium, Blue tansy, frankincense, sandalwood, neroli, rosewood (Carrier: Almond oil)	Diffuse; *Liver*, heart, *chest*, face, ears, neck, thymus, wrists; Sacral chakra; Perfume	
Aroma Life	Cypress, marjoram, helichrysum, ylang ylang (Carrier: Sesame seed oil)	Heart; Vita Flex heart points—under left ring finger, under left ring toe, above left elbow, arteries; Spine	
Aroma Siez	Basil, marjoram, lavender, peppermint, cypress	Muscles; Neck; Heart; Vita Flex points; Full body massage; Bath	Dilute 1:1
Australian Blue	Blue cypress, ylang ylang, cedarwood, Blue tansy, White fir	Diffuse; Perfume; Forehead	CS, SI
Awaken	Oil Blends of Joy, Forgiveness, Dream Catcher, Present Time, Harmony	Diffuse; Chest, heart, *forehead*, neck, temples, wrists; Perfume; Full body massage; Bath	
Believe	Balsam fir, rosewood, frankincense	Diffuse; *Heart, forehead, temples*; Perfume	Dilute 1:1
Brain Power	Cedarwood, sandalwood, frankincense, melissa, Blue cypress, lavender, helichrysum	Diffuse; Neck, throat, nose; Inside of cheeks; Perfume	
Chivalry	Oil Blends of Valor, Joy, Harmony, Gratitude	Diffuse; *Heart, forehead, temples*; Perfume	Dilute 1:1
Christmas Spirit	Orange, cinnamon bark, spruce	Diffuse; Crown; Perfume; Place on pine boughs or fireplace logs; Add to potpourri	CS*, SI* Dilute 1:1
Citrus Fresh	Orange, tangerine, mandarin, grapefruit, lemon, spearmint	Diffuse; Ears, heart wrists; Perfume; Full body massage; Bath; Purify drinking water	SI*, PH* Dilute 1:1
Clarity	Basil, cardamom, rosemary verbenon, peppermint, rosewood, geranium, lemon, palmarosa, ylang ylang, bergamot, Roman chamomile, jasmine	Diffuse; Forehead, neck, temples, wrists; Perfume; Bath	SI, P, PH*

Blend Name	Single Oil Contents	Uses/Application Areas	Safety Data
Di-Gize	Tarragon, ginger, peppermint, juniper, anise, fennel, lemongrass, patchouli	Vita Flex points—feet and ankles; stomach; abdomen, bottom of throat; Compress	P, E
Dragon Time	Clary sage, fennel, lavender, jasmine, yarrow	Vita Flex points; Diffuse; Abdomen, lower back, location	P
Dream Catcher	Sandalwood, bergamot, ylang ylang, juniper, Blue tansy, tangerine, Black pepper, anise	Diffuse; Forehead, eye brows, *temples*, ears, throat chakra; Perfume; Pillow; Bath or sauna	PH
Egyptian Gold	Frankincense, lavender, Balsam fir, myrrh, spikenard, hyssop, cedarwood, rose, cinnamon bark	Diffuse; Wrists, ears, neck, temples; Perfume	SI, E Dilute 1:4
En-R-Gee	Rosemary cineol, juniper, nutmeg, fir, Black pepper, lemongrass, clove	Diffuse; Wrists, ears, neck, temples, feet; Full body massage; Perfume	SI*, E Dilute 1:1
EndoFlex	Spearmint, sage, geranium, myrtle, nutmeg, German chamomile (Carrier: Sesame seed oil)	Thyroid, kidneys, liver, pancreas, glands; Vita Flex points	SI, E
Envision	Spruce, sage, rose, geranium, orange, lavender	Vita Flex points; Diffuse; Wrists, *temples*; Bath; Massage	HBP, E, P
Evergreen Essence	Colorado Blue spruce (*Picea pungens*), Ponderosa pine (*Pinus ponderosa*), pine, Red fir (*Abies magnifica*), cedar (*Cedrus canadensis*), White fir, Black pine (*Pinus nigra*), Pin: on pine (*Pinus edulis*), Lodge Pole pine (*Pinus contorta*)	*Diffuse*; Hands, bottoms of feet	CS, SI Dilute 1:1
Exodus II	Cinnamon bark, cassia, calamus, myrrh, hyssop, frankincense, spikenard, galbanum (Carrier: Olive oil)	Vita Flex points; Spine (dilute well)	CS*, SI*, P* Dilute 1:1
Forgiveness	Frankincense, sandalwood, lavender, melissa, angelica, helichrysum, rose, rosewood, geranium, lemon, palmarosa, ylang ylang, bergamot, Roman chamomile, jasmine (Carrier: Sesame seed oil)	Diffuse; *Navel*, heart, ears, wrists; Perfume	
Gathering	Galbanum, frankincense, sandalwood, lavender, cinnamon bark, rose, spruce, geranium, ylang ylang	Diffuse; *Forehead, heart, temples*, neck, thymus, face, chest; Perfume	
Gentle Baby	Rose geranium, rosewood, palmarosa, lavender, Roman chamomile, ylang ylang, rose, lemon, bergamot, jasmine	Diffuse; Ankles, lower back, abdomen, feet, face, neck; Massage; Perfume; Bath	

Blend Name	Single Oil Contents	Uses/Application Areas	Safety Data
GLF	Grapefruit, helichrysum, celery seed, ledum, hyssop, spearmint.	Liver; Vita Flex points on feet	
Gratitude	Balsam fir, frankincense, rosewood, myrrh, galbanum, ylang ylang	Diffuse; *Heart, forehead, temples*; Perfume	Dilute 1:1
Grounding	Juniper, angelica, ylang ylang, cedarwood, pine, spruce, fir	Diffuse; *Brain stem, back of neck, sternum*, temples	SI
Harmony	Hyssop, spruce, lavender, frankincense, geranium, ylang ylang, orange, sandalwood, angelica, sage lavender, rose, rosewood, lemon, palmarosa, bergamot, Roman chamomile, jasmine	Diffuse; Each chakra; Ears, feet, heart; *Energy meridians*, crown; Perfume	P, E*, HBP, PH
Highest Potential	Oil Blends of Australian Blue, Gathering, and Single Oils of ylang ylang and jasmine	Diffuse; *Heart, forehead, temples*; Perfume	Dilute 1:1
Hope	Melissa, myrrh, juniper, spruce (Carrier: Almond oil)	Diffuse; *Ears*; Chest, heart, temples, solar plexus, neck, feet, wrists; Perfume	
Humility	Geranium, ylang ylang, frankincense, spikenard, myrrh, rose, rosewood, melissa, neroli (Carrier: Sesame seed oil)	Diffuse; *Heart, neck, temples*	
ImmuPower	Cistus, frankincense, hyssop, ravensara, Mountain savory, oregano, clove, cumin, Idaho tansy	Diffuse; Throat, chest, spine, feet; Thymus; Veins in neck, under arm pits	SI, P, E Dilute 1:1
Inner Child	Orange, tangerine, jasmine, ylang ylang, spruce, sandalwood, lemongrass, neroli	Diffuse; *Navel, chest, temples, nose*	SI
Inspiration	Cedarwood, spruce, rosewood, sandalwood, frankincense, myrtle, mugwort	Diffuse; *Horns*, crown, shoulders, back of neck	
Into the Future	Frankincense, jasmine, Clary sage, juniper, Idaho tansy, fir, ylang ylang (Carrier: Almond oil)	Diffuse; Bath; Heart, wrists, neck; Compress; Full body massage	
Joy	Lemon, mandarin, bergamot, ylang ylang, rose, rosewood, geranium, palmarosa, Roman chamomile, jasmine	Diffuse; *Heart*, ears, neck, thymus, temples, forehead, wrists; Bath; Compress; Massage; Perfume	PH*
Juva Cleanse	Helichrysum, celery seed, ledum	Liver; Vita Flex points on feet	SI

Blend Name	Single Oil Contents	Uses/Application Areas	Safety Data
JuvaFlex	Fennel, geranium, rosemary cineol, Roman chamomile, Blue tansy, helichrysum (Carrier: Sesame seed oil)	Vita Flex points; Feet, spine, LIVER; Full body massage	SI Dilute 1:1
Lady Flash	Geranium, fennel, sage, Clary sage, ylang ylang, peppermint, cypress, jasmine, Roman chamomile, bergamot, rosewood, lemon, palmarosa	Vita Flex points; Feet, ankles; Compress over abdomen	PH
Lady Love	Mandarin, bergamot, palmarosa, geranium, sage, Clary sage, ylang ylang, jasmine, Roman chamomile, rosewood, lemon	Massage; Bath; Compress over abdomen; Diffuse; *Perfume*	PH
Lady Sclareol	Rosewood, vetiver, geranium, orange, Clary sage, ylang ylang, sandalwood, sage lavender, jasmine, Idaho tansy	On Location (by male partner); Massage; Bath; Compress over abdomen; Diffuse, *Perfume*	
Lazarus	Peppermint, cardamom, basil, ginger, juniper, frankincense, cinnamon, lemongrass	Feet, heart; Diffuse, Perfume or cologne	CS, SI, Dilute 1:4
Legacy	(See LEGACY in Blend section for complete list of 90 single oils)	Diffuse; Forehead, wrists, sternum, feet; Perfume	CS, SI Dilute 1:4
Live with Passion	Melissa, helichrysum, Clary sage, cedarwood, angelica, ginger, neroli, sandalwood, patchouli, jasmine	Wrists, *temples, chest, forehead*; Bath; Perfume or cologne	
Longevity	Thyme, orange, clove, frankincense	Internally as Dietary Supplement;	CS, SI, PH Dilute 1:4
M-Grain	Basil, marjoram, lavender, peppermint, Roman chamomile, helichrysum	DIFFUSE; Forehead, crown, shoulders, neck, temples; Vita Flex points; Massage	Dilute 1:1
Magnify Your Purpose	Sandalwood, nutmeg, rosewood, cinnamon bark, ginger, sage	Vita Flex points; Feet, wrists, *temples*; Diffuse; Bath; Massage	E, P, CS, SI
Melrose	Melaleuca (*alternifolia* & *quin-quenervia*), rosemary cineol, clove	Diffuse; Forehead, liver; Topically on location	CS, SI Dilute 1:1
Mister	Sage, fennel, lavender, myrtle, yarrow, peppermint (Carrier: Sesame seed oil)	Vita Flex points; Ankles, lower pelvis, prostate (dilute); Compress	P*, E
Motivation	Roman chamomile, ylang ylang, spruce, lavender	Diffuse; Chest, neck; *Solar plexus*, sternum, feet, navel, ears; wrists, palms; Perfume	
PanAway	Wintergreen, helichrysum, clove, peppermint	Compress on spine; Vita Flex on feet; Topically on location	Dilute 1:1

Blend Name	Single Oil Contents	Uses/Application Areas	Safety Data
Peace & Calming	Tangerine, orange, ylang ylang, patchouli, Blue tansy	Diffuse; Navel, nose, neck, feet; Bath; Perfume	PH
Present Time	Neroli, spruce, ylang ylang (Carrier: Almond oil)	*Thymus*; Neck, forehead	
Purification	Citronella, lemongrass, rosemary cineol, melaleuca, lavandin, myrtle	Diffuse; Vita Flex points; Ears, feet, temples; Topically on location	CS, SI
Raven	Ravensara, *Eucalyptus radiata*, peppermint, wintergreen, lemon	Diffuse; Vita Flex points; Lungs, throat; Pillow; Suppository (diluted)	SI Dilute 1:1
RC	4 eucalyptuses (E. globulus, E. radiata, E. australiana, E. citriodora), myrtle, marjoram, pine, cypress, lavender, spruce, peppermint	DIFFUSE; Chest, back, feet; Sinuses, nasal passages; Ears, neck, throat; Compress; Massage	
Release	Ylang ylang, lavandin, geranium, sandalwood, Blue tansy (Carrier: Olive oil)	*Compress on liver*; Ears, feet, Vita Flex points; Perfume	Dilute 1:1
Relieve It	Spruce, Black pepper, hyssop, peppermint	Apply on location of pain	SI, P, E, HBP Dilute 1:1
Sacred Mountain	Spruce, ylang ylang, Balsam fir, cedarwood	Diffuse; *Solar plexus, brain stem,* crown, neck, ears, thymus, wrists; Perfume	SI
SARA	Blue tansy, rose, lavender, geranium, orange, cedarwood, ylang ylang, White lotus (Carrier: Almond oil)	*Energy centers*; Vita Flex points; *Temples, nose*; Places of abuse	
SclarEssence	Clary sage, peppermint, sage lavender, fennel	Internally as Dietary Supplement	
Sensation	Rosewood, ylang ylang, jasmine	Diffuse; Apply on location; Massage; Bath	
Surrender	Lavender, Roman chamomile, German chamomile, angelica, Mountain savory, lemon, spruce	*Forehead, rim of ears, nape of neck, chest, solar plexus*; Bath	P, SI
Thieves	Clove, lemon, cinnamon bark, *Eucalyptus radiata*, rosemary cineol	Diffuse; Feet, throat, stomach, intestines; Thymus, arm pits (Dilute well for topical uses!)	CS*, SI*, P Dilute 1:4
3 Wise Men	Sandalwood, juniper, frankincense, spruce, myrrh (Carrier: Almond oil)	Diffuse; *Crown of head*; Neck, forehead, solar plexus, thymus; Perfume	
Transformation	Lemon, peppermint, sandalwood, frankincense, Clary sage, Balsam fir, rosemary cineol, cardamom	Diffuse; *Forehead, heart*	

Blend Name	Single Oil Contents	Uses/Application Areas	Safety Data
Trauma Life	*Citrus hystrix* (Leech Lime), davana, geranium, spruce, helichrysum, rose, sandalwood, frankincense, lavender, valerian	Diffuse; Spine; Feet, chest, ears, neck, forehead	
Valor	Spruce, rosewood, Blue tansy, frankincense (Carrier: Almond oil)	*FEET*; Diffuse; Heart, wrists, solar plexus, neck to thymus, spine; Perfume	
White Angelica	Geranium, spruce, myrrh, ylang ylang, hyssop, bergamot, melissa, sandalwood, rose, rosewood (Carrier: Almond oil)	Diffuse; *Shoulders*, crown, chest, ears, neck, forehead, wrists; Bath; Perfume	PH*

Note: Italicized application areas represent the most effective areas for **emotional applications**. Refer to the safety data legend shown previously (following the Single Oil Summary Information chart).

GLOSSARY OF TERMS

Topic	Definition
Topic	**Definition**
Acne	Acne is a blockage of a skin pore by dead skin cells, tiny hairs, and oil secreted by the sebaceous glands located near hair follicles in the face, neck, and back. This blockage occurs deep within the skin. Acne is not caused by dirt on the face or by eating certain foods. Over scrubbing the face may actually make acne worse. For more information, visit the website of the American Academy of Dermatologists at www.aad.org, or the National Institute of Arthritis and Musculoskeletal and Skin Diseases at http://www.niams.nih.gov/hi/topics/acne/acne.htm.
ADD/ADHD	Attention Deficit Disorder or Attention Deficit/Hyperactive Disorder is a psychological condition characterized by inattentiveness, restlessness, and difficulty concentrating. For more information, visit www.help4adhd.org/
Alcoholism	Alcoholism is an increasing dependency on alcohol that interferes with health, career, or family and social interactions. This problem affects between 5-10% of all people who use alcohol. Alcoholism has also been defined as any irresponsible drinking (such as binge drinking, or drunk driving).
Allergies	An allergy is an immune response to a harmless substance that most people don't react to. Allergies can cause sneezing, stuffy or runny noses, hives, itching, red eyes, breathing problems, stomach cramps, or vomiting.
Alopecia Areata	Alopecia Areata is an autoimmune disease where the body's immune system attacks fast-growing cells in the hair follicles, causing patches of hair, or all of the hair to fall out. For more information, visit the National Institute of Arthritis and Musculoskeletal and Skin Diseases: http://www.niams.nih.gov/hi/topics/alopecia/alopecia.htm
Analgesic	A substance that acts as a pain reliever
Anemia	Anemia is a lack of red blood cells in the body resulting in weakness and impaired motor and mental development. It is most common in infants and small children and is often (although not always) caused by a deficiency of iron in the diet. For more information, visit www.cdc.gov.
Aneurysm	A swelling or dilation of a blood vessel in the area of a weakened blood vessel wall.
Anorexia	A psychological disorder where an individual is addicted to depriving themselves of food.
Arteriosclerosis	A thickening or hardening of the artery walls due to high blood pressure, calcification, or fatty deposits.
Arthritis	Arthritis is any painful swelling of a joint.
Asthma	Asthma is a disease that causes the lung's airways to narrow, making it difficult to breath. Episodes (or attacks) of asthma can be triggered by any number of things, including smoke, pollution, dust mites, and other allergens. For more information, visit www.cdc.gov/nceh/airpollution/asthma/faqs.htm
Autism	Autism is a disorder caused by an abnormality in the brain which makes it difficult for an individual to communicate or interact with other people. For more information, visit www.cdc.gov/ncbddd/dd/ddautism.htm
Baldness	Baldness is usually caused by the hair follicles in the scalp failing to replace the hair when it falls out. This failure to replace the hairs is typically attributed to either aging, hormone imbalance, or an increase in the male hormone testosterone.
Boils	Boils (furuncles) are infections of the upper layers of the skin by staphylococcus or streptococcus bacteria. These infections often become filled with pus and dead cells, causing painful pea to golf ball sized swellings
Bronchitis	Inflammation of the bronchi (the tubes that lead from the trachea to the lungs).
Bruises	A bruise is an injury to tissue that results in blood capillaries breaking and spilling blood into the tissue.
Bulimia	Bulimia is a chronic psychological desire to purge the body of recently eaten foods either through vomiting or through the abuse of laxatives.
Calluses	A callus is a thickening of the outer layer of skin in a small area caused by friction or rubbing. Calluses can sometimes lead to serious infections.
Cancer	Cancer is when damaged or abnormal DNA causes a cell to divide out of control, resulting in clumps of rapidly dividing cells, or tumors, within healthy tissue.
Cataracts	A cataract is a clouding of the lens of an eye, causing blurriness, double-vision, or blindness. Cataracts can be caused by medications, injury, disease, or the natural aging process.
Catarrh	Chronic inflammation of the mucus membranes in the nose and throat.

Cellulite	Fat deposits.
Charley Horse	A Charley horse, or painful muscle spasm in the calf, is often caused by overuse, dehydration, or a lack of potassium, sodium, calcium, or magnesium in the body. Stretching the muscle and applying an initial hot compress, followed by a cold compress or ice pack once the pain starts to subside can often alleviate the pain associated with a muscle spasm.
Chiggers	Chiggers are the parasitic larvae of certain types of mites found in wooded areas, or areas of high grass. When chiggers bite, they cause red, severely itching bumps to appear.
Cholera	Cholera is a bacterial illness that can cause severe diarrhea, vomiting, and leg cramps. The most important treatment for cholera is to re-hydrate the body by drinking large amounts of an oral rehydration solution. (In an emergency when no commercially prepared re-hydration solution is available, mix 6 tsp. sugar, ½ tsp. salt, and 1 liter of water and drink.)
Chorea	Involuntary twisting, jumping, dancing, or other coordinated body movements that interfere with normal movement. Often caused by a previous strep (streptococcus) infection. A sign of rheumatic fever.
Colic	Periods of loud crying in young infants that seem to be caused by pain in the abdomen.
Colitis	Inflammation of the large intestine.
Conjunctivitis	Also called "pinkeye" or "red eye", conjunctivitis is an inflammation of the membrane that covers the whites of the eyes and the inside of the eyelid due to infection, allergies, or irritation.
Convulsions	Uncontrolled rapid contracting and relaxing of muscles, usually caused by a seizure (sudden random electrical activity in the brain).
Corns	A small, sometimes painful, callus caused by the friction between a bone and an outside pressure (such as a shoe) on the intermediate tissues.
Cortisone	A natural hormone created in the outer layers of the adrenal gland that has anti-inflammatory and anti-arthritic properties. Cortisone has also been synthetically developed as a drug for rheumatoid arthritis.
Crohn's Disease	A disease that causes chronic ulceration (either mild or severe) of the large and sometimes the small intestine.
Cushing's Disease	(or Cushing Syndrome) describes many different symptoms (including weight gain, weakness, bruising, & osteoporosis) caused by an overabundance of the cortisol hormone. This disease is often caused by taking artificial cortisone or cortisone-like substances
Cystic Fibrosis	Cystic fibrosis is a potentially deadly genetic disease that causes an excess of mucus to build up, inhibiting pancreas function and slowly clogging the airways.
Dermatitis	Dermatitis is redness, itching or soreness of the skin caused either by an allergic reaction or contact with a skin irritant.
Diaper Rash	Irritation of the skin in the area covered by the diaper caused by infection, sweat, friction, or allergic reactions.
Diphtheria	Diphtheria is a rare bacterial infection that causes sore throat, low fevers, and swelling of the neck and throat that can possibly lead to airway obstruction and other complications.
Diuretic	Any substance that causes an increase in the amount of urine created by the body.
Down Syndrome	Down Syndrome is a genetic condition characterized by an extra chromosome 21. This extra chromosome causes the formation of various distinguishing physical attributes, and slight to severe mental disabilities or retardation.
Dysentery	Dysentery is a painful intestinal inflammation due to an infection of the intestine by an ameba, causing severe cramping, diarrhea, vomiting, and bloody stools. Rehydration is critical to anyone suffering from dysentery.
Eczema	Itchy or painful patches of inflamed skin caused by allergic reactions, irritating substances, infection, or disease.
Edema	A swelling in the body caused by the accumulation of water, blood, or other fluids.
Electrolytes	Any substance that acquires the ability to conduct electricity when it is dissolved in a solution. Sodium, calcium, and potassium are three electrolytic substances that play an important role in the body. Low levels of any of these substances in the blood can lead to muscle cramps and other problems.
Emphysema	Damaged or burst air sacs in the lungs caused by smoking or a long-lasting lung infection.
Enzymes	An enzyme is any biological agent that mediates the speed or frequency of chemical reactions.
Fatigue	Being unable to work or think at full capacity.
Fiber	Complex carbohydrates that cannot be digested by the body. Fiber serves to help clean the colon and regulate bowel movements. Fiber can be found in fruits, vegetables, whole grain breads and cereals.
Fibroids	A benign tumor found in the uterus that can cause pain, reproductive problems, or heavy menstrual bleeding.

Fever	A fever is defined as any body temperature above 98.6 degrees F. A fever is the body's natural way of fighting disease (many pathogens cannot survive, or are weakened in these elevated temperatures). High fevers (over 104 degrees F.), however, can cause convulsions and other undesired effects.
Fibrositis	(See Fibromyalgia)
Flu	(See also Influenza) Any of several viral diseases that cause fever, nausea, fatigue, soreness, impaired breathing, and other cold-like symptoms.
Gangrene	Localized decay of body tissue caused by a loss of blood to that area. Gas gangrene is caused by bacteria invading a deep wound that has lessened the blood supply, or cut it off entirely. The bacteria create gases and pus in the infected area, causing severe pain and accelerating decay of the tissue
Gingivitis	A gum disease that results in sore gums that bleed easily. This condition can sometimes be corrected with more frequent/longer brushing and flossing.
Glaucoma	Glaucoma is an increasing eye pressure caused by a slowing in fluid drainage from the eye. Glaucoma can cause damage to the optical nerve or loss of sight over time.
Goiter	An enlarged thyroid gland. Goiter is often attributed to a deficiency of iodine in the body (found in iodized salts). While this is one possible cause, goiter is often a symptom of any of several diseases or conditions.
Gout	Gout is a painful inflammation of a joint caused by a buildup of uric acid crystals deposited in the joint. Uric acid is formed during the natural breakdown of dead tissues in the body. An excess of uric acid in the bloodstream can lead to the formation of crystals in the joints or kidneys (kidney stones). Some good ways to prevent the formation of uric acid crystals include maintaining a healthy body weight (which leaves less body tissue to be broken down), exercise, and drinking plenty of water.
Grave's Disease	Toxicity of the thyroid gland which leads to goiter, an autoimmune skin disease, and an eye disease that often causes bulging of the eyes.
Hashimoto's Disease	An autoimmune disease of the thyroid gland, leading to goiter and a decreased ability of the thyroid to produce essential hormones.
Heartburn	A burning pain in the chest caused by stomach acid rising up into the esophagus.
Hemorrhaging	Any internal or external bleeding.
Hepatitis	Hepatitis is a liver disease caused by one of five different Hepatitis viruses. The symptoms and seriousness of the disease depend on the type of virus causing the disease. www.cdc.gov/ncidod/diseases/hepatitis/
Hernia	A hernia is the protrusion of any tissue or organ outside of the cavity in which it is normally contained.
High Blood Pressure	Blood pressure that is consistently higher than 140 over 90. Chronic high blood pressure can cause severe health problems. High blood pressure can often be reduced by losing weight if overweight, cutting back on salty foods, and regular exercise.
Hodgkin's Disease	Hodgkin disease is a cancer that develops in the lymph system, causing enlarged lymph nodes, fever, sweating, fatigue, and loss of weight.
Inflammation	Inflammation is the body's response to infection, irritation, or injury in a localized area. The tissue becomes inflamed due to dilation of the blood vessels (which allows greater blood flow into the affected area).
Insomnia	Lack of adequate sleep. Insomnia is caused by a variety of factors, including stress, disease, the environment, overuse of caffeine and other stimulants, and changes in sleeping times or behaviors.
Irritable Bowel Syndrome	Chronically irregular bowel movements that result in frequent bouts of constipation and diarrhea.
Jet Lag	Jet lag is caused by the hypothalamus (the body's internal clock) trying to re-adjust the body's schedule to differing environmental cues (such as when the sun rises) after a person has traveled rapidly across different time zones.
Laryngitis	Inflammation of the larynx due to viral or bacterial infection. Often causes hoarseness, or voice loss.
Lice	Lice are any of three varieties of small, parasitic insects that are found either on the head, body, or pubic hair. Lice can be passed to another person through personal contact or by sharing bed linens, clothing, hats, hair ribbons, scarves, combs or brushes.
Lou Gehrig's Disease	Lou Gehrig's disease (or ALS) is caused by the atrophy of certain nerve cells in the body that control voluntary movement. This atrophy leads to weakness in the muscles controlled by these nerve cells. Lou Gehrig's disease usually leads to death within several years due to opportunistic infections overcoming an already weakened body.
Lyme Disease	Lyme disease is a disease caused by an infection of B. Burgdorferi bacteria transmitted by the bite of a deer tick. Symptoms of Lyme disease include a red circular rash, arthritis, neurological problems, and possible heart

irregularities. For more information on Lyme disease, visit:
www.niaid.nih.gov/publications/lyme/contents.htm

Malaria	Malaria is a disease caused by one of four types of parasites transmitted to humans from several species of mosquitoes. Symptoms can include muscle pains, headaches, fevers, sweating, and chills. More serious cases involve anemia and kidney failure that can lead to death. www.cdc.gov/malaria/
Melanoma	A type of malignant skin cancer that presents itself as a rapidly growing/spreading, irregularly shaped mole. This type of cancer can be very dangerous if not detected and treated early.
Menopause	The natural cessation of menstruation in women associated with a decline in the ovary hormones estrogen and progesterone.
Metabolism	The entire range of chemical processes that build up and break down substances within the body.
Migraine Headaches	A throbbing headache caused by spasms in the brain's blood vessels. Sometimes accompanied by an "aura"—perception of lights, or sounds that do not exist.
Mold	Mold is a type of fungus that grows in damp, warm conditions. The CDC recommends using a weak bleach solution (1 part bleach, 10 parts water) to remove any mold growths within the house. www.cdc.gov/nceh/airpollution/mold/moldfacts.htm
Mononucleosis	Mononucleosis—an illness characterized by fever, sore throat, fatigue, and swollen lymph nodes—is caused by an infection of the Epstein-Barr virus during adolescence or early adulthood. The Epstein-Barr virus is very common in humans (it can be found in 95% of people over the age of 40), and many people acquire the virus with few or no symptoms during infancy and early childhood. When an individual acquires the virus during adolescence and early adulthood, it can sometimes develop into mononucleosis (about 35-50% of the time). www.cdc.gov/ncidod/diseases/ebv.htm
Mumps	Mumps is a viral disease that causes fever, sore muscles, headache, and swelling of the lymph nodes by the jaw. www.cdc.gov/nip/diseases/mumps/default.htm
Muscular Dystrophy	Any of several genetic diseases that cause gradual weakening of the skeletal muscles.
Myelin Sheath	The myelin sheath is the fatty protective layer that surrounds the nerve fibers allowing nerve cells to transmit their signals properly. It is composed of lipids (70%), and proteins (30%). It is produced by oligodendrocyte cells surrounding the nerve fibers.
Neuritis	Inflammation of the nerve cells.
Neuropathy	Any nerve malfunction or disease.
Pancreatitis	Inflammation of the pancreas, often associated with alcohol or gallstones.
Parkinson's Disease	A neurological disease that over time causes progressively worse shaking, muscle weakness, and other symptoms.
Pharyngitis	(See also Sore Throat) Inflammation of the Pharynx (throat).
Phlebitis	Inflammation or swelling of a vein, usually caused by a blood clot.
Plague	Plague is a potentially deadly bacterial disease that is caused by the Yersinia pestus bacteria transmitted to humans and animals through close contact or bites from fleas that have previously bitten infected animals. Symptoms include fever, headaches, and extremely swollen and hot lymph nodes. If left untreated, plague can quickly invade the lungs causing severe pneumonia, high fever, bloody coughing, and death. www.cdc.gov/ncidod/dvbid/plague/index.htm
Pleurisy	Pleurisy is the inflammation of one or both of the two protective layers that surround the lungs. This inflammation causes sharp pains that are intensified by breathing. Pleurisy can be caused by infection, injury, blood clots, or disease.
Poison Oak/Ivy	These two plants create a chemical that is caustic to the skin, causing inflammation, redness, itching, and pain in the areas it comes in contact with.
Polyps	An outgrowth of tissue on the inside of hollow organs.
Progesterone	A female hormone produced by the ovaries responsible for regulating the lining of the uterus.
Psoriasis	Psoriasis is a chronic skin disease that causes skin cells to be rotated to the surface before they are mature, resulting in inflamed patches of scaly, red skin that either itch or are sore. About 20% of the time, psoriasis also causes arthritis in adjoining joints. Psoriasis occurs when T cells (white blood cells that help fight infections) become unnecessarily active, triggering inflammation and causing skin cells to rotate to the surface before they are mature. One possible treatment for the itching and soreness is to soak for 15 minutes in a bath with Epsom or dead sea salts, oiled oatmeal, or oil, followed by application of a moisturizer on the affected areas. www.niams.nih.gov/hi/topics/psoriasis/psoriafs.htm

Radiation	Radiation is any of several different forms of energy that may or may not be harmful to the human body. Common forms of radiation include light, radio waves, and x-rays. The three types of radiation considered most dangerous to humans include alpha particles (large, slow moving particles that typically bounce off the skin, and are not dangerous unless the source of these particles is ingested into the body), beta particles (tiny, fast moving particles that can penetrate deep within the body when emitted within several thousand feet), and gamma rays (bursts of energy that can penetrate deep within the body). Each of these types of radiation can change the chemical state or break chemical bonds of molecules they collide with, potentially damaging vital life processes within a cell. www.epa.gov/radiation/
Rheumatic Fever	An illness that causes pain in the joints, fever, nausea, and vomiting. This disease follows an infection by the streptococcus bacteria or scarlet fever. Rheumatic fever can cause severe damage to the heart, joints, and brain. Rheumatic fever often returns once a person develops it.
Ringworm	Ringworm is a skin disease cause by a fungus that can result in ring-shaped red rashes that can be itchy, crusty or scaly.
Scabies	Scabies is an infestation of a microscopic mite (Sarcoptes scabei) that burrows into your skin, leaving pimple-like burrows that itch. www.cdc.gov/ncidod/dpd/parasites/scabies/default.htm
Sciatica	Lower-back/upper-leg pain caused by irritation of the sciatic nerve (a large nerve that extends from the lower back down into the legs). The cause of this irritation is often a herniated disk pressing on the nerve, but it can also be caused by inflammation or other irritants.
Scoliosis	Scoliosis is a sideways curving of the spine. www.niams.nih.gov/hi/topics/scoliosis/scochild.htm
Scurvy	A disorder caused by a lack of vitamin C that causes bleeding in the gums, anemia, and bumpy skin.
Shingles	(See "Shingles" in the Personal Guide section of this book) www.cdc.gov/nip/diseases/varicella/faqs-gen-shingles.htm
Spurs, Bone	Outgrowths of bone (typically in the heel or sole of the feet) that cause inflammation of the surrounding tendons, making movement painful. Ice packs on the inflamed tendons can help reduce pain and swelling.
Staph Infections	Staph infections are any type of infection caused by the Staphylococcus bacteria. While skin infections caused by the staphylococcus bacteria are very common, and usually require no treatment, they can become very serious—especially when they occur in surgical wounds, or open bed sores. www.cdc.gov/ncidod/hip/ARESIST/mrsafaq.htm
Strep Throat	Strep throat is an infection caused by the streptococcal bacteria in the throat that causes a sore throat and fever. www.cdc.gov/ncidod/dbmd/diseaseinfo/groupastreptococcal_g.htm
Tendonitis	Tendonitis is the painful inflammation of the tendons (the tissue that connects muscles to bones) due to injury, overuse, or disease.
Thrush	Thrush is an overgrowth of the fungus Candida (found normally on the skin and mucus membranes) caused by an imbalance in the environment in the mouth or throat that results in white patches in the mouth and potentially painful swallowing. www.cdc.gov/ncidod/dbmd/diseaseinfo/candidiasis_opc_g.htm
Tinnitus	Tinnitus, or a ringing in the ears, is caused by many different things, including: ear damage from loud noises, excess ear fluid, infections, diseases, and some medications.
TMJ	TMJ (temporomandibular joint) disorder or syndrome is characterized by chronic pain in the joint connecting the jawbone to the skull and in the surrounding area. This pain is often caused by clenching or grinding the jaw due to stress or habit. It can also be caused by an injury to the joint or arthritis.
Tonsillitis	Inflammation of the tonsils due to infection or disease.
Tuberculosis	Tuberculosis is a disease caused by bacteria that can attack the lungs, resulting in a severe, bloody cough, chest pains, fever, chills, and loss of appetite. www.cdc.gov/nchstp/tb/faqs/qa.htm
Tumors	An abnormal growth of tissue. A tumor may be either cancerous (malignant) or non-cancerous (benign).
Typhoid	Typhoid is a bacterial disease that causes a high, sustained fever, weakness, stomach pains, headache, and loss of appetite. If untreated, the fever may last for weeks, or even months, and could result in death. www.cdc.gov/ncidod/diseases/submenus/sub_typhoid.htm
Vasodilator	Any agent that causes the blood vessel walls to relax, increasing the diameter of the blood vessel and allowing more blood to flow through.

Vertigo	A feeling that the environment is spinning around you, or that you are spinning. Typically caused by a problem in the inner ear.
Warts	A small outgrowth of skin caused by a virus.
Whiplash	Over stretching or tearing the muscles and tendons in the neck and head due to a collision pushing the body in one direction, while the head's tendency is to remain in the same place, causing the head to quickly rock in the opposite direction the body is going.
Whooping Cough	Whooping cough (or pertussis) is caused by Bordetella pertussis bacteria. This highly contagious disease causes severe bouts of coughing, whooping, and vomiting; and in small children and infants can lead to seizure, apnea (closure of airways), pneumonia, malnutrition, and other serious complications. www.cdc.gov/health/pertussis.htm

Sources (besides those listed above):
www.MedTerms.com
Center for Disease Control (www.cdc.gov)
Environmental Protection Agency (www.epa.gov)
Medline Plus Medical Encyclopedia (www.nlm.nih.gov/medlineplus/ency)

TAXONOMICAL INFORMATION

The following chart is the taxonomical breakdown of the plant families for each of the essential oils found in this book. On the pages following this division chart, there is further information for each family, including the plants within that family that essential oils are derived from, the body systems affected by these essential oils, the properties of these oils, and general uses for these oils.

Division: Embryophyte Siphonogama (plants with seeds)
    Subdivision: Gymnosperm (plants with concentric rings, exposed seeds, & resinous wood)
        Class: Coniferae (cone-bearing plants) & Taxaceae (yew-like plants)
            Family: **Pinaceae** (Trees or shrubs with cones and numerous "scales")
                    Genus: Abies (firs, balsam trees), Cedrus (cedars), Pinus (pines), Picea (spruces), Pseudotsuga (false hemlock), Tsuga (hemlocks)
            Family: **Cupressaceae**
                    Genus: Callitris (blue cypress), Cupressus (cypresses), Juniperus (junipers), Thuja (Arbor vitae or cedars)
    Subdivision: Angiosperm (highly evolved plants with seeds enclosed by fruits)
        Class: Monocotyledons (plants with one-leaf embryos)
            Family: **Gramineae, Zingiberaceae**
        Class: Dicotyledons (plants with multiple-leaf embryos)
            Family: **Anacardiaceae, Annonaceae, Betulaceae, Burseraceae, Cistaceae, Compositae, Ericaceae, Geraniaceae, Guttiferae, Labiatae, Lauraceae, Myristicaceae, Myrtaceae, Oleaceae, Piperaceae, Rosaceae, Rutaceae, Santalaceae, Styracaceae, Umbelliferae, Valerianaceae**

ANACARDIACEAE (consists of about 850 species in 73 genera of mostly subtropical and tropical resinous trees, shrubs, and climbers; drupe type fruit.)
Body Systems: Lymphatic System, Respiratory System, Water balance
Properties: detoxifying, astringent action
General Uses: congestion (lymphatic, respiratory), hypotension, arthritis, psoriasis
Schinus molle: California pepper tree (Pink pepper)

ANNONACEAE (shrubs, trees, climbers; fragrant flowers; 128 genera, 2000 species; mostly tropical, found in Old World & rain forest)
Body Systems: Cardiovascular System, Nervous System (calming), Hormonal System (aphrodesiac)
Properties: extreme fire and water; nervous sedative, balancing
General Uses: depression, frigidity, impotence, palpitations, skin care
Cananga odorata; two forms exist:
        var. odorata (var. genuina., *Unona odorantissimum*): ylang-ylang
        var. macrophylla: cananga

BETULACEAE (shrubs, trees; fruit is one-seeded nut, often winged; includes birches, alders, hornbeams and hazels; 6 genera, 150 species; from northern hemisphere to tropical mountains)
Body Systems: Digestive and Respiratory Systems, Muscles and Bones
Properties: analgesic, draining (lymph), purifying
General Uses: auto intoxication, muscle pain
Betula alleghaniensis: yellow birch
Betula lenta: sweet birch

BURSERACEAE (means "dry fire"; resinous tropical timber trees; drupe or capsule fruit; 21 genera, 540 species)
Body Systems: Respiratory System (secretions), Emotional Balance (psychic centers),
Skin **Properties:** cooling, drying, fortifying
General Uses: anti-inflammatory, expectorant, scar tissue (reducing), ulcers, wounds (healing)
Boswellia carterii: frankincense
Bursera graveolens: palo santo
Canarium luzonicum: elemi
Commiphora myrrha: myrrh

CISTACEAE (low shrubs, few herbs; capsule fruit; Cistus species have large flowers; 7 genera, 175 species; Mediterranean, Europe, central Asia and America)
Body Systems: Emotional Balance, Skin (care)
Properties: calming, fortifying, healing
General Uses: anxiety, depression, stress-related disorders, wound healing
Cistus ladanifer: labdanum, cistus

COMPOSITAE (ASTERACEAE) (largest family of flowering plants; inflorescence, small flowers; 1317 genera, 21,000 species; found everywhere, especially around Mediterranean)
Body Systems: Digestive System, Skin
Properties: "perfect balance of etheric and astral forces, promoting realization, reorganization, structure" [Lavabre, *Aromatherapy Workbook*]; adaptive, calming, regeneration (note: because of the large variety of plants withing this family, the therapeutic activity is very diversified; some plants are neurotoxic)
General Uses: infections, inflammation, regeneration
Achillea millefolium: yarrow
Artemisia dracunculus: tarragon
Artemisia pallens: davana
Artemisia vulgaris: mugwort
Chamaemelum nobile: Roman chamomile
Conyza canadensis: Canadian fleabane
Helichrysum angustifolium (var. *Italicum*): helichrysum
Matricaria recutita: German chamomile
Solidago odora (*Solidago canadensis*): goldenrod
Tanacetum annum: blue tansy
Tanacetum vulgare: wild tansy

CUPRESSACEAE (conifer cypress family, needle-like leaves and cones; 17 genera, 113 species, most in northern temperate zones)
Body Systems: Hormonal, Respiratory, and Nervous Systems
Properties: appeasing, reviving, tonic, warming
General Uses: anti-rheumatic, astringent, cellulite (reduces), insomnia, nervous tension (reduces), respiration (when taken through inhalation), stress-related conditions
Callitris intratropica: blue cypress
Cupressus sempervirens: cypress
Juniperus communis: juniper
Juniperus scopulorum (*J. osteosperma*): Rocky Mountain juniper
Thuja occidentalis: cedarleaf
Thuja plicata: Western red cedar (leaf)

ERICACEAE (shrubs and small trees with leathery evergreen leaves, fruit berry, drupe or capsule; 103 genera, 3350 species; cosmopolitan centered in northern hemisphere)
Body Systems: Cardiovascular and Digestive Systems

Properties: detoxifying
General Uses: hypertension, kidney and liver stimulant
Ledum groenlandicum: Labrador tea
Gaultheria procumbens: wintergreen

GERANIACEAE (herbs or low shrubs, 14 genera, 730 species; temperate and tropical zones)
Body Systems: Hormonal System, Digestive System (kidneys - excretion, liver & pancreas - metabolism), Nervous System, Emotional Balance
Properties: balancing (nervous system)
General Uses: burns, depression, diabetes, hemorrhage, nervous tension, skin, sore throat, ulcers, wounds
Pelargonium graveolens: geranium, rose geranium (*P. x asperum*)

GRAMINEAE (or **POACEAE**) (nutritious grass family; used for ground covering and food (wheat, rice, corn, barley); large root systems; 737 genera, 7950 species; distributed throughout the world)
Body Systems: Cardiovascular System, Digestive System (stimulant), Respiratory System, Skin
Properties: air purifier, calming, refreshing, sedative
General Uses: air deodorizer, calm digestion, cleanse and balance skin (acne)
Cymbopogon flexuosus: lemongrass
Cymbopogon martinii: palmarosa
Cymbopogon nardus: citronella
Vetiveria zizanoides: vetiver

GUTTIFERAE (or **HYPERICACEAE**) (trees and shrubs; many useful for timber and edible fruits; 47 genera, 1350 species; tropics)
Body Systems: Muscles and Bones, Skin
Properties: anti-inflammatory, analgesic
General Uses: infections, muscle pain, wounds
Calophyllum inophyllum: tamanu

LABIATE (**LAMIACEAE**) (herbs or low shrubs with quadrangular stems; largest of all essential oil producing plant families; oils are mostly non-toxic and non-hazardous; some antiseptic oils; some oils used for flavoring; most oils helpful for headaches, congestion, muscular problems (analgesic, anti-inflammatory), and stimulate one or more body systems; 224 genera, about 5600 species; main distribution in tropical and warmer temperate regions)
Body Systems: Digestive and Respiratory Systems
Properties: appeases overactive astral body [Lavabre, *Aromatherapy Workbook*], curative, stimulates, warms
General Uses: anemia, diabetes, digestion (poor), headaches, respiratory problems; "good for people with intense psychic activity to prevent exhaustion and loss of self" [Lavabre, *Aromatherapy Workbook*]
Hyssopus officinalis: hyssop
Lavandula angustifolia: lavender
Lavandula x hybrida: lavandin
Melissa officinalis: melissa
Mentha piperita: peppermint
Mentha spicata: spearmint
Ocimum basilicum: basil
Origanum majorana: marjoram
Origanum vulgare: oregano
Pogostemon cablin: patchouli
Rosmarinus officinalis: rosemary several varieties
        var. *officinalis*: common rosemary; numerous cultivars and forms;
                chemotypes: CT I: camphor; CT II: cineole; CT III: verbenone
Salvia lavendulifolia: Spanish sage
Salvia officinalis: sage *Salvia sclarea*: clary sage
Satureja montana: winter savory
Thymus vulgaris: thyme
        chemotypes: linalool; thymol (or geraniol)
Vitex negundo: vitex

LAURACEAE (trees and shrubs with evergreen leaves and aromatic oils; some valued for timber, as ornamentals, or for oils or spices; 45 genera, 200-2500 species; found in tropics and sub-tropics in Amazona and South-east Asia)

Body Systems: Cardiovascular System (cardiac-stimulates, pulmonary-stimulates), Nervous System (regulates), Hormonal System (aphrodisiac), Skin (cellular-regenerates)
Properties: anti-fungal, anti-viral, anti-bacterial, stimulant, tonic (some oils in this family are irritant)
General Uses: depression, headache, hypotension, scars, sexual debility
Aniba roseodora var. amazonica: Brazilian rosewood, bois de rose
Cinnamomum cassia: cassia
Cinnamomum zeylanicum (*C. verum*): cinnamon bark
Laurus nobilis: laurel
Ravensara aromatica: ravensara

MYRISTICACEAE (plants whose bark produces watery, blood-like exudate; fruit is fleshy with one large seed; 19 genera, about 400 species; found throughout tropics, centered in Malaysia lowland rain forest)
Body Systems: Digestive, Hormonal, and Nervous Systems, Emotional Balance
Properties: analgesic, aphrodisiac, circulation, nervous system stimulant
General Uses: digestion, fatigue (mental and physical), impotence, nervousness, rheumatism
Myristica fragrans: nutmeg

MYRTACEAE (mainly tropical and sub-tropical plants with dotted leaves and oil glands; fruit is woody capsule or berry with one or many seeds; some have ornamental or showy flowers; many produce valuable timber; 121 genera, 3850 species; found in tropical and warm regions, especially Australia)
Body Systems: Respiratory and Immune Systems
Properties: "balances interaction of four elements (earth, air, fire, water)" [Lavabre, *Aromatherapy Workbook*], antiseptic, stimulant, tonic
General Uses: antiseptic, energy (balances), respiratory (infections), stimulant, tonic
Backhousia citriodora: lemon myrtle
Eucalyptus citriodora: lemon-scented eucalyptus
Eucalyptus dives: peppermint eucalyptus
Eucalyptus globulus: eucalyptus
Eucalyptus polybractea: blue leaved mallee
        chemotype: cineole
Eucalyptus staigeriana: lemon-scented ironbark
Eugenia caryophyllata (*Syzygium aromaticum*): clove bud
Leptospermum scoparium: manuka
Melaleuca alternifolia: tea tree
Melaleuca ericifolia: rosalina
Melaleuca leucadendra: cajeput
Melaleuca quinquenervia: niaouli
Myrtus communis: myrtle (two sub-species exist: green and red)

OLEACEAE (trees or shrubs; including olive and ash; used for timber; 24 genera, 900 species; widely distributed, centered on Asia)
Body Systems: Emotional Balance, Hormonal System (aphrodisiac)
Properties: calming, soothing, uplifting
General Uses: anxiety, depression, frigidity, impotence, stress *Jasminum officinale*: jasmine

PINACEAE (ABIETACEAE) (conifers with male and female cones; 9 genera, 194 species; found in northern hemisphere, temperate climates)
Body Systems: Hormonal, Nervous, and Respiratory Systems; signifies air element
Properties: antiseptic, appeasing, reviving, tonic, warming
General Uses: arthritis, congestion (inhaled), oxygen deficiency, respiratory disorders, rheumatism, stress
Abies alba: fir, silver fir
Abies balsamea: balsam fir
Abies grandis: white fir, giant fir
Cedrus atlantica: Atlas cedarwood
Picea mariana: black spruce
Pinus ponderosa: ponderosa pine
Pinus sylvestris: Scotch pine
Pseudotsuga menziesii: Douglas fir
Tsuga canadensis: hemlock spruce (or tsuga)

PIPERACEAE (pepper family; small trees, shrubs and climbers; small fleshy drupe with single seed; some widely cultivated for condiments; 4 genera, over 2000 species; found throughout tropics, mostly in rainforests)
Body Systems: Cardiovascular, Digestive, and Nervous Systems; root chakra
Properties: drying, heating, stimulant, tonic
General Uses: fevers, indigestion, pain (muscle, tooth), grounding
Piper nigrum: black pepper

ROSACEAE (trees, shrubs, and herbs; some edible fruits; many cultivated for fruits (almond) or flowers (rose); 107 genera, 3100 species; found in temperate climates throughout the world)
Body Systems: Hormonal System (female reproductive); heart chakra
Properties: aphrodisiac, harmonizing, tonic, uplifting
General Uses: emotional shock, frigidity, grief, impotence
Rosa canina: rosehip
Rosa damascena: Bulgarian rose

RUTACEAE (aromatic trees and shrubs; sometimes thorny; dotted, compound leaves with aromatic glands; includes citrus fruits; 161 genera, about 1650 species; found in tropical and warm temperate regions, especially Australia and South Africa)
Body Systems: Digestive (kidneys, liver) and Nervous Systems, Skin
Properties: cooling, refreshing, secretion (fruits), sedative (flowers)
General Uses: inflammation, over-sensitivity, water balance
Citrus aurantifolia: lime
Citrus aurantium: neroli (var. *bigaradia*), petitgrain
Citrus bergamia: bergamot
Citrus hystrix: leech-lime
Citrus limon: lemon
Citrus nobilis: tangerine
Citrus x paradisi: grapefruit
Citrus reticulate: mandarin
Citrus sinensis: orange

SANTALACEAE (herbs, shrubs and trees which are semi-parasitic on roots and stems of other plants; 36 genera, about 500 species; found in tropical and temperate regions)
Body Systems: Digestive System (excretory-balances, genito-urinary-disinfects), Nervous System (balances), and Respiratory System (balances)
Properties: balancing, calming, constriction, grounding
General Uses: genito-urinary tract infections, impotence, lung congestion, stress-related disorders
Santalum album: East Indian sandalwood, Mysore sandalwood, sandalwood

STYRACACEAE (trees and shrubs with resinous bark used medicinally; used for incense, obtained by wounding tree; 12 genera, 165 species; found in tropical and warm temperate climates in Americas, Malaysia, Mediterranean, and South-east Asia)
Body Systems: Cardiovascular and Nervous Systems; first chakra
Properties: calming, grounding, soothing
General Uses: hyper-activity
Styrax benzoin: benzoin, onycha

UMBELLIFERAE (APIACEAE) (herbs and a few shrubs, flowers borne in umbels (flowers radiating from a central point, like an umbrella); some important as food (carrot, celery), while others are very poisonous; some have medicinal actions; 420 genera, 3100 species; found throughout the world, mainly in norther temperate regions)
Body Systems: Digestive System (balances), Hormonal System (stimulates uterus), Respiratory System, Skin (regenerates)
Properties: air element; accumulation (elimination, excretion), secretion
General Uses: gas, glandular problems, spasms
Anethum graveolens: dill
Angelica archangelica: angelica
Apium graveolens: celery
Carum carvi: caraway
Coriandrum sativum: coriander
Cuminum cyminum: cumin

Daucus carota: <u>carrot seed oil</u>
Ferula galbaniflua: <u>galbanum</u>
Foeniculum vulgare: <u>fennel</u>
Pimpinella anisum: <u>aniseed</u>

VALERIANACEAE (herb family; fruit is dry; roots often used medicinally (valium); 17 genera, 14 species; found throughout the world (except Australia))
Body Systems: Nervous System (calming)
Properties: grounding, sedative; balances upper and lower body
General Uses: anxiety, insomnia, nervous headaches, palpitations, stomach; living in one's head
Nardostachys jatamansi: <u>spikenard</u>
Valeriana officinalis: <u>valerian</u>

ZINGIBERACEAE (ginger family comprising rhizomatous herbs; 53 genera, 1200 species; found mostly in rain forests throughout the tropics, but mainly in Indo-Malaysia)
Body Systems: Digestive and Hormonal Systems, Muscles and Bones
Properties: analgesic, fever reducing, scurvy (prevents), stimulant, tonic, warming
General Uses: digestive (stimulant), rheumatism, sexual tonic
Elettaria cardamomum: <u>cardamom</u>
Zingiber officinale: <u>ginger</u>

Index

The following index has been manually verified and adjusted to increase its effectiveness and reduce its length. Due to the extent that the single oils are listed throughout this reference guide, we thought it best to list only the most relevant page numbers for each single oil listing. The single oils are all listed in bold print to make it easy to identify them. All other page numbers that are listed in bold print, are the most relevant for their respective listing.

C

D

F

I

P

Q

R

S

T

Bibliography

Balch, M.D., James, and Phyllis Balch, C.N.C. *Prescription for Nutritional Healing.* Garden City Park, NY: Avery Publishing Group, 1990.

Becker, M.D., Robert O. *The Body Electric.* New York, NY: Wm. Morrow, 1985.

Burroughs, Stanley. *Healing for the Age of Enlightenment.* Auburn, CA: Burroughs Books, 1993.

Burton Goldberg Group, The. *Alternative Medicine: The Definitive Guide.* Fife, WA: Future Medicine Publishing, Inc., 1994.

DeVita, Sabina M. *Electromagnetic Pollution. A Hidden Stress to Your System.* Marble Hill, MO: Stewart Publishing Company, 2000.

--------------. *Essential Oils Desk Reference.* Essential Science Publishing. Third Edition, First Printing March 2004.

Fischer-Rizzi, Suzanne. *Complete Aromatherapy Handbook.* New York, NY: Sterling Publishing, 1990.

Foley, Marcy. *Embraced by the Essence! Your Journey into Wellness Using Pure Quality Essential Oils.* Boulder, Colorado: Holistic Wellness Foundation I, April 2000.

Gattefosse, Ph.D., Rene-Maurice. *Gattefosse's Aromatherapy.* Essex, England: The C.W. Daniel Company Ltd., 1937 English translation.

Green, Mindy. *Natural Perfumes: Simple Aromatherapy Recipes.* Loveland CO: Interweave Press Inc., 1999.

--------------. *Integrated Aromatic Medicine.* Proceedings from the First International Symposium, Grasse, France. Essential Science Publishing, March 2000.

Lawless, Julia. *The Encyclopaedia of Essential Oils.* Rockport, MA: Element, Inc., 1992.

Lee, M.D., John R. *Natural Progesterone: The Multiple Roles of a Remarkable Hormone.* Sebastopol, CA: BLL Publishing, 1995.

Maury, Marguerite. *Marguerite Maury's Guide to Aromatherapy.* C.W. Daniel, 1989.

Pènoël, M.D., Daniel and Pierre Franchomme. *L'aromatherapie exactement.* Limoges, France: Jollois, 1990.

Price, Shirley, and Len Price. *Aromatherapy for Health Professionals.* New York, NY: Churchill Livingstone Inc., 1995.

Price, Shirley, and Penny Price Parr. *Aromatherapy for Babies and Children.* San Francisco, CA: Thorsons, 1996.

Rose, Jeanne. *The Aromatherapy Book: Applications and Inhalations.* Berkeley, CA: North Atlantic Books, 1992.

Ryman, Danièle. *Aromatherapy: The Complete Guide to Plant & Flower Essences for Health and Beauty.* New York: Bantam Books, 1993.

Sheppard-Hanger, Sylla. *The Aromatherapy Practitioner Reference Manual.* Tampa, FL: Atlantic Institute of Aromatherapy, Twelfth Printing February 2000.

Stewart, Ph.D., R.A., David. *A Statistical Validation of Raindrop Technique.* Marble Hill, MO: Care Publications, 2003

Tisserand, Maggie. *Aromatherapy for Women: a Practical Guide to Essential Oils for Health and Beauty.* Rochester, VT: Healing Arts Press, 1996.

Tisserand, Robert. *Aromatherapy: to Heal and Tend the Body.* Wilmot, WI: Lotus Press, 1988.

Tisserand, Robert. *The Art of Aromatherapy.* Rochester, VT: Healing Arts Press, 1977.

Tisserand, Robert, and Tony Balacs. *Essential Oil Safety: A Guide for Health Care Professionals.* New York, NY: Churchill

Livingstone, 1995. Valnet, M.D., Jean. *The Practice of Aromatherapy: a Classic Compendium of Plant Medicines and their Healing Properties.*

Rochester, VT: Healing Arts Press, 1980.

Watson, Franzesca. *Aromatherapy Blends & Remedies.* San Francisco, CA: Thorsons, 1995.

Wilson, Roberta. *Aromatherapy for Vibrant Health and Beauty: a practical A-to-Z reference to aromatherapy treatments for health,*

skin, and hair problems. Honesdale, PA: Paragon Press, 1995.

Worwood, Valerie Ann. *The Complete Book of Essential Oils & Aromatherapy.* San Rafael, CA: New World Library, 1991.

Young, N.D., D. Gary. *An Introduction to Young Living Essential Oils.* Payson, UT: Young Living Essential Oils, 2000.

Young, N.D., D. Gary. *Aromatherapy: The Essential Beginning.* Salt Lake City, UT: Essential Press Publishing, 1995.

Young, Ph.D., Robert O. *One Sickness, One Disease, One Treatment.* Alpine, UT: Self-published, 1995.

Video Listing

---------------. Essential Tips for Happy, Healthy Pets. The Vision Firm, LLC, 2000.

Eaton, Cathy. Raindrop Therapy. Health is Your Wealth Enterprises, 1997.

Woloshyn, Tom. Vita Flex Instruction. Vita-Gem Enterprises, 1998.

Young, ND, D. Gary. Raindrop Technique. Young Living Essential Oils, 2000.

Products Available from Abundant Health

Health Related Books

1001 Reference Guide for Essential Oils
by Connie and Alan Higley

The November 2006 edition contains 560 pages of comprehensive information about pure, therapeutic quality essential oils in a readily accessible reference guide format. This coil-bound reference gives you detailed information about *Science & Application, Single Oils, Oil Blends, Personal Care Products, Bath & Shower Gels, Tinctures, Massage Oils,* and *Supplements* available from Young Living Essential Oils. It even includes a *Personal Guide* which is alphabetized by health condition. This book is perfect for those beginning their journey into the scent-sational world of essential oils and aromatherapy!

1002 Quick Reference Guide for Using Essential Oils
by Connie and Alan Higley

Designed as a convenient pocket guide, this book contains the *Personal Guide* section of the *Reference Guide for Essential Oils,* the Vita Flex Feet Chart and other summary information. With information on over 650 health conditions, it is probably one of the most comprehensive and concise books of its kind on the market today (*November 2006 Edition, 213 pgs, coil-bound*).

1000 Reference Guide Bundle
Buy both of the fantastic books listed above and receive a special bundle discount price!

Essential Oils Desk Reference & Pocket Reference
(3rd Edition) by Essential Science Publishing

9048 Desk Reference
9047 Pocket Reference
9049 Bundle: *Save when purchaseing these two books together!*

Much of the material contained in these books is derived from the research, lectures, and workshops of D. Gary Young, N.D. and the work of other practitioners and physicians at the forefront of understanding the clinical potential of essential oils (*Desk Reference: 513 pgs, hardcover; Pocket Reference: 268 pgs, coil-bound*).

8903 Essential Oils Integrative Medical Guide
by D. Gary Young, ND

This essential oil reference book by D. Gary Young is a must have for those who are serious about therapeutic application of pure essential oils. Dr. Young combines years of scientific research on the use and application of essential oils, and blends it into an easy to use guidebook. This book includes detailed instructions on how to apply the oils, information on Dr. Young's journeys across the world, and recipes for 25 special oil blends (*610 pgs, hardcover*).

Chart   *Chart Detail*

1200 Premium Essential Oils Cross-Reference Chart
1201 Portable Essential Oils Cross-Reference Chart

Quickly find the right essential oil to use for different health conditions with these easy-to-use charts! Each chart cross-references 75 different essential oils with 120 different health conditions so you can quickly see which oils have been used to help with a specific condition. Also included is a color coding that quickly shows which oils might need to be diluted before applying, and information about photosensitizing oils. Each chart measures 26" x 38" for easy reading, and adds a professional touch to any office. These charts are coated for durability, and include a slide-rule for easy matching of the correct oil to the desired condition.

For additional products, current prices and ordering information:

Phone: 1-888-718-3068 / 1-801-798-0642   **Website:** www.AbundantHealth4u.com

Aromatherapy Books

9046

9046 **Healing Oils of the Bible** by David Stewart Ph.D.
This book documents more than 500 scriptural references to thirty-three species of essential oils.

9066

9066 **Saving Face** by Dr. Sabina DeVita
Enjoy the benefits of using essential oils with this easy to follow guidebook.

9019 **Healing with Aromatherapy** by Marlene Ericksen
This book contains step-by-step instructions and recipes for beauty treatments.

9074 **Holistic Aromatherapy for Animals**
by Kristen Leigh Bell
This comprehensive guide focuses on safety and common uses of essential oils for animals.

9035

9035 **Releasing Emotional Patterns with Essential Oils**
by Carolyn L. Mein, DC
This book tells how to apply Young Living Essential Oil blends for emotional healing.

9062

9062 **Making Aromatherapy Creams & Lotions**
by Donna Maria
Create exciting and unique body products using all-natural ingredients and aromatherapy.

9036 **What To Do When Antibiotics Don't Work**
by Dirk Van Gils
Discover the secrets of treating the most frequently-occurring infectious diseases naturally.

9004

9004 **Healing Oils, Healing Hands** by Linda L. Smith
A complete look at healing in the early Christian Church, including anointing with aromatic oils.

9073 **Aromatherapy for the Healthy Child**
by Valerie Ann Worwood
Scientifically proven remedies, along with complete charts of essential oils for children's health.

9044 **The Chemistry of Essential Oils Made Simple**
by David Stewart Ph.D.
An essential addition to the library of anyone serious about understanding how essential oils work!

9044

9014 **Advanced Aromatherapy—The Science of Essential Oil Therapy** by Kurt Schnaubelt, Ph. D.
Broad-based research that demonstrates how essential oils interact with different body systems.

9015

9015 **Medical Aromatherapy—Healing with Essential Oils**
by Kurt Schnaubelt
Kurt Schnaubelt shows that for hundreds of years, essential oils have been used for healing.

9012

9012 **Statistical Validation of Raindrop Therapy**
by David Stewart
This booklet summarizes the experiences of more than 14,000 sessions of the Raindrop Technique.

More Aromatherapy Books

9006

9006 500 Formulas for Aromatherapy
by Carol Schiller & David Schiller
Create your own personal aromatic oils for every use—healing, pleasure, and beauty.

8902 Clinical Aromatherapy by Jane Buckle
Highlights how aromatherapy can enhance care and the role of the health care professional.

8909 Discovery of the Ultimate Superfood
by D. Gary Young, Ronald Lawrence, MD, & Marc Schreuder
Research behind a food showing potential for promoting health—the Ningxia wolfberry.

8911

8911 Aromatherapy Workbook by Marcel Lavabre
This classic book on aromatherapy is the perfect guide for beginners and advanced users alike.

9050

9050 Essential Oil Safety by Robert Tisserand & Tony Balacs
An excellent book for those who needs to be familiar with the appropriate and safe use of oils.

9029 The Complete Book of Essential Oils & Aromatherapy by Valerie Ann Worwood
More than 500 recipes using oils as alternatives to health, beauty, and cleaning products.

9029

9028 Natural Home Health Care Using Essential Oils
by Daniel Pénoël, M.D., & Rose-Marie Pénoël
This unique work is filled with wonderful insights on how to heal with essential oils.

9028

8904 The Aromatherapy Practitioner Reference Manual by Sylla Sheppard-Hanger
This manual is one of the most comprehensive, well-researched books on essential oils.

9034 Aromatherapy Soothing Remedies to Restore, Rejuvenate, and Heal by Valerie Gennari Cooksley, RN
This guide provides all the tools necessary to use the curative power of essential oils.

9034

9033 Aromatherapy and Massage for Mother and Baby
by Allison England
This guide provides advice on using oils in massage, baths, compresses, lotions, and inhalations.

9033

8906 Raindrop Technique by D. Gary Young, ND.
This wonderful booklet takes you step by step through the Raindrop Technique.

8901 Clinical Aromatherapy for Pregnancy and Childbirth by Denise Tiran
The safe, effective and appropriate administration of essential oils in pregnancy and labor.

8906

Other Health Related Books

9030

9031

9065

9077

9043

9061

9038

9061

9080

8941

9030 Feelings Buried Alive Never Die ... by Karol K Truman
Learn why you feel the way you feel, then learn how to easily transform those undesirable feelings.

9031 Healing Feelings... From Your Heart
by Karol K Truman
Learn to discover the indicators of your feelings and to free yourself from self-imposed restrictions.

9052 Electromagnetic Pollution
by Dr. Sabina M. DeVita, RN, EdD
Learn about the electromagnetic pollution that surrounds you and how it can affect your life.

9065 Liver Cleansing Handbook by Rhody Lake
Combining up to the minute research, full color photographs, and tons of great recipes.

9077 Prozac, Panacea or Pandora? by Ann Blake Tracy, PhD
Learn more than most professionals know about the SSRI antidepressants.

9043 Alkalize or Die by Theodore A Baroody
This powerful title carries an important message about personal pH that can benefit everyone.

8937 Vibrational Medicine by Richard Gerber, M.D.
This book offers new insights into the physical and spiritual perspectives of health and disease.

9061 Rub a Dub, Dub...Is Cancer in your Tub?
by Network News and Publications.
DEA—found in over 600 products—has been linked to cancer. Find out more in this brochure!

9038 How's Your pH? by Network News and Publications.
Sparkling clear pool water is all about optimum pH levels. Your body works the same way.

9016 Pregnenolone by D. Gary Young, ND
Learn about some of the amazing benefits of the "Master Hormone," Pregnenolone.

9080 Alternative Medicine – The Definitive Guide
by The Burton Goldberg Group
Everything you must know about effective therapies and self-help cures for you and your family.

9081 Definitive Guide to CANCER
by W. John Diamond MD, W. Lee Cowden MD, & Burton Goldberg
Cancer can be REVERSED by using clinically proven complementary and alternative therapies.

9003 Is Your Child's Brain Starving?
by Dr. Michael R. Lyon, MD, & Dr. G. Christine Laurell, PhD
How to improve brain function and health in children and adults by changing diets, not drugs.

8941 Your Aura and Your Chakras by Karla McLaren
A clear and comprehensive text for the restoration and maintenance of your subtle energy system.

For additional products, current prices and ordering information:

Phone: 1-888-718-3068 / 1-801-798-0642   **Website:** www.AbundantHealth4u.com

Diffusers

9320

9371

9315

9360

9340 **Optima Model Diffuser**
This is one of our most powerful and quietest diffusers yet!

9320 **Economy Model Diffuser**
Our most economical model with a fixed low output and fairly quiet operation.

9371 **Well & Jet Diffuser**
This diffuser has got to be the most powerful and versatile diffuser on the market today.

9310 **Battery Operated Diffuser**
Features an ultra-quiet fan that blows cool air through a pad to disperse the oil into the air.

9315 **The "FanFuser™"**
This is the easiest-to-use diffuser you'll ever find. Powerfully and quickly disperses the oils.

9360 **Programmable Diffuser Timer**
This mechanical timer can be set for any 15-minute increment over a 24-hour period!

Vita Flex Products

9040 **Healing for the Age of Enlightenment**
by Stanley Burroughs
Contains a detailed explanation of the "Master Cleanser" and the entire system of Vita Flex.

9302 **Video: Vita Flex Instruction** with Tom Woloshyn
Teaches the proper Vita Flex technique and illustrates the Vita Flex points over the entire body!

9301 **Vita Flex Roller or "Relax-a-Roller"**
A roller designed by Stanley Burroughs to create a pressure point massage similar to Vita Flex.

Videos

9202   9214

9227 **Essential Tips for Happy, Healthy Pets**
Demonstrations of using the oils on pets, including application of the raindrop technique.

9202 **Raindrop Technique** by D. Gary Young, ND
D. Gary Young, the inventor of Raindrop Technique, walks you through this valuable treatment.

9214 **Healing Oils of the Bible** by David Stewart, Ph.D.
Dr. David Stewart demonstrates how to effectively carry out a community Bible Oils Program.

Electromagnetic Field (EMF) Protection

9700 **Digital Cell Phone Diode**
This highly concentrated formula, combined with the energies of the stone, provides excellent protection against EMF's generated by cellular phones, hair dryers, and other small appliances.

For additional products, current prices and ordering information:

Phone: 1-888-718-3068 / 1-801-798-0642   **Website:** www.AbundantHealth4u.com

Glass & Plastic Products

9102 1/6 Dram Sample Vials w/ Dabber Cap
These sample vials are great for giving samples of oil as gifts!

9102

9100

9100 5/8 Dram Amber Glass Vials w/ Orifice Reducers
These small bottles are wonderful for creating samples and portable oil kits! .

Amber Glass Bottles w/ Reducer & White Caps
9155 5 ml amber
9156 10 ml amber
9157 15 ml amber
Protect your oil with these dark bottles that feature a Euro-style orifice reducer for easy dispensing.

9155-9157

Glass Vials w/ Dropper Caps
9160 2 Dram Amber
9180 1 Ounce Amber
These vials include a dropper cap and are excellent for making blends or for diluting an oil.

9160   9180

9123 Spray Top for 1 oz. Amber Glass Bottle
Great for turning your glass bottles into spray-bottles for spritzes and room sprays!

9193 Nasal Inhalers
These small inhalers are the perfect size to carry your favorite aroma in your pocket, purse, or bag!

9193

9193 1/3 oz. (10 ml) Roll-On Bottles
Quick and easy "roll-on" application of your favorite oils. Clear glass bottle with applicator and cap.

Syringes
9251 1 ml
9253 5 ml
9260 20 ml rectal
Create blends, dispense oils, and fill vials easily with these essential oil dispensing syringes.

9253 & 9271

9271 Adapta-Cap™ Bottle Adapters
Use with syringes for quick, mess-free dispensing. *(Size A—fits our 5, 10, & 15 ml bottles).*

9190 2 oz. Plastic Bottles w/ Dispensing Cap
Ideal for travel and for storing shampoos, bath gels, massage oils, and base oils.

9190

Carrying Cases and Storage/Display Racks

9550 Essential Bags—Carrying Case for 16 5-15 ml vials
These beautifully sewn, padded, cloth carrying cases hold 16 bottles (from 5 ml to 15 ml.).

9560 Carrying Case for 16 vials (5/8 dram)
This case holds 16 of our 5/8-dram vials in a zippered, flat pouch.

9560

Essential Oil Portfolios
9535 Holds 32 vials - 11½"x11½"x1¾"
9530 Holds 64 vials - 11¼"x10¾"x2¾"
These portfolios make a professional statement while conveniently carrying your essential oils.

9573 Premium Solid Oak Storage/Display Shelves
These beautiful shelves are made from solid oak. The bottom shelves slide out for easy access.

9573

For additional products, current prices and ordering information:

Phone: 1-888-718-3068 / 1-801-798-0642   **Website:** www.AbundantHealth4u.com

About the Cover Painting and the Artist

Can you identify the plants in this painting?
The answers are at the bottom of the page.

This painting was created by **_Valerieann J. Skinner_**, artist and author from Georgetown, Idaho. For nineteen years, Valerieann has taught others how to heal, better know themselves and express their uniqueness through art. This and painting professionally for over twenty years, has taught her much—especially about color and its affect on people. She has discovered the importance of using color consciously. You can learn how to use it more effectively in your own life by reading her book, Cashing in on the "Simple Magic" of Color. Get a FREE copy by visiting her website.

Her newest book, The World of Mirrors—A Bridge to Knowing and Being Your "True" Self, is a self-empowering book that gives the reader a life changing perspective on everything happening in their life and world. Read this book and your world will come alive with the answers, guidance and healing you are seeking. **Valerieann's books, handmade "essential oil" greeting cards, and art prints are available through Abundant Health.**

Do you need a cover for your book, CD or creation?
Contact Valerieann and discuss your ideas with her.

Inner Light Creations
Website: www.valerieann.com
E-mail: valerieann@valerieann.com

1. Tansy 2. Lavender 3. Chamomile 4. Rose 5. Echinacea 6. Geranium
7. Goldenseal 8. Hyssop 9. Nutmeg 10. Clove 11. Coriander 12. Lotus 13. Pine